DVD Contents

Approximate run time 265 mins

Atlas of Abdominoplasty

Atlas of Abdominoplasty

JOSEPH P. HUNSTAD, MD, FACS
The Hunstad Center for Cosmetic Plastic Surgery
Charlotte, NC, USA

and

REMUS REPTA, MD
Advanced Aesthetic Associates, LLC Phoenix, AZ, USA

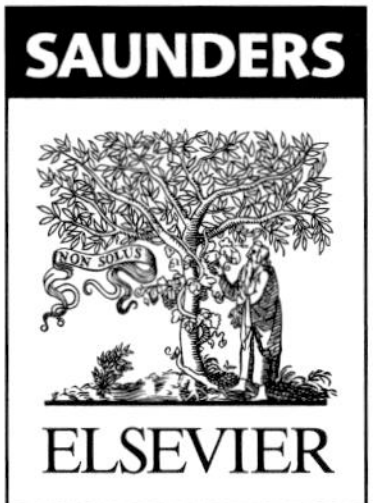

SAUNDERS
ELSEVIER
is an affiliate of Elsevier Inc.

First published 2009

ISBN: 978 1416040804

British Library Cataloguing in Publication Data
A catalogue record for this book is available from the British Library

Library of Congress Cataloging in Publication Data
A catalog record for this book is available from the Library of Congress

Notice
Medical knowledge is constantly changing. Standard safety precautions must be followed, but as new research and clinical experience broaden our knowledge, changes in treatment and drug therapy may become necessary or appropriate. Readers are advised to check the most current product information provided by the manufacturer of each drug to be administered to verify the recommended dose, the method and duration of administration, and contraindications. It is the responsibility of the practitioner, relying on experience and knowledge of the patient, to determine dosages and the best treatment for each individual patient. Neither the Publisher nor the author assume any liability for any injury and/or damage to persons or property arising from this publication.

The Publisher

For Elsevier
Commissioning Editor: *Sue Hodgson*
Development Editor: *Sharon Nash*
Project Manager: *Andy Palfreyman*
Design: *Stewart Larking*
Illustration Manager: *Merlyn Harvey*
Illustrator: *Ethan Danielson*
Marketing Manager (USA): *Radha Mawrie*, (UK): *John Camelon*

The Publisher's policy is to use **paper manufactured from sustainable forests**

Printed in China
Last digit is the print number: 9 8 7 6 5 4 3 2 1

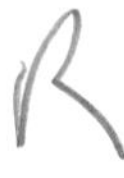

Contents

Foreword

Writing a foreword for this book in abdominoplasty by Dr. Joseph Paul Hunstad gives me great personal pleasure and satisfaction. I am very impressed with his great contributions to abdominoplasty and aesthetic body contouring surgery. Abdominoplasty has been an ongoing source of fascination for me for over 50 years now. Dr. Hunstad has prepared this book carefully on the basic topics of this procedure and ancillary procedures. He reviews the history of abdominoplasty that is always interesting to remember the contributions that pioneers have made in the past.

Reviewing the anatomy contained in this text allows us, as plastic surgeons, to perform a more precise procedure. Liposuction came to be the procedure that substitutes occasionally for abdominoplasty and in many occasions serves as a great complement to the procedure. At the present time minimally invasive plastic surgery is popular, therefore it is helpful to know when it is indicated to use endoscopic abdominoplasty as is discussed herein. Revision of postoperative care is very necessary to know especially to avoid complications. Likewise, for the occasional patient where mini abdominoplasty is a suitable procedure, Dr. Hunstad has described it perfectly.

The combination of abdominoplasty and liposuction is thoroughly covered and at the present time has become the procedure that is utilized more frequently. For obese exaggerated patients circumferential abdominoplasty is the best procedure and it has also been included in this valuable book. When mammary ptosis and supra umbilical abdominal wall adiposis and relaxation exist reverse abdominoplasty is the best procedure and has been covered as well.

All plastic surgeons can have complications and therefore the description of prevention and treatment of complications is extremely valuable. This charming book is one that plastic surgery residents in their first years, when they are beginning to operate, should master. Plastic surgeons with experience also have now a great book to review the present status of abdominoplasty and ancillary procedures. This book is sound and practical. It is based on the comprehensive experience of the author: it will give the reader an opportunity to learn and see plastic surgery of the abdominal wall through the mind and the hands of a superb plastic surgeon.

Jose Guerrerosantos, MD

Foreword

I was offered by Joseph P. Hunstad, MD, the privilege to write a foreword for his book on abdominoplasty. After having familiarized myself with its content and his impressive CV, I was delighted to turn this into a mission possible.

Only a select group of plastic surgeons around the world are able to aggregate such experience in body contouring surgery, including, obviously, the abdominal wall cosmetic surgeries. I am an eyewitness. I was able to attend to his presentations several times. In addition, Dr. Hunstad has contributed his experience and efforts to administrative committees, has made more than 200 scientific presentations, as well as several surgical performances around the world, has been granted several awards and is responsible for approximately 45 domestic and international articles. With such an active and restless personality, associated with his great creativity and accurate observational capacity, Dr. Hunstad now offers the plastic surgery community his 23-year experience summarized in this text on Abdominoplasty.

We all know that the anterior abdominal wall is one of the body areas most affected by aging, body weight variations, non disciplined life style, adipose tissue anomalous accumulations, celiotomies and pregnancies. For decades, these dysmorphisms have led many men and women to pursue exercise, physiotherapy, sports, dietary regimens and all sorts of non invasive treatments to solve their physical problems, of which the anterior abdominal wall is one of the most important. And in face of the very limited and unsatisfactory results achieved, the best solution turned out to be cosmetic abdominoplasty.

Due to the wide and diversified range of cosmetic problems involving the abdominal wall, a great number of techniques were simultaneously created, improved, discarded and recovered with a view to reducing surgical aggressiveness, improving the quality of the results and allowing reproducibility by experienced hands. This process also allowed the creation of several types of incisions and their peculiar scars, duly described by literature according to the nature of the problem.

Dr. Hunstad is lead author of all chapters of this book, but the sixth one, which was written by Dr. Ruth Graf. In this chapter she describes the abdominoplasty operation in simultaneous combination with liposuction including the epigastrium and the hypochondria, something no one has ever accepted or thought of before. Once again, medicine has proved to be the art of the transient truths.

Readers will be impressed with Dr. Hunstad's wide experience. He discusses everything from the traditional abdominoplasty to the leading edge refinements, including hip-trunk remodeling by the body contouring surgery and the most selective and less aggressive procedures, such as the mini-abdominoplasty. A comprehensive study on complications and solutions is also richly illustrated with specific discussions, thus providing readers with more important tips on what to avoid, what to do and how to perform when facing unacceptable problems. Also, to complete the information list, a selected number of DVDs on the different types of surgery is included to enrich the didactic nature of this text.

As we have already stated, the surgical techniques are neither static nor permanent. We are sure Dr. Hunstad will soon provide readers with new procedures aimed at increasingly improving the cosmetic results of the body contouring procedure and its reproducibility by other plastic surgeons' experienced hands. It was a pleasure to record my thoughts in this foreword.

Ricardo Baroudi, MD

Preface

It is a great honor to be a plastic surgeon. In this field we are entrusted with a patient's desired change in appearance, enhancement in form and physique, and often, most importantly, the patient's view of self. Aesthetic body contouring surgery provides improvement and transformation of a patient's body to one with desirable shape and contour while simultaneously achieving the elevation of a patient's spirit.

Abdominoplasty has been performed for more than 110 years. During this time, many significant advancements of this procedure have been developed. This operation is no longer simply an excision and closure removing unwanted redundant lower abdominal skin. It is now a family of procedures that addresses each individual patient's body habitus, personal desires and health status to provide for maximal benefit in shape and contour.

My purpose for writing this book was to share with my plastic surgery colleagues, in training, and those first entering practice, as well as experienced practicing surgeons my abdominoplasty and body contouring experience over the last 20 years. This text began as a thorough evaluation of the abdominoplasty procedure by itself and then expanded to include procedures to address adjacent areas of body contouring much as one does surgically to achieve smooth flowing harmonious contours.

A critical attempt to provide consistent pre- and post-operative photography was a key element for evaluating results. Including many intra-operative photographs and artistic renderings is intended to further enhance the understanding of the individual steps necessary to achieve optimal results.

Each chapter includes Key Presentation Points and a Summary Box. Patient Selection is emphasized for each procedure and appropriate examples are shown. Preoperative History and Considerations covers the item unique to the individual procedures. The Operative Approach is the key element of each chapter and includes a step-by-step description of the individual procedures. Included within this section are the majority of the text, images, tables, and pearls for success. Postoperative Care is subsequently emphasized to ensure appropriate follow-up. References are given specifically for each chapter and a large group listed as suggested reading.

Each specific technique of abdominoplasty is covered in its own chapter from endoscopic abdominoplasty through extended and circumferential abdominoplasty. The *Anatomic Considerations* chapter should be reviewed together with the comprehensive chapter on *Complications*. Understanding the changes in vascularity during these procedures is repeatedly illustrated and critical to minimize complications. Individual chapters on *The Umbilicus* and *Management of Existing Scars* emphasize the importance of these two entities.

Complete Revision Abdominoplasty reviews the main reasons for patient disappointment following previous abdominoplasty, including residual excess adiposity, skin excess, and abdominal wall/myofascial laxity. Correction of these unsatisfactory results is achieved by performing concurrent thorough tumescent liposuction, subscarpal fat resection, strong myofascial plication, and appropriate skin excision. This revision operation can transform a disappointed patient to one who is ecstatic with their final shape and contour.

Liposuction in Abdominal Contouring is an important chapter describing an important component necessary to achieve excellent results for most abdominoplasty procedures in a safe consistent manner. Methods to safely perform thorough concurrent liposuction are explained in detail.

Complications – Prevention and Treatment thoroughly reviews all entities that can go awry during abdominoplasty. Understanding these complications and providing effective treatment, and as importantly their prevention, is thoroughly emphasized.

Liposuction Abdominoplasty, and *Reverse Abdominoplasty*, were written with two prominent Brazilian colleagues, Drs. Graf and Deos, emphasizing the most current state-of-the-art for these procedures.

Plastic surgery is very much a visual endeavor. In composing this text, I visualized the specific procedures and described each element of these procedures in chronological fashion. Photographic documentation of each of these important steps is provided throughout each procedure. Combining photographic images with the specific steps, described in the text, provides for a readily usable description that can be incorporated into a surgical plan.

Achieving consistent, highly desirable results with minimal complications is a goal of all surgical procedures. By incorporating the technical specifics included in this treatise on abdominoplasty, high – quality results should be obtained, and surgeon and patient satisfaction should be enhanced. I sincerely hope that all readers will find the information contained herein to be useful and valuable in their practices, and will provide for them and their patients highly – satisfactory results.

Joseph P. Hunstad

Dedication

I dedicate this book to my wonderful family; Sherry, Lauren, Megan, and Biscuit.

Acknowledgments

I assisted on my first abdominoplasty procedure as a resident in 1981. I assisted my program chief Dr. John Beernink and Dr. W. David Moore. Both gentlemen freely shared aesthetic facial and body contouring procedures with me. I was excited and amazed with the tissue undermining, muscle plication, umbilical transposition, and skin excision. It was the most dramatic procedure I had ever witnessed. I remain excited and amazed today by the procedure in its entirety and the individual elements comprising it.

On entering practice in 1987, I began performing abdominoplasty. I performed a significant skin resection, concurrent modest liposuction, and a tight myofascial closure. I performed my first body lift or circumferential abdominoplasty in 1988. Although I had never seen this procedure, I reviewed the currently available world literature to formulate an appropriate plan to deliver the desired result. The results were very good and my patient was very pleased and has had additional aesthetic procedures with me over the last 20 years. Although my patients were pleased with their results at that time, I was seeking enhanced thinning, waistline enhancement, and an overall more dramatic result.

I began performing concurrent liposuction developed by Dr. Illouz with abdominoplasty at this time. I utilized the wet technique of Dr. Hetter and my results were improved with a decreased blood loss. I expanded my infiltration with greater amounts of wetting solution and further reduced the blood loss during liposuction performing the superwet technique championed by Fodor. I began performing more aggressive skin resections and closing all layers of the tissue including the Scarpa's or superficial fascia as the layer of maximum tension in 1988. This was consistent with Lockwood's subsequent description which validated this concept.

By 1992 I became aware of and utilized tumescent infiltration as described by Klein. When the virtual absence of bleeding was noted during liposuction, this technique immediately replaced all of my previous methods of infiltration. I developed an improved formula for the tumescent fluid that was Lactated Ringers-based instead of normal saline and most importantly was warmed. Dr. Gerald Pitman was very interested in the tumescent technique as well and he and I taught many teaching courses together and largely introduced the tumescent technique to the plastic surgery community. Also in 1992 I was elected as a member of the Board of Directors of the Lipoplasty Society. As a member of the board I was privileged to become friends with many great contributors to body contouring surgery.

I have shared the "Breakfast with the Experts" table and become good friends with Yves-Gerard Illouz. This allowed me to have a thorough understanding of the true development of liposuction and the brilliant simplicity of the blunt tipped cannula. His development of liposuction in 1977 was a milestone in body contouring.

As program chairman of the annual Lipoplasty meeting, I invited Dr. Jeff Klein to participate and together we gave an instructional course on the tumescent technique and have subsequently exchanged ideas. Dr. Ted Lockwood's enormous contribution of the understanding of the superficial fascia in body contouring is a critical element in achieving a high tension closure with a high-quality fine line incision scar. Prior to his untimely death, he was a guest at our home and we taught together at many international congresses.

It has been an honor to become acquainted with Professor Ivo Pitanguy and Dr. Fred Grazer, both inspirational leaders. As co-chairman with Dr. Jack Friedland of the combined Lipoplasty Society and ASAPS meeting in Tahoe, we honored both of these gentlemen for their considerable contributions to body contouring surgery. We have had many informative conversations together as faculty at national and international meetings discussing the history of body contouring and current innovations which helped further enhance the techniques that are presented herein. I was pleased to contribute to Fred Grazer's edition of the Clinics in Plastic Surgery. When I filmed the PSEF's DVD on Circumferential Abdominoplasty, I had the opportunity to visit Fred Grazer one last time prior to his death.

My understanding of liposuction was further enhanced by the teachings of my dear friends Dr. Ewaldo Bolivar de Souza Pinto and Dr. Sergio Luis Toledo. We have taught together at many symposia throughout the world, and their understanding of body contouring has been a great inspiration to me. Superficial liposuction and body shaping was taught to me by these gentlemen as well as by Dr. Carson Lewis and Dr. Marco Gasparotti.

By 1992, I had been performing very thorough liposuction throughout the entire abdominoplasty flap, flanks, hips, and mons. I was doing this successfully with an extremely low rate of ischemia or necrosis. The benefit of tumescent infiltration to minimize ischemia and necrosis cannot be overestimated. Professor Jim May and I have discussed the protective nature of this technique and I reinforce this concept throughout this text. I have been advocating this method of thorough liposuction during abdominoplasty now for 16 years. This technique differs from more conservative teachings by Dr. Alan Matarasso and others whom I respect. The safety of concurrent tumescent liposuction in abdominoplasty is documented in this Atlas.

I first performed subscarpal fat resection in 1993. I was unaware of anyone else performing this at that time. I was pleased when I presented this at the Vail Winter symposium in 1994 that Dr. Gilbert Gradinger concurred and had also been performing the procedure without any difficulties. I subsequently spoke to many physicians internationally regarding the use of subscarpal resection that has improved results without compromising vascularity.

In 1993 I presented at the annual meeting of the American Society of Plastic Surgeons Circumferential Abdominoplasty. This was well received and it was suggested that I consider a teaching course at the Aesthetic Society's annual meeting. Subsequently I have given the Advanced Abdominoplasty Teaching Course with Dr. Lee Colony, my close friend and colleague for many years. I have also given the teaching course on Circumferential Abdominoplasty for almost 8 years.

In 1992 with the development of the tumescent technique in plastic surgery, again advocated by Dr. Gerald Pitman and myself, there was a real need for instrumentation to provide for tumescent fluid infiltration. Dr. Ted Lockwood suggested that I take my ideas to Mr. Byron Economidy, president of Byron Medical. Byron put my ideas into production of an infiltration handle, infiltration cannulas, and a pressurized infusion device. According to Byron, this has become the most widely used instrument line for tumescent infiltration worldwide. Byron has become a true friend of mine and my wife Sherry, and I applaud him for his innovations in medical devices. Mr. Todd Lane, current president of Byron Medical, has been highly influential in my practice providing us current instrumentation for liposuction, fat grafting, and ultrasonic liposuction. We are currently in collaboration working on a number of other products. It has been a pleasure working with Byron and Todd.

Over the last 14 years, during my development of many body contouring procedures and enhancements in Liposuction surgery I have worked closely with my anesthesiologist, Dr. Philip Walk. He has been innovative as well, and always focused on safety in patient care. Working together we have published a number of articles on Outpatient Anesthesia and Anesthetic Considerations for Liposuction and Body Contouring. He has been a dear friend and colleague and has been very influential in my practice. He tolerates the time requirements for intraoperative photography, the silence necessary for video filming, working with multiple fellows with varying degrees of ability, and my emotional volatility and arcane musical interests.

I frequently discussed anesthesia considerations with my brother, Dr. David Hunstad an anesthesiologist, who encouraged me throughout the writing of this book. His intimate knowledge of physiology and patient care help me formulate important protocols that are included in this book. I am grateful to Dr. Tolbert "T" Wilkinson for his recommendation of me for an abdominoplasty book project to Elsevier. I appreciate Dr. Robert Ersek's support of the concepts and techniques that I've presented over the years.

My surgical nurses and surgical technicians have provided me unending support and tolerance. Mina Patel, Kim Butler, Stacie Jorishie, Heather Baerga, Casey Darling, and Melissa Earls are always focused first on patient safety and care. Their excellent work at improving efficiency and streamlining the practice of our surgical center is very much appreciated. They tolerate repeated clinical studies, data gathering, a steady stream of new fellows and visitors, and consistently work with me during difficult times. I wish to express heartfelt thanks for their understanding during difficult and challenging moments in the operating room. I also thank them for their enthusiasm and appreciation when they see our positive patients' results. My administrative staff deserves special thanks as well. Denise Poland, Jessica Rose, and Danai Garay are responsible for consultations and maintain order at the front desk. Ashley Helms and Rosalie Natoli, the center surgery schedulers, keep the schedule full and handle the many patient concerns regarding upcoming surgery. My aestheticians, Marti DeCoste and Tammy Ledford, provide excellent postoperative care including lymphatic drainage, Endermologie, and ultrasound treatments. Samantha and Annie Mason ensure smooth running of the Medi-Spa and Surgical Center respectively.

I would like to thank Elsevier and their talented staff, particularly Ms. Sue Hodgson and Ms. Sharon Nash. They were both more than supportive and provided the encouragement I needed during the difficult months working on this manuscript. Their never ending enthusiasm and encouragement helped make this come together.

Sincere thanks to Dr. Remus Repta who worked with me as a fellow and in the capacity of a colleague and friend. His many suggestions and challenging questions provided a more comprehensive and thoughtful book. I wish him the best of luck in his new practice in the Phoenix area.

My family is extraordinarily important to me. During the writing of this book and with other pending plastic surgery projects, I have been more absent than present. My parents Freda and Norman Hunstad encouraged me throughout my life but most importantly during those important developmental years of high school and college. They supported me during challenging times and always demonstrated and promoted excellence. Their acknowledgment of my uniqueness and encouragement of my goals are traits that I've tried to apply in my life and to my children.

My wife Sherry has stood by me during many difficult times. Her support of me personally and in my practice is really more than I deserve. We have grown together and share many wonderful friendships throughout the world that came about because of the travels that plastic surgery has provided us. My daughters Lauren and Megan understand the time requirements of plastic surgery and have both voiced interest in the field of medicine. It has been a delight to see them take interest in my practice, observe surgical procedures, and positively interact with all the members of my staff. The very special love in a family cannot be easily described but would be terribly missed.

CHAPTER 1

History

Joseph P. Hunstad and Remus Repta

The American history of abdominoplasty begins with Kelly's first report in 1899,[1] in which he coined the term 'abdominal lipectomy.' During this first procedure, lower abdominal tissue was excised much as one 'takes a slice lengthwise of a watermelon.' This visually understandable description set the stage for many modifications and enhancements of this procedure. The tissue resection was quite substantial, weighing 7450g and measuring 90 × 31 × 7 cm! In 1910 he reported his eight-patient experience at the Johns Hopkins Hospital, where the incision extended across the central abdomen onto the flanks.[2] This transverse wedge excision of skin and subcutaneous tissue, with possible hernia repair, was performed without undermining. He was the first to note 'cosmetic benefit' from this procedure.

Prior to that, in 1890, the French surgeons Demars and Marx had performed significant skin and fat resection from the abdomen. In 1905 Gaudet and Morestin performed a resection of significant excess skin and underlying fat, repair of a large umbilical hernia, and umbilical preservation. In 1931, Passot included undermining with the resection.

German contributions included the transverse elliptic incision in abdominoplasty as described by Morestin,[3] who also published notably on the correction of prominent ears, breast lift, and breast reduction. Weinhold, in 1909, combined a vertical and transverse cloverleaf resection, and in 1911 Jolly[4] first reported the low transverse incision for abdominal tissue resection. A vertical resection was championed by Babcock[5] in 1916.

Thorek's textbook *Plastic Surgery of the Breast and Abdominal Wall* in 1924[6] described umbilical preservation. In 1939, Thorek[7]coined the term 'plastic adipectomy' for the resection of 'fat aprons.' He described his resection technique as a wedge resection eliminating dead space when the skin edges were closed. He removed the umbilicus with the tissue specimen and then replanted it as a graft in a new, fitting location. He also postulated on alternative methods of circumscribing the umbilicus and leaving it attached by its stalk to the abdominal wall, bringing it through the skin at the end of the procedure.

Foged, in 1949,[8] emphasized the importance of hemostasis. Gillies and Millard,[9] in their 1957 textbook *Principles and Art of Plastic Surgery,* were the first to describe the 'Jack-knife' position, and recommended postoperative knee flexion to reduce the tension on the transverse closure.

Barsky, in 1964,[10] was the first to describe the use of a postoperative abdominal binder. The standard abdominoplasty incision was lengthened circumferentially by two notable surgeons, namely Somalo in 1941[11] and Gonzalez-Ulloa in 1960.[11a] Gonzalez-Ulloa coined the term 'belt lipectomy.' This was subsequently expanded upon by Kamper et al.,[12]who in 1972 recognized the value of circumferential resection after massive weight loss. These concepts are current today and widely used for the treatment of massive weight loss.

Vernon, an American surgeon, was the first to publish umbilical transposition and relocation with extensive undermining in 1957.[13] Also during the 1950s, dermolipectomy procedures were being performed on the abdomen with increased frequency, notably in South America. Pitanguy's landmark article in 1967[14] described 300 abdominal lipectomies and attracted considerable interest. This technique used a transverse incision which curved down at both ends.

The W technique was described by Regnault, from Montréal, Canada, in 1972.[15,16] This involved resection of the upper hair-bearing mons with lateral incisions along the inguinal folds.

Baroudi[17] published his significant experience in 1974 and 1975, drawing particular attention to the importance of an aesthetic appearance of the umbilicus. His many significant contributions to all techniques in body contouring are well known. The use of quilting sutures was championed by Baroudi as well, and is used extensively to minimize or eliminate seroma and to lessen or eliminate the need for drains in reverse abdominoplasties (Chapter 10) and lipoabdominoplasty (Chapter 6).

During this time Grazer[18] first described rectus plication, which he first learned from Pitanguy (personal discussion, 2001) and which is still in routine use today. His contributions to body contouring are numerous, including gull-wing modification of the Pitanguy abdominoplasty and dermatolipectomies of the extremities, liposuction, and body contouring for the massive weight loss patient. He also performed critical reviews of the American history of abdominoplasty, and by using survey techniques established frequently cited risks and complications.[19]

In 1977 Illouz[20] first performed blunt-tipped liposuction, which ushered in a completely new concept for body contouring. Previous techniques used sharp cutting devices which resulted in significant tissue trauma and scarring. Illouz's technique has certainly stood the test of time. The simple brilliance of a blunt-tipped cannula protecting important neurovascular structures is now one of the most popular cosmetic plastic surgery procedures worldwide. Illouz states that 'It is now rare that an abdominoplasty be performed without the assistance of adipoaspiration. Not only is adipoaspiration a useful complement, but it also allows undisputedly good refinements.' This concept will be described in detail throughout this text as an important adjunctive procedure.

Also in 1977, Rebello[21] described the reverse abdominoplasty, a useful technique for selected patients that have a small amount of soft-tissue laxity primarily located in the supraumbilical abdomen.

Converse (personal communication 2008) was the first to use the concept of hydrodissection which was further expanded by Illouz and Hetter.[22,23] The process of injecting so-called 'wetting' solutions was again greatly expanded upon by Klein,[24] who coined the term 'tumescent' for large-volume infiltrations. These concepts resulted in a substantial reduction in blood loss during liposuction procedures, allowing much greater volumes of liposuction to be performed without the need for transfusion. These concepts are equally appropriate for both local and general anesthesia and are used concurrently with the majority of abdominoplasty procedures.

Toranto,[25] in 1988, expanded on Pitanguy's and Grazer's concepts for rectus plication by bringing together not only the medial borders of the rectus muscle anterior rectus sheath but often the lateral borders as well. This was noted to dramatically improve the waistline and posture of the abdominoplasty patient.

A very important concept in body contouring was set forth by Lockwood[26] in 1991, with his emphasis on the superficial fascial system (SFS). Wounds closure by maximum tension at the level of the superficial fascia allowed the skin closure to be performed under minimal tension, which helps to achieve a fine-line high-quality scar.[26] Lockwood further described a high-lateral tension abdominoplasty which was designed to improve the waistline.

In the mid-1990s endoscopic techniques were being applied to aesthetic procedures of the face, breast and body. The concept of an endoscopic abdominoplasty was introduced, which consisted of abdominal liposuction with endoscopically assisted muscle plication.[27] This is a useful technique for patients with only a small amount of soft tissue laxity and whose abdominal contour irregularity is largely a result of myofascial laxity.

In the recent years, Hunstad[28] has used many of the above concepts in a combined fashion, including high-lateral tension, SFS closure, wide rectus abdominis plication, subscarpal fat resection, and thorough concurrent tumescent liposuction, to achieve desirable and predictable results.

Continuous improvement in body contouring procedures in general, and in abdominoplasty techniques in particular, has been observed since the very first procedures were performed more than 100 years ago. Future improvements and innovation will undoubtedly be introduced as the current and future generations of plastic surgeons continue to refine the practice of body contouring surgery.

References

1. Kelly HA. Report of gynecological cases excessive growth of fat. Johns Hopkins Med J 1899; 10: 197.
2. Kelly HA. Excision of the fat of the abdominal wall lipectomy. Surg Gynecol Obstet 1910; 10: 299.
3. Morestin A. La restauration de la paroi abdominate par résection enteudue des téguments et de la graisse souscutúee et le plissement des apouéurises superficielles envisagé comme complément de la cure radicule des hernies omblicales. Thése Paris 1911.
4. Jolly IT. Abdominoplasty. Berl Klin Wschr 1911; 48: 1317.
5. Babcock W. On diseases of women and children. Am J Obstet Gynecol 1916; 74: 596.
6. Thorek M. Plastic surgery of the breast and abdominal wall. Springfield, Ill: Charles C Thomas, 1924.
7. Thorek M. Plastic reconstruction of the female breast and abdomen. Am J Surg 1939; 43: 268.
8. Foged J. Operative treatment of abdominal obesity, especially pendulous abdomen. Br J Plast Surg 1949; 1: 274–283.
9. Gillies H, Millard DR Jr. The principles and art of plastic surgery, Vol 2. Boston, MA: Little Brown, 1957.
10. Barsky AJ, Kahn S. Principles and practices of plastic surgery. New York: McGraw-Hill, 1964.
11. Somalo M. Dermolipectomia circular del tronco. Cir Plast II Arch Chir Exp 1941; 1: 404.

11a. Gonzalez-Ulloa M. Belt lipectomy. Br J Plast Surg 1960; 13: 179.

12. Kamper MJ, Galloway DV, Ashley F. Abdominal panniculectomy after massive weight loss. Plast Reconstruct Surg 1972; 50: 441.
13. Vernon S. Umbilical transplantation upward and abdominal contouring in lipectomy. Am J Surg 1957; 94: 490.
14. Pitanguy I. Abdominal lipectomy: An approach to it through an analysis of 300 consecutive cases. Plast Reconstruct Surg 1967; 40: 384.
15. Regnault P. Abdominoplasty by the ‘W’ technique. Plast Reconstruct Surg 1975; 55: 265.
16. Regnault P. The history of abdominal dermolipectomy. Aesthet Plast Surg 1978; 2: 113.
17. Baroudi R, Keppke EM, Tozzi-Netto F. Abdominoplasty. Plast Reconstruct Surg 1974; 54: 161.
18. Grazer FM. Plastic operation on the abdomen. Calif Med 1973; 119: 64.
19. Grazer FM. Abdominoplasty. Plast Reconstruct Surg 1973; 51: 617.
20. Illouz YG. History and current concepts of lipoplasty. Clin Plast Surg 1996; 23: 721.
21. Rebello C, Franco T. Abdominoplasty through a submammary incision. Int Surg 1977; 62: 462.
22. Illouz YG. Illouz's technique of body contouring by lipolysis. Clin Plast Surg 1984; 11: 409.
23. Hetter GP, Lipoplasty. The theory and practice of the blunt suction lipectomy, 2nd edn. Boston: Little, Brown, 1990.
24. Klein JA. Tumescent technique for liposuction surgery. Am J Cosmet Surg 1987; 4: 263.
25. Toranto IR. Resolution of back pain with the wide abdominal rectus plication abdominoplasty. Plast Reconstruct Surg. 1988; 81: 777.
26. Lockwood TE. Superficial facial system SFS of the trunk and lower extremities: A new concept. Plast Reconstruct Surg 1991; 87: 1009.
27. Eaves FF III, Nahai F, Bostwick J III. Endoscopic abdominoplasty and endoscopically assisted miniabdominoplasty. Clin Plast Surg 1996; 23: 599.
28. Hunstad JP. Advanced abdominoplasty concepts. In: Saleh M, ed. Perspectives in plastic surgery, Vol. 12. New York: Thieme, 1999; 13–38.

CHAPTER 2

Anatomic Considerations in Abdominal Contouring

Joseph P. Hunstad and Remus Repta

IN THIS CHAPTER

KEY POINTS/SUMMARY

When performing abdominal contouring procedures, it is necessary to understand the anatomy of the abdominal region and how it relates to the specific surgical operation being performed. The vascularity of the abdominal soft tissue is particularly important, considering the large area that is often undermined during abdominoplasty, the common use of concurrent liposuction, and the fact that the tissue is often closed under tension. Understanding the muscular and fascial components of the abdominal wall is important for myofascial plication and hernia repair. The sensory distribution is also important when considering incision placement for abdominal body contouring procedures. Specific caveats of the abdominal anatomy are important to note, as they play an important role in simplifying and safely achieving excellent aesthetic results in abdominal contouring procedures.

Introduction

The anatomy of the abdominal wall and overlying soft tissues is both straightforward and elegant. This chapter will review the relevant anatomy of abdominal contouring procedures, including topography, superficial structures, deep structures, vascular supply, the lymphatic system, and the innervation of the abdominal soft tissue. Important aspects of each of these categories as they pertain to abdominal contouring procedures will be discussed.

Topography (Box 2.1)

Patients who present for abdominoplasty or abdominal contouring procedures do so with a variety of different body types and levels of fitness. Some may have excess skin laxity and little excess adiposity; others may have extensive excess adiposity; and yet others may have neither or both, along with various degrees of abdominal myofascial laxity. The topography of the abdominal area will differ among these different patients, but it is always important to identify and visualize the pertinent anatomy in order to properly plan and execute the desired abdominal contouring procedure.

There are a number of important bony and soft-tissue landmarks that should be identified during preoperative marking (**Fig. 2.1**). The bony landmarks include the paired anterior–superior iliac crests, the pubic symphysis, the xiphoid, and the costal margins bilaterally. These landmarks can usually be palpated in all

Box 2.1 Topography

- The aesthetic result is determined largely by the preoperative marking/surgical plan.
- Preoperative marking begins by identifying key landmarks, including the xiphoid, anterosuperior iliac spines, and the pubic symphysis.
- The soft-tissue structures, including linea alba, paired linea semilunares, and the tendinous insertions of the rectus abdominus, are particularly important when lipo-etching is planned.

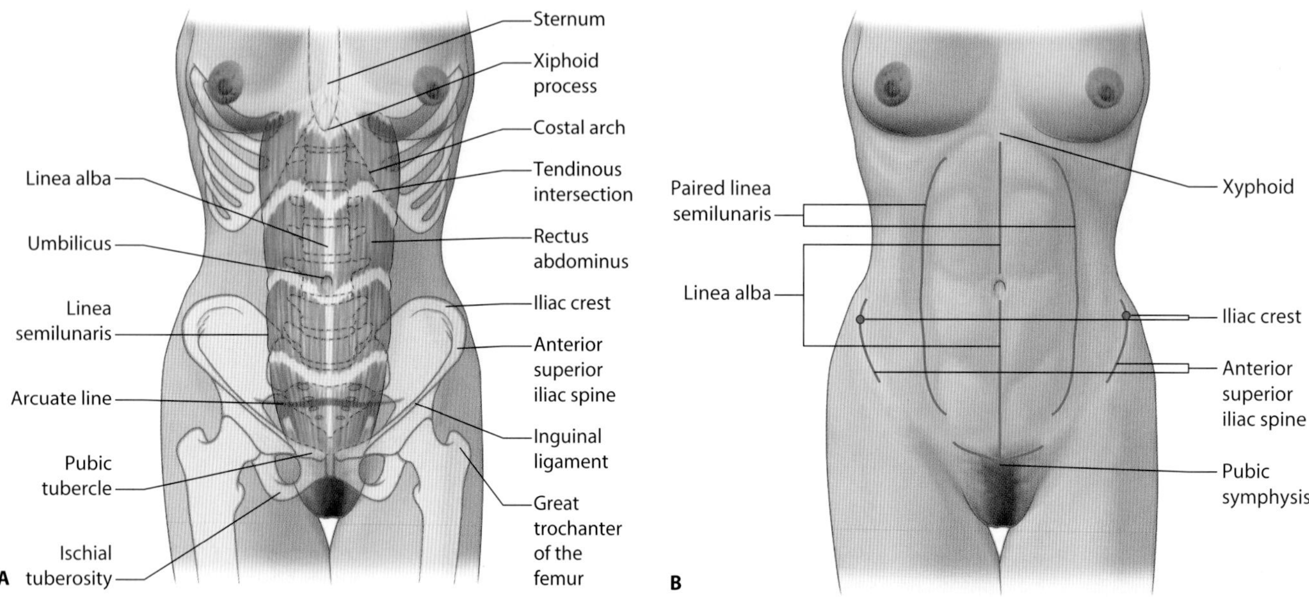

Fig. 2.1 A, B Topographically, a handful of bony and soft tissue landmarks can be identified. The bony landmarks include the xiphoid, pubic symphysis, the anterior superior iliac spine, and the iliac crest. These landmarks are useful in orienting and ensuring the symmetry of the transverse incision in abdominoplasty procedures as well as during myofascial plication and umbilical inset.

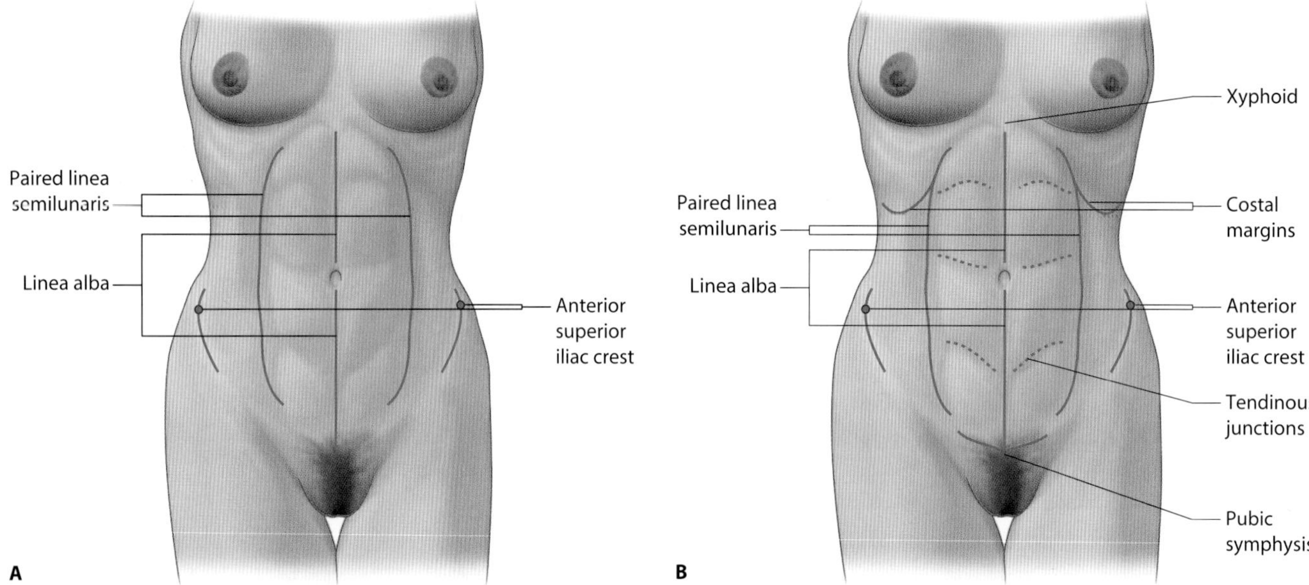

Fig. 2.2 A, B The soft-tissue landmarks may not be easily visualized in patients with excess adiposity. These landmarks include the linea alba, the paired linea semilunares, and the tendinous junctions or insertions of the rectus abdominis muscles. These landmarks become especially important in patients undergoing abdominal contouring with lipo-etching. The aesthetically pleasing abdomen often has these soft-tissue landmarks noticeable to a certain extent.

patients regardless of body mass index (BMI) or habitus, although it may be somewhat more difficult in patients who are significantly overweight. These bony landmarks will serve as the initial reference points for the preoperative markings to identify the midline and to ensure the symmetry of the final planned incision. It is important to note that the marks on the skin may shift considerably relative to the bony landmarks, especially in patients with significant soft-tissue laxity. This is why it is important for the preoperative marking to be performed with the patient standing.

The soft-tissue landmarks include the linea alba, the paired linea semilunaris, and the transverse tendinous junctions of each rectus abdominis muscle (**Fig. 2.2**). It is interesting to

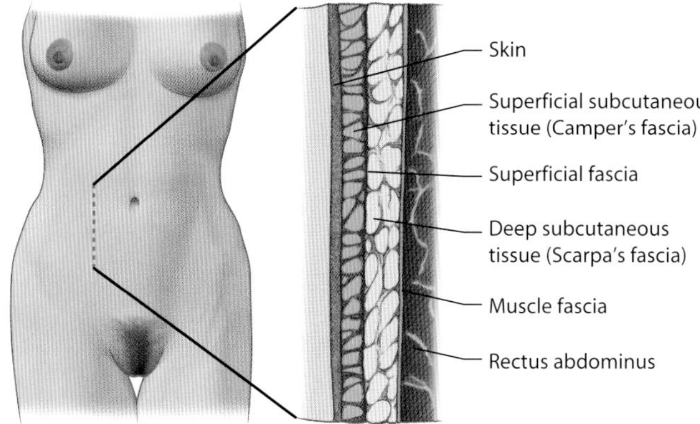

Fig. 2.3 The superficial structures of the abdominal wall are contained in the soft-tissue apron. From superficial to deep, these structures include the skin, superficial fat and investing Camper's fascia, Scarpa's fascia, and the sub-Scarpa's fascia fat. Knowledge and appreciation of Scarpa's fascia (superficial fascia of the abdomen) is critical to performing any abdominoplasty procedure. Resection of soft tissue during an abdominoplasty procedure is dependent on placing the tension of the closure on the Scarpa's fascia. This allows the skin to be closed with relatively little tension to avoid poor healing or poor scar formation. The deep fat or sub-Scarpa's fascia fat tends to be less fibrous and organized than the superficial fat.

note how much of the aesthetic appeal of a healthy, fit abdomen is attributed to these landmarks that are primarily associated with the anatomical architecture of the rectus abdominis muscles. These landmarks are particularly important in fairly thin or fit patients who desire improved abdominal definition. Abdominal liposuction for improved definition, especially when it involves lipo-etching, relies on knowledge and identification of these landmarks.

Superficial Structures

For the purpose of discussing anatomy in the context of abdominal body contouring procedures, the abdominal layers can be separated into superficial and deep structures. The superficial structures include skin, the superficial subcutaneous fat associated with Camper's fascia, Scarpa's fascia or the superficial fascial system of the abdomen (SFS), and the deep subcutaneous fat or sub-Scarpa's fat (sub-Scarpal fat) (**Fig. 2.3**). The proportion of the superficial to the deep fat layer is variable among patients, depending on their BMI and body habitus. The sub-Scarpal fat is usually less compact, with less fibrous architecture than the fat superficial to Scarpa's fascia.[1] Scarpa's fascia, or the superficial fascia system of the abdomen (SFS), is an important anatomic layer in body contouring in general, and in abdominoplasty procedures in particular. Scarpa's fascia is the structure that allows surgical closure in abdominoplasty procedures to be performed under remarkably high tension without vascular compromise to the skin.[2] As most of the tension of the closure is placed on the SFS, and the skin closure is subjected to considerably less tension, a good-quality scar can be achieved.

Deep Structures

The deep structures include the deep muscular fascia overlying the abdominal wall musculature and the abdominal wall muscles themselves, with all of the corresponding layers of investing fascia (**Fig. 2.4 A–C**). The anatomy of the rectus sheath is of considerable importance because the majority of myofascial plication methods involve approximating this tissue. The three components of the lateral abdominal wall – the external oblique, internal oblique, and transverse abdominis – come together medially as fascial extensions to form the anterior and posterior rectus sheath. Superior to the arcuate line, the anterior rectus sheath is composed of the fascial extensions of the external oblique and half of the internal oblique. The fascial extension of the internal oblique muscle splits around the rectus abdominis above the arcuate line and reforms at the linea alba. Inferior to the arcuate line the anterior rectus sheath is composed of the fascial extensions of all three muscular layers, with the tissue posterior to the rectus abdominis consisting of only the peritoneum (**Fig. 2.4 E and F**). One can also include the intra-abdominal fat as one of the deep abdominal structures, as for some patients the presence of extensive amounts of such fat can play a role in the final aesthetic result, limiting how much flattening of the abdomen can be accomplished.

The three components of abdominal contouring that are routinely addressed include reduction of excess adiposity by liposuction, elimination of soft-tissue laxity by resection, and correction of abdominal wall laxity by myofascial plication. The latter deals with the deeper structures directly. The term myofascial plication is used throughout this book because it describes more accurately the process of correction of abdominal wall laxity through plication. Classically, abdominal wall plication was described as plication of the rectus abdominis muscles in conjunction with plication of the anterior rectus sheath, because of the presence of rectus abdominis diastasis, seen as linea alba widening. Although rectus abdominis diastasis is frequently seen in abdominoplasty candidates, it is the global laxity of the abdominal wall/fascia that is important. The main purpose of myofascial abdominal wall plication is **correction of global abdominal wall laxity as well as rectus diastasis**. In so doing, the waistline is narrowed on AP view and abdominal convexity is corrected on lateral profile.

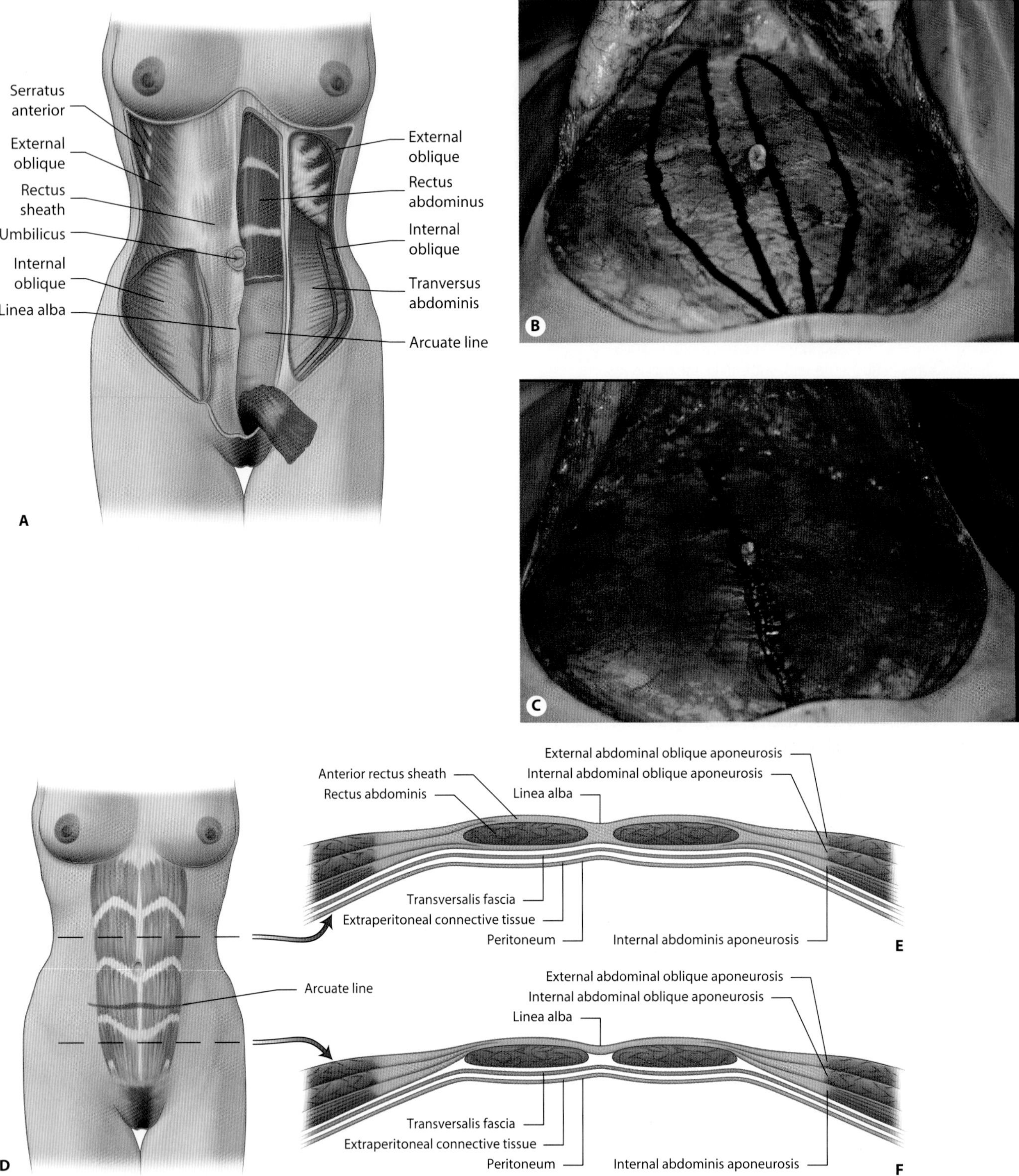

Fig. 2.4 A–F The deep structures of the abdominal wall include all of the abdominal wall muscles and the investing fascia. (A) Once the abdominal soft tissue is elevated, the fascia, the rectus abdominis muscles medially and the external obliques laterally are seen. The fascia overlying the rectus abdominis is substantially thicker. Above the arcuate line it is composed of the continuation of the external oblique and half of the internal oblique fascia. (E) Below the arcuate line, the entire fascia from the external and internal oblique muscles as well as the transverse abdominis muscles forms the anterior rectus sheath. (F) Most abdominoplasty procedures involve myofascial plication. Traditionally, this is described as rectus abdominis muscle plication. Although some degree of rectus diastasis is usually seen, most of the abdominal wall laxity is a result of global fascial laxity. Myofascial plication reduces this laxity by imbricating the anterior rectus sheath, narrowing the linea alba and bringing the linea semilunares closer together. In doing so, the fascial laxity of the abdominal wall is pulled in and reduced (B,C).

Box 2.2 Vascular anatomy

- The abdominal soft tissue has an extensive vascular network.
- The three main vascular sources to the abdominal soft tissue include perforators from the deep epigastric arcade, the superficial epigastric and circumflex vessels, and the continuation of the intercostal and subcostal vessels bilaterally.
- Most standard abdominoplasty procedures, including full, extended, and circumferential, result in an abdominal soft tissue flap that is supplied by the intercostal and subcostal vessels.

Box 2.3 Lymphatics

- The superficial abdominal lymphatic system is contained within the abdominal soft tissue above the muscular/deep fascia.
- Most of the lymphatics superior to the umbilicus drain to the axillary lymph node basin. Most of the lymphatics inferior to the umbilicus drain to the superficial inguinal lymph node basin.
- A significant portion of the lower abdominal tissue associated with lymphatic disruption during abdominoplasty procedures is resected.

Vascular Anatomy (Box 2.2)

The vascular perfusion of the abdominal wall, subcutaneous tissue, and abdominal skin, comes from three separate sources.[3,4] The primary blood supply comes from rectus perforators that originate from the deep epigastric arcade supplied by both the deep superior and deep inferior epigastric vessels, the superficial inferior and superficial superior epigastric vessels, the superficial circumflex vessels, and several intercostal and subcostal vessels (**Fig. 2.5**). An intimate knowledge of the vascular supply of the abdominal soft tissue is critical because abdominoplasty procedures involve soft-tissue undermining with division of at least one or more of these vascular sources. With the sole exception of abdominal liposuction, all abdominoplasty procedures, including endoscopic, mini, full, extended, reverse, and circumferential techniques, divide at least one of the vascular sources to the abdominal soft tissue. Endoscopic and reverse abdominoplasty techniques usually divide the perforators from the deep epigastric vascular arcade coursing through the rectus muscle. Full abdominoplasty, extended abdominoplasty, and circumferential abdominoplasty techniques also divide the superficial inferior epigastric and superficial circumflex vascular supply. In essence this creates a bipedicled abdominal soft-tissue flap based on the intercostal and subcostal vessels[5] (**Fig. 2.6**).

Lymphatics (Box 2.3)

The lymphatics of the abdominal wall can be categorized into superficial and deep vessels. The superficial lymphatic vessels are located in the abdominal soft tissue above the deep muscular fascia, and the deep lymphatic vessels are those associated with the abdominal wall musculature. In large part, abdominal contouring procedures involve the superficial lymphatic vessels. Although myofascial plication involves the deep fascia, the deep lymphatics are not encroached upon by standard abdominoplasty procedures.

The abdominal soft tissue lymphatics are a latticework of lymph vessels that drain primarily into the axillary and superficial inguinal lymph nodes, with the umbilicus serving as the watershed between these two lymphatic tributaries[6] (**Fig. 2.7**). Cephalic to the umbilicus the superficial lymphatic vessels coalesce and drain into the axillary lymph node basin. There is also some lymphatic flow to the parasternal lymph node basin, but this is a minor portion. Caudal to the umbilicus the lymphatic vessels coalesce and drain into the superficial inguinal lymph node basin.

Abdominal contouring procedures inevitably disturb some of these superficial lymphatic vessels. Depending on the technique used, some or most of the superficial inferior lymphatic flow may be disturbed. Fortunately, most abdominoplasty techniques also involve resection of the inferior skin and subcutaneous tissue that has undergone disruption of the lymphatics. Lymphatic preservation may be possible by performing extensive deep liposuction of the inferior abdominal region, which is then left in place during flap elevation and resection. These concepts of liposuction abdominoplasty are addressed in Chapter 6.

Nerves (Box 2.4)

The cutaneous innervation of the abdomen includes dermatomes T4–L1 (**Fig. 2.8**).[6] The lateral and anterior cutaneous branches of the intercostal and subcostal nerves supply much of the innervation to the abdominal soft tissue (**Fig. 2.9**). The anterior branches of the intercostal and subcostal nerves travel between the internal oblique and the transverse abdominis muscles. The cutaneous portions of these nerves travel through the rectus abdominis muscles to emerge from the anterior rectus sheath and supply sensation to the midline abdomen. The cutaneous distribution of the anterior branches of the intercostals and subcostals mirrors the vascular supply of the deep epigastric arcade discussed above. These nerves are seen as they are transected during the process of abdominal soft-tissue elevation.

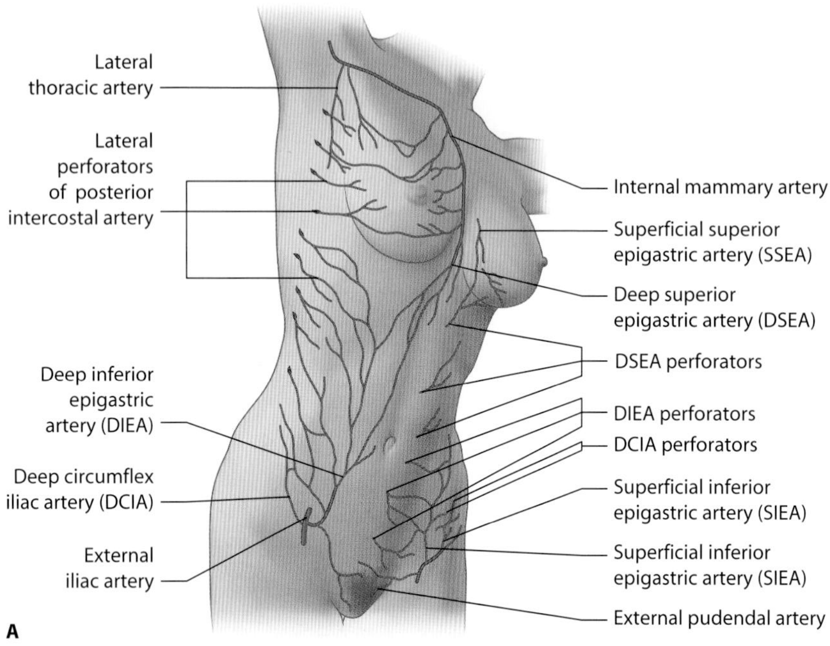

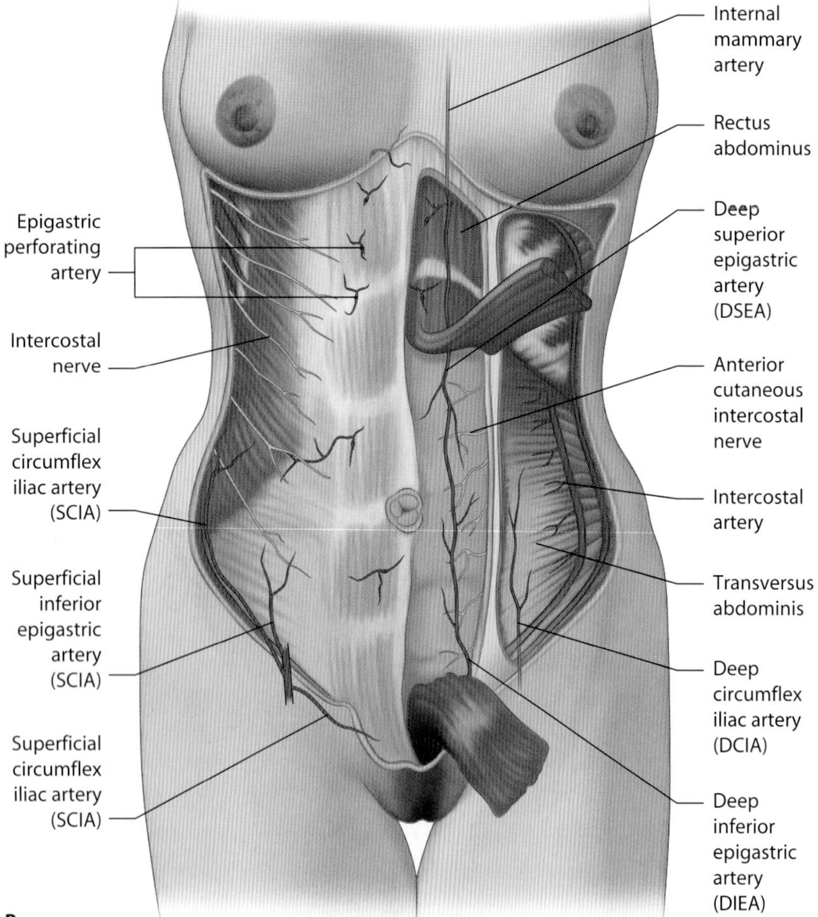

Fig. 2.5 A, B The abdominal wall has an extensive blood supply. Although the soft tissue vascular plexus is extensive and interconnected, the vascular contribution can be grouped into three separate sources based on the primary source of the perforators. In the midline of the abdomen, multiple perforators from the deep epigastric vessels course through the rectus abdominis muscles and supply the overlying soft tissue. The continuation of the internal mammary vessels and the deep inferior epigastric vessels form an anastomosis deep to the rectus abdominis muscles. The superficial superior epigastric vessels may also contribute a small component in the midline superiorly. Laterally, the continuation of the intercostals and subcostal vessels bilaterally contribute to the soft-tissue vascular plexus. In the lower half of the abdomen, the superficial inferior epigastric and superficial circumflex vessels join the soft-tissue vascular plexus.

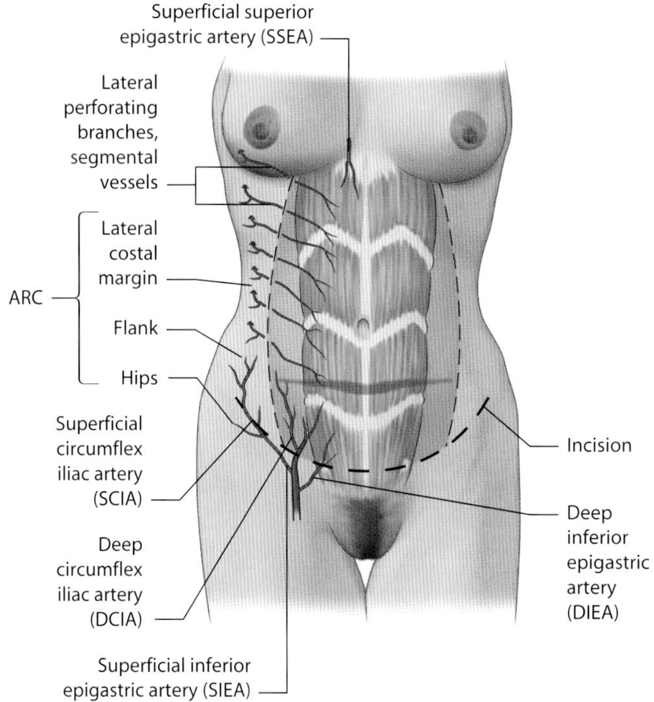

Fig. 2.6 Most abdominal contouring procedures, apart from liposuction, disrupt at least one vascular source to the abdominal soft tissue. All abdominoplasty procedures that involve myofascial plication disrupt the perforators from the deep epigastric vessels. Abdominoplasty procedures, including extended and circumferential abdominoplasty and potentially full abdominoplasty techniques, also disrupt the superficial inferior epigastric and superficial circumflex perforators. With these techniques, the abdominal soft tissue is essentially a bipedicled flap with perforators from the intercostal and subcostal perforators bilaterally.

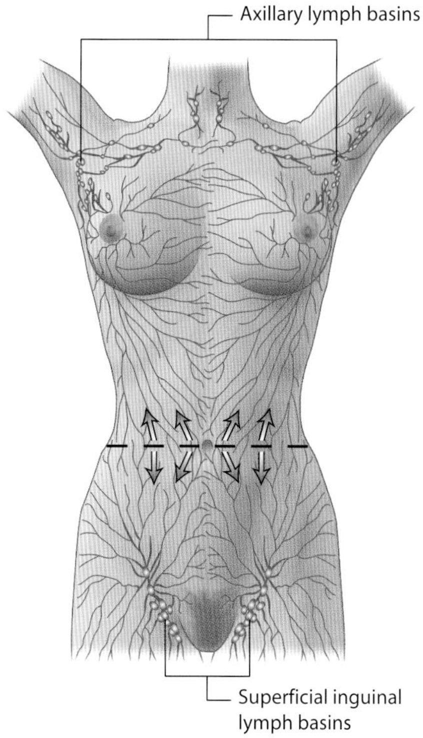

Axillary lymph basins

Superficial inguinal lymph basins

Fig. 2.7 The abdominal soft-tissue lymphatics drain largely into the axillary and superficial inguinal lymph basins. The lymphatic network is located within the soft tissue apron, with the umbilicus serving as a watershed point. The soft-tissue lymphatics above the umbilicus drains primarily into the axillary lymph basin while those below the umbilicus drain primarily into the superficial inguinal lymph basin.

Box 2.4 Nerves

- Lower abdominal numbness is common following most abdominoplasty procedures because ascending branches of the ilioinguinal nerve are divided.
- The lateral femoral cutaneous nerve is at risk when the transverse incision is placed very low.
- Patients should be instructed not to use excessive heat or cold on the abdomen postoperatively, as their altered abdominal sensation cannot protect them from thermal injury.
- Branches of the ilioinguinal nerve are divided as they course superiorly from the mons following cesarean section or abdominoplasty.

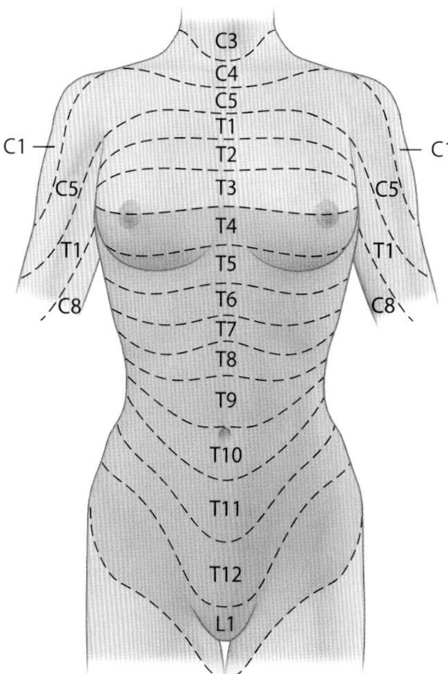

Fig. 2.8 The abdominal skin and soft tissue receives its innervation from the continuation of intercostal and subcostal nerves, T4–L1.

The lateral branches of the intercostal and subcostal nerves emerge through the oblique muscles laterally near the midaxillary line and travel superficial to the external oblique (**Fig. 2.9**). These nerves are visible when dissection is performed laterally over the external oblique muscles. The lower intercostal and subcostal cutaneous connections of these nerves

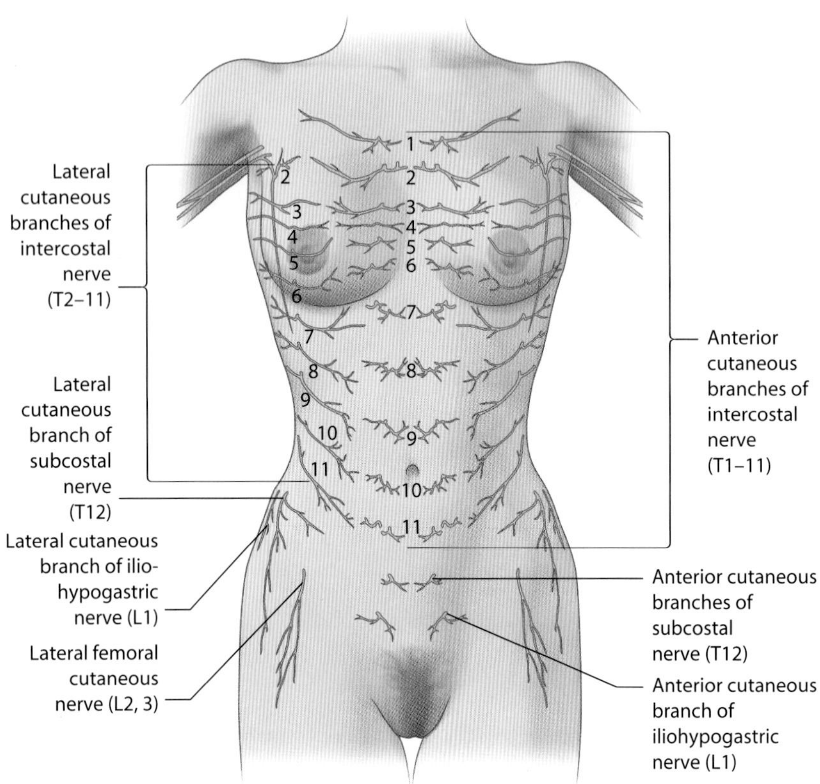

Fig. 2.9 The anterior branches of the intercostal and subcostal nerves supply sensation to the midline abdomen. These nerves travel between the internal oblique muscles and the transverse abdominis muscles. They pass through the rectus abdominis muscles and emerge through the anterior rectus sheath to supply the overlying skin and soft tissue. The lateral branches of the intercostal and subcostal nerves exist through the oblique muscles near the midaxillary line and travel superficially to the external obliques to supply sensation to the overlying skin and soft tissue laterally. The continuation of the subcostal nerve and L4 – which is the iliohypogastric nerve – supply sensation of the skin and soft tissue over the iliac crest and lateral thigh. The lateral femoral cutaneous nerve emerges from the muscular fascia below the inguinal ligament near the midpoint of the inguinal ligament, classically described as the junction between the lateral one-third and the medial two-thirds of the inguinal ligament.

may also be transected during dissection, whereas the upper (T4–T8) intercostal nerves usually remain intact.

The most inferior abdominal skin is innervated by the ilioinguinal nerve, which courses superiorly through the mons. Many patients presenting for abdominoplasty have had a previous Pfannenstiel incision or a cesarean section, and have numbness of the lower abdominal skin because superiorly coursing branches of the ilioinguinal nerve have been divided. Abdominoplasty procedures that have the transverse incision very low near or slightly below the inguinal fold must be performed with care to avoid damage to the lateral femoral cutaneous nerve. This usually exits the muscular fascia just below the inguinal ligament near its midpoint. Although all standard abdominoplasty procedures produce temporary numbness of the lower abdominal skin, injury to the lateral femoral cutaneous nerve will result in numbness of the anterior thigh on that side. This can be more bothersome to patients than abdominal numbness, perhaps because the sensation is different between the left and right anterior thighs.

Summary

The anatomy of the abdominal wall is both straightforward and elegant. A thorough knowledge of the vascular source, the innervation, the lymphatics, as well as the deep and superficial structures of the abdominal wall is important for performing abdominoplasty and abdominal contouring procedures. Most importantly, knowledge of the vascular supply to the abdominal soft tissue as well as the superficial soft-tissue structures, specifically Scarpa's fascia, is critical to safely achieve an optimum aesthetic result.

Clinical Caveats: Anatomical considerations in abdominal contouring

- The anatomy of the abdominal wall is both straightforward and elegant. A thorough understanding of vascular supply, fascial planes, nerves, and lymphatics is critical to safely achieve excellent aesthetic results while minimizing morbidity.
- Identifying key topographic landmarks, including the anterior superior iliac spines, the pubic symphysis, the costal margins, and the xiphoid, during preoperative marking facilitates accurate and symmetric surgical design.
- Understanding the superficial fascia (SFS) or Scarpa's fascia is important in achieving safe and aesthetically pleasing results in abdominoplasty procedures. Significant tension can be placed on Scarpa's fascia, allowing considerable soft tissue resection without undue tension on the skin. The final skin contour will be smooth and even because of this. Failure to close the specific anatomic layer will lead to a result similar

to that following a cesarean section, namely a bulge superior to, a depression at, and a bulge inferior to the final scar.

- Traditional abdominoplasty procedures, including full, extended, and circumferential abdominoplasty, divide the deep inferior epigastric perforators as well as some or all of the deep superior perforators, leaving the abdominal soft tissue as a bipedicled flap based on the intercostal and subcostal vessels bilaterally.
- Although the lymphatics of the lower abdominal soft tissues are interrupted during dissection, most of this soft-tissue area is resected at the completion of the case.
- Most abdominoplasty techniques result in disturbance of some of the innervation to the central and lower abdomen. Extra care should be taken in dissection near the inguinal fold when the transverse abdominoplasty incision is placed very low to avoid injury to the lateral femoral cutaneous nerve.

References

1. Markman B, Barton FE. Anatomy of the subcutaneous tissue of the trunk and lower extremity. Plast Reconstruct Surg 1987; 80: 248.
2. Lockwood T. Superficial fascia system (SFS) of the trunk and extremities: a new concept. Plast Reconstruct Surg 1991; 87: 1009.
3. Boyd JB, Taylor GI, Corlett RJ. The vascular territory of the superficial and the deep inferior epigastric arteries. Plast Reconstruct Surg 1984; 73: 1.
4. Taylor GI, Palmer JH. The vascular territories (angiosomes) of the body: experimental study and clinical applications. Br J Plast Surg 1987; 40: 113.
5. Mayr M, Holm C, Höfter E, et al. Effects of aesthetic abdominoplasty on abdominal wall perfusion: a quantitative evaluation. Plast Reconstruct Surg 2004; 114: 1586.
6. Moore KL, Dalley AF. Clinically oriented anatomy. Baltimore: Lippincott Williams & Wilkins, 2006.

Suggested Reading

Farah AB, Nahas FX, Ferreira LM, et al. Sensibility of the abdomen after abdominoplasty. Plast Reconstruct Surg 2004; 114: 577.

Grevious MA, Cohen M, Shah SR, Rodriguez P. Structural and functional anatomy of the abdominal wall. Clin Plast Surg 2006; 33: 169.

Moore KL, Dalley AF. Clinically oriented anatomy. Baltimore: Lippincott Williams & Wilkins, 2006.

Rozen WM, Ashton MW, Taylor GI. Reviewing the vascular supply of the anterior abdominal wall: redefining anatomy for increasingly refined surgery. Clin Anat 2008; 21: 89.

Suami H, O'Neill JK, Pan WR, Taylor GI. Perforating lymph vessels in the canine torso: direct lymph pathway from skin to the deep lymphatics. Plast Reconstruct Surg 2008; 121: 31.

Tregaskiss AP, Goodwin AN, Acland RD. The cutaneous arteries of the anterior abdominal wall: a three-dimensional study. Plast Reconstruct Surg 2007; 120: 442.

CHAPTER 3

Liposuction in Abdominal Contouring

Joseph P. Hunstad and Remus Repta

IN THIS CHAPTER

KEY POINTS

Liposuction is an important part of abdominoplasty and abdominal contouring procedures. It should be performed in a well thought-out and organized manner in order to optimize safety and the aesthetic result. It can be used concurrently with abdominoplasty procedures to appropriately thin the abdominal flap while maintaining vascularity. If the patient is actively smoking or has other potential healing issues, less aggressive liposuction, less tension during closure, or both should be performed. Smoking cessation is strongly preferred.

Introduction

Liposuction plays an integral role in abdominal contouring procedures. Most patients presenting for abdominal contouring benefit from the concurrent use of liposuction. Whether liposuction is used to thin the abdominal flap, to contour adjacent areas such as the hips and thighs, or to contour the posterior trunk, it is indispensable in achieving an optimum aesthetic result. The goal of most body contouring procedures is not only to improve the contour and shape of the abdomen, but to achieve a smooth, flowing, harmonious contour by improving the overall silhouette and appearance of the region. In this chapter we will discuss the specific caveats of liposuction in abdominoplasty, including the technical aspects of tumescent infiltration, power-assisted liposuction (PAL), ultrasound-assisted liposuction (UAL), and a review of the instruments and techniques used to achieve optimal results.

Preoperative Preparation

There are several decisions that must be made before the patient is brought to the operating room. Among these are the preoperative markings that will guide the surgeon as to the areas and extent of liposuction, the entry sites, whether UAL will be needed, the volume of tumescent fluid needed, concentration of lidocaine and epinephrine per liter of infiltration fluid, as well as patient positioning. Addressing these decisions preoperatively will facilitate efficient use of the operating room and staff, reduce the overall time the patient is under anesthesia, and optimize safety, and provide superior results.

Patient Positioning and Intraoperative Precautions

Patient positioning depends on the area or areas that need to be treated, other procedures the patient will be undergoing, the patient's body habitus/BMI, and surgeon preference. If the patient is scheduled to undergo liposuction of the abdominal flap as well as the lumbar area, then both prone and supine positioning is usually recommended. Some surgeons prefer using the left and right lateral decubitus positions instead of a combination of prone and supine.

One caveat with regard to patient positioning is that it is better to have sufficient and efficient positioning and achieve the optimum aesthetic result during the initial surgery than to have to return to the operating room for revisions and correction of contour irregularities. With that said, we believe that the prone and supine positioning offers the best opportunity to achieve symmetry by simultaneously evaluating the left and right sides of all body areas, and reduces the need for revision. Certain areas, such as the lateral trunk, hips, and thighs, may be amenable to supine-only positioning, but we prefer to ensure symmetry and perform these procedures with the patient in both the prone and the supine positions, allowing better contouring of the areas from several access points and from different directions. It is import-ant to keep the patient well padded at all pressure points and safely positioned. In addition, placing lower extremity compression devices, keeping the patient warm, and placing a urinary catheter when appropriate should all be on the preoperative checklist before surgery can proceed.

Tumescent Infiltration (Box 3.1)

The use of infiltration fluid containing epinephrine has become obligatory when performing liposuction. The three types of infiltration methods – wet, superwet, and tumescent – differ largely according to the volume of fluid used and infiltration/aspiration ratios. All three methods involve infiltration of physiologic intravenous fluid (lactated Ringer's solution is preferred) containing lidocaine and epinephrine. The wet infiltration method involves injecting 200–300 mL of solution per area to be treated; the superwet and tumescent techniques use larger volumes than the wet technique and have essentially become the methods of choice. The superwet technique involves injecting a volume of infiltrate that is roughly equal to the amount of aspirate that is proposed to be suctioned out. The ratio of infiltration to aspiration is approximately 1:1.5. The tumescent technique uses a larger amount of infiltrate than the anticipated amount of fat to be removed.[1] The ratio of infiltration fluid to aspirate volume is roughly 1:1 for large-volume suctioning; for smaller procedures the ratios are higher. Small areas, such as touch-up liposuction, can have an infiltration-to-aspirate ratio of 10:1, i.e., 1000 mL of infiltrate to 100 mL of aspirate. The amount of blood loss per aspirate is comparable for both superwet and tumescent methods at approximately 1–2%.

Box 3.1 Tumescent infiltration

- Tumescent solution should be at or slightly above body temperature to avoid heat loss.
- Epinephrine should be added to the solution just prior to infiltration to reduce the time the epinephrine is exposed to heat and light which degrades it.
- The amount of lidocaine per kg patient weight should be determined preoperatively. Large-volume liposuction will benefit from using a modified tumescent solution of 12.5 mg lidocaine per liter in order to avoid surpassing the safe maximum dose.
- The amount of solution needed should be judged by clinical examination, including tissue rigidity and the presence of a fountain sign.
- Sufficient time should be allowed between infiltration and liposuction to achieve maximum vasoconstriction.

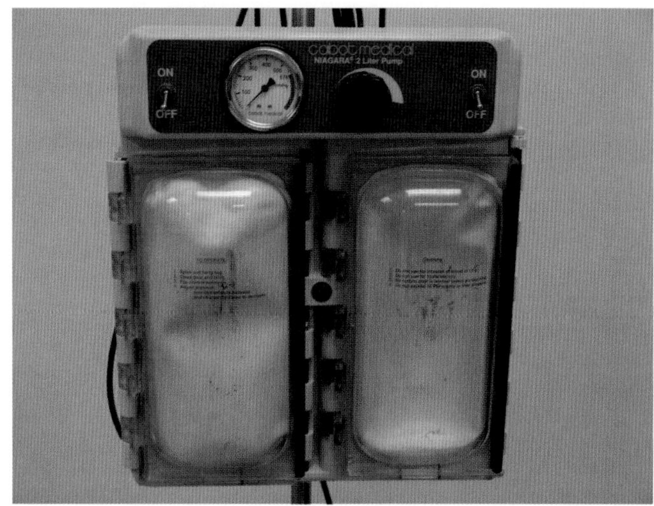

Fig. 3.1 A variety of infiltration machines exist. We use a common air-pressurized machine that holds two 1 L bags and can be rapidly switched from one bag to another. The goal is to have an infiltration set-up that allows infiltration to be performed rapidly and efficiently, minimizing the time the patient is exposed to anesthesia.

For efficient tumescent infiltration we use a pneumatic pressurized pump (**Fig. 3.1**). This gives us continuous uninterrupted infiltration while the tumescent fluid bags are changed. This is the most efficient technique. The composition of the infiltration fluid depends on the amount of liposuction anticipated. The amount of epinephrine generally remains the same at one ampule (1 mL) per liter (1: 1 000 000) of Lactated Ringer's, and we modify the lidocaine

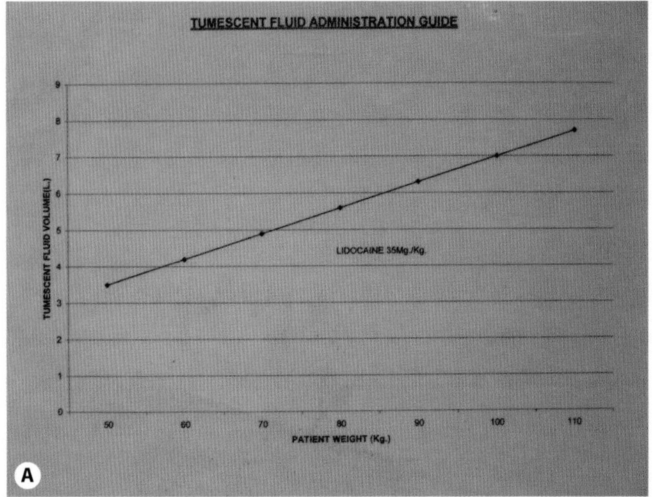

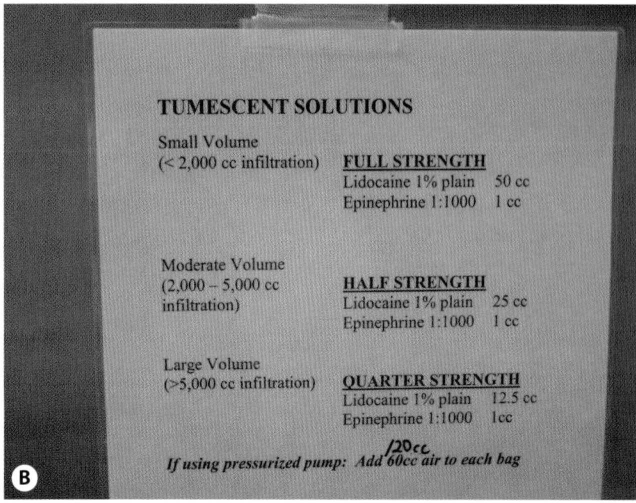

Fig. 3.2 A, B The tumescent infiltration fluid is made using predetermined formulas for lidocaine concentration. Two tables are available in the operating room near the infiltration fluid that show the amount of lidocaine per liter, number of liters used, and maximum safe lidocaine concentration levels per patient, as well as the appropriate infiltration mixture formulas for the volume of liposuction planned. This simplifies and improves safety in relation to lidocaine concentration.

Table 3. 1 The modified Hunstad tumescent solution mix. For larger-volume liposuction cases the amount of lidocaine per liter of infiltrate is reduced to avoid exceeding the maximum accepted safe levels of lidocaine

Modified Hunstad Tumescent Fluid Solutions		
	Half-Strength Solution (Normal Mixture)	Quarter-Strength Solution (Large-Volume Mixture)
Lactated Ringer's solution	1000 ml	1000 ml
1% Lidocaine plain	25 ml	12.5 ml
Epinephrine 1:1000	1 ml	1 ml
Final concentrations (fluid warmed to 38°C)	Lidocaine: 0.05% Epinephrine 1:1,000,000	Lidocaine: 0.0125% Epinephrine 1:1,000,000

concentration depending on the amount of proposed liposuction to keep the dosage below the accepted maximum of 55 mg/kg.[2] We routinely keep the lidocaine dosage below 35 mg/kg, as this has an extremely good margin of safety (**Fig. 3.2**). When large-volume liposuction is planned it is beneficial to use a modified, more dilute tumescent mixture in order to avoid exceeding the safe level of lidocaine (**Table 3.1**).

Lactated Ringer's is superior to normal saline for tumescent infiltration for many reasons. The pH is relatively neutral at 6.5, whereas normal saline is quite acidic at pH 5.0. Because of this neutral pH, it is not necessary to add sodium bicarbonate to Lactated Ringer's-based tumescent fluid, as it is with normal saline-based fluid. Ringer's Lactate is more physiologic than saline and is very useful for fat grafting.

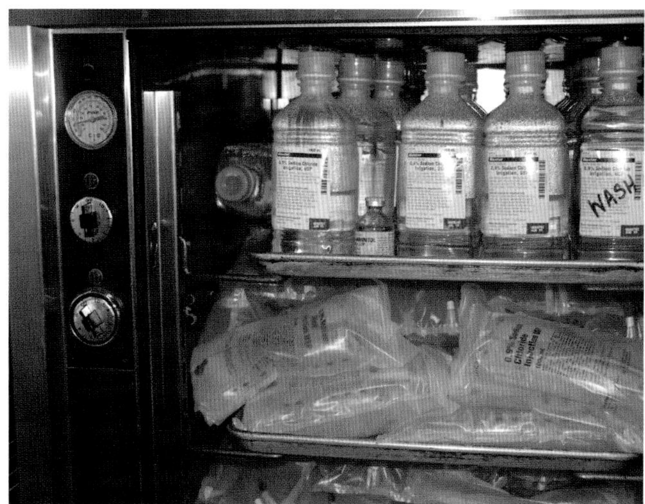

Fig. 3.3 Liposuction infiltration fluid should be maintained at or slightly above body temperature in order to reduce heat loss for the patient (38°C is ideal). Lidocaine and epinephrine are added to the solution prior to infiltration to minimize the amount of time the epinephrine is exposed to light and heat.

There is 3.5 mEq/L less sodium in Lactated Ringer's than in normal saline. All of our liposuction solutions are kept at a temperature of 38°C or 100°F (**Fig. 3.3**).

A few key points about infiltration fluid are worth emphasizing. The first is that although it is important for the fluid to be warm so as to help maintain the patient's core body temperature, it must not be too hot. In addition to the physical trauma created by fluid that is too warm, one must remember that epinephrine is susceptible to degradation at elevated temperatures. Epinephrine has a recommended

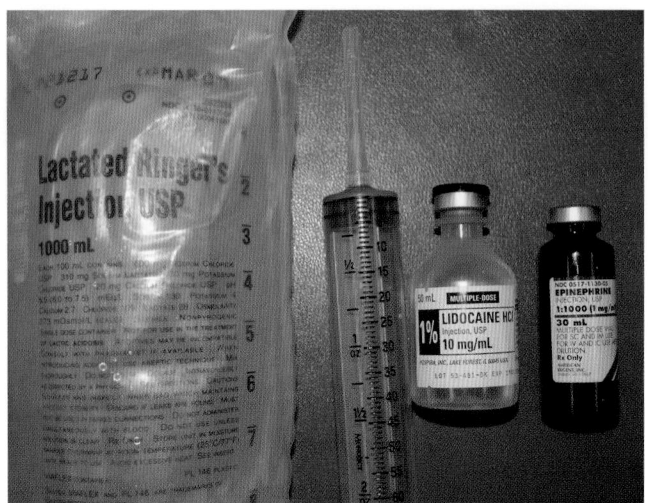

Fig. 3.4 The tumescent liposuction infiltration is made by adding lidocaine and epinephrine to lactated Ringer's solution based on the amount of liposuction planned. The epinephrine is added just before infiltration to minimize the amount of time the solution is exposed to light and heat.

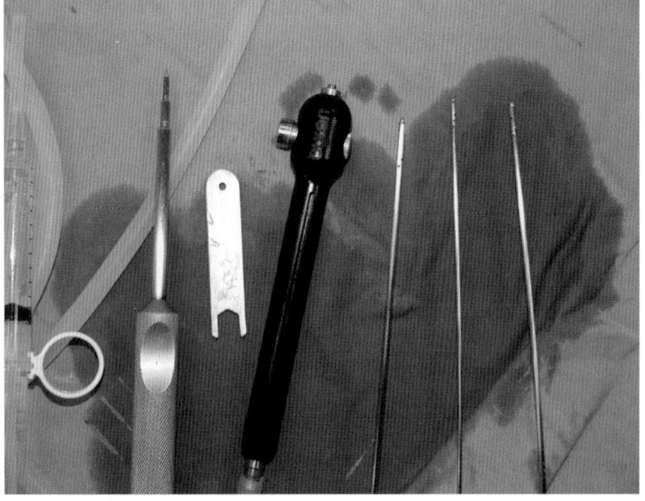

Fig. 3.5 The instruments used for tumescent infiltration are basic and include a Hun-Han infiltration handle to control the infiltration fluid flow, blunt-tipped infiltration cannulas of sufficient length to reach the areas to be suctioned from the planned access sites, a skin entry device, and an automatic stainless steel skin stapler (Byron Medical). The skin entry device we use is the Enter-Ease. It allows entry sites to be made with minimal bleeding. The stainless steel stapler is used to close the entry sites after infiltration to prevent the fluid escaping.

storage temperature of 15–25°C (59–77°F),[3] and should be protected from light as well as from freezing. It is difficult to know at what temperature the clinical effects of degradation are noted. Our infiltration fluid is roughly body temperature at 38°C, and importantly, **the epinephrine is added to the Lactated Ringer's solution just before it is infiltrated** (**Fig. 3.4**). We have noticed a reduction in the effect of

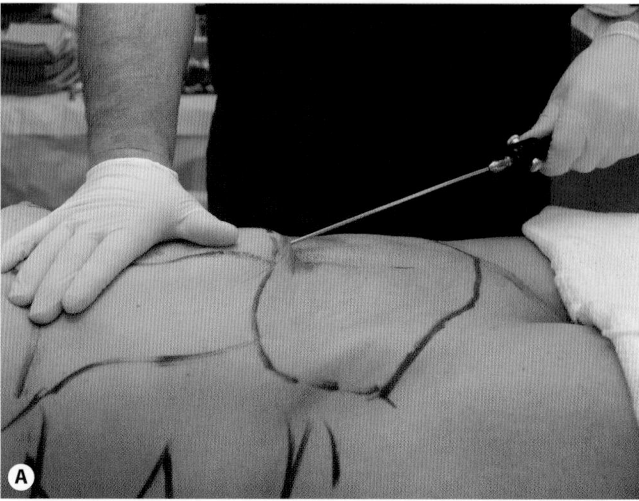

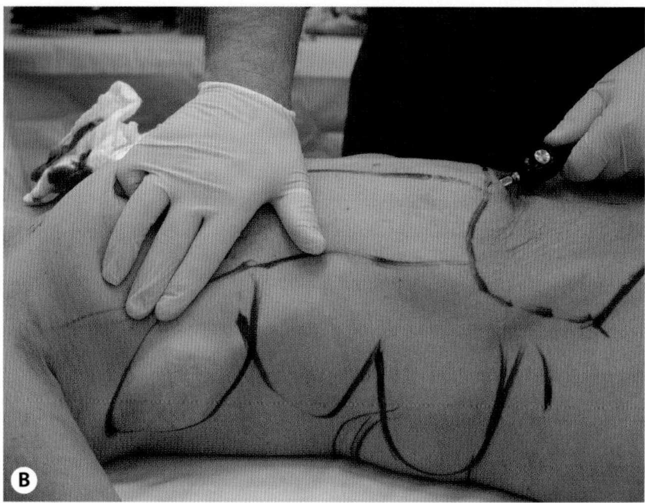

epinephrine due to prolonged fluid warming; and we have experienced poor vasoconstriction with the use of epinephrine from certain manufacturers. We cannot be sure why this occurred, but we believe that the epinephrine may have been exposed to prolonged elevated temperatures in transit from the supplier to our office. Epinephrine should be stored in a cool, dark location without direct sun exposure.

Infiltration is performed through the preoperatively designated assess sites. Entry into the access sites can be performed in a variety of ways. Using the Enter-Ease device reduces dermal bleeding from the skin puncture site (**Fig. 3.5**). The desirable interval between infiltration and surgery corresponds to the time necessary for patient preparation and draping, approximately 20 minutes. This stepwise design is time efficient and allows the epinephrine to be maximally effective (**Fig. 3.6**). Tumescent fluid is placed superficially first, and then at successively deeper levels (**Fig. 3.7**). The amount of infiltration performed

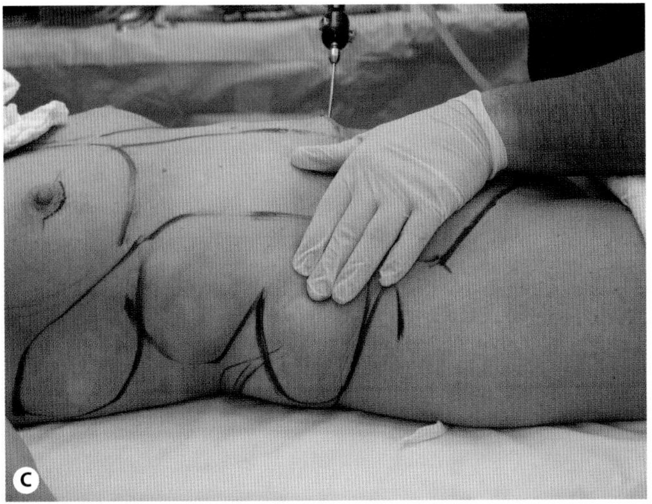

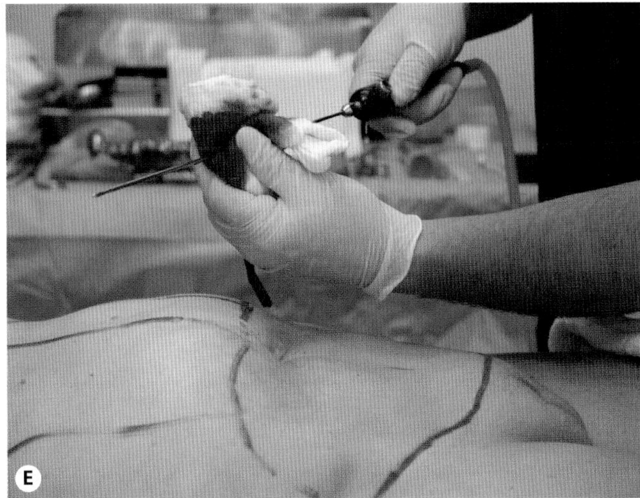

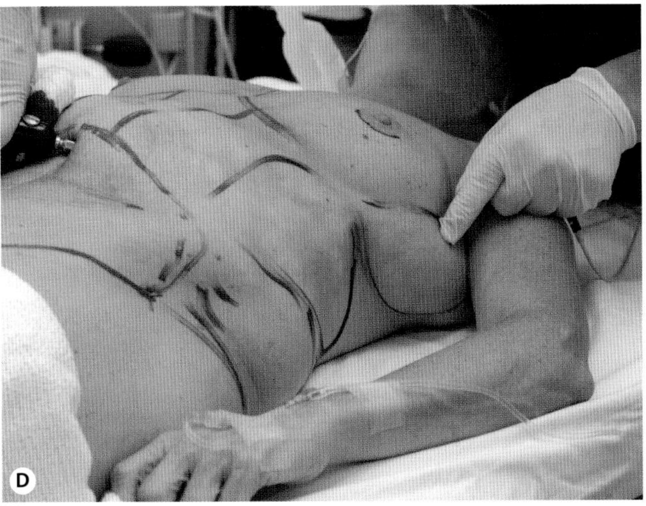

Fig. 3.6 A–E Infiltration is performed **before** preparation and draping, to allow ample time for the epinephrine to achieve proper vasoconstriction before the start of the procedure. During infiltration, the skin entry site and infiltration cannula are wiped with a Betadine-soaked surgical sponge. We have noticed no increase in the incidence of infection when performing infiltration in this manner. Infiltration of all of the liposuction areas is performed via the preoperatively marked entry sites.

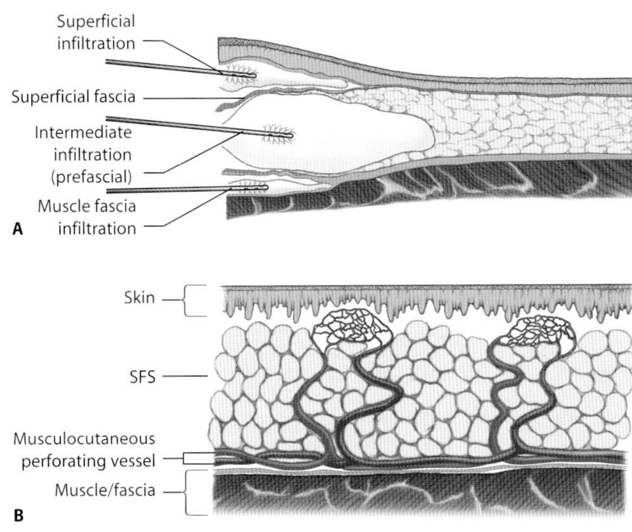

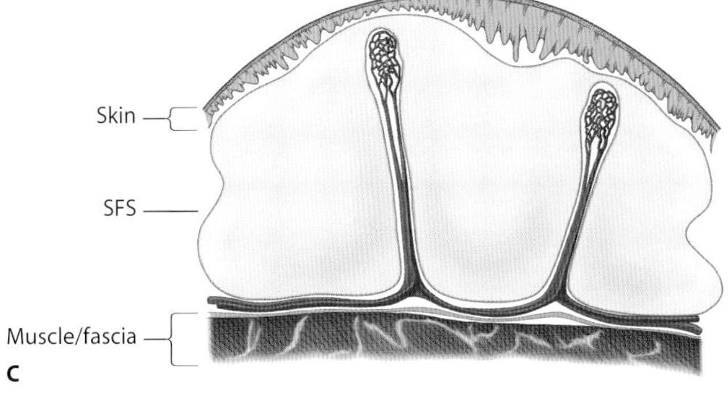

Fig. 3.7 Well-hydrated tissue after tumescent infiltration.

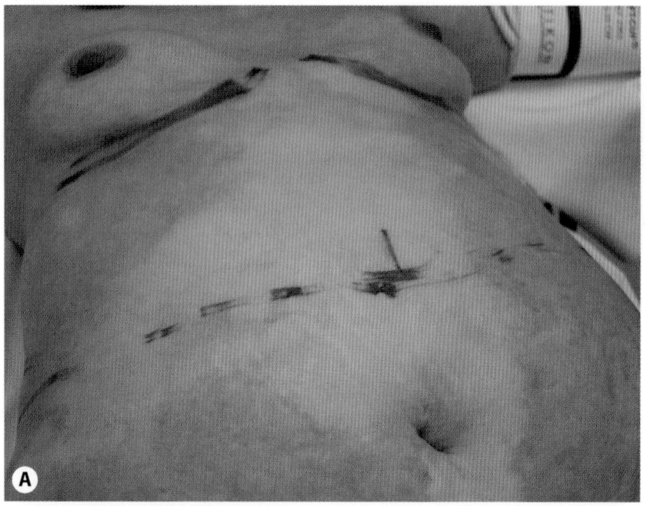

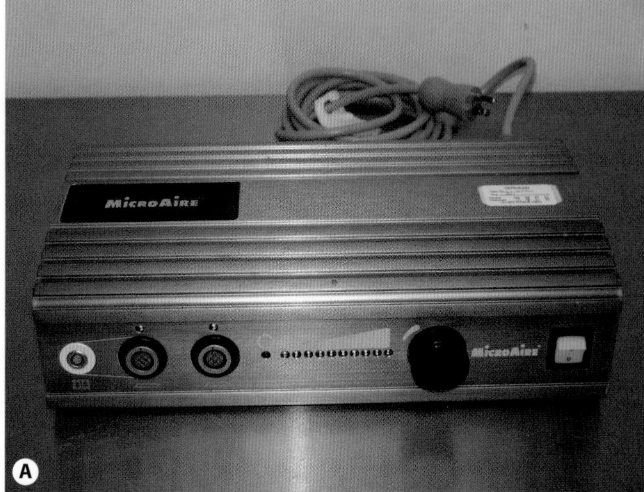

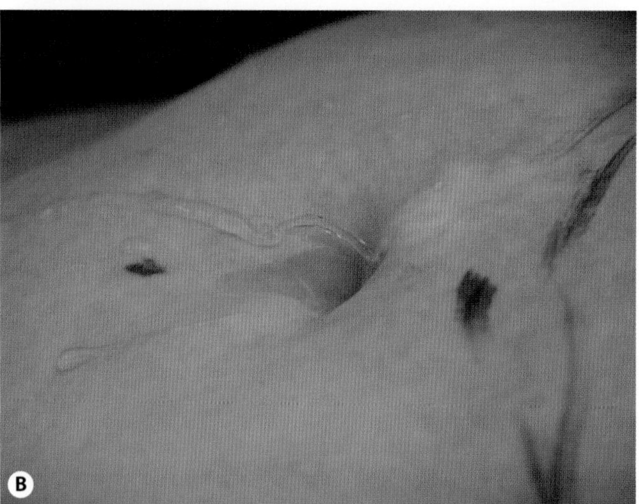

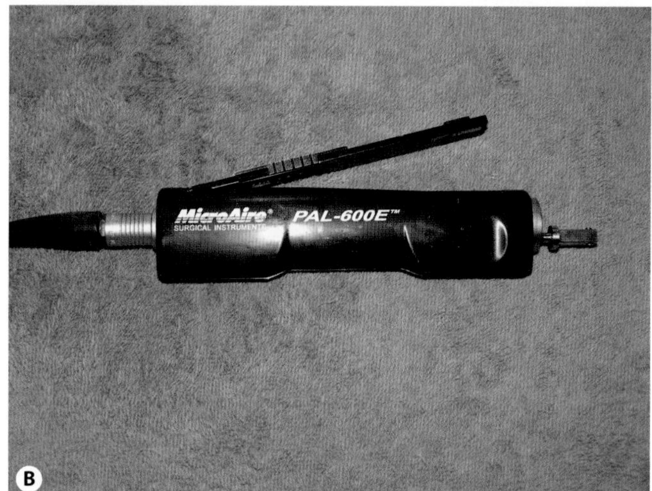

Fig. 3.8 A, B When infiltration is performed using the tumescent technique the amount of fluid needed is determined by noting several clinical signs. The first is tissue turgor, i.e., when the area being infiltrated becomes firm to palpation. The second sign is peau d'orange and blanching of the overlying skin. The third is the fountain sign, which is when the infiltration cannula is withdrawn and some of the infiltration fluid escapes.

is determined intraoperatively. Several clinical signs can be relied on to verify that the appropriate amount of infiltration has been given, including tissue turgor, blanching of the overlying skin, and the 'fountain sign' (**Fig. 3.8**).

Power-assisted Liposuction

The use of regular suction-assisted liposuction or power-assisted liposuction (PAL) is a matter of surgeon preference. PAL involves a motorized handle that reciprocates the liposuction cannula, making it easier to pass back and forth through the tissues, thereby reducing operator fatigue. The principle behind the technology is analogous to trying to push your hand through a bag of sand. A direct straight-line advancement of your hand runs into resistance early, until a slight alteration of the direction is made. This movement is constantly made by PAL to allow the tip of the cannula to find the path of least resistance. On smaller cases this may not be significantly advantageous, but for larger cases and over the course of the day it results in a significant reduction in the amount of energy expended by the surgeon. It further allows the surgeon to spend more time performing liposuction, thereby achieving better results.

A series of cannulas are available for PAL. The machine handle and cannulas currently employed are shown in **Figure 3.9**. This MicroAire device has been reliable and user-friendly. (We have no financial involvement with this company.)

Ultrasound-assisted Liposuction

Ultrasound-assisted liposuction can be very useful in abdominal contouring procedures,[4–6] especially for treating

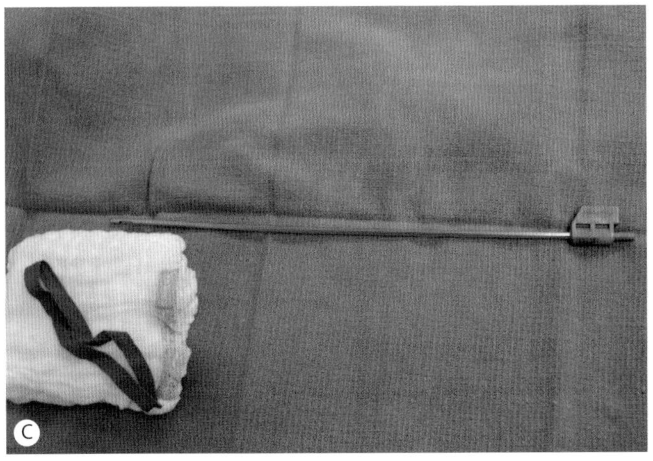

Fig. 3.9 A–C Power-assisted liposuction is valuable tool in abdominoplasty. The technology reduces the amount of force exerted by the surgeon to advance the cannula, lessening surgeon fatigue and improving efficiency. Given this, it is reasonable to assume that a more thorough liposuction can be performed. Cannulas for PAL are comparable to regular SAL cannulas in terms of hole configuration, diameter, and length. We often perform much of the liposuction in abdominal contouring concurrently with abdominoplasty procedures using a 4 mm cannula, Mercedes or reverse pyramid design.

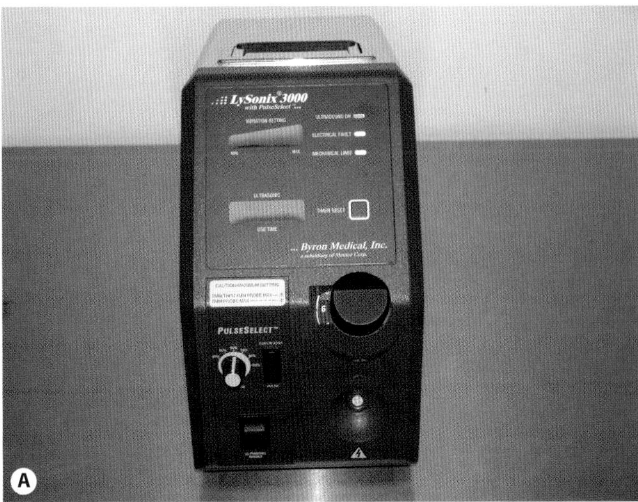

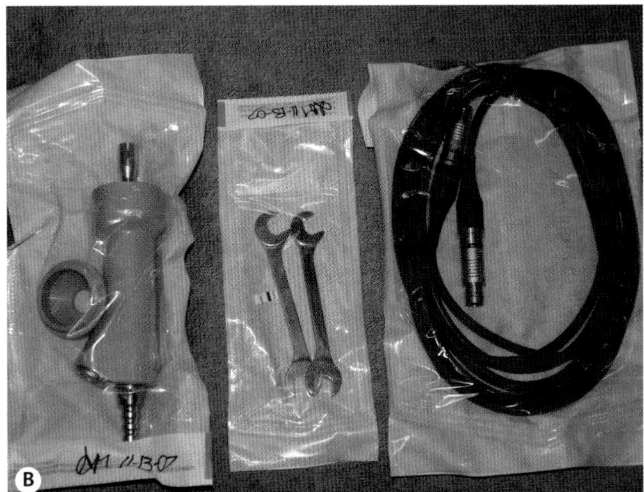

Fig. 3.10 A, B Ultrasound-assisted liposuction is beneficial when fibrous or scar tissue may be present. Indications for UAL include male gender, the upper back, and a history of previous liposuction. There are numerous UAL machines available. We use LySonix and have found it to work well.

fibrous areas and for secondary procedures where previous abdominal liposuction has resulted in scar tissue formation. Specific indications for UAL include male gender, and areas where fibrous tissue is likely to be present. The chest, in males and the upper back in both males and females, often has a greater preponderance of fibrous tissue, making the use of UAL beneficial.

The instruments used in UAL include the machine itself, the handle with the crystal stack, cannulas, and skin protection devices. A number of UAL machines are currently in use throughout the world. We use the Lysonix 3000 (**Fig. 3.10**), which we have found to be both reliable and easy to use. Although a pulsed mode is available, we find a continuous mode most beneficial. Several choices for UAL cannulas also exist. We prefer to use solid-tipped cannulas to perform UAL first, and then use PAL to remove the lipoaspirate (**Fig. 3.11**). When UAL is used it is beneficial to keep track of the amount of time spent on each area. Avoiding end hits and protecting the skin near the access site is also very important. Some type of skin entry protection device is beneficial when UAL is used: we use a device that simply screws into the skin entry site (**Fig. 3.12**). Placing a towel between the skin and the external portion of the UAL cannula is also helpful in avoiding thermal damage to the skin.

Perioperative Data

There are three sets of data that are beneficial to have when performing body contouring and liposuction. Two of these are preoperative and postoperative weight and photographs. The third set comes from the operating room. During the liposuction component of the case an accurate ongoing summary of the amount of infiltration fluid used, total aspirate removed, and total fat removed both per area and as a grand total, is critical for patient safety as

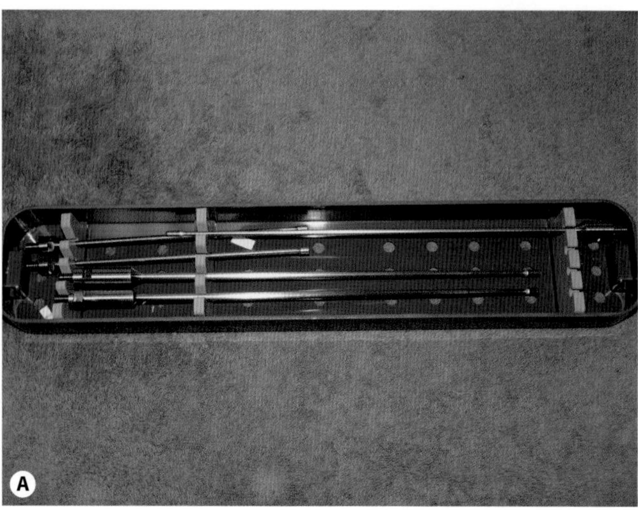

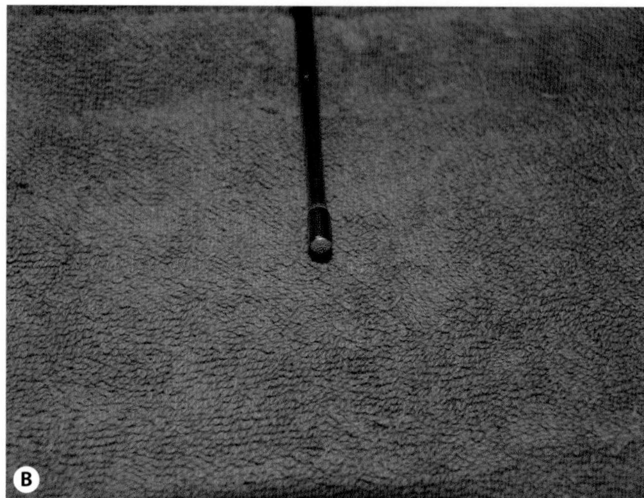

Fig. 3.11 A, B There are a variety of cannulas available for UAL. One of the key decisions to be made about UAL is whether suction will be performed concurrently, or whether UAL will be performed alone first and liposuction with regular SAL or PAL afterwards. As the presence of water is beneficial to the efficiency of UAL, we prefer to perform it separately with solid cannulas and then go back through each area with PAL and complete the liposuction. Timing the amount of UAL per area is beneficial in achieving symmetric results.

Table 3.2 Intraoperative data tracking volume of infiltration, aspirate, and fat removed are carefully cataloged during surgery and recorded in the patient's chart postoperatively

	1	2	3	4	5	6	7	8	9
Total container volume (TV)									
Intranatant tumescent fluid (TF)									
Fat volume in container (FAT)									
Ultrasonic time (UAL)									
Liposuction area (SITE)									

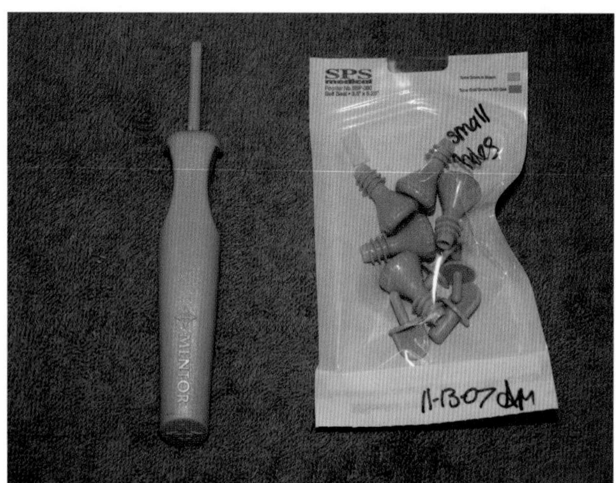

Fig. 3.12 The use of UAL requires that the skin be protected. There are a number of devices available to accomplish this. We use the Pathway Introducer by Mentor, which screws into the infiltration access sites. It is efficient and does not require further skin trauma. A surgical lap sponge is placed on the skin under the UAL cannula to further protect it from inadvertent thermal injury.

well as for achieving symmetry (**Table 3.2**). The use of all three data sets also allows accurate assessment of the final aesthetic results. The surgeon can frequently look at this board to assess the progress of the procedure: he does not need to inquire as to specific numbers as they are always available.

There is only one chance to obtain a preoperative weight for the patient. Patients must be weighed before surgery so that one can be certain that they have attained an appropriate weight after surgery that will truly demonstrate the results of the liposuction. Weight gain following surgery is common and can only be documented against the preoperative weight. The liposuction aspirate weighs approximately 2 lb/L of the fat component. We provide a goal weight for each patient undergoing body contouring: this is their preoperative weight minus the weight of the tissue removed during surgery. This information is calculated and recorded in the patient's chart. With each postoperative visit we weigh the patient and tell them their current weight and goal weight, providing an incentive for them to reach their target; the procedures performed will be truly affected by this target. If they don't reach their goal weight, by 3 or 4 months postoperatively, they have gained weight. This is discussed preoperatively.

Drains

Drains are usually placed whenever a large area has been liposuctioned, whether by PAL or by UAL, to facilitate postoperative fluid evacuation and seroma prevention. Drain use is planned when liposuction of the abdominal flap is performed during an abdominoplasty. We also use a drain in the lumbar area when the lumbar area or back is suctioned. An easy way to place the drain is simply to advance the liposuction cannula through one access site and out the other, at which point the drain tubing is slipped onto the cannula and pulled backwards to exit the skin.

Postoperative Considerations

Compression garments are beneficial following liposuction procedures. An appreciable degree of soft-tissue edema may remain in the treated area for many months after surgery. During this time, reassurance and education are very important for patient understanding. A preoperative weight, intraoperative measurement of liposuctioned tissue, and a postoperative weight are all important for an accurate evaluation of the final aesthetic result. We use non-adherent foam between the skin and the garment to provide even, uniform compression for all areas suctioned. This foam is used for liposuction alone and in combination with body contouring procedures.

Liposuction of the Abdominal Flap (Box 3.2)

There has been much discussion about the pros and cons of concurrent liposuction with full abdominoplasty (or any other abdominoplasty method).[7–10] As a general rule, if the patient stands to benefit aesthetically from thinning of the abdominal flap, we perform concurrent abdominal liposuction.

The importance of thorough tumescent infiltration of all areas to be suctioned cannot be overstated. When ample infiltration is performed – normally 4–6 L for a full abdominoplasty – the tissues achieve a tumescent state. The tissues become firm and evenly blanched. The tumescent fluid creates an internal exsanguination by compressing the blood vessels in the infiltrated area. These compressed, elongated vessels are exposed to the dilute epinephrine, which then can exert its maximal vasoconstrictive effect. The exsanguination of the tissue to be suctioned eliminates all stagnant blood that can be detrimental to flap survival. It also compresses the vessels, which makes them a smaller target and less likely to be traumatized by concurrent liposuction. The sensory nerves are also stretched, allowing the accompanying lidocaine to be effective as well. Small-cannula liposuction is used in a method that parallels the vascular course, minimizing devascularization.

Box 3.2 Liposuction of the abdominal flap

- Liposuction of the abdominal flap and the surrounding area is a powerful tool in maximizing the aesthetic result of abdominoplasty procedures.
- Patients with excess adiposity benefit from concurrent use of liposuction.
- Appropriate use of tumescent infiltration will help exsanguinate the soft tissue and produce profound vasoconstriction.
- The umbilicus provides an excellent access site for abdominal liposuction.
- Uniform liposuction at all layers of the abdominal soft tissue, starting superficially and progressing deeper, will produce a thinned and smooth abdominal flap.

Tumescent infiltration is performed with a solution containing 1 ample of epinephrine per liter of LR (1:1,000,000) either 12.5 or 25 mL 1% lidocaine/L, depending on the volume infiltrated. The combination of properly performed thorough infiltration, where the tissues are fully hydrated, with appropriate time allowed for epinephrine vasoconstriction to take place, and the inherent safety of the blunt-tipped liposuction cannulas to preserve vessels and nerves, allows thorough liposuction to be performed in all areas of the abdominal flap without a deleterious effect on healing. This is our finding and that of many other plastic surgeons worldwide.

We do not perform aggressive liposuction with abdominoplasty on smokers. Caution should be exercised in treating these patients and others with suspected wound healing difficulties.

Clinical caveats: Liposuction in abdominal contouring

- Liposuction is an integral part of abdominoplasty and abdominal contouring procedures.
- The use of liposuction should be tailored to each patient.
- Patients with excess adiposity are appropriate candidates for concurrent liposuction because it allows the abdominal flap to be thinned, enhancing the overall result.
- The maximum dose of lidocaine for each patient should be calculated and tracked as infiltration proceeds. A modified tumescent solution, with a reduced lidocaine dose, should be used for large-volume liposuction.

- Proper use of tumescent infiltration produces profound vasoconstriction and exsanguination of the soft tissue.
- An organized and accurate account of intraoperative infiltration, aspirate, and fat volume is important to maximize safety and aesthetic results.
- Postoperative use of drains and garments helps speed up recovery, reduce swelling and bruising, and increase patient comfort.

References

1. Klein JA. Tumescent technique for liposuction surgery. Am J Cosmet Surg 1987; 4: 263.
2. Ostad A, Kageyama N, Moy RL. Tumescent anesthesia with a lidocaine dose of 55 mg/kg is safe for liposuction. Dermatol Surg 1996; 22: 921–927.
3. Physicians' desk reference, 61st edn. Montvale, NJ: Thompson, 2007; 1702.
4. Kenkel JM, Rohrich RJ. Ultrasound-assisted lipectomy using the solid probe: a retrospective review of 100 consecutive cases. Plast Reconstruct Surg 2000; 105: 2178–2179.
5. Rohrich RJ, Raniere J Jr, Beran SJ, Kenkel JM. Patient evaluation and indications for ultrasound-assisted lipoplasty. Clin Plast Surg 1999; 26: 269.
6. Graf R, Auersvald A, Damasio RC, et al. Ultrasound-assisted liposuction: an analysis of 348 cases. Aesthet Plast Surg 2003; 27: 146–153.
7. Hafezi F, Nouhi A. Safe abdominoplasty with extensive liposuctioning. Ann Plast Surg 2006; 57: 149.
8. Hunstad JP, Aitken ME. Liposuction: techniques and guidelines. Clin Plast Surg 2006; 33: 13.
9. Dillerud E. Abdominoplasty combined with suction lipoplasty: A study of complications, revisions, and risk factors in 487 cases. Ann Plast Surg 1990; 25: 333.
10. Matarasso A. Abdominoplasty: A system of classification and treatment for combined abdominoplasty and suction-assisted lipectomy. Aesthet Plast Surg 1991; 15: 1432.

Suggested Reading

Abramson DL. Ultrasound-assisted abdominoplasty: combining modalities in a safe and effective technique. Plast Reconstruct Surg 2003; 112: 898–902.

Ali-Eed MD. Mega-liposuction: Analysis of 1520 patients. Aesthet Plast Surg 1999; 23: 16.

Apfelberg DB, Rosenthal S, Hunstad JP, et al. Progress report on multicenter study of laser-assisted liposuction. Aesthet Plast Surg 1994; 18: 259.

Cardenas-Camarena L, Gonzales LE. Large-volume liposuction and extensive abdominoplasty: A feasible alternative for improving body shape. Plast Reconstruct Surg 1998; 102: 1698.

Dillerud E, Haheim LL. Long-term results of blunt suction lipectomy assessed by a patient questionnaire survey. Plast Reconstruct Surg 1993; 92: 35.

Gargan TJ, Courtiss EH. The risks of suction lipectomy: Their prevention and treatment. Clin Plast Surg 1988; 11: 457.

Grazer FM, de Jong RH. Fatal outcomes from liposuction: census survey of cosmetic surgeons. Plast Reconstruct Surg 2000; 105: 436.

Hunstad JP. Tumescent and syringe liposculpture: a logical partnership. Aesth. Plast Surg 1995; 19: 321.

Hunstad JP. The tumescent technique facilitates hair micrografting. Aesthet Plast Surg 1996; 20: 43.

Hunstad JP, Aitken ME. Liposuction and tumescent surgery. Clin Plast Surg 2006; 33: 39.

Illouz YG. Body contouring by lipolysis: a 5 year experience with over 3000 cases. Plast Reconstruct Surg 1983; 72: 591.

Illouz YG. History and current concepts of lipoplasty. Clin Plast Surg 1996; 23: 721.

Iverson RE, Lynch DJ. Practice advisory on liposuction. Plast Reconstruct Surg 2004; 113: 1478.

Kesselring UK. Regional fat aspiration for body contouring. Plast Reconstruct Surg 1983; 72: 610.

Klein JA. Tumescent technique for regional anesthesia permits lidocaine doses of 35 mg/kg for liposuction. J Dermatol Surg Oncol 1990; 16: 248.

Klein JA. Tumescent technique for local anesthesia improves safety in large volume liposuction. Plast Reconstruct Surg 1993; 92: 1085.

Mentz HA 3rd, Gilliland MD, Patronella CK. Abdominal etching: differential liposuction to detail abdominal musculature. Aesthet Plast Surg 1993; 17: 287.

Rao RB, Ely SF, Hoffman RS. Deaths related to liposuction. N Engl J Med 1999; 340: 1471.

Rohrich RJ, Broughton G 2nd, Horton B, et al. The key to long-term success in liposuction: a guide for plastic surgeons and patients. Plast Reconstruct Surg 2004; 114: 1945–1953.

Rohrich RJ, Smith PD, Marcantonio DR, Kenkel JM. The zones of adherence: role in minimizing and preventing contour deformities in liposuction. Plast Reconstruct Surg 2001; 107: 1562–1569.

Rohrich RJ, Kenkel JM, Janis JE, Beran SJ. An update on the role of subcutaneous infiltration in suction-assisted lipoplasty. Plast Reconstruct Surg 2003; 111: 926.

de Jong RH, Grazer FM. Perioperative management of cosmetic liposuction. Plast Reconstruct Surg 2001; 107: 1039.

Shiffman MA. Task force on ultrasound-assisted lipoplasty. Plast Reconstruct Surg 1997; 100: 1931.

Teimourian B, Adham MN. A national survey of complications associated with suction lipectomy: what we did then and what we do now. Plast Reconstruct Surg 2000; 105: 1881–1884.

Teimourian B. Complications associated with suction lipectomy. Clin Plast Surg 1989; 16: 385.

Trott SA, Beran SJ, Rohrich RJ, et al. Safety considerations and fluid resuscitation in liposuction: An analysis of 53 consecutive patients. Plast Reconstruct Surg 1998; 102: 2220–2229.

CHAPTER **4**

Endoscopic Abdominoplasty

Joseph P. Hunstad and Remus Repta

IN THIS CHAPTER

KEY POINTS

Endoscopic abdominoplasty has very specific indications. Good to excellent skin quality combined with excess adiposity and diastasis recti is a treatable condition (signs and symptoms). This procedure consists of thorough abdominal liposuction combined with correction of muscular diastasis, performed under endoscopic control through easily concealed and usually invisible umbilical and pubic incisions.

Introduction

Endoscopic abdominoplasty is a minimally invasive procedure, usually without visible scars performed on selected patients. It is indicated for those few patients with excess abdominal adiposity and muscular diastasis, but without excessive skin laxity. Appropriate candidates represent less than 5% of patients seeking body contouring.[1] This procedure requires endoscopic instrumentation and the ability to perform endoscopically controlled suturing at a distance. For patients that meet the criteria of excess adiposity, and muscular diastasis, without significant skin laxity, this procedure can offer pleasing results without visible scarring.

Patient Selection (Box 4.1)

Patients who are appropriate candidates for endoscopic abdominoplasty are usually close to their ideal body weight but may have excess abdominal adiposity, muscular diastasis, and minimal skin and soft-tissue laxity (**Fig. 4.1**). These patients represent a small number of those seeking abdominal contouring, and often present interested in liposuction unaware of the option of endoscopic abdominoplasty. Appropriate candidates should be counseled as to the availability of this procedure. Patients with excessive skin and soft-tissue laxity are not good candidates for this procedure and can experience a worsening of their condition, requiring subsequent skin resection.

Box 4.1 Relative contraindications for endoscopic abdominoplasty

The relative contraindications for all abdominal contouring procedures where the abdominal soft tissue is elevated and there is myofascial plication are similar.

Excess soft-tissue laxity that would benefit from formal resection is the most common contraindication to endoscopic abdominoplasty. These patients are better served by a mini or full abdominoplasty where excess skin and soft tissue can be resected inferiorly.

Endoscopic abdominoplasty patients are usually younger and healthier than patients undergoing full or circumferential abdominoplasty. The following is a list of relative contraindications:

- Smoking
- Diabetes mellitus
- Malnutrition
- Wound-healing disorders
- Bowel/bladder dysfunction
- Immune deficiency
- Medications that inhibit blood coagulation
- A significant history of pulmonary or deep vein thrombosis
- Lower extremity lymphedema/venous insufficiency
- Significant medical problems, including COPD/pulmonary issues, renal insufficiency, anemia, and other systemic issues that may make abdominal tightening surgery dangerous

Note: Age alone should not be a contraindication to abdominoplasty procedures if the patient is in good health. Patients who have a history of chronic pain should also be approached cautiously, as postoperative care may be significantly affected.

Preoperative History and Considerations (Box 4.2)

The extent of excess abdominal adiposity, skin condition and quality, including the presence and extent of striae, and the degree of muscular diastasis must all be taken into account when performing endoscopic abdominoplasty.

Because these patients are usually considering only abdominal liposuction they are probably unaware of the presence of their abdominal muscle laxity or diastasis since their skin quality is reasonably good. These patients usually believe that the lower abdominal fullness is secondary to excess adiposity only, not the combination of excess adiposity *and* myofascial laxity. They are often also unaware of the availability of endoscopic muscle plication. When patients are told that endoscopic abdominoplasty can accomplish abdominal tightening and flattening as well as thinning, they are often interested in achieving these improved results, especially without noticeable scars.

Liposuction alone can thin the abdominal soft tissue, but without correction of rectus abdominis muscle diastasis and abdominal wall tightening, complete correction of the abdominal convexity will not be achieved. Because of this, liposuction only patients may be disappointed by surgery because of residual abdominal laxity and poor abdominal contour on lateral profile. These patients will have a thin – *but not a flat* – abdomen. If they have reasonably good skin quality and are close to their ideal body weight, but have excess adiposity and muscular laxity and/or diastasis recti, they are reasonable candidates for endoscopic abdominoplasty.

Box 4.2 Preoperative recommendations for endoscopic abdominoplasty

Most abdominal contouring procedures have similar preoperative requirements. Because the abdominal soft tissue in endoscopic abdominoplasty maintains a greater blood supply, the danger of healing problems and perfusion issues is less than with full/extended or circumferential abdominoplasty.

- Smoking cessation/avoidance of nicotine exposure for 4–6 weeks prior to surgery is preferred. For more extensive abdominal contouring procedures this is a strict requirement
- Multivitamin daily
- Stop aspirin/other blood thinning products with primary care doctor's permission
- Abstain from all dietary/herbal supplements not approved by the surgeon
- Basic laboratory work should be tailored to each patient. It may include a pregnancy test, complete blood count (CBC), basic metabolic panel (BMP/Chem7), and standard coagulation profiles (PT/PTT/INR)
- Medical clearance if needed
- Wearing abdominal binder for 2 weeks before surgery
- Shower with a gentle antimicrobial soap the night before and day of surgery

Surgical diagrams depicting the areas for liposuction and the incision locations for endoscopic rectus plication and suction drain placement are helpful to facilitate patient discussion and education.

Operative Approach

Preoperative markings are made as for a complete abdominal liposuction procedure. They should be made with the patient standing. The areas that will undergo liposuction, including the mons, lower abdomen, epigastric region, hip rolls, flanks and lateral breast, are marked. Surgical incisions in the periumbilical and mons areas and drain locations should also be marked. Additional inframammary liposuction incisions to address the axilla are usually not necessary. Incision placement vertically within the hair-bearing mons and within the umbilicus should be marked, as well as the lateral borders of the rectus abdominis muscle. This is the internal extent of undermining (**Fig. 4.2**, **Table 4.1**).

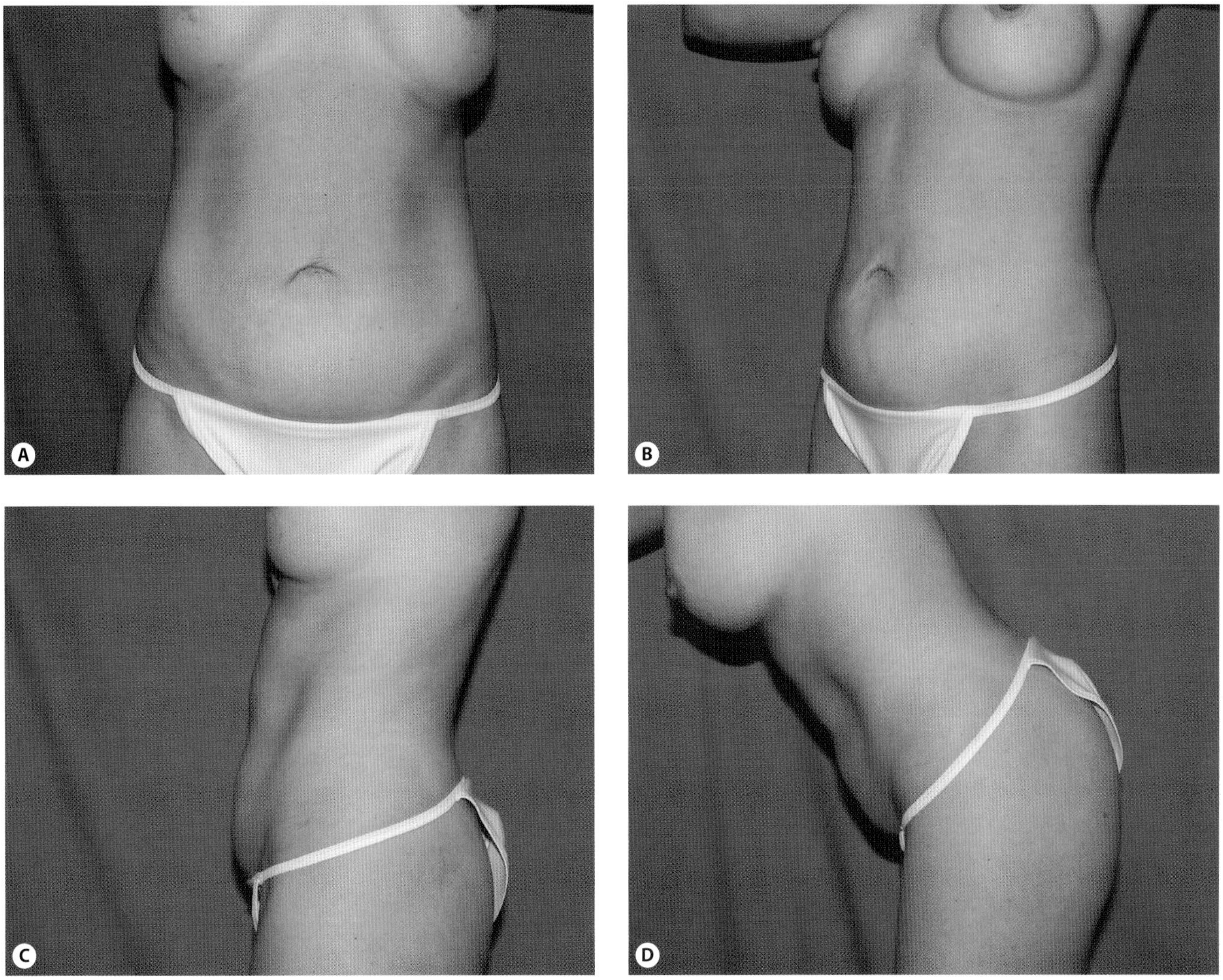

Fig. 4.1 The ideal endoscopic abdominoplasty patient has myofascial abdominal wall laxity with little or moderate skin redundancy and excess adiposity. Skin quality is usually good.

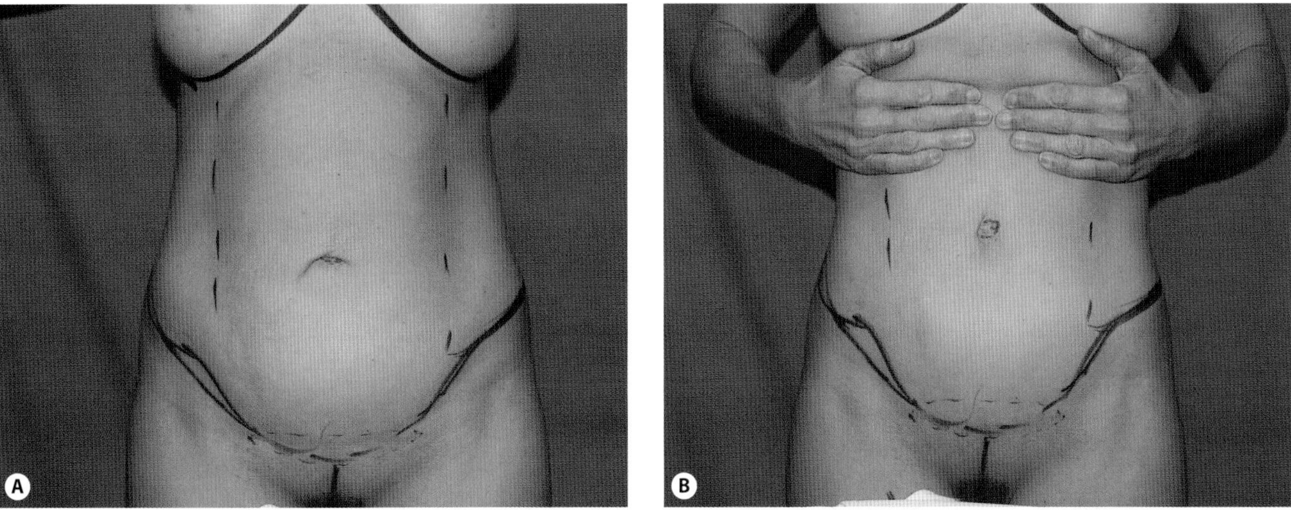

Fig. 4.2 Preoperative markings are performed with the patient standing. The areas designated for liposuction are outlined and the incision sites that will facilitate dissection are identified and marked. Two main access points are marked for the abdominal wall plication. One is a vertical incision in the midline hair-bearing mons, and the other is a periumbilical incision. The lateral borders of the rectus are marked indicating the extent of lateral undermining.

General, epidural, or dissociative anesthesias are all reasonable options. Muscular relaxation is desirable during this procedure to allow proper myofascial plication to be performed. Because of this requirement, general anesthesia is preferred. Sequential compression pumps are placed prior to the induction of anesthesia.

In the supine position tumescent infiltration is performed throughout all areas of subcutaneous fat to be suctioned (**Fig. 4.3**). The normal tumescent infiltration volume is between 3 and 5 L, depending on the amount of subcutaneous fat. Sufficient time should be allowed between infiltration and liposuction to optimize the vasoconstrictive effect of the epinephrine. This will minimize blood loss during liposuction.

An easy way to perform this is to infiltrate the patient prior to preparation and draping. This is easily performed by painting the entry sites with Betadine, making entry site openings, and frequently wiping the infiltration cannula with Betadine during the infiltration. This allows approximately 20 minutes between tumescent infiltration and the beginning of the surgical procedure, which ensures that the epinephrine has had enough time to achieve excellent vasoconstriction and hence minimize blood loss. This technique is used for all liposuction and body contouring procedures.

Very thorough liposuction is then performed in all areas to be treated. A very thin, even layer of residual subcutaneous fat should remain below the dermis to minimize the chance of irregularities and avoid skin adherence to the underlying abdominal wall fascia with healing. When the endpoint of liposuction has been achieved, muscle plication follows.

A vertical mons incision is used first, and under direct vision undermining, using electrocautery for dissection and hemostasis, is performed superiorly to the level of the umbilicus (**Fig. 4.4**). At this point, the umbilical incision is

Table 4.1 Instrumentation specific for endoscopic abdominoplasty

Zero-degree endoscope
Light source, camera, monitor
Lighted retractor
Regular and extended electrocautery
Endoscopic needle holder
Insulated endoscopic electrocautery
Defogging agent
Suction (connected to endoscopic electrocautery or extended cannula)
Plication suture

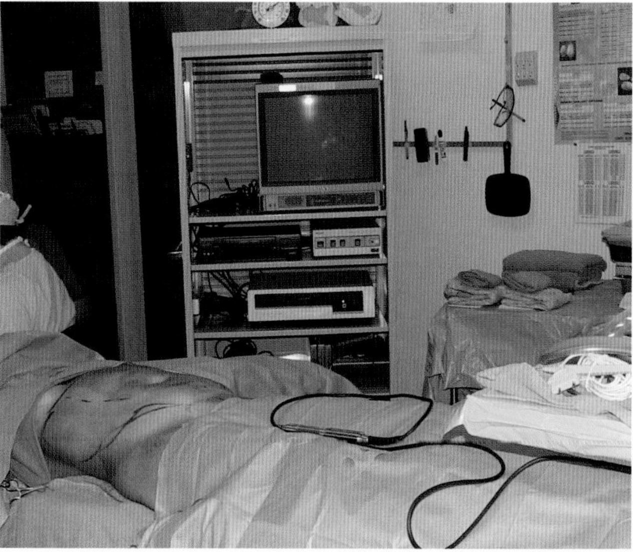

Fig. 4.3 The patient is placed supine, sequential compression leg pumps are placed, and anesthesia is administered. Tumescent infiltration is performed in all of the areas that will be liposuctioned.

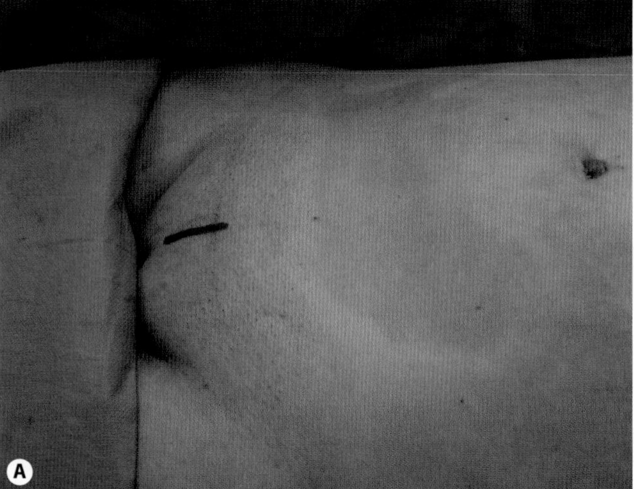

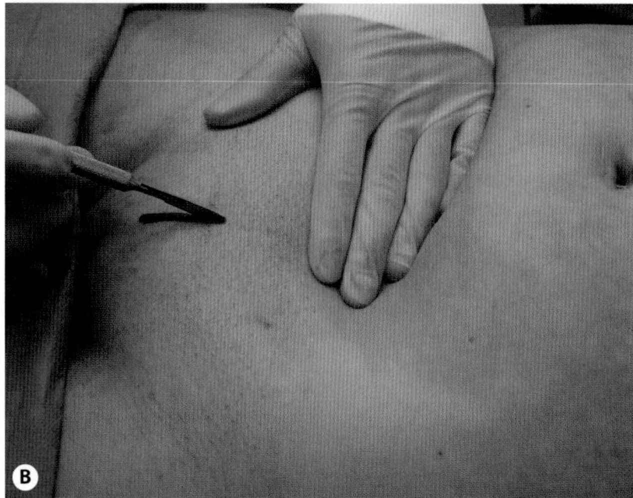

Fig. 4.4 The incision that facilitates dissection up the level of the umbilicus is made vertically in the midline of the mons. This allows ample exposure up to the level of the umbilicus and heals with an essentially invisible scar. Use of a standard lighted retractor similar to that used in breast cases facilitates the infraumbilical dissection.

made. This completely encircles the umbilicus and frees it from the surrounding skin. Additional dissection can be performed under direct vision inferiorly and superiorly through the periumbilical incision (**Fig. 4.5**). This is facilitated with lighted retractors commonly employed for breast augmentation and other procedures.

The endoscope is then used for visualization superior to the umbilicus (**Fig. 4.6**). It is in this region that the subcutaneous tissue becomes more adherent to the underlying anterior rectus sheath and the linea alba. Great care must be taken to avoid dissection into or through the anterior rectus sheath between the umbilicus and xiphoid. Undermining is usually performed laterally to the level of the lateral border of the anterior rectus sheath and superiorly to the xiphoid. Meticulous hemostasis should be achieved under direct or endoscopic vision.

Myofascial plication is performed next. This is performed with the use of the endoscope and a continuous size 0 double-stranded looped nylon suture and a large tapered needle (**Fig. 4.7**). A continuous loop suture obviates the need to tie a knot at the level of the xiphoid. This type of suture is very strong, and in the author's experience over many years of use has never broken. The plication begins at the xiphoid and runs in a continuous fashion to the level

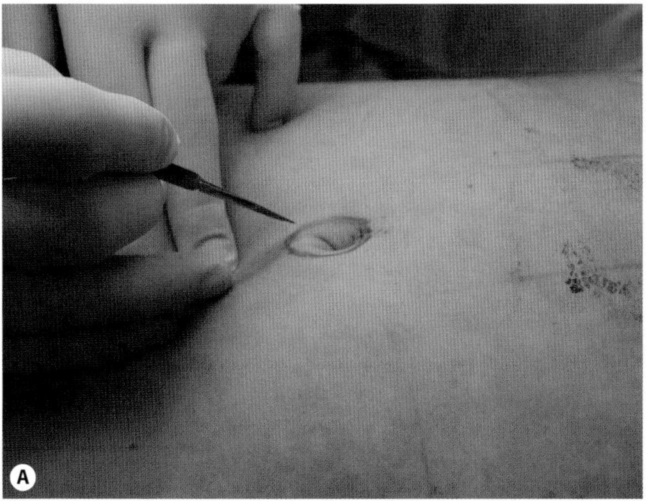

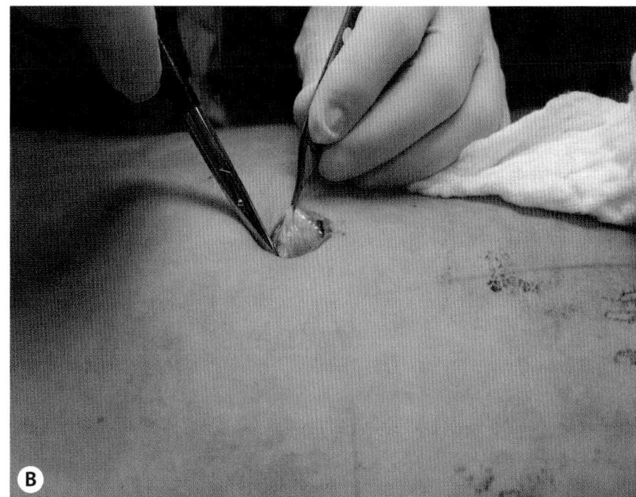

Fig. 4.5 The umbilicus is released via a complete circumumbilical incision. It is dissected free from the surrounding soft tissue to allow access to the abdomen superior to the umbilicus to the level of the xiphoid, in preparation for myofascial plication. The initial supraumbilical dissection is performed under direct vision using a lighted retractor.

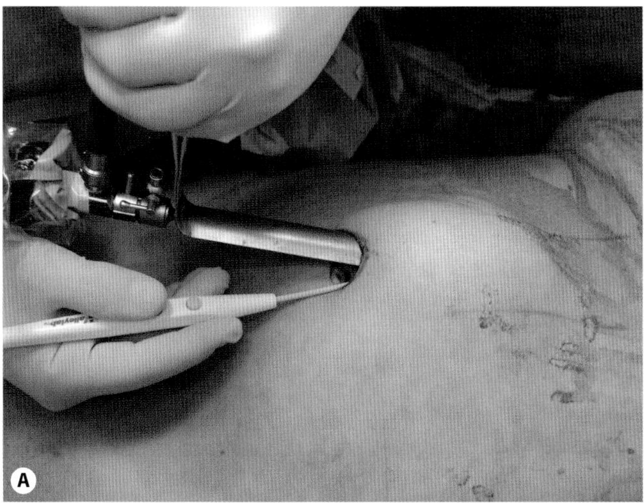

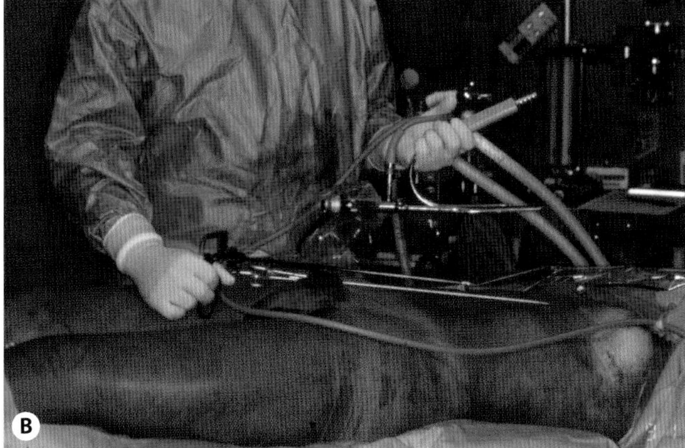

Fig. 4.6 The remainder of the supraumbilical dissection and all of the myofascial plication in the upper half of the abdomen is performed using the endoscope. Meticulous hemostasis is important for proper visualization while using the endoscope.

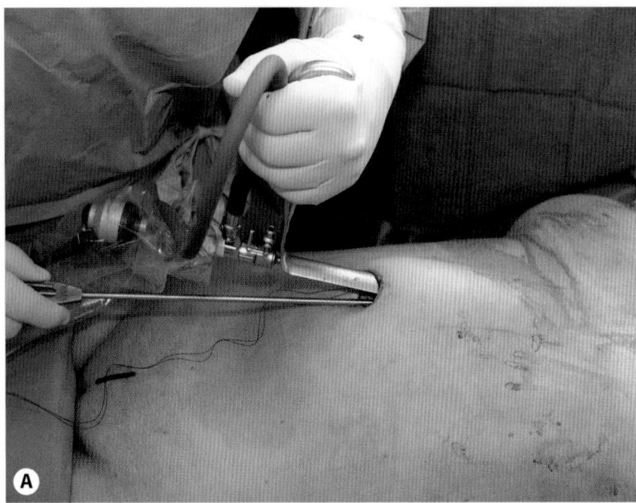

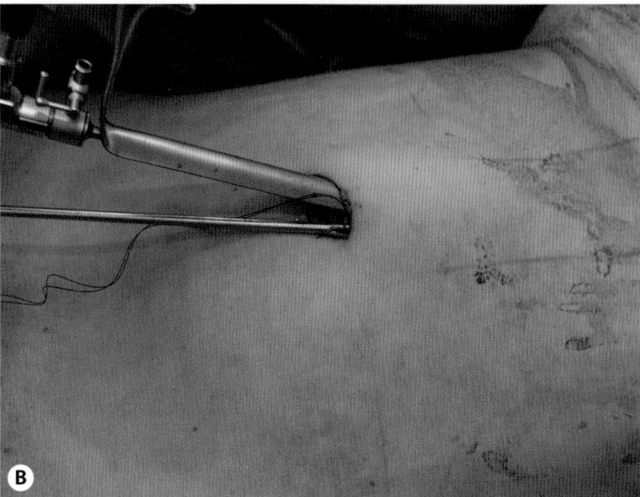

Fig. 4.7 Myofascial plication above the umbilicus is performed using the endoscope and under direct visualization below the umbilicus. Plication is performed in a running fashion with a size 0 double-stranded looped nylon suture that allows strong myofascial plication without the need for a knot at the xiphoid. The suture is temporarily run on one side of the rectus sheath when the umbilicus is reached. Plication resumes below the umbilicus down to the pubic symphysis.

of the umbilicus. The suture is then run along the lateral edge of the umbilicus until its inferior edge is reached. At this point plication resumes and continues down to the level of the pubic symphysis. Only the plication superior to the umbilicus is performed under endoscopic control. The remaining plication is performed under direct vision facilitated by lighted retractors.

A single or double layer of plication is performed, depending on the muscular diastasis and laxity of the abdominal wall. The knot at the pubis symphysis is buried to minimize postoperative palpability. Bupivacaine is injected into the rectus sheath and peripherally to reduce postoperative discomfort. A suction drain is placed and brought out, usually through the mons area to minimize scar deformity. The umbilical and mons incisions are closed in layers with intracuticular absorbable sutures. Light compressive dressings and an abdominal binder are then placed.

Postoperative Care (Box 4.3)

Early ambulation is recommended. Patients may prefer to maintain a partially flexed waist position until it is comfortable to assume a normal erect posture, usually between 7 and 10 days. Postoperative evaluation should be performed within a day or so to be sure that the garments are being worn properly and that the skin is smooth and even. A suction drain should be maintained until less than 30–50 mL of drainage occurs during a 24-hour period. Normal physical activity can usually be resumed by 6 weeks. The incisions should be protected from the sun until all redness is gone.

Box 4.3 **Postoperative instructions for endoscopic abdominoplasty**

The postoperative instructions for most abdominal contouring procedures that involve myofascial plication are similar. Endoscopic abdominoplasty patients are usually younger and healthier and often more eager to resume their normal activity and exercise regimen before their body has had a chance to heal properly.

- Maintain a partially flexed position at the waist for the first 7–10 days
- Wear the abdominal binder at all times, except when showering
- Make sure the binder is maintained low enough on the abdomen
- Verify that there are no significant creases, folds, or drain tubes underneath the binder
- Avoid smoking or exposure to nicotine-containing products
- Breathe deeply and use the incentive spirometer frequently
- Drink plenty of fluids
- Move legs frequently while resting, and walk regularly
- Drain care as instructed
- Continue to take multivitamin daily. Resume medications as instructed
- No vigorous activity or heavy lifting for 4–6 weeks

Preoperative and postoperative photographs are shown in **Figs 4.8 and 4.9**.

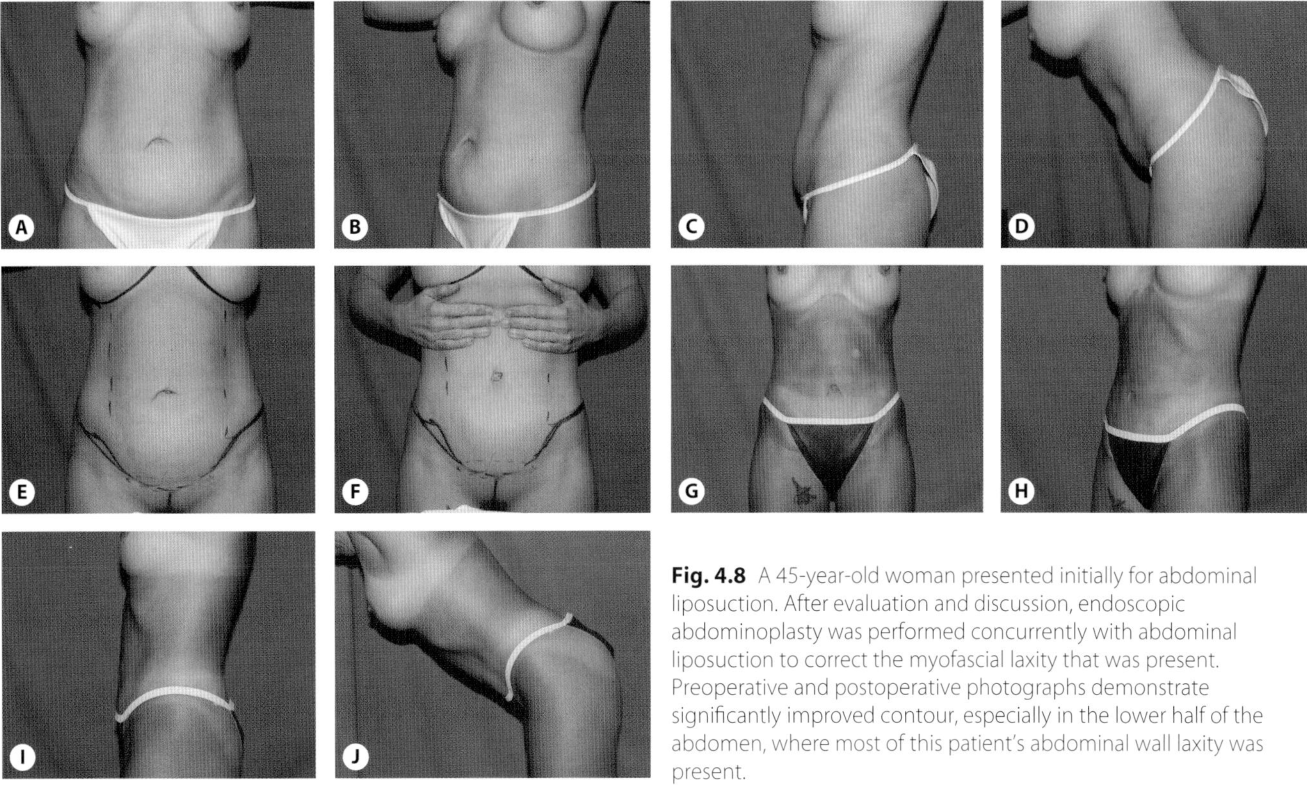

Fig. 4.8 A 45-year-old woman presented initially for abdominal liposuction. After evaluation and discussion, endoscopic abdominoplasty was performed concurrently with abdominal liposuction to correct the myofascial laxity that was present. Preoperative and postoperative photographs demonstrate significantly improved contour, especially in the lower half of the abdomen, where most of this patient's abdominal wall laxity was present.

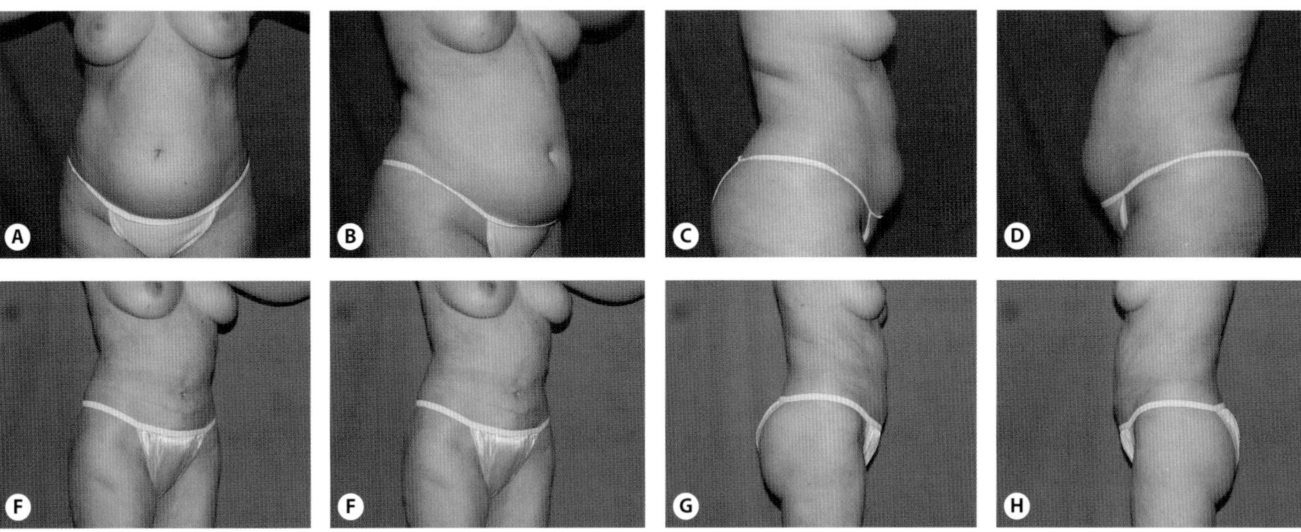

Fig. 4.9 A 46-year-old woman also requested abdominal liposuction initially. The presence of abdominal wall laxity was noted and discussed with the patient, who wanted a better abdominal contour with a flatter, more toned appearance. She underwent endoscopic abdominoplasty with concurrent abdominal liposuction as well as liposuction of her saddlebag areas. Preoperative and postoperative photographs demonstrate a thinner and tighter abdomen, with a better overall contour and silhouette.

Summary

Endoscopic abdominoplasty is a unique abdominal contouring procedure representing less than 5% of abdominoplasty procedures. It is ideal for the patient who presents with relatively normal weight, excess abdominal adiposity, muscular laxity and diastasis, and little or no soft-tissue laxity. For these patients, endoscopic abdominoplasty can achieve very positive results. The ability to perform muscle plication with completely concealable scars is the highlight of this procedure. For this reason, patient satisfaction is often very high.

Clinical caveats: Endoscopic abdominoplasty

- Endoscopic abdominoplasty is ideal for a select group of patients who have little soft-tissue laxity, good skin quality/tone, mild to moderate excess adiposity, and myofascial laxity.
- Because myofascial plication will contribute significantly to the overall aesthetic result, proper dissection for good visualization and strong reliable myofascial plication are key to the success of this procedure.
- Keeping the incision hidden in the hear-bearing mons and within the circumference of the umbilicus is very important, as these patients are in good shape and expect to wear two-piece swimsuits and revealing clothing. This may be more important than for full abdominoplasty patients.
- Preoperative instructions/requirements must be methodically followed to maximize safety.
- Preoperative markings and photographs should be performed standing and are invaluable to achieve the best possible results.
- Concurrent liposuction of the abdominal soft-tissue apron and the surrounding area is of great benefit and enhances the final result.
- Injection of bupivacaine into the rectus sheath and peripherally will help reduce postoperative discomfort, which facilitates deep breathing and reduces the postoperative use of pain medication.
- Although overnight care in an accredited facility is not required for endoscopic abdominoplasty, as opposed to more extensive body contouring procedures, it will allow better fluid status management and better pain control, and reduce the chance of DVT with the use of pneumatic compression devices and ambulation.
- Early postoperative evaluation and regularly over the next week will allow proper intervention if postoperative care issues arise.

Reference

1. Eaves FF 3rd, Nahai F, Bostwick J 3rd. Endoscopic abdominoplasty and endoscopically assisted miniabdominoplasty. Clin Plast Surg 1996; 23: 599.

Suggested Reading

Cardoso de Castro C, Marica Branco Cupello A, Cintra H. Limited incisions in abdominoplasty. Ann Plast Surg 1987; 19: 436.

Eaves FF 3rd, Price CI, Bostwick JH 3rd, et al. Subcutaneous endoscopic plastic surgery using a retractor-mounted endoscopic system. Perspect Plast Surg 1993; 7: 1.

Ferraro FJ, Zavitsanos GP, Van Buskirk ER, et al. Improving the efficiency, ease, and efficacy of endoscopic abdominoplasty. Plast Reconstruct Surg 1997; 99: 895–898.

Jackson TL, Jackson RF, Freeman L. Minimally invasive abdominoplasty: surgical technique development and report of three cases. Surg Laparosc Endosc 1995; 5: 301–305.

O'Brien JJ, Glasgow A, Lydon P. Endoscopic balloon-assisted abdominoplasty. Plast Reconstruct Surg 1997; 99: 1462.

CHAPTER **5**

Mini Abdominoplasty (Short Scar Abdominoplasty)

Joseph P. Hunstad and Remus Repta

IN THIS CHAPTER

KEY POINTS

The mini abdominoplasty procedures is highly variable, depending on the clinical findings and patient desire. Such procedures usually encompass a shortened scar, a smaller skin excision, and no umbilical transposition as in a full abdominoplasty. Mini abdominoplasty is ideal for younger patients with lower abdominal soft-tissue laxity that is not significant enough to allow a full abdominoplasty skin resection. Thorough abdominal liposuction is usually an important component of this procedure, as well as strong myofascial plication.

Introduction

The mini or short scar abdominoplasty is an important procedure for patients with mild to moderate skin laxity, excess adiposity, and muscular diastasis. The term mini abdominoplasty is often used to refer to any abdominoplasty procedure where the length of the transverse incision is smaller than that typically used in a full abdominoplasty, as well as avoiding the use of umbilical translocation. The option of a short scar is very appealing, especially to younger women. Even with a short scar, however, excellent myofascial plication and concurrent thorough liposuction can be performed to achieve a very desirable result. The umbilical stalk may be released during undermining and secured or repositioned to the rectus fascia. The umbilicus may be left intact, but this makes supraumbilical myofascial plication more difficult. With this procedure, no external umbilical scar is created and the vertical position of the umbilicus is minimally changed at the completion of the case. The exact length of the transverse incision that designates a mini abdominoplasty is somewhat variable and based on clinical findings, patient desires, and surgeon preference. A mini abdominoplasty involves the removal of a smaller amount of skin and subcutaneous tissue than a full abdominoplasty.

This procedure is much less commonly performed than full abdominoplasty because most patients presenting for abdominal contouring have gained significant weight and/or have had several pregnancies, resulting in significant excess skin laxity, striae, and muscular diastasis. The mini abdominoplasty represents a spectrum of surgical procedures depending on the deformity present.

Patient Selection (Box 5.1)

The ideal patient for a mini abdominoplasty is usually a young woman between the ages of 25 and 50, who has had a number of children but never suffered from significant weight gain. These patients often have mild to moderate excess adiposity, mild to moderate skin laxity, and striae. They are generally relatively thin and their abdominal skin is usually in good condition. Any striae present are usually located in the inferiormost portion of the infraumbilical skin. Myofascial laxity in this patient population is variable.

Patients with moderate excess soft-tissue laxity may be candidates for either mini or full abdominoplasty. Because the soft-tissue resection will not incorporate the umbilicus, a full abdominoplasty resection will result in a vertical midline scar (previous umbilical location) at or near the low transverse incision (**Fig. 5.1**).

Preoperative History and Considerations (Box 5.2)

In general, candidates for mini abdominoplasty are usually younger, healthier, and fitter than patients requiring more extensive procedures. However, with all forms of abdominoplasty that include myofascial plication, any personal or family history of deep vein thrombosis (DVT) and/or pulmonary embolism (PE) is very important, and standard precautions should be taken.[1–3]If this is noted, laboratory testing should be performed to rule out a hypercoagulable state. Basic or specific preoperative laboratory tests may be obtained as indicated by each patient's medical history. For a healthy patient taking no medications, basic preoperative laboratory analysis should be considered and may include a pregnancy test, complete blood count (CBC), basic metabolic panel (BMP/Chem7), and standard coagulation profiles (PT/PTT/INR). Patients taking

Box 5.1 Patient selection

- The ideal mini abdominoplasty candidate has isolated soft-tissue laxity of the lower (infraumbilical) abdomen
- These patients may have variable amount of excess adiposity and myofascial laxity, but the skin at and above the umbilicus is usually free of striae
- Many mini abdominoplasty candidates may be reasonable candidates for other abdominal contouring procedures, such as abdominal liposuction, endoscopic abdominoplasty, or full abdominoplasty, depending on the degree of soft-tissue laxity and the presence of excess adiposity and myofascial laxity
- Appropriate evaluation and discussion with the patient about the anticipated final result and the scars associated with the abdominoplasty are especially important for the mini abdominoplasty candidate

Box 5.2 Preoperative considerations

- The preoperative evaluation for mini abdominoplasty is comparable to that performed for full abdominoplasty
- Although these patients are usually younger and relatively fit, standard preoperative tests are recommended, and additional tests and clearances should be obtained as appropriate
- Smoking cessation is important for all abdominoplasty procedures. If the mini abdominoplasty candidate cannot stop smoking preoperatively, omission of concurrent abdominal liposuction should be considered
- PE/DVT precautions are the same as for all of the other abdominoplasty techniques. Any history of PE/DVT or other blood clotting disorders should be properly evaluated by a specialist prior to the abdominal contouring procedure

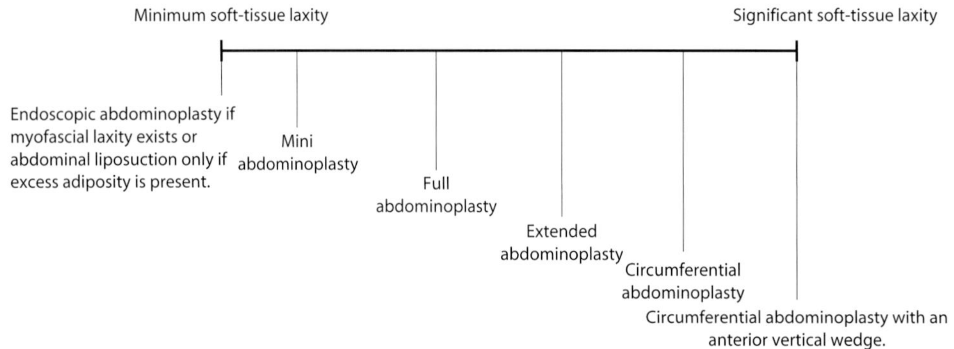

Fig. 5.1 The ideal abdominoplasty procedure for each patient depends on many factors, including the degree of soft-tissue laxity. The mini abdominoplasty occupies a specific niche between endoscopic abdominoplasty or abdominal liposuction and full abdominoplasty.

birth control medication are at an increased risk of DVT/PE. Discontinuation of such medication 2 weeks before surgery will reduce or perhaps even eliminate this increased risk.[4–6]

Smoking cessation is an important part of all abdominoplasty procedures,[7, 8] and should be begun several weeks before and continue after the procedure. Cessation of 6 or more weeks is probably ideal; however, patients with a long smoking history will still be at increased risk of ischemia. Those who do not stop smoking should be deferred, or the procedure should be performed in a more conservative fashion, for example a lipoabdominoplasty procedure (see Chapter 6).

Patients must understand that although this is a 'mini' procedure compared to a full abdominoplasty, the recovery can often be very similar. Oral and transdermal medications are suggested to help prevent postoperative nausea and vomiting.

Operative Approach

Standard preoperative photographs in nine cardinal views are suggested with the patient standing (**Fig. 5.2**). The incision for a mini abdominoplasty should be kept as low as possible because there is no concern about removing all of the infraumbilical skin. Whenever possible, the incision should be placed inferior to existing scars so as to eliminate them with the skin resection. The location and length of the incision are negotiable between the patient and surgeon and agreed upon prior to surgery. Normally the patient is asked to forcefully lift the lower abdominal skin and the inferior incision is marked at the level of the symphysis pubis (**Fig. 5.3**). It then courses laterally toward the anterior superior iliac crest in a natural skin fold. The patient can also be asked to wear revealing swimwear, and the incision can be marked appropriately so that it will be hidden by the garment (**Figs 5.4 and 5.5**). Preoperative markings should be reviewed by the patient in a mirror before surgery, to be certain that the position and length of the final scar is acceptable.

The primary variable for this procedure is the length of the incision. Patients almost always desire the shortest scar possible, yet their anatomy will often dictate the incision length. Some patients request a short scar abdominoplasty but have moderate skin laxity. A short incision combined with removal of significant amounts of skin can easily be associated with lateral dog-ears, which are undesirable and should be avoided. A physical demonstration of this by bimanual palpation of the lower abdominal skin will demonstrate to the patient the need for a longer incision. Seeing this demonstrated on their own skin is very educational and helps the patient understand the limitations of short scar

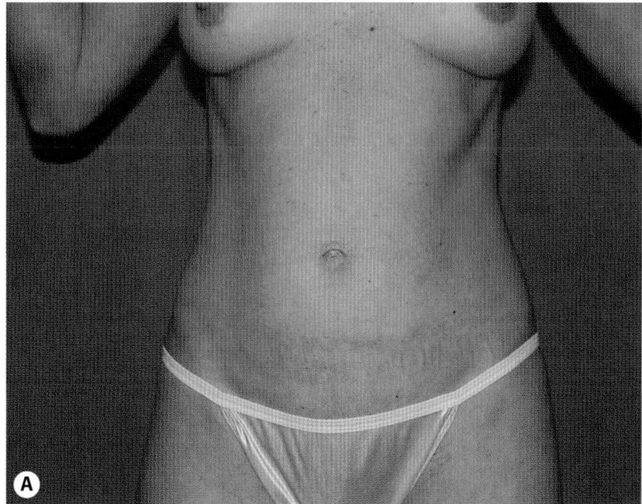

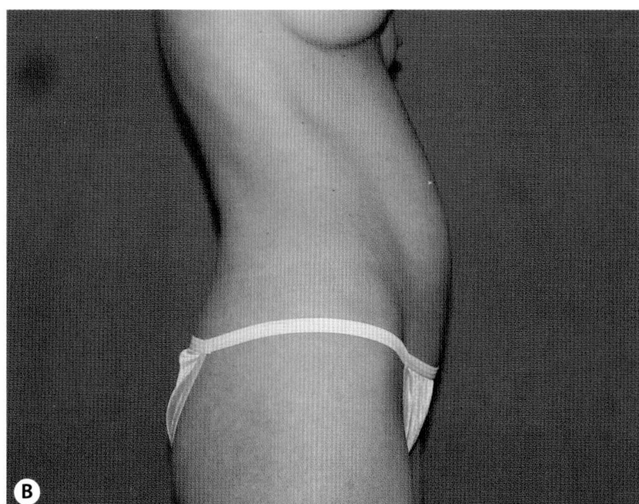

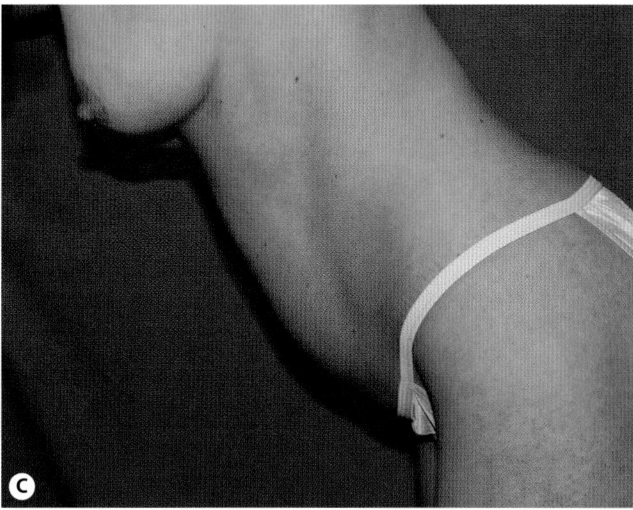

Fig. 5.2 A–C Ideal mini abdominoplasty candidates have soft-tissue laxity isolated to the lower, infraumbilical abdomen. These patients are often younger, thinner, and fitter than candidates for full abdominoplasty. There may be variable amount of adiposity and myofascial laxity, but the skin at and above the umbilicus is usually good quality and free of striae.

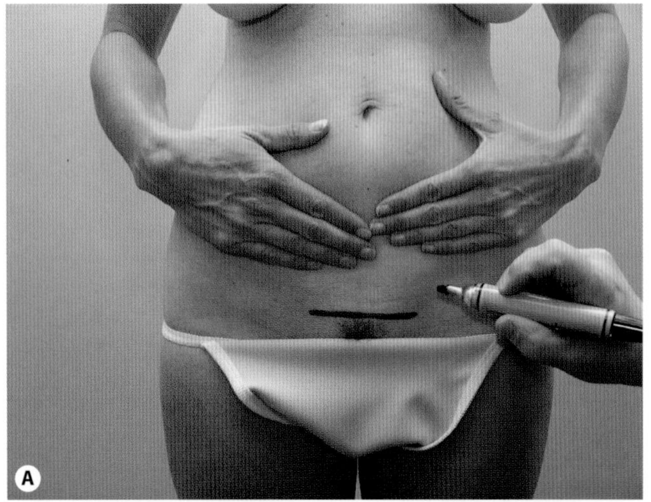

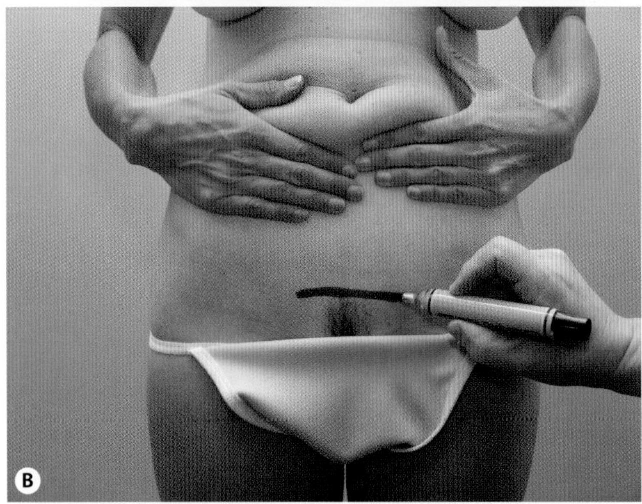

Fig. 5.3 A, B Preoperative marking is performed with the patient standing. The transverse incision is marked while the patient pulls up on the lower abdominal soft tissue. This ensures that the final transverse scar is kept as low as possible.

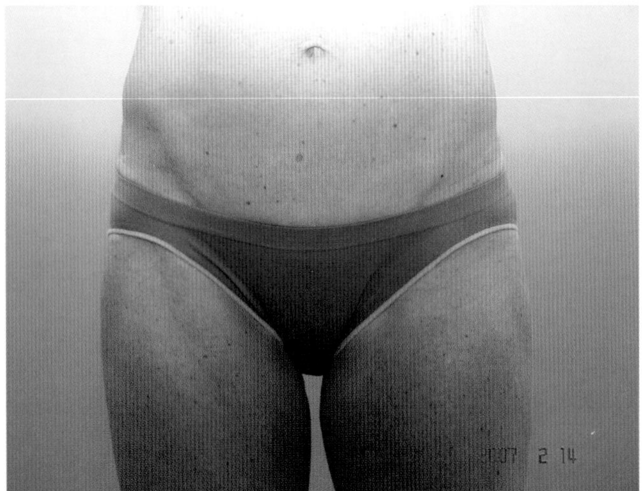

Fig. 5.4 Another method to make sure the final transverse scar will be well hidden is to have the patient bring their smallest, most revealing underwear or swimsuit.

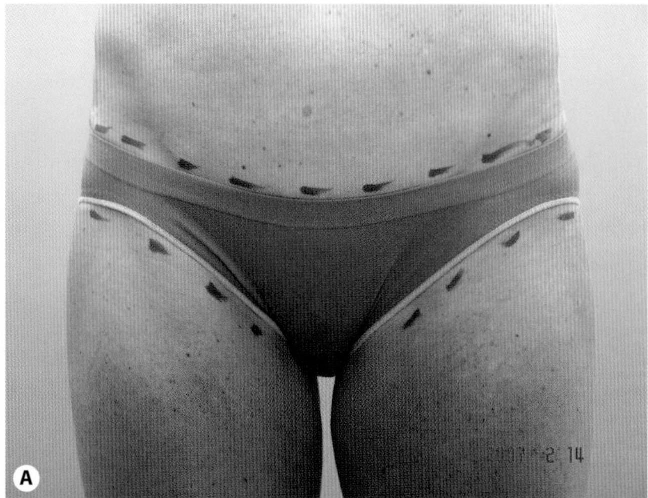

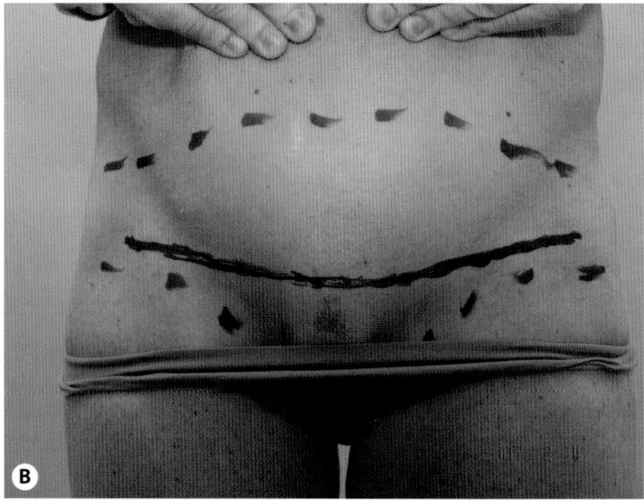

Fig. 5.5 A, B The borders of the undergarment are outlined. The center of the transverse incision is similarly marked by having the patient pull up on the lower abdominal soft tissue.

abdominoplasty. In general, patients tolerate a longer incision in order to achieve an excellent result (**Fig. 5.6**).

Patients should be counseled that a mini abdominoplasty may not be the ideal procedure for them and a longer incision, or possibly full abdominoplasty, would be more appropriate. If this option is properly presented, patients who could benefit from a full abdominoplasty may become more accepting of the scar, particularly if it can be placed low, where it can be hidden by swimwear or clothing.

Another important consideration for patients requesting mini or short scar abdominoplasty, but who really would benefit from a more significant procedure, is to disclose preoperatively that if the results of a mini abdominoplasty are undesirable, conversion to a full abdominoplasty is possible. Preoperative discussion of the necessary additional costs, recovery, and risks and complications is recommended (**Box 5.3**)

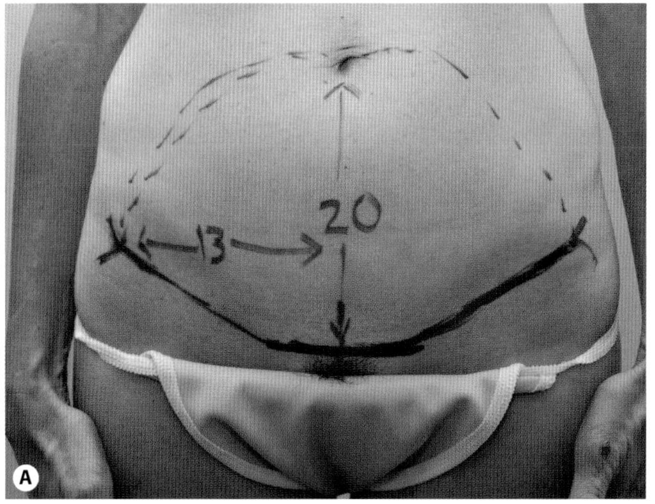

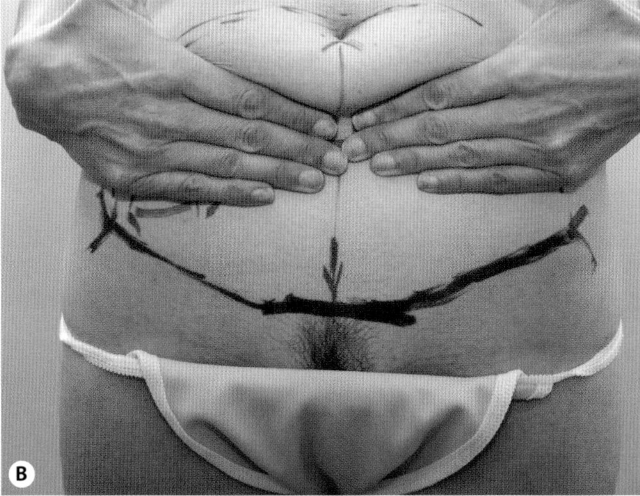

Fig. 5.6 A, B The transverse mark is continued in a natural skin crease towards the anterior superior iliac crest bilaterally. The exact length is estimated based on the amount of soft-tissue laxity present and the amount of resection planned.

Box 5.3 Extent of soft-tissue dissection

- The extent of the abdominal soft-tissue dissection and undermining for a mini abdominoplasty depends directly on the source of the abdominal contour irregularity and the desired aesthetic result
- Elevation of the abdominal soft tissue up to the level of the xiphoid is almost always appropriate for proper myofascial plication. Myofascial plication is one of the most important components in achieving a desirable outcome for the mini abdominoplasty
- When there is significant abdominal wall laxity, full myofascial plication from xiphoid to pubic symphysis is performed. To accomplish this, the umbilical stalk should be released and dissection completed up to the xiphoid and costal margins

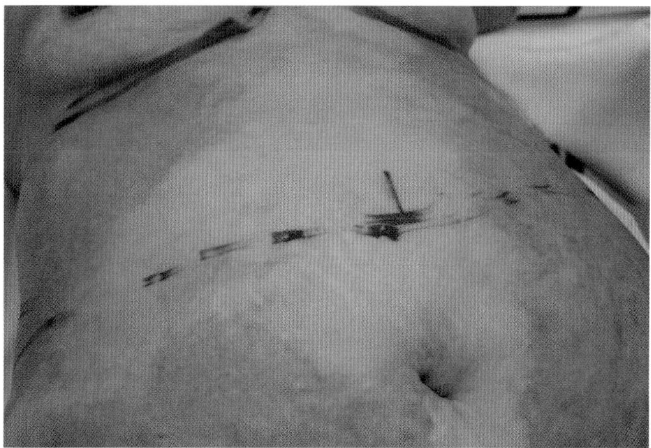

Fig. 5.7 When concurrent abdominal liposuction is planned, tumescent infiltration is performed prior to prepping and draping the patient so as to maximize the vasoconstriction effect of the epinephrine. Infiltration should be performed to the costal margins, inframammary fold, the flanks, hips, and mons.

If the degree of abdominal skin laxity is minimal and the majority of the excess adiposity and skin laxity can be corrected by a minimal excision, the incision can be kept short. This is an unusual scenario most commonly seen in younger patients who have never been significantly overweight. Most patients' deformity in the category of excess adiposity and mild to moderate skin laxity is usually secondary to changes following pregnancy.

Concurrent Liposuction

Once the incision line is drawn, marking should be made for concurrent liposuction that will address all areas of excess adiposity and usually include the entire abdomen, lateral breasts, flanks, and mons area (**Fig. 5.7**). Liposuction is a key element in the majority of mini or short scar abdominoplasties. Rarely will a patient present without excess adiposity where liposuction will not be a significant benefit. A thorough liposuction of this subcutaneous fat will significantly enhance the final outcome.

For liposuction during the average mini abdominoplasty procedure, 3–5 L of infiltration of the subcutaneous fat using a epinephrine- and lidocaine-containing solution allows for thorough liposuction while minimizing bleeding (see also Chapter 3, Liposuction in Abdominal Contouring). Entry sites are ideally placed within the skin to be resected and within the umbilicus. If excess adiposity is present lateral to the breast area and in the flank, an entry site in the inframammary crease is well concealed and allows direct access to these areas for treatment.

The patient is brought to the operating room where sequential compression devices are placed on the lower

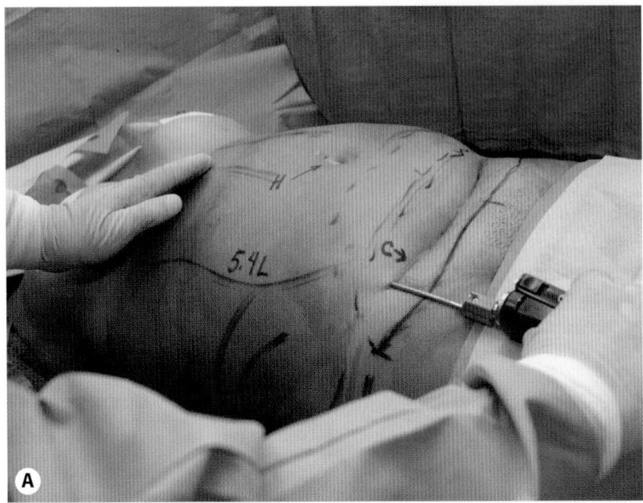

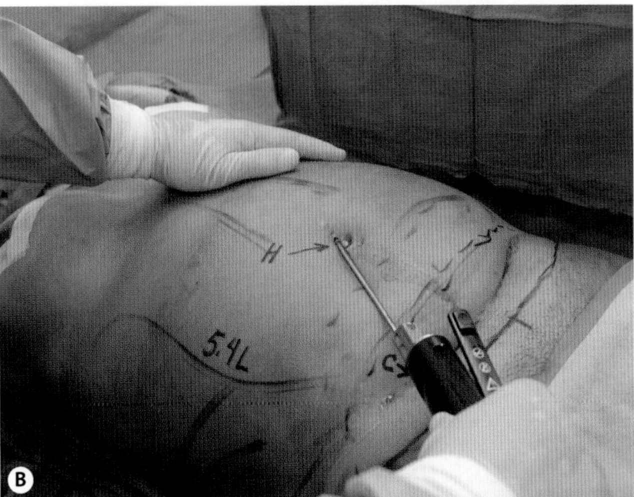

Fig. 5.8 A, B When concurrent abdominal liposuction is planned, it is performed first prior to the abdominoplasty component of the case. Infiltration is performed through entry sites within the abdominal skin resection and within the umbilicus. Liposuction is performed through the same entry sites throughout all areas of the abdomen, most commonly to the level of the xiphoid, inframammary fold, flanks, hips, and mons.

extremities, and general endotracheal anesthesia is begun. A Foley catheter may be beneficial to properly monitor fluid status and to ensure an empty bladder, which is helpful for muscle plication. Nitrous oxide inhalation agents may cause visceral distension and should probably be avoided for most abdominoplasty procedures. IV antibiotics are administered routinely.

Thorough infiltration of all subcutaneous tissue to be suctioned is then performed prior to full prepping and draping to allow time for maximal vasoconstriction (see Chapter 3, Liposuction and Abdominal Contouring). Entry sites are placed within the planned surgical resection area and umbilicus (**Fig. 5.8**). The usual infiltration volume is between 3 and 5 L.

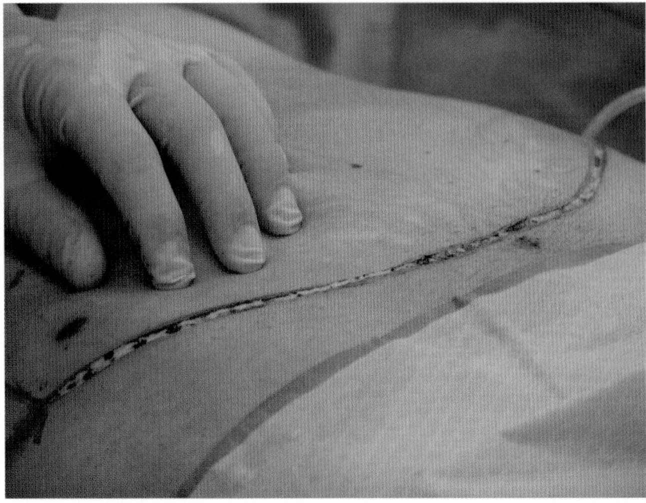

Fig. 5.9 The initial transverse incision is made partially through the dermis using a number 10 scalpel. It is then completed with the use of electrocautery to minimize bleeding from the skin edges.

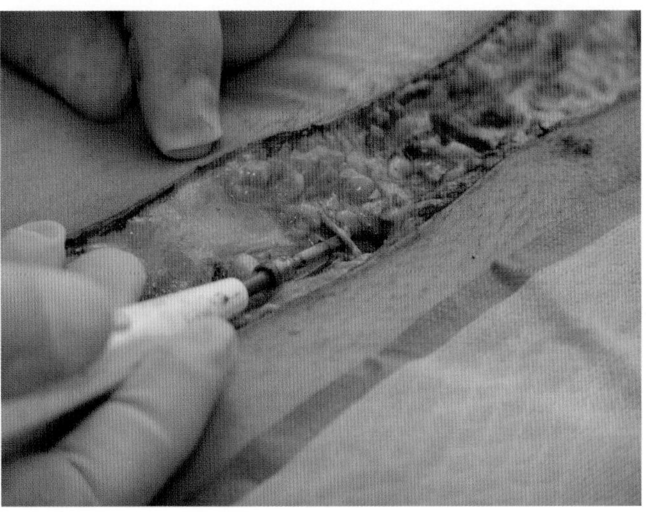

Fig. 5.10 The superficial inferior epigastric vessels should be identified and controlled as they are a potential source of postoperative hematoma. The tumescent infiltration hydrates and distends the tissues and helps identify the vessels more easily.

The lower transverse incision is made first using a number 10 scalpel partway through the dermis (**Fig. 5.9**). The electrocautery is used to complete the skin incision so as to minimize bleeding from the skin margin. The electrocautery device is used to continue the dissection (**Fig. 5.10**). The initial dissection down to the abdominal wall fascia should proceed with care, as many patients have a scar from a cesarean section that creates fibrosis, altering the normal anatomy. Additional care should be taken to identify and control the superficial inferior epigastric and the superficial circumflex vessels, as these are likely to be encountered in most mini abdominoplasty patients and can be a source of postoperative

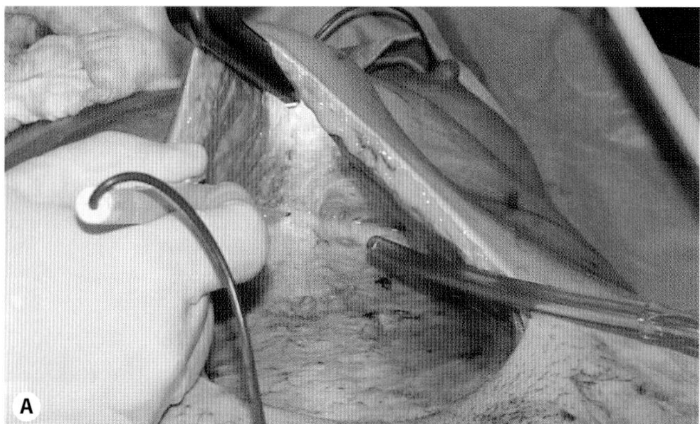

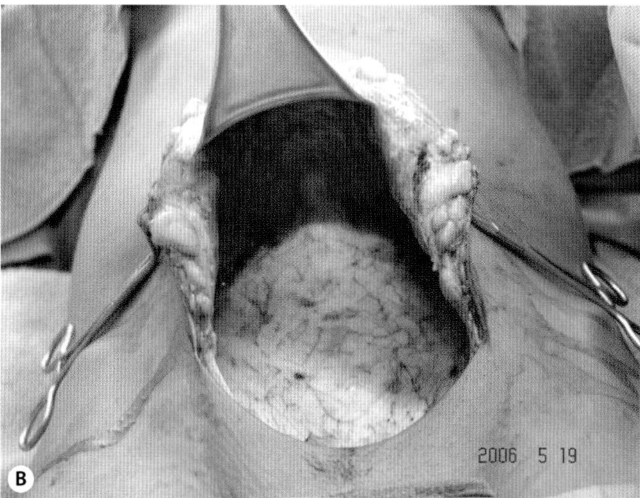

Fig. 5.11 A, B Dissection of the abdominal soft tissue up to the level of the umbilicus is performed with electrocautery. Additional care is warranted in patients who have had lower abdominal surgery or a history of hernia, otherwise the dissection is straightforward.

hematoma unless properly controlled (see Chapter 2, Anatomical Considerations in Abdominal Contouring). Dissection continues with electrocautery under direct vision to the level of the umbilicus. All perforators must be carefully controlled during this dissection (**Fig. 5.11**). Once the umbilicus is reached, it is either divided at its base, left intact, or – rarely – circumscribed as in a full abdominoplasty. Dissection continues to the xiphoid and costal margins to complete the undermining (**Fig. 5.12**).

Umbilical Considerations

Mini or short scar abdominoplasty has significant challenges, particularly in relation to treatment of the umbilicus. An improved umbilical appearance can often be achieved with a mini abdominoplasty not requiring umbilical repositioning. With smaller skin resections the umbilical location can be left unchanged, and this is usually desirable. Often in this scenario additional superior umbilical hooding is created

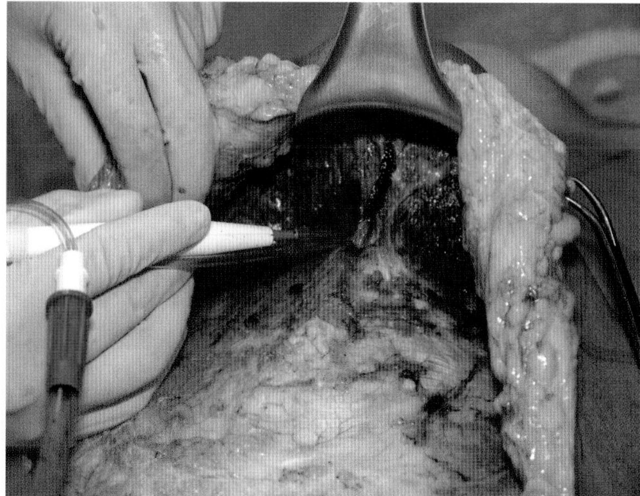

Fig. 5.12 When myofascial plication is planned, the dissection should be performed up to the level of the xiphoid and costal margins. To accomplish this, the umbilical stalk is usually released at its base from the abdominal wall fascia.

by inferior skin migration, which can be attractive. A more vertically oriented umbilicus with a deeper appearance is frequently achieved without any umbilical relocation as the stalk is pulled inwardly following muscle plication.

With more significant skin resections, options of umbilical float or repositioning with a residual midline scar may be necessary. It is unusual in a mini abdominoplasty to be able to resect all of the skin between the lower incision and the umbilicus. This usually requires a longer scar and changes the nature of the procedure to a full abdominoplasty. If the patient's body habitus allows for this – which is very unusual – it may be an ideal scenario for a short scar abdominoplasty.

In patients with significant supraumbilical skin laxity a mini abdominoplasty procedure will probably not correct this deformity because of the umbilical tethering. Conversion to a full abdominoplasty is more likely to correct this supraumbilical skin laxity. Reverse abdominoplasty is a procedure that can be of benefit to this subgroup of patients as well (see Chapter 10).

In the event that umbilical relocation is necessary, a decision whether to close the umbilical site vertically or transversely must be made. In our experience, a vertical closure as apposed to a transverse closure usually heals without a residual dog-ear deformity.

Umbilical Float

Umbilical float deserves special attention. During this procedure the base of the umbilicus is detached from the midline abdominal wall. Muscle plication is then performed and the umbilical stalk is reattached to the midline in a location inferior to its original site. When increasing amounts of skin are excised, it becomes more difficult to reattach the umbilicus within a normal range, i.e., within 2 cm.If the umbilicus is attached more than 2 cm inferior to its original location, an unnatural and undesirable appearance often results. This must be avoided. Correction of this deformity is difficult and usually requires umbilical excision and the creation of a neoumbilicus at a more normal location (see Chapter 13).

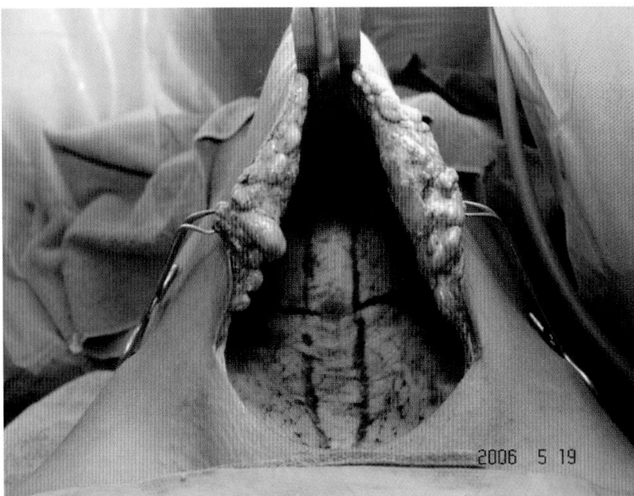

Fig. 5.13 The vertical level of the umbilical stalk connection is marked with methylene blue ink for future reference. Methylene blue is also used to mark the borders of the rectus diastasis and/or the estimated amount of myofascial plication. Note the small amount of fat protruding from the divided umbilical stalk. The small hernia is closed with interrupted absorbable suture.

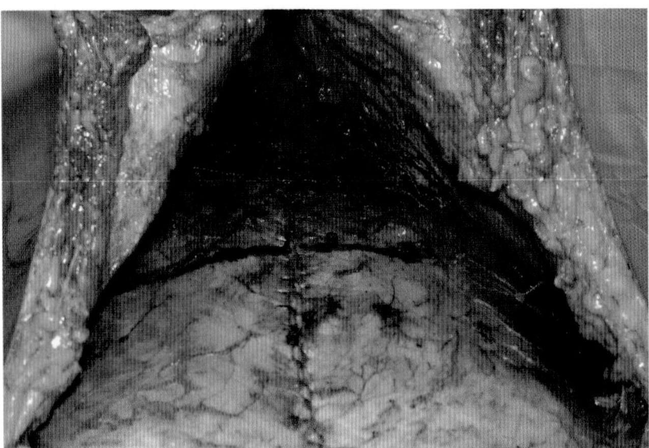

Fig. 5.14 Myofascial plication is performed with size 1 or 0 looped nylon on a tapered needle. Because the umbilical stalk has been released there is no need to modify the plication process near the periumbilical area; instead, myofascial plication proceeds from xiphoid to pubic symphysis in a continuous running fashion. The level of the umbilicus should be marked transversely, because with the muscle plication the umbilical origin is internalized and may be difficult to identify. Failure to do so could lead to an undesirable inferior umbilical location.

A much more desirable and commonly used approach is to detach the umbilical stalk, continue undermining to the xiphoid, perform xiphoid-to-symphysis pubis plication, and then reattach the stalk at its native or original level (see **Fig. 5.12**). When the stalk is detached from the abdominal wall, a transverse mark at this level should be made with indelible ink such as methylene blue (**Figs 5.13 and 5.14**). This will permit the umbilicus to be reattached at the correct level after muscle plication, which internalizes the previous stalk attachment point. This is a highly desirable technique because it avoids inferior umbilical displacement and allows for continuous muscle plication without suture interruption. An inferior skin excision creates the most desirable umbilical appearance because the stalk remains at its normal location but the umbilicus is often deepened, made more vertical, and with greater superior hooding.

Small umbilical hernias are frequently seen and are easily repaired with umbilical stalk division and reinforced with the muscle plication. This technique does not jeopardize umbilical perfusion (**Fig. 5.13**).

Muscle Plication (Box 5.4)

Muscle plication during mini or short scar abdominoplasty should be performed in a similar manner as for a full abdominoplasty to achieve the best results. This is as important in mini abdominoplasty as in all other techniques. The umbilical stalk should never be in the way because it can be easily divided and reinserted in its native location, floated, or transposed. The best technique appears to be division of the umbilical stalk with continuous muscle plication from the xiphoid to the symphysis pubis, and reattachment of the umbilical stalk at its original level.

A number 1 or 0 loop nylon suture on a large tapered needle is very effective for a running myofascial plication (**Figs**

Box 5.4 Myofascial plication

- Myofascial plication during a mini abdominoplasty is performed from xiphoid to pubic symphysis in similar fashion as described for the other abdominoplasty techniques
- A size 1 or 0 looped nylon suture is used to perform the plication in running fashion
- Plication of the infraumbilical abdominal wall only may result in compensatory supraumbilical abdominal wall bulging, and is rarely advised
- In order for full myofascial plication to be performed, complete elevation of the abdominal soft tissue up to the xiphoid and costal margins is necessary
- The umbilical stalk should be re-secured to the abdominal wall after plication is complete to help create an 'inny' and augment the periumbilical depression.

5.13 and 5.14). The knot should be buried at the symphysis pubis to prevent postoperative palpability (**Fig. 5.15**).

Following a strong myofascial plication with limited undermining, an undermining ridge may be present bilaterally. Using the Lockwood dissector, this ridge can be eliminated by tissue mobilization, which maintains excellent perfusion. Undermining of the ridge creates multiple septa within which neurovascular structures are intact (**Fig. 5.16**). Bupivacaine is injected into the sheath and throughout the entire area of undermining (**Fig. 5.17**). The umbilicus is then replaced in its previous location or slightly inferior to this using interrupted 2/0 Vicryl sutures (**Fig. 5.18**).

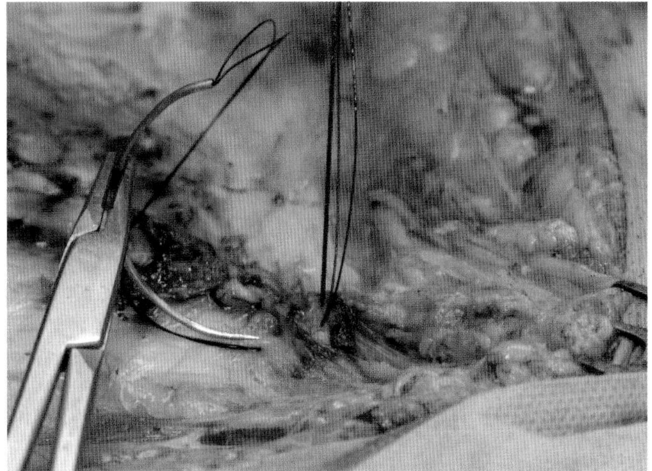

Fig. 5.15 The suture knot is buried between the plicated edges at the completion of myofascial plication at the pubic symphysis to avoid palpability.

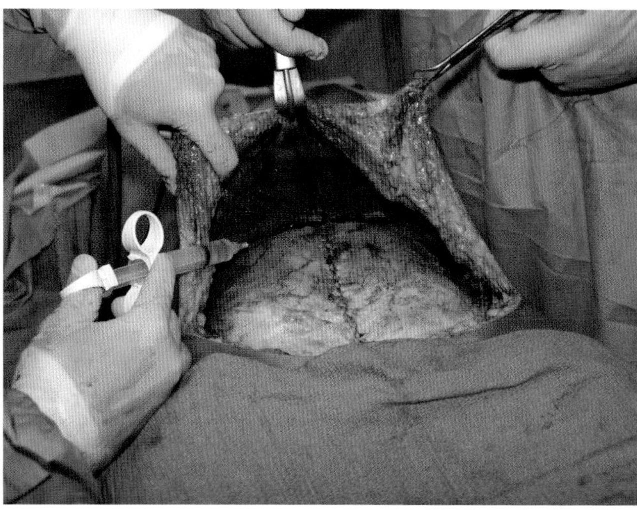

Fig. 5.17 Bupivacaine is routinely used to lessen the postoperative discomfort associated with the myofascial plication. It is infiltrated under the anterior rectus sheath bilaterally as well as throughout the periphery of the undermining.

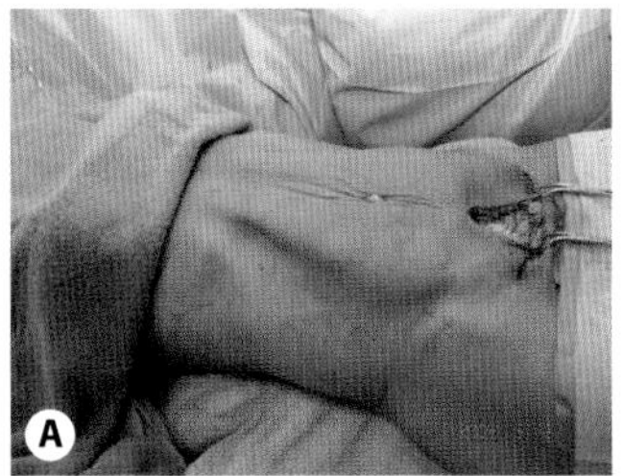

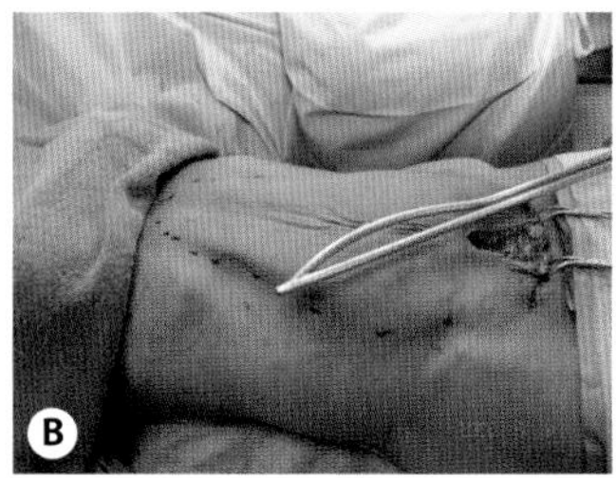

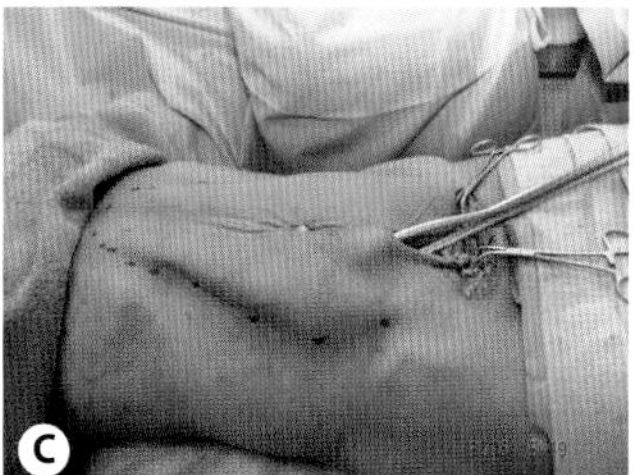

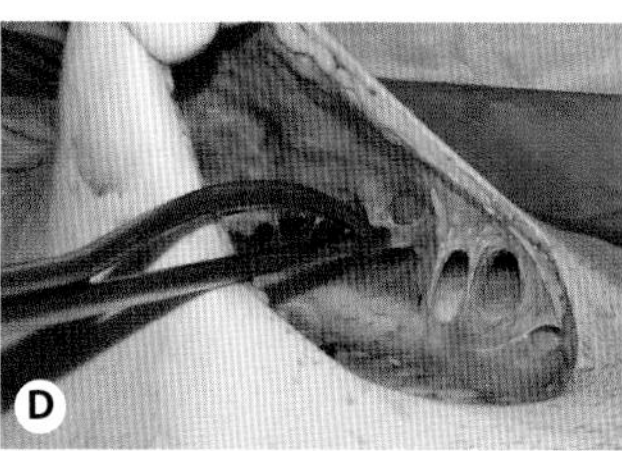

Fig. 5.16 A–D Any soft-tissue tethering noted at the completion of the plication process is released bluntly using the Lockwood dissector. These undermining ridges are clearly seen and are brought medially by the strong muscle plication. The Lockwood dissector thoroughly mobilizes this undermining edge, allowing the tissue to release and become smoother, flattened, and mobilized. The intervening septa that are created are clearly seen, within which are the important vascular structures that are maintained to ensure flap viability and sensitivity.

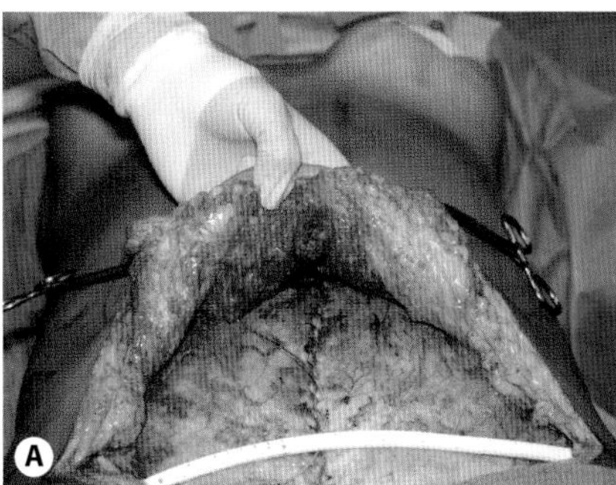

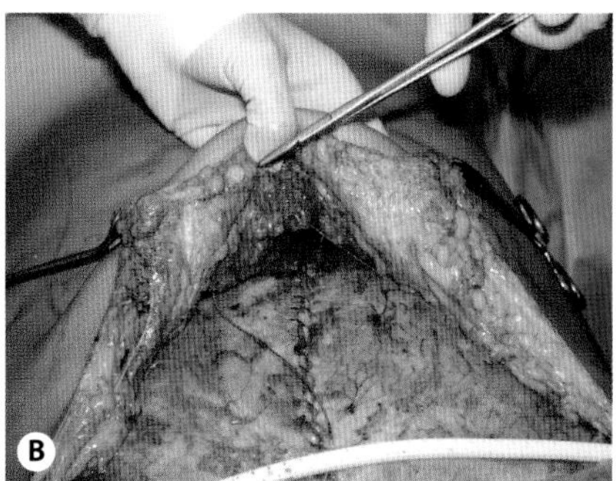

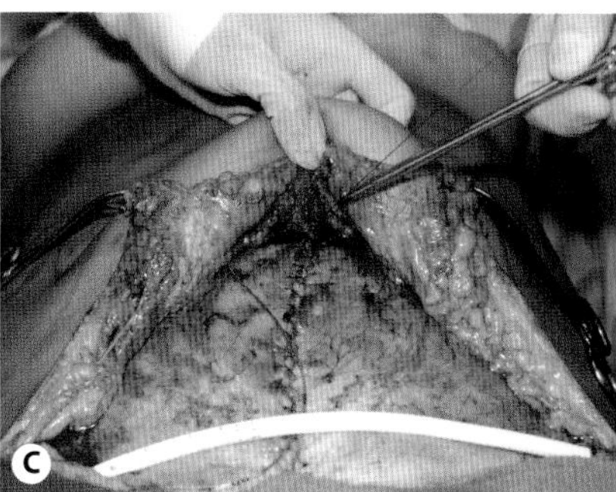

Fig. 5.18 A–C The umbilical stalk is re-secured to the abdominal wall fascia. This maneuver augments the periumbilical depression and helps create a ideal recessed umbilical shape, commonly referred to as an 'inny.' Two 2/0 Vicryl sutures are used.
The transverse mark made to identify the normal location of the umbilical stalk will facilitate placement. Additional care should be taken to make sure the umbilicus is re-secured in the midline.

Tissue Demarcation and Closure

If a pain pump is going to be used, it should be placed and secured prior to reattachment of the umbilicus. Following muscle plication and umbilical reattachment, tissue demarcation is best performed using the Pitanguy demarcator. The midline is demarcated and the tissue divided and temporarily closed. Penetrating towel clips are placed on each side of this, and with moderate traction caudally, the Pitanguy demarcator is used to identify the amount of tissue to be resected (**Fig. 5.19**).

If there is a significant thickness of subscarpal fat, it can be removed prior to umbilical replacement and closure (**Fig. 5.20**). This may thin the abdominal flap by an additional one-third without compromising vascularity. A pain pump catheter and a drain are placed in the normal fashion (**Fig. 5.21**).

The operating table is flexed and placed into the semi-Fowler's position. Skin closure for this procedure is critical to avoid the occurrence of a dog-ear. These are much more common with a mini than with a full or extended abdominoplasty, and are completely eliminated by a circumferential abdominoplasty. The abdominal skin flaps must be very strongly advanced from the lateral aspects medially. This can be advanced in three layers, with the superficial fascia strongly bringing the tissue medially, the deep dermis also bringing the tissue strongly medially, and finally the intracuticular suture advancing the upper incision line medially. If any dog-ear is left after the deep dermal

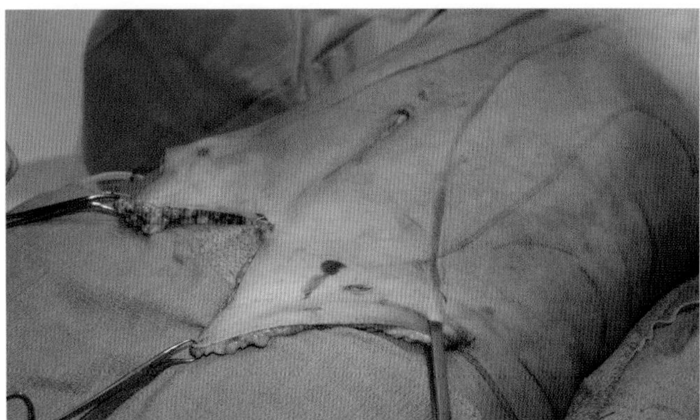

Fig. 5.19 The process of soft-tissue resection is facilitated by placing the patient in a partially flexed position and using the Pitanguy demarcator to determine the proper amount of resection. The flap is first divided in the midline at a point determined by the demarcator and temporarily stapled. Towel clips are then equally placed and tensioned as the demarcation is performed.

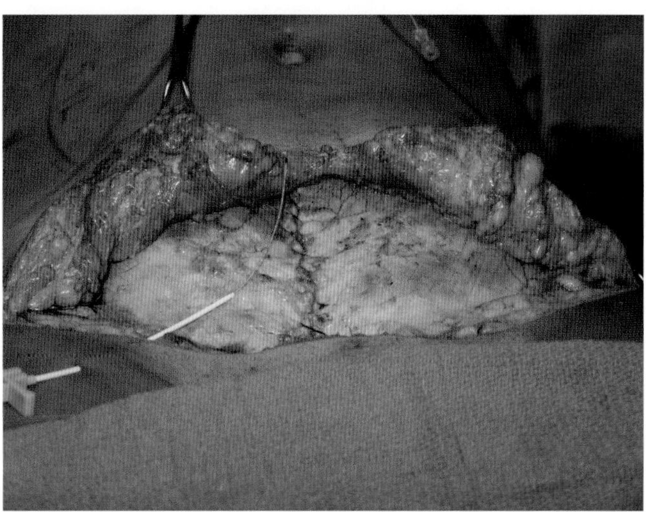

Fig. 5.21 A pain pump can be introduced and secured at this time. It is secured in the midline over the myofascial plication with a few 4/0 Vicryl sutures and brought out laterally below the inferior skin margin. We use lidocaine as a continuous drip to help reduce the discomfort associated with myofascial plication.

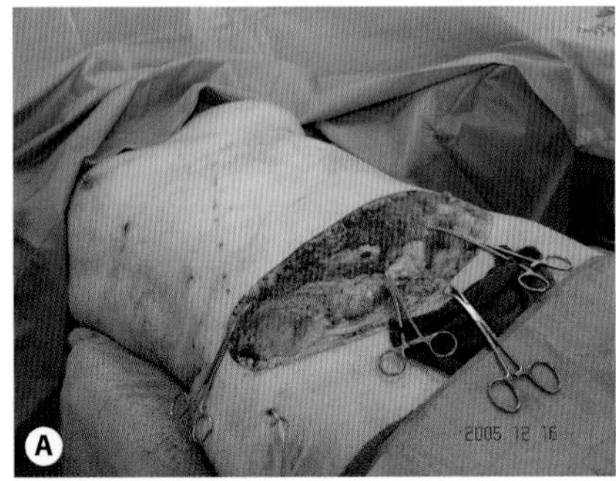

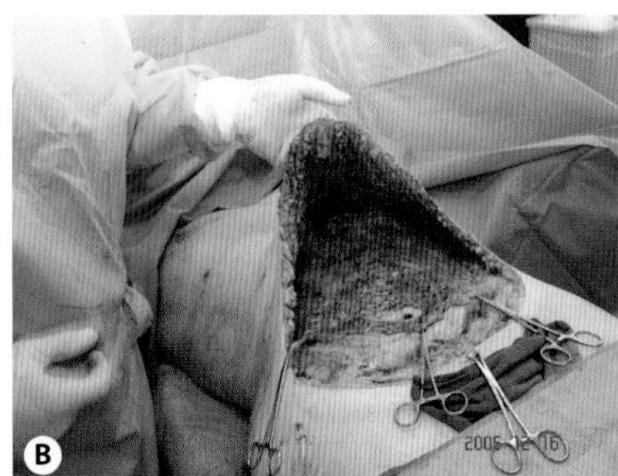

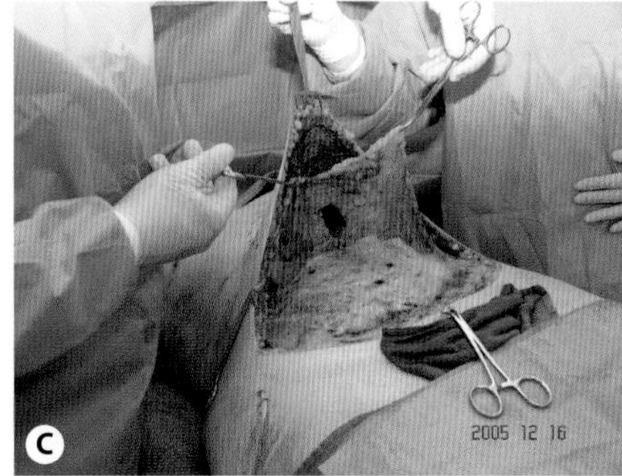

Fig. 5.20 A–C Sub-Scarpal fat resection can be performed if deemed beneficial to the final aesthetic result. This can be performed up to the level of the dissection if necessary. Frequently the layer of subscarpal fat in the mini abdominoplasty patient is fairly thin and resection is usually not necessary.

closure, additional skin trimming should be performed, otherwise a persistent dog-ear will remain, requiring subsequent correction (**Fig. 5.22**).

Following wound closure, skin adhesive is applied. The patient is placed in a compressive binder and taken to the recovery room.

Postoperative Care (Box 5.5)

The postoperative care for mini abdominoplasty is comparable that of as for a full abdominoplasty. Care should be taken to minimize the risk of postoperative nausea and vomiting, as this will cause great anxiety to the patient, with significant abdominal wall discomfort, increased blood pressure, abdominal swelling, and possible hematoma formation. Careful inspection in the recovery room is important to ensure there is no kinking or folding of the binder, which could result in ischemia or necrosis. The caregivers should be instructed to release the binder if it feels too tight to the patient. It should also be released, smoothed and repositioned every few hours. During the early postoperative period it should be worn only snugly, not tight. Arrangements for postoperative inspection should be made, usually within a few days of the procedure. Patients are allowed to shower from the second postoperative day. Vigorous activity and heavy lifting are restricted for the first 3 weeks. We find that most patients will slowly increase their activity at a reasonable pace as they recover.

In the early postoperative period it is advisable to connect the abdominal drain to high-vacuum wall suction, which

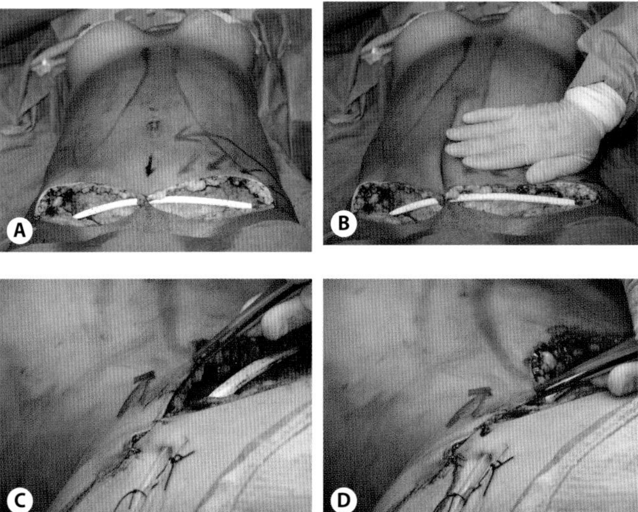

Fig. 5.22 A–D The transverse incision is closed in a similar fashion to other abdominoplasty procedures using 0 Vicryl at the superficial fascia level, 2/0 Vicryl buried deep dermally, and 4/0 Monocryl running intradermally. The upper tissue is strongly advanced bilaterally toward the midline with each layer of closure to reduce the chance of lateral dog-ears. This greatly enhances the waistline achieved.

Box 5.5 Postoperative care

- Postoperative care following mini abdominoplasty is comparable to that for other abdominoplasty procedures (i.e. full abdominoplasty)
- A partially flexed position, early ambulation, proper hydration, and appropriate use of an abdominal binder are all key components
- The patient is allowed to shower starting the second postoperative day
- Activity is restricted for 3–4 weeks. No vigorous or strenuous activity is allowed during this period
- The drain(s) is removed when output decreases to 25–30 mL/24 h

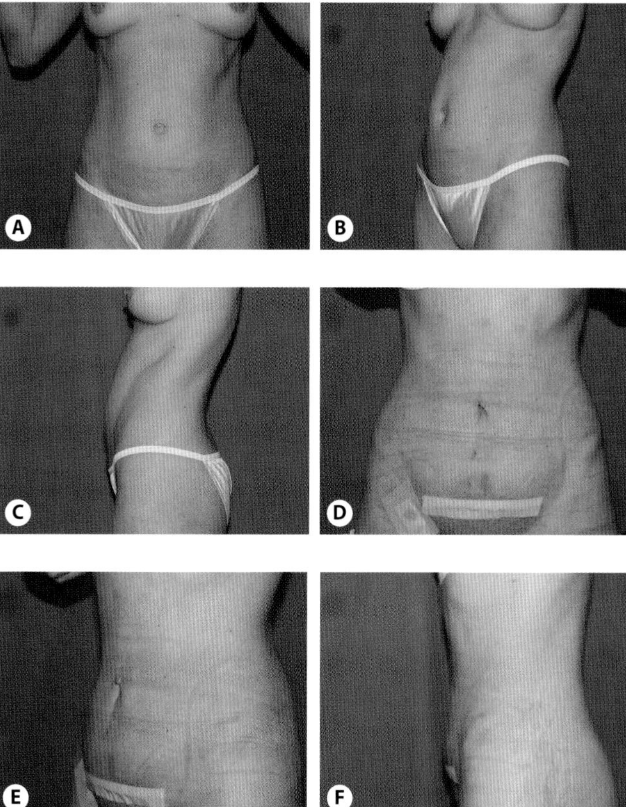

Fig. 5.23 A–F This 30-year-old woman complained about a persistent bulging-in of her lower abdomen despite proper diet and exercise. She was not a candidate for endoscopic abdominoplasty because of the presence of appreciable lower abdominal soft-tissue laxity. Because of this, however, she was an ideal candidate for a mini abdominoplasty, and underwent this procedure with full myofascial plication from xiphoid to pubic symphysis. Postoperative photographs show improved contour, particularly on lateral profile, with a very short transverse incision and no umbilical scar. With thorough infiltration and gentle tissue handling virtually no bruising should be expected.

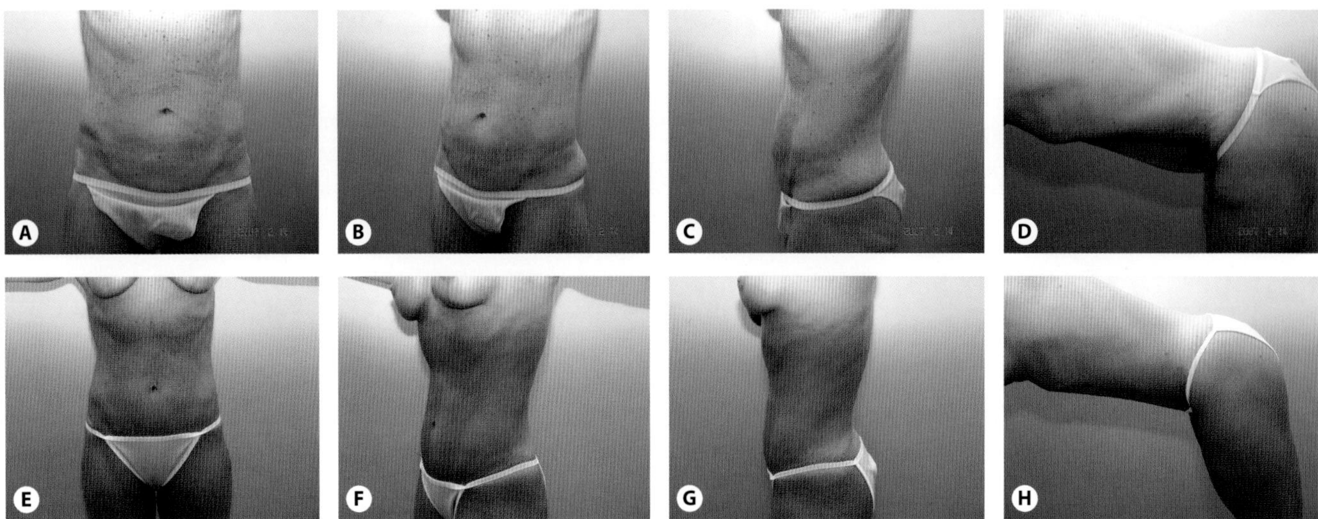

Fig. 5.24 A–H This 35-year-old woman complained of loose skin and soft tissue in her lower abdomen as well as lower abdominal bulging, despite exercising regularly. She noted that this was worse when she bent over. A mini abdominoplasty was performed with full myofascial plication and resection of excess soft tissue from the infraumbilical area. Her postoperative photographs show improved contour, particularly on the diver's view. (The diver's view is a standard plastic surgery photographic term used to describe the patient's position when they are leaning strongly forward, usually with their hands against a door, allowing their abdominal tissue to hang down. It is the most dramatic before and after view which demonstrates the tightening, thinning, and flattening following abdominoplasty.) Here, the lower abdominal laxity has been completely eliminated, achieving a more youthful attractive silhouette.

will help remove most of the residual tumescent fluid. Drains are removed when drainage is less than 30–50 mL over a 24-hour period. The patient is instructed to maintain a flexed position, and can usually straighten up between 7 and 10 days postoperatively. Preoperative and postoperative photos are shown in **Figs 5.23 and 5.24**.

Conclusion/Summary

The mini abdominoplasty is a highly effective procedure for patients with mild to moderate excess abdominal adiposity, skin laxity, and muscular diastasis. Thorough concurrent liposuction, strong myofascial plication, appropriate skin excision, and proper wound closure are all important elements for this procedure. When properly designed, with important patient input, a very pleasing and gratifying result can be obtained for both patient and surgeon.

Clinical Caveats: Mini abdominoplasty

- Candidates for mini abdominoplasty comprise a small and specific segment of the overall abdominal contouring population
- Ideal candidates have soft-tissue laxity isolated to their lower abdomen. There may be variable adiposity and myofascial laxity, but the skin around and above the umbilicus is usually good quality and free of striae
- Concurrent abdominal liposuction and full myofascial plication can be performed if needed
- These patients benefit from the shorter transverse scar and the absence of an umbilical scar provided by the mini abdominoplasty
- Appropriate discussion with the patient is particularly important, as some patients are more reasonable candidates for other type of abdominal contouring procedure (i.e., abdominal liposuction, endoscopic abdominoplasty, or full abdominoplasty)

References

1. McDevitt NB. Deep vein thrombosis prophylaxis. American Society of Plastic and Reconstructive Surgeons. Plast Reconstruct Surg 1999; 104: 1923.
2. Davison SP, Venturi ML, Attinger CE, et al. Prevention of venous thromboembolism in the plastic surgery patient. Plast Reconstruct Surg 2004; 114: 43.
3. Broughton G 2nd, Rios JL, Rohrich RJ, Brown SA. Deep venous thrombosis prophylaxis practice and treatment strategies among plastic surgeons: survey results. Plast Reconstruct Surg 2007; 119: 157.
4. Seeger JD, Loughlin J, Eng PM, et al. Risk of thromboembolism in women taking ethinylestradiol/drospirenone and other oral contraceptives. Obstet Gynecol 2003; 110: 587.

5. Blickstein D, Blickstein I. Oral contraception and thrombophilia. Curr Opin Obstet Gynecol 2007; 19: 370.
6. van Vlijmen EF, Brouwer JL, Veeger NJ, et al. Oral contraceptives and the absolute risk of venous thromboembolism in women with single or multiple thrombophilic defects: results from a retrospective family cohort study. Arch Intern Med 2007; 167: 282.
7. Krueger JK, Rohrich RJ. Clearing the smoke: the scientific rationale for tobacco abstention with plastic surgery. Plast Reconstruct Surg 2001; 15: 108–1063.
8. Manassa EH, Hertl CH, Olbrisch RR. Wound healing problems in smokers and nonsmokers after 132 abdominoplasties. Plast Reconstruct Surg 2003; 111: 2082.

Suggested Reading

Boyd BJ, Taylor GI. The vascular territories of the superior epigastric and deep inferior epigastric systems. Plast Reconstruct Surg 1984; 73: 1.

Cooper MA. Mini-abdominoplasty. Plast Reconstruct Surg 1988; 81: 473–475.

Dillerud E. Abdominoplasty combined with suction lipoplasty: A study of complications, revisions, and risk factors in 487 cases. Ann Plast Surg 1990; 25: 333.

Ferraro GA, Rossano F, Miccoli A, et al. Modified mini-abdominoplasty: navel transposition and horizontal residual scar. Aesthet Plast Surg 2007; 31: 663–665.

Greminger RF. The mini-abdominoplasty. Plast Reconstruct Surg 1987; 79: 356–365.

Hunstad JP. Addressing difficult areas in body contouring with emphasis on combined tumescent and syringe techniques. Clin Plast Surg 1996; 23: 57.

Nguyen TT, Kim KA, Young RB. Tumescent mini abdominoplasty. Ann Plast Surg 1997; 38: 209–212.

Matarasso A. Abdominolipoplasty: a system of classification and treatment for combined abdominoplasty and suction-assisted lipectomy. Aesthet Plast Surg 1991; 15: 111–121.

Peltier M. Musculoaponeurotic plication in abdominoplasty: How durable are its effects? Aesthet Plast Surg 1995; 19: 531.

Pitanguy I. Evaluation of body contouring surgery today: a 30-year perspective. Plast Reconstruct Surg 2000; 105: 1499.

Shestak KC. Marriage abdominoplasty expands the mini-abdominoplasty concept. Plast Reconstruct Surg 1999; 103: 1020–1031; discussion 1032–1035.

Sozer SO, Agullo FJ, Santillan AA, Wolf C. Decision making in abdominoplasty. Aesthet Plast Surg 2007; 31: 117–127.

Spiegelman JI, Levine RH. Abdominoplasty: a comparison of outpatient and inpatient procedures shows that it is a safe and effective procedure for outpatients in an office-based surgery clinic. Plast Reconstruct Surg 2006; 118: 517.

Stewart KJ, Stewart DA, Coghlan B, et al. Complications of 278 consecutive abdominoplasties. J Plast Reconstruct Aesthet Surg 2006; 59: 1152–1155.

Wilkinson TS. Mini-abdominoplasty. Plast Reconstruct Surg 1988; 82: 917–918.

CHAPTER 6

Lipoabdominoplasty: Safe Innovations

Ruth Graf, André R. D. Tolazzi & Maria Cecília C. Ono

IN THIS CHAPTER

Introduction

Many surgical techniques are currently available for abdominal contouring. Based on the individual characteristic of the patients' anatomy and their goals, these abdominal contouring procedures include, liposuction, mini abdominoplasty, and full abdominoplasty. According to the American Society for Aesthetic Plastic Surgery's 2004 Cosmetic Surgery National Data Bank, during the previous 7 years the number of abdominoplasty procedures performed increased by 344%.[1] In 2006, a survey study of randomly chosen members of the American Society of Plastic Surgeons[2] evaluated the frequency of various abdominal contour techniques and complications. There were 497 respondents, and a total of 20029 procedures reported. Regarding the types of abdominal contouring procedures performed, 35% (7010) were liposuction of the abdomen, 10% (2003) were limited abdominoplasties, and 55% (11016) were full abdominoplasties.

The advent of liposuction dramatically altered the field of body contouring surgery and vastly improved our ability to contour the abdomen (see Chapter 3). There has been much debate about performing liposuction on an undermined abdominoplasty flap, the use of wetting solutions, and the safety of combining plastic surgery procedures with abdominal contouring surgery. Since the first publication on lipoplasty by Illouz in 1980,[3] liposuction has increasingly been associated with abdominoplasty resections. Initially, liposuction was rarely performed at the same time as classic abdominoplasty, because of the fear of compromising blood supply to the flap, and also of accumulating fluids under the flap, thereby increasing seroma rates. Matarasso's[4,5] publication describing the safety areas for lipoplasty in the abdominal region – the epigastric and mesogastric areas – did not recommend lipoplasty at the same time as classic abdominoplasty. Hunstad and Stevens[6,7] and others have used liposuction in these areas without ischemic consequences.

Because of these concerns, abdominoplasty and liposuction have often been performed together, albeit with a reduced skin resection superior to the mons or by limiting liposuction to the flank and dorsal areas.[4,5] Unfortunately, these approaches have limitations, either because of inadequate skin resection, leaving residual laxity in the supraumbilical area, or as a result of limited or absent abdominal liposuction, leaving residual excessive central abdominal thickness.

The technique of 'lipoabdominoplasty' was described by Saldanha in 2003.[8,9] This combines liposuction of the entire abdomen and flanks, reduced undermining, complete midline aponeurotic plication, and traditional abdominal skin flap resection. This new approach offers some advantages and may reduce the most common complications of ischemia and seroma seen with classic abdominoplasty. The wide undermining of the abdominal flap in traditional abdominoplasty is believed by some to be a cause of complications. Distal skin ischemia and necrosis can be reduced in lipoabdominoplasty by the limited skin flap undermining and by preserving most of the peri- and supraumbilical perforator vessels to the abdominal skin. The incidence and volume of seromas was also shown to be reduced because of the reduced undermining, and by using space-obliterating 'quilting sutures' between the undersurface of the elevated skin and fat and the abdominal wall. The supraumbilical flap undermining (tunnel), however, was made wide enough to allow for myofascial plication to correct rectus diastasis from the xiphoid to the mons. Closure was facilitated with quilting sutures described by Baroudi,[10] and no suction drains are used.

Patient Selection

We select patients for this procedure based on the clinical classification of Bozola: type I, fat deposit, normal musculoaponeurotic layer and no skin excess; type II, mild skin excess, normal musculoaponeurotic layer, fat may or may not be in excess; type III, mild skin excess, laxity of the infraumbilical area of the musculoaponeurotic layer, fat may or may not be present; type IV, mild skin excess, laxity in the whole extension of the musculoaponeurotic layer, fat may or may not be in excess; and type V, large skin excess, laxity of the musculoaponeurotic layer with or without hernias, fat may or may not be in excess.[11]

The procedure of lipoabdominoplasty with traditional abdominal flap resection is indicated for types III–V. Ideal candidates are those with indications for traditional abdominoplasty with rectus diastasis, skin laxity, and significant excess adiposity requiring liposuction, particularly in the supraumbilical area.

Preoperative History and Considerations

The preoperative considerations for lipoabdominoplasty are similar to those for full abdominoplasty (see Chapter 7). Because of the more limited undermining and preservation of important perforating vessels, the need for absolute smoking cessation is reduced. Preoperative history and physical examination are performed. A previous history of DVT/PE would require hematologic evaluation and work-up prior to surgery. Existing scars and the presence of any hernia should be evaluated. For a healthy patient taking no medications, basic preoperative laboratory analysis should be considered.

Operative Approach

The skin is marked with the patient in the standing position. The midline and the proposed suprapubic incision line are marked. The lower incision line is extended laterally towards the anterior superior iliac spine. Existing scars and natural creases are used to place the incisions. (**Figs 6.1 and 6.2**). The superior line is marked as a bicycle handlebar incision as described by Baroudi.[12,13] The areas for liposuction are marked, including all of the upper abdomen to the level of the inframammary crease superiorly and laterally to the flanks (**Figs 6.1 and 6.2**).

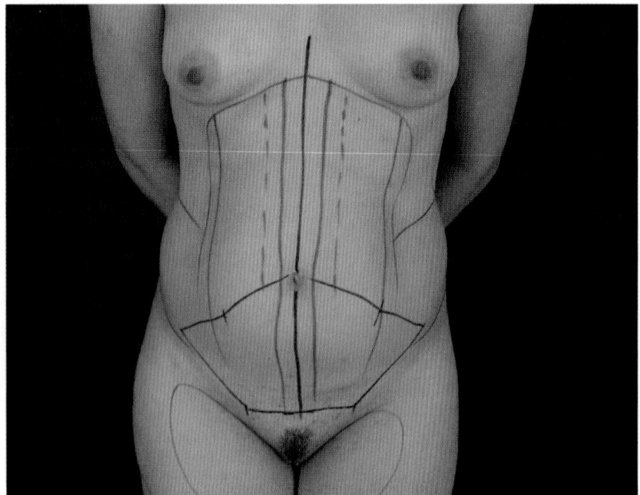

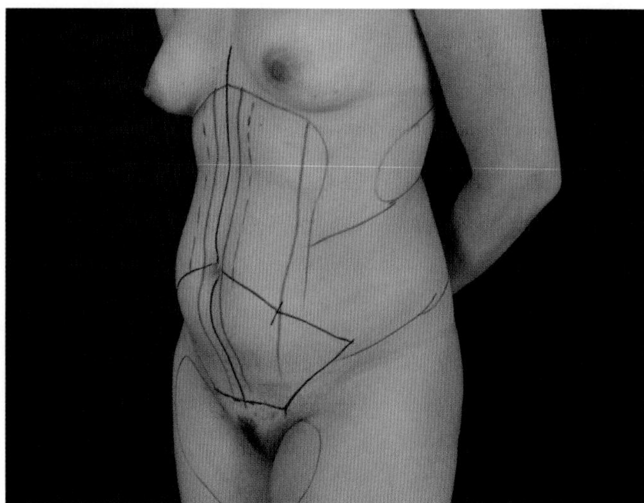

Figs 6.1 and 6.2 Skin markings showing the liposuction areas (abdomen, flaks and inner thighs) and the resection area in the lower abdomen. Preoperative markings are performed with the patient standing. The low midline transverse incision is extended bilaterally into a natural skin groove to the level of the anterior superior iliac crest. The Baroudi bicycle handle marks are then made from the ends of this incision to the umbilicus. The rectus muscles are outlined in red. The plication tunnel is marked with interrupted purple lines coursing 1.5 cm lateral to the medial edge of the rectus muscles. The areas for concurrent liposuction are marked in blue.

Intermittent compression stockings are worn prior to the beginning of surgery and continued until 6 hours afterwards. Epidural anesthesia is used for the majority of procedures, with some selected cases performed under general anesthesia. Infiltration for liposuction is performed using the superwet technique with an epinephrine concentration of 1:500 000; liposuction is performed with 3.0 and 3.5 mm cannulas, beginning initially in the deep subcutaneous layer and then superficially in the flanks and upper abdomen, except in the area superior to the umbilicus. Liposuction in the central supraumbilical area is performed only in the deep layer (**Fig. 6.3**). When the liposuction is complete, the lower abdominal flap is undermined using electrocautery up to the umbilicus, the skin around it is incised, and the flap is split from the umbilicus inferiorly (**Figs 6.4–6.7**).

Two different methods of umbilicoplasty are used for thin and obese patients. For those with a thin layer of abdominal subcutaneous tissue, the original umbilicus is preserved as a fishtail-shaped triangle, and reattached to the skin of the abdominal flap through an inverted Y incision **Figs 6.8–6.11**.

For heavier patients or those with thick subcutaneous tissue, the umbilicus is excised. A neoumbilicus is created by completely defatting the undersurface of the abdominal flap

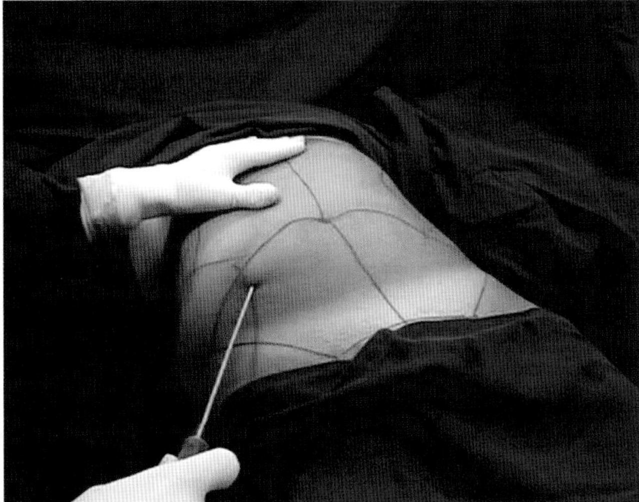

Fig. 6.3 Concurrent thorough liposuction is performed in all areas marked after superwet infiltration is performed. The central abdomen to suction deeply and the lateral flanks and hip rolls are suctioned deeply and superficially.

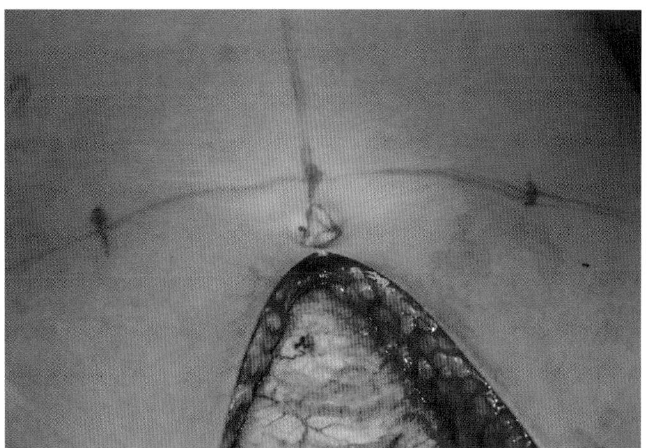

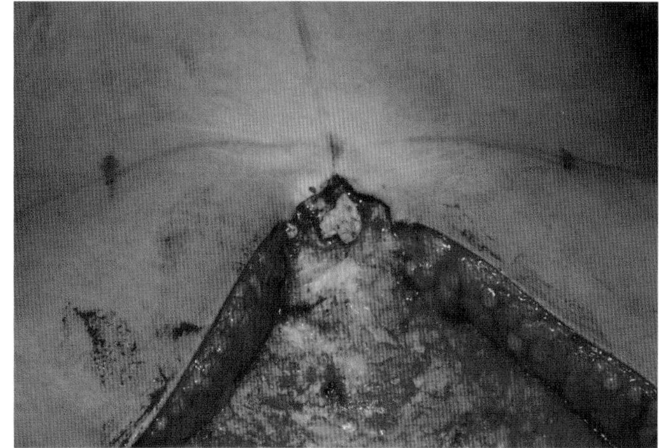

Figs 6.7–6.8 The umbilical scar is kept as an inferiorly based triangle, and sutured to the abdominal wall.

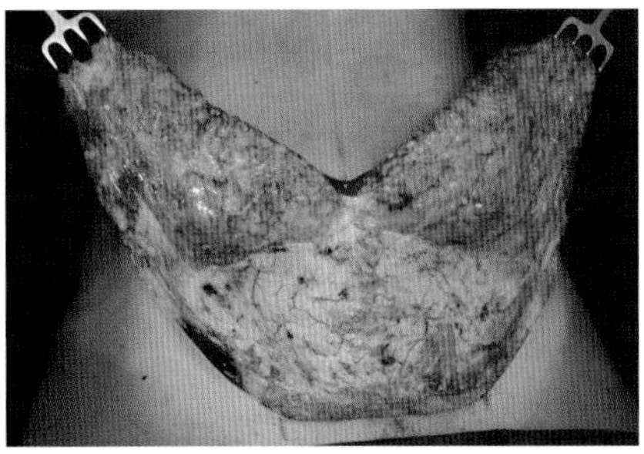

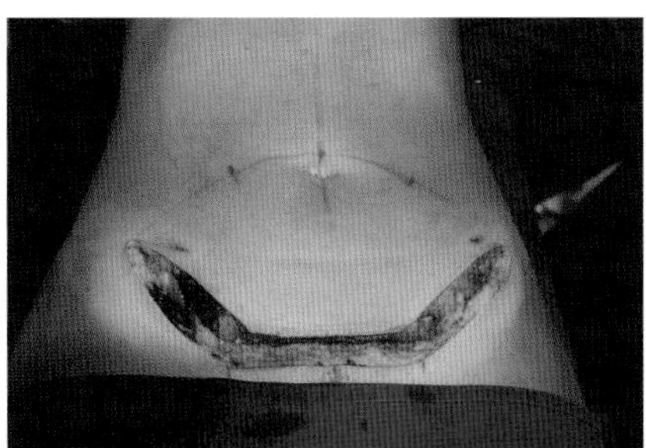

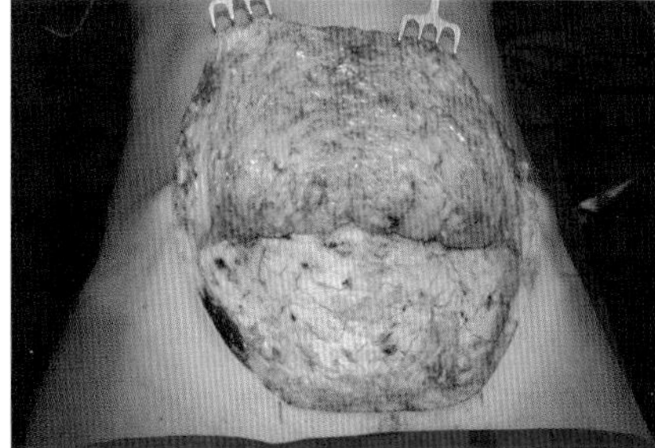

Figs 6.4–6.6 The incision is made on the line drawn and deepened through the subcutaneous tissue to the underlying abdominal wall. Dissection is performed superiorly to the level of the umbilicus with electrocautery. At this point, the raised abdominal flap is split to facilitate proper dissection and umbilical treatment.

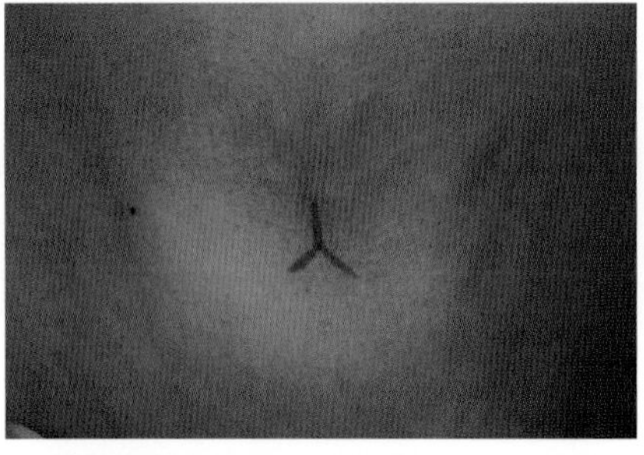
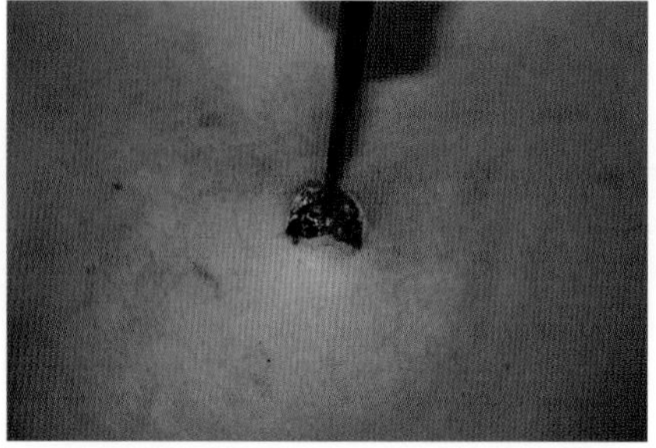
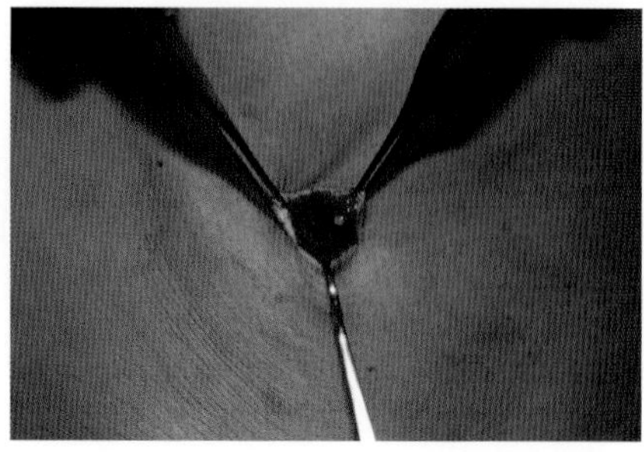

Figs 6.9–6.11 The neoumbilical site in the skin flap is incised as an inverted Y. The corners between triangular flaps are sutured to the umbilical scar and to the abdominal wall with absorbable sutures.

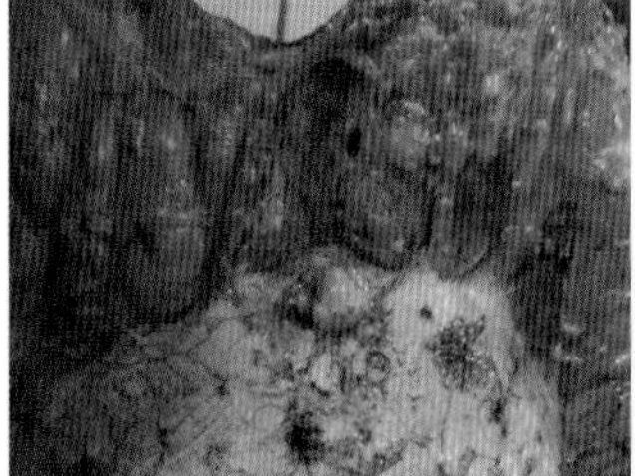
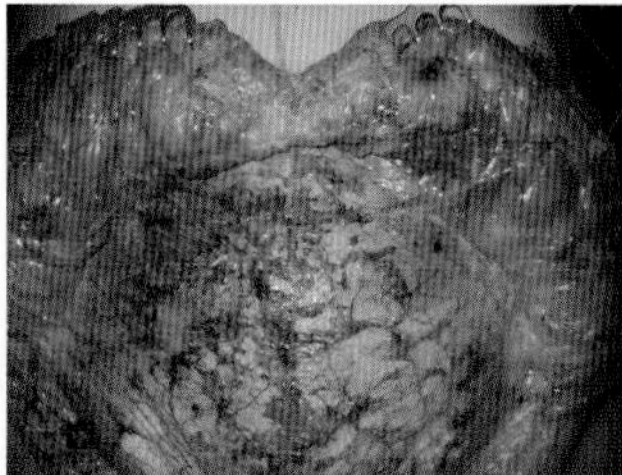
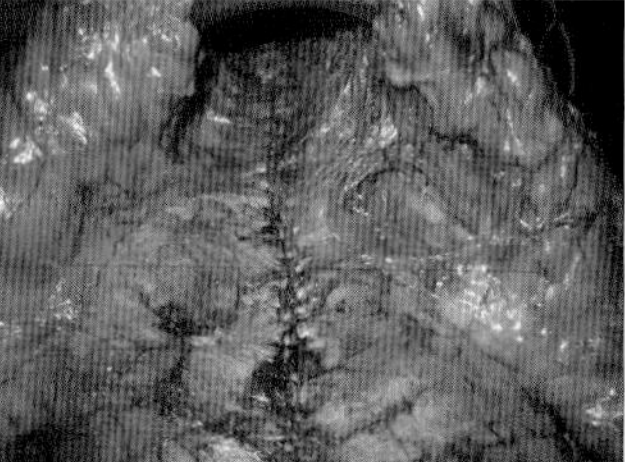
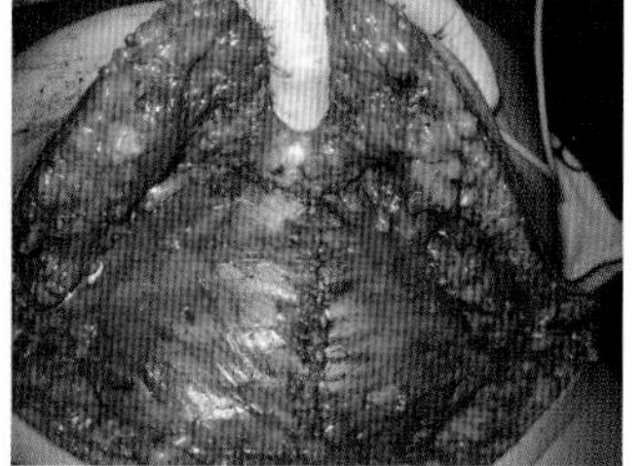

Figs 6.12–15 For patients with relatively thick subcutaneous tissue, a neoumbilicoplasty is suggested. This is a neoumbilicoplasty without scars. Figure 6.12 shows an umbilical hernia after complete resection of the umbilical scar. Figures 6.13 and 6.14: before and after supraumbilical tunnel dissection and abdominal wall plication. Figure 6.15: abdominal flap being defatted to expose the dermis that will be fixed to abdominal wall.

at the desired new location, and strongly suturing the undersurface of the dermis of the flap to the midline aponeurosis with five interrupted 3/0 nylon sutures (**Figs 6.12–6.15**). The final appearance is like a true umbilical depression, without any original scar or incision line (**Fig. 6.16**). This approach should only be used for patients with thick subcutaneous tissue, because in thin patients the umbilicus becomes flat.

The supraumbilical undermining is performed as a midline tunnel, releasing only 1.5 cm laterally to the medial border of the rectus abdominis muscle bilaterally to the level of the xiphoid. This limited undermining allows for moderate rectus plication and preservation of the perforators. The plication is performed in two layers with a running 2/0 nylon suture. In the lower abdomen inferior to the umbilicus, the plication continues with a two-layer running 2/0 nylon suture to the level of the symphysis pubis (**Figs 6.17–6.20**).

The patient is placed in the semi-Fowler's position and Baroudi quilting sutures are placed, securing the undersurface of the subcutaneous tissue of the tunnel to the abdominal fascia. These sutures are placed from the xiphoid to the umbilicus in the midline, thereby obliterating the tunnel (**Figs 6.21–6.23**).

Traction is then placed on the abdominal tissue and the umbilicus is positioned and secured. The distal excess of the flap is resected (**Fig. 6.24**). Additional quilting sutures are placed throughout the remaining area of undermining to the level of the incision (**Figs 6.25–6.27**). The final incision

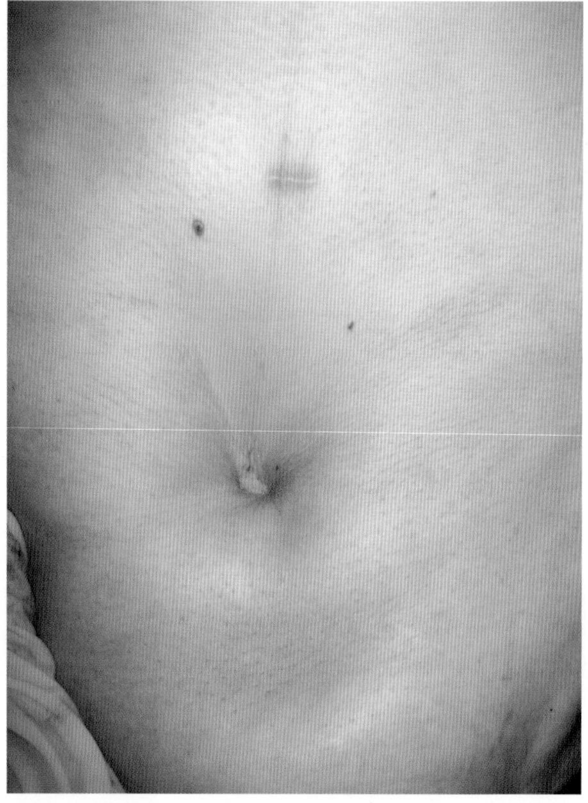

Fig. 6.16 Immediate neoumbilical result, with significant depression of the flap but no previous scar or wound to heal. The final appearance of the neoumbilicoplasty is demonstrated. This achieves a very natural shape with no scar.

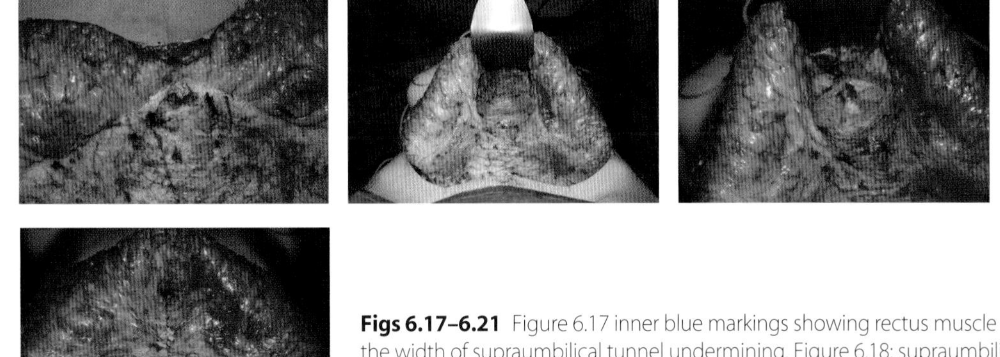

Figs 6.17–6.21 Figure 6.17 inner blue markings showing rectus muscle diastasis, outer markings illustrating the width of supraumbilical tunnel undermining. Figure 6.18: supraumbilical tunnel dissected. Figures 6.19–6.21: Myofascial plication is performed with 2/0 continuous running nylon suture in two separate layers. The plication begins at the xiphoid and runs continuously to the symphysis pubis. This plication results in a significant narrowing of the undermining tunnel.

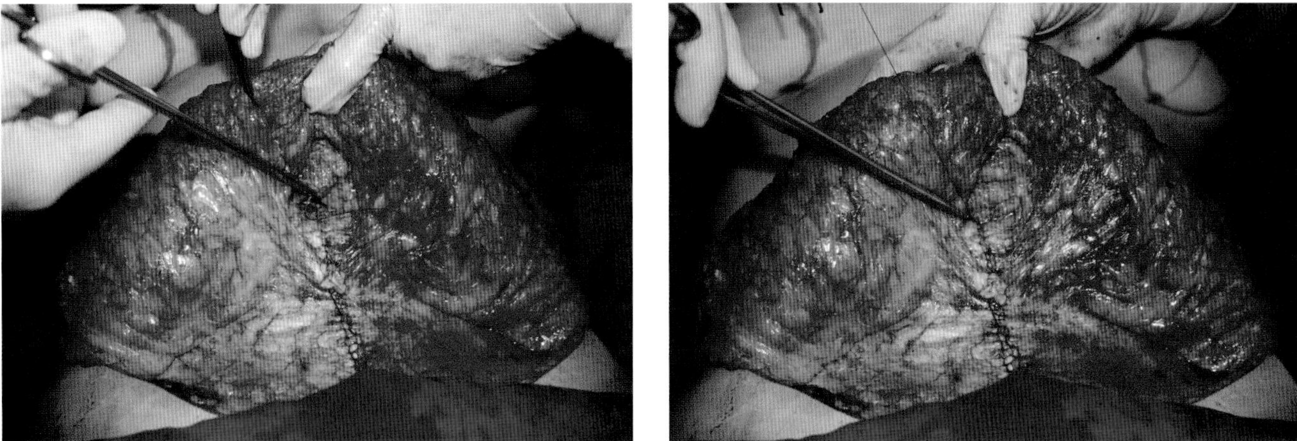

Figs 6.22 and 6.23 Baroudi quilting sutures are demonstrated: absorbable interrupted sutures from the subcutaneous of the flap to the abdominal fascia are performed from the xiphoid appendix down to the umbilicus. These sutures are used to obliterate the entire tunnel from the xiphoid to the umbilicus.

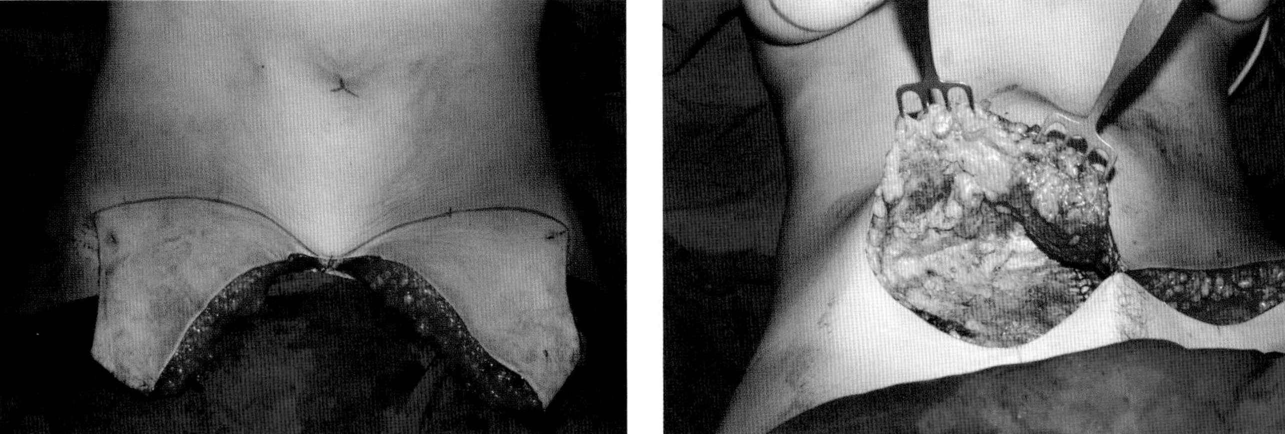

Figs 6.24 and 6.25 Distal excess of the flap is marked and resected, leaving minimal tension on the final incision line.

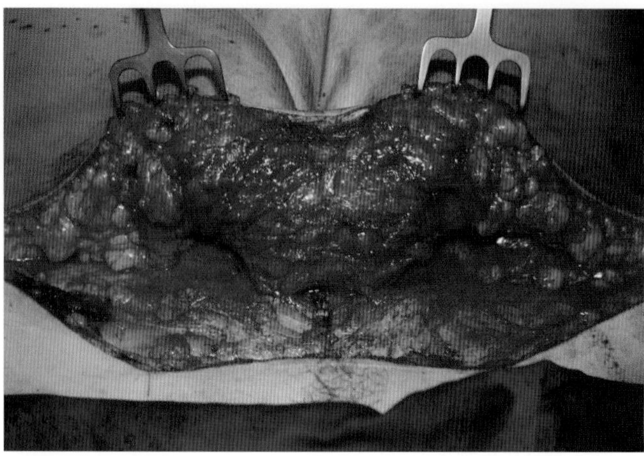

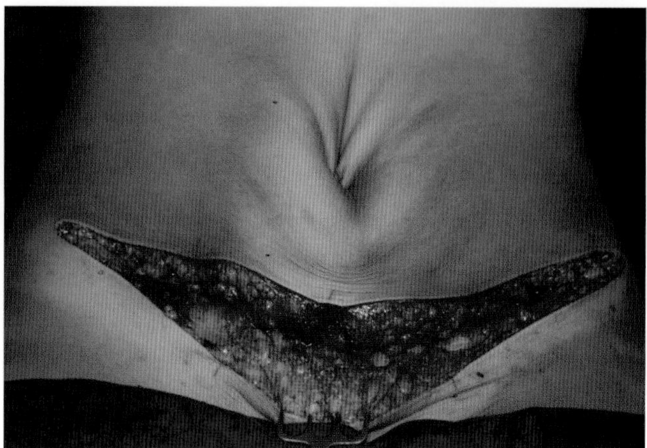

Figs 6.26 and 6.27 Additional Baroudi quilting sutures are then placed throughout the entire remaining area of undermining inferior to the umbilicus. This completely eliminates all dead space and fixes the skin, shifting the tissue flap down to the abdominal wall and eliminating the need for drain placement. The sutures also decreased tension on the final incision line.

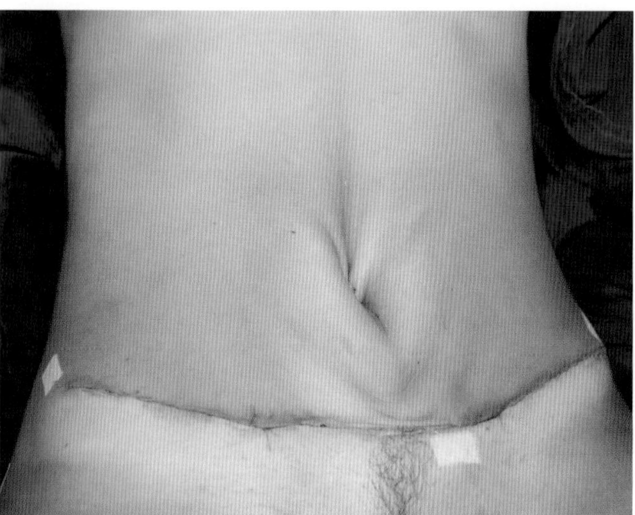

Fig. 6.28 Final appearance following lipoabdominoplasty.

is closed in layers with 3/0 and 4/0 absorbable sutures (**Fig. 6.28**). No drains are placed.

Postoperative Care

Patients stay overnight in our facility, where they can be cared for by nursing staff, and begin walking the next day. Our patients wear compressive stockings from 1 hour preoperatively until 1 week postoperatively. Patients are examined the evening following surgery and the next morning. Following discharge they are seen again in the surgical center between 5 and 7 days postoperatively. Patients are asked to maintain the flexed position at the waist for the first week to 10 days after surgery. An abdominal binder is placed following surgery – snugly not tightly – and released and readjusted every few hours to avoid a crease or fold. Diet is advanced as tolerated, and exercise is increased according to patient tolerance. For patients undergoing liposuction of more than 3 L, DVT prophylaxis is prescribed for 1 week postoperatively. Results following this procedure are pleasing. (**Figs 6.29 and 6.30**).

Conclusion

Lipoabdominoplasty can be performed in patients with significant abdominal skin laxity and fat deposition. Liposuction reduces subcutaneous thickness and releases or mobilizes the skin flap from musculoaponeurotic tissues without sacrificing large perforator vessels, allowing the flap to move inferiorly. We have performed Doppler flowmetry to identify and measure the perforator vessels and quantify blood flow to the flap. The findings have confirmed the preservation of perforator arteries greater than 1 mm in the periumbilical area. The caliber of the arteries was augmented by 9%, increasing the blood flow by more than 50% in the branches identified.

With lipoabdominoplasty, we have noticed a significant reduction in seroma, hematoma, and distal flap necrosis. For the last 2 years we have not used any drainage system for this procedure. This became feasible because of the reduced flap undermining and the use of Baroudi's quilting sutures, thereby reducing dead space. These sutures help to prevent seroma and also assist in flap fixation, maintaining the final scar in a lower position.

Final outcomes obtained with one-stage lipoabdominoplasty are similar to those seen after two-stage procedures (abdominoplasty and isolated liposuction), achieving good body contour and reducing the number of additional procedures. The technique of lipoabdominoplasty has provided excellent aesthetic outcomes with low morbidity. Good body contouring has been possible even in obese patients with this single and safe operation. The lower rate of complications is related to the reduced abdominal flap undermining and preservation of perforator vessels.

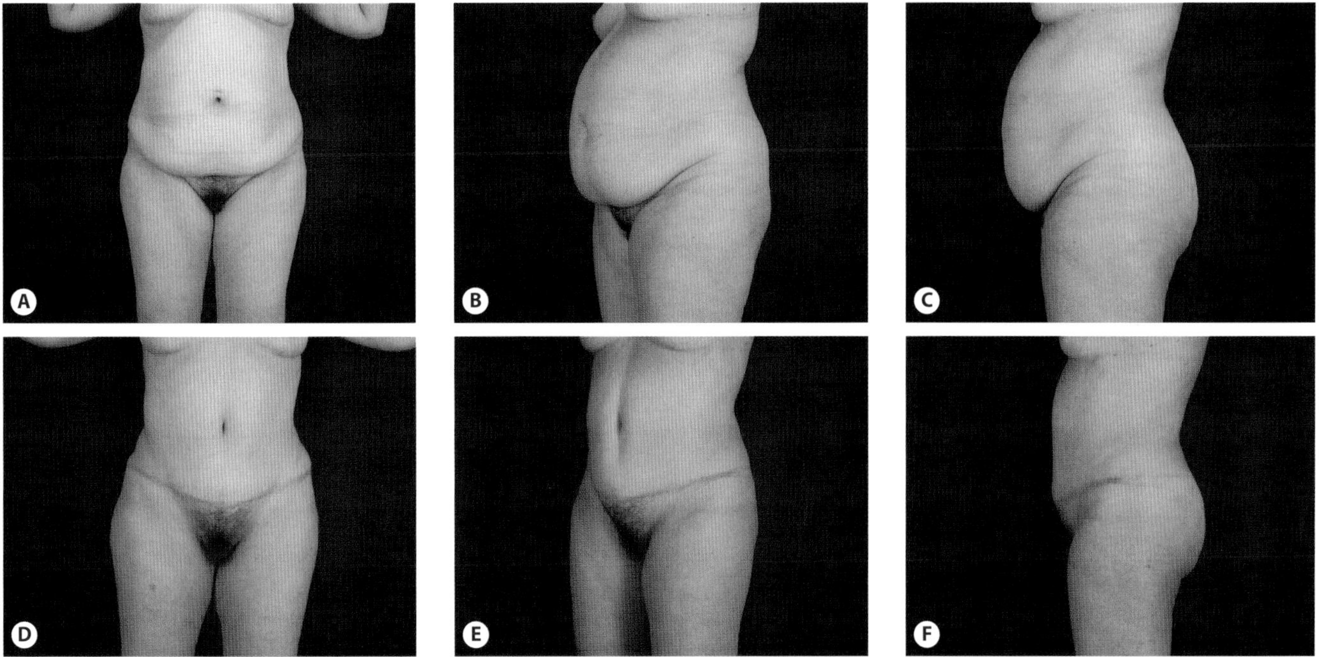

Fig. 6.29 A–F This 53-year-old woman underwent lipoabdominoplasty with 4250 mL infiltration, 4600 mL of liposuction aspirated, and 2160 g of skin and subcutaneous tissue resected. A no-scar neoumbilicoplasty was performed (the previous umbilical scar was completely resected). **A–C** Preoperative photos. **D–F** Postoperative photos at 8 months.

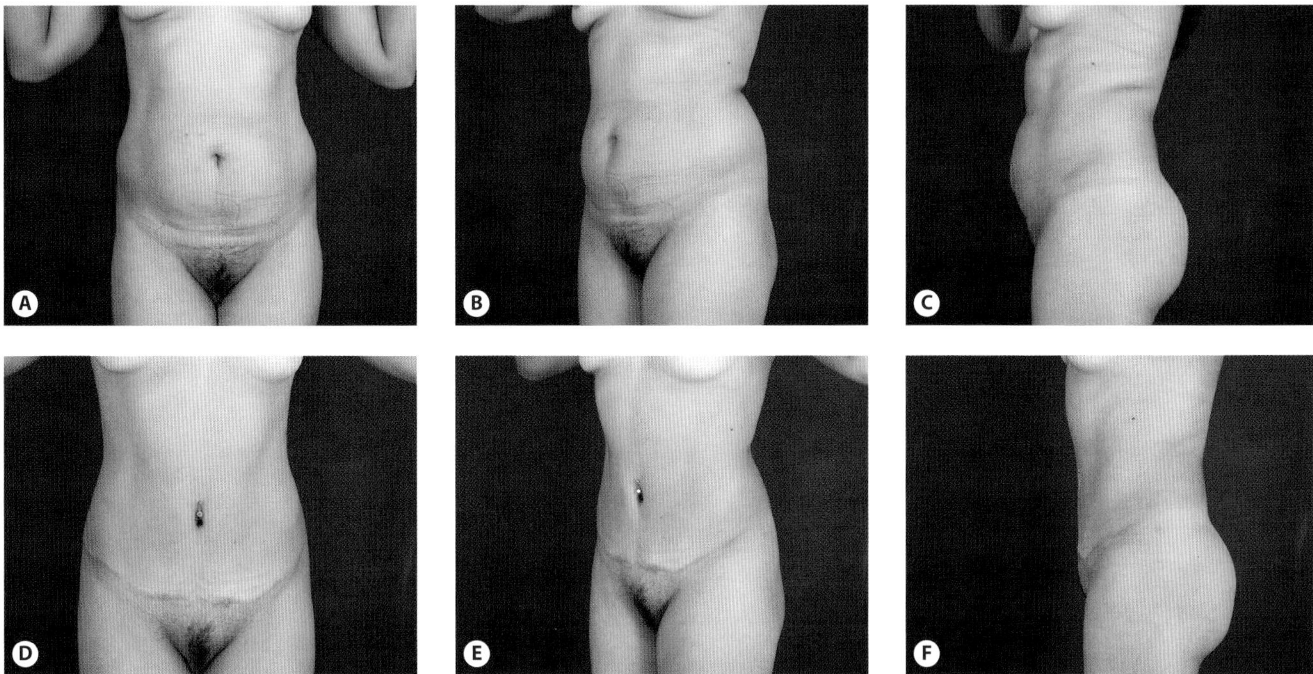

Fig. 6.30 A–F This 37-year-old woman underwent lipoabdominoplasty with 1200 mL infiltration, 1500 mL of liposuction aspirated, and 1240 g of skin and subcutaneous tissue resected. This umbilicoplasty technique maintained the original umbilical scar as an inferiorly based triangle, fixing it to the abdominal flap through an inverted Y incision. **A–C** Preoperative photos. **D, E** Postoperative photos at 2 years.

Clinical Caveats: Lipoabdominoplasty

- Candidates for lipobdominoplasty include most patients deemed appropriate for full abdominoplasty procedures
- Thorough abdominal liposuction is a key component to this procedure
- Reducing the undermining preserves many central abdominal perforating vessels, thereby maintaining skin viability. The undermining tunnel is limited yet sufficient to allow for moderate myofascial plication
- The use of extensive Baroudi quilting sutures eliminates dead space throughout the entire abdomen and plication tunnel, significantly reduces seroma formation, and has eliminated the need for drain placement
- For patients with relatively thick subcutaneous tissue a neoumbilicoplasty is preferable, and by removing the umbilicus, rectus plication is facilitated and continuous

References

1. American Society for Aesthetic Plastic Surgery 2004 Cosmetic Surgery National Data Bank. Available at www.surgery.org. Accessed May 2005.
2. Matarasso A, Swift RW, Rankin M. Abdominoplasty and abdominal contour surgery: a national plastic surgery survey. Plast Reconstruct Surg 2006; 117: 1797–1808.
3. Illouz YG. Une nouvelle technique pour les lipodystrophies localisées. Rev Chir Esthét Franç 1980; 6.
4. Matarasso A. Abdominoplasty: A system of classification and treatment for combined abdominoplasty and suction-assisted lipectomy. Aesthet Plast Surg 1991; 15: 111.
5. Matarasso A. Liposuction as an adjunct to full abdominoplasty. Plast Reconstruct Surg 1995; 95: 829–836.
6. Hunstad JP. Advanced abdominoplasty concepts. Perspect Plast Surg 1999; 12: 13–38.
7. Stevens WG, Cohen R, Vath S, et al. Does liposuction really add morbidity to abdominoplasty? Revisiting the controversy with a series of 406 cases. Aesthet Surg J 2005; 25: 353–358.
8. Saldanha OR, Souza Pinto EB, Matos WM, et al. Lipoabdominoplasty without undermining. Aesthet Surg J 2001; 21: 518–526.
9. Saldanha OR, Souza Pinto EB, Matos WM, et al. Lipoabdominoplasty with selective and safe undermining. Aesthet Plast Surg 2003; 27: 322–327.
10. Baroudi R, Ferreira CAA. Seroma: how to avoid it and how to treat it. Aesthet Surg J 1988; 18: 439.
11. Avelar JM. Abdominoplasty: A new technique without undermining and fat layer removal. Arq Catarin Med 2000; 29: 147–149.
12. Boyd JB, Taylor GI, Corlett RJ. The vascular territories of the superior epigastric and the deep inferior epigastric systems. Plast Reconstruct Surg 1984; 73: 1–14.
13. Baroudi RA. Bicycle handlebar type of incision for primary and secondary abdominoplasty. Aesthet Plast Surg 1995; 19: 307–320.

Suggested Reading

El-Mrakby HH, Milner RH. The vascular anatomy of the lower anterior abdominal wall: A micro dissection study on the deep inferior epigastric vessels and the perforator branches. Plast Reconstruct Surg 2002; 109: 539–547.

Fisher M, Bark A, Loureiro ALRS, et al. Doppler flowmetry in the flap of abdominoplasty. Arq Catarin Med 2003; 32: 173–178.

Grazer FM. Suction-assisted lipectomy, lipolysis, and hypexeresis. Plast Reconstruct Surg 1983; 72: 620–623.

Hakme F. Technical details in lipoaspiration associated with liposuction. Rev Bras Cir 1985; 75: 331–337.

Shestak KC. Marriage abdominoplasty expands the mini-abdominoplasty concept. Plast Reconstruct Surg 1999; 103: 1020–1031.

Taylor GI, Watterson PA, Zelt RG. The vascular anatomy of the anterior abdominal wall: The basis for flap design. Perspect Plast Surg 1991; 5: 1.

Willkinson TS, Swartz BE. Individual modifications in body contour surgery. The 'limited' abdominoplasty. Plast Reconstruct Surg 1986; 77: 779–784.

CHAPTER 7

Full Abdominoplasty

Joseph P. Hunstad & Remus Repta

IN THIS CHAPTER

KEY POINTS

The full abdominoplasty procedure is suitable for the majority of patients seeking abdominal contouring. This procedure addresses and corrects excess abdominal adiposity and soft-tissue laxity, rectus diastasis and abdominal wall laxity, and skin striae. A significant number of full abdominoplasty candidates present after having had children as well as after failed attempts at weight loss. Patients often have the desired goal of returning to their pre-pregnancy or pre-weight gain abdominal contour.

Introduction

The full or complete abdominoplasty is the most commonly performed method of abdominoplasty.[1] This is because the majority of abdominal contouring patients present with a combination of excess adiposity, significant soft-tissue laxity, diastasis recti, and abdominal striae. This procedure offers the most significant correction for these problems in the majority of cases. A full or complete abdominoplasty incision usually extends across the abdomen laterally to a point corresponding to each anterior superior iliac spine. This length is necessary to achieve the best results by facilitating complete removal of the infraumbilical skin and soft-tissue laxity that bothers these patients. Undermining the abdominal soft-tissue apron to the xiphoid process allows for correction of rectus diastasis and strengthening of the myofascial components of the abdominal wall. This procedure can offer a lifetime improvement, particularly for patients who maintains their weight following the procedure.

This chapter will emphasize a number of technical points that can enhance the final result, including the concurrent use of tumescent liposuction, subscarpal fat resection, and wide rectus abdominis muscle plication techniques.

Patient Selection (Box 7.1)

The majority of patients presenting for abdominal body contouring are candidates for full abdominoplasty. They are usually good candidates if they are not significantly overweight and do not present with prohibitory health issues. Healthy patients with infraumbilical striae, moderate excess adiposity, skin and

Box 7.1 Relative contraindications for full abdominoplasty

- Smoking
- Diabetes mellitus
- Malnutrition
- Various wound-healing disorders
- Bowel/bladder dysfunction
- Immunodeficiency
- Medications that inhibit blood coagulation
- A significant history of pulmonary or deep vein thrombosis
- Lower extremity lymphedema/venous insufficiency
- Significant medical problems, including COPD/pulmonary issues, renal insufficiency, anemia, and other systemic issues that may make and abdominal tightening surgery dangerous

Note: Age alone should not be a contraindication to abdominoplasty procedures if the patient is in good health. Patients who have a history of chronic pain should also be approached cautiously, as postoperative care may be significantly affected.

soft-tissue laxity, and rectus diastasis or myofascial laxity are ideal candidates for full abdominoplasty. Patients who are significantly overweight, with a BMI >30–35, may also be candidates, but would benefit from better preoperative weight management.[2,3] Patients more than 100lb over ideal body weight, referral for bariatric surgery should be considered.

Diabetes is a significant relative contraindication to this procedure, but with careful planning, limited liposuction, and attention to detail, a safe and successful result can be achieved.[4–6] Patients with respiratory difficulties are potentially also of increased concern, because myofascial plication results in a transient increase in intra-abdominal pressure which may be a source of postoperative respiratory difficulties. For these patients, muscle plication could be deferred and a more conservative approach to soft-tissue resection may also be considered.

Smoking is of great concern for all abdominoplasty procedures, particularly when thorough concurrent tumescent liposuction, subscarpal fat resection, and strong muscle plication is being considered. Active smokers are at increased risk of ischemia and necrosis, particularly midline in the infraumbilical area above the transverse incision.[5,7] Also at risk is the remaining subcutaneous fat, which can undergo necrosis due to vasoconstriction-induced ischemia secondary to smoking. In our practice, we suggest complete smoking cessation for 6 weeks preoperatively for patients wishing to undergo the complete full abdominoplasty. This will allow the patient's physiology to return to a more normal level and hopefully eliminate many of the deleterious effects on healing that smoking creates. The changes associated with long-term chronic smoking can be improved but may not be completely corrected, and we stress that there is always some continued increased risk for patients with a history of smoking.

Possible future pregnancy should be discussed with the patient and, if this is anticipated, it is suggested that abdominoplasty be performed following the last pregnancy.[8] Bowel or bladder dysfunction should be considered a relative contraindication to myofascial plication, as this could worsen the patient's preoperative condition.

Preoperative History and Considerations: (Box 7.2)

Abdominal scars from previous operations should be carefully examined and discussed with the patient (see Chapter 14, Management of Pre-existing Abdominal Scars). A right subcostal cholecystectomy scar should be treated with great care, because undermining to the level of the scar can result in ischemia and/or necrosis of the residual tissue medially, from the cholecystectomy scar to the midline. It is important to explain to the patient that limited dissection is necessary to preserve perforating vessels to the tissue medial to the subcostal scar. Because of this, the amount of undermining will be reduced and the final tension on the incision will also be less, so as to minimize the risk of ischemia and/or necrosis. This may result in some residual laxity at the end of the procedure. It is easy for the patient to accept this when a proper explanation has been given preoperatively, but very difficult if the explanation and discussion take place postoperatively.

Box 7.2 Preoperative, recommedations for full abdominoplasty

- Smoking cessation/avoidance of nicotine exposure for 4–6 weeks prior to surgery
- Multivitamin daily
- Stop aspirin/other blood thinning products with primary care doctor's permission
- Abstain from all dietary/herbal supplements not approved by the surgeon
- Basic laboratory tests should be tailored to each patient and may include CBC, Chem 7, Factor V Leiden, and PT/PTT/INR
- Medical clearance if needed
- Wearing abdominal binder for 2 weeks before surgery
- Shower with a gentle antimicrobial soap the night before and day of surgery

A vertical midline incision is not a contraindication to surgery and can often be improved with scar revision. Importantly, if transverse laxity exists, additional tissue transversely can be removed, further enhancing the procedure with no increased risk for ischemia. This allows for transverse tightening during abdominoplasty, in addition to the vertical tightening associated with lower abdominal soft-tissue excision. The vertical tissue excision also allows for removal of some of the most poorly perfused tissue in the midline following undermining. If significant transverse laxity exists it is possible to remove a large amount of central abdominal tissue, which can minimize or virtually eliminate areas for potential fat necrosis or ischemia.

Appendectomy or laparoscopy incisions are usually of minimal concern. The appendectomy scar is often included in the tissue resection. Laparoscopic surgery scars are usually short and do not interfere with undermining, but they can be associated with an unrecognized hernia discovered intraoperatively (see Chapter 15, Complications). This should be taken into account during liposuction and with soft-tissue elevation. All scars, particularly a vertical midline scar, can be associated with an incisional hernia. The most common location for an incisional hernia is in the midline, particularly in patients following massive weight loss. Hernias not associated with an incision are most commonly seen in

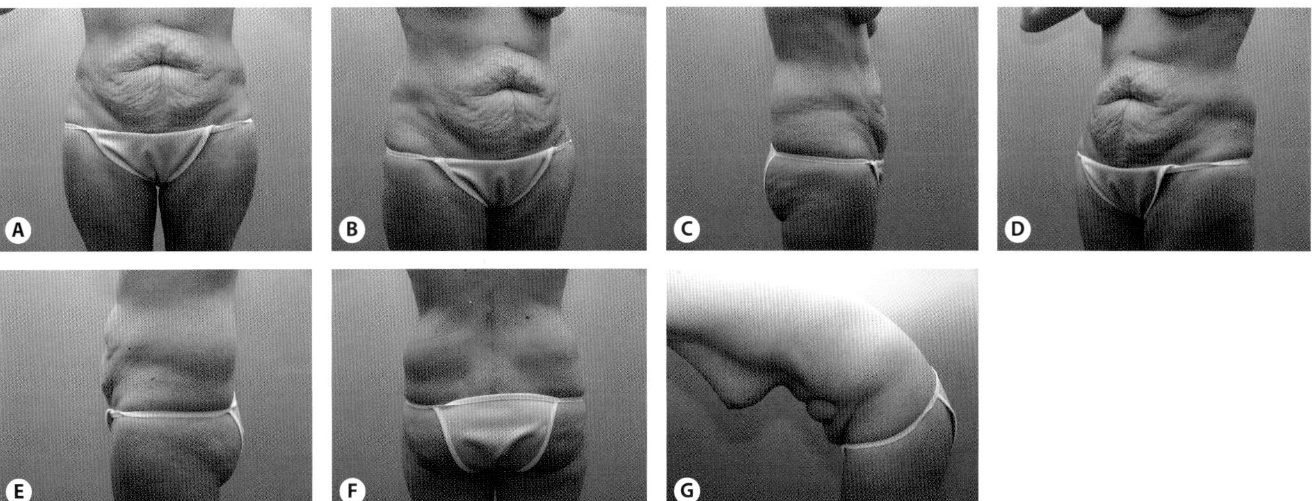

Fig. 7.1 (**A–G**) Abdominal contouring photos are usually taken in nine cardinal views. The patient should be relaxed to eliminate tightening of the abdomen and rectus muscles and permit accurate evaluation of contour and shape. All photographs should include the area from the inframammary folds to the mid-thigh, because some thigh elevation will occur with this procedure (**A**). (**B** and **D**) Left and right oblique views demonstrating the waist, extent of abdominal laxity, and the anterior thighs and hips. (**C** and **E**) Left and right lateral views, which further demonstrate abdominal contour. The posterior view (**F**) is helpful in evaluating the buttocks and hip rolls. (**G**) The 'diver' view, which shows the extent of abdominal laxity. A left and right posterior oblique view complete the nine cardinal views (not pictured).

the periumbilical region and should be evaluated for during the preoperative examination. These hernias are easy to deal with intraoperatively, but should be kept in mind during liposuction and soft-tissue elevation.

Preoperative laboratory analysis is dependent on the facility where the procedure is to be performed, surgeon and anesthesiologist preference, and existing health issues. For an otherwise healthy patient, basic preoperative laboratory analysis should be considered and may include a pregnancy test, complete blood count (CBC), basic metabolic panel (BMP/Chem7), and standard coagulation profiles (PT/PTT/INR).

Prophylaxis for pulmonary embolism (PE) and deep vein thrombosis (DVT) is an important consideration. Patients taking birth control medications or hormone replacement therapy are at an increased risk for DVT and PE, and this should be discussed preoperatively.[9,10] Discontinuing such medications for 2 weeks preoperatively will reduce the associated risks to a normal level. In some cases, however, it may not feasible to stop these medications and the patient needs to be informed of the increased risk of DVT/PE. A personal or family history of DVT or PE is of even greater concern. If there is such a history, preoperative laboratory analysis to evaluate the patient's coagulation profile including a factor V Leiden and to search for possible familial tendencies for hypercoagulability is recommended. A hematology consultation should be considered to evaluate for this.

The abdominal wall plication performed with full abdominoplasty can result in increased intra-abdominal pressure and potential interference with venous return and pulmonary ventilation volumes. Because of this, we recommend placing all abdominoplasty patients in a tight abdominal binder for 2 weeks preoperatively. We ask them to wear the binder both day and night, which may help them accommodate to the increased intra-abdominal pressure changes associated with myofascial plication,[11,12] and have documented a consistent reduction in abdominal circumference at the level of the anterior superior iliac crest, umbilicus, and xiphoid in patients who consistently wore the binder.

Operative Approach

Preoperative photographs are taken in nine cardinal views (**Fig. 7.1 A–G**) anterior, posterior, left and right oblique, left and right lateral, and left and right posterior oblique, and diver's view. These last two views are more appropriate if posterior or posterolateral work is done, such as when concurrent liposuction is performed. These views are important because the reduction of the fullness at the waistline is often most evident from a posterior or posterolateral view.

Markings are made with the patient standing. We ask the patient to place their hands together and strongly lift the lower abdominal skin vertically (**Fig. 7.2 A**). The central portion of the initial transverse incision is then marked at the superior level of the pubic symphysis. This normally removes the upper third of the hair-bearing mons (**Fig. 7.2 B**). This mark is continued laterally, following a natural skin fold (**Fig. 7.2 C**). The length and location of this

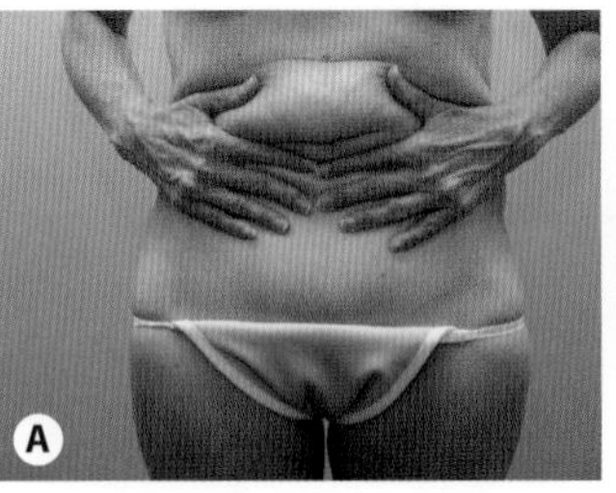
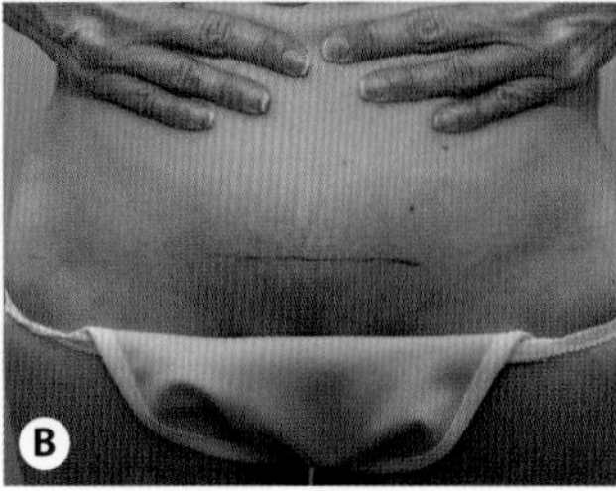
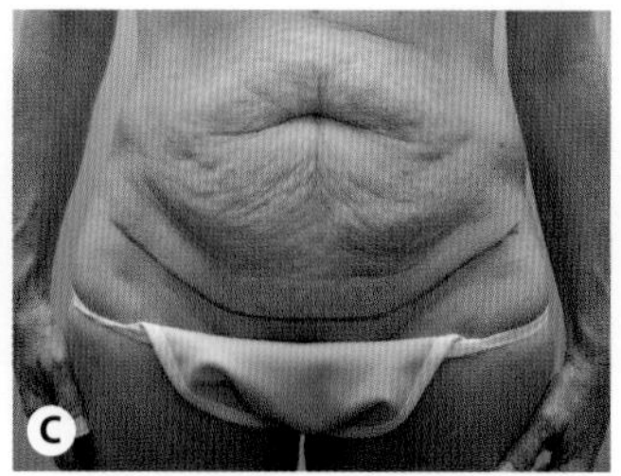
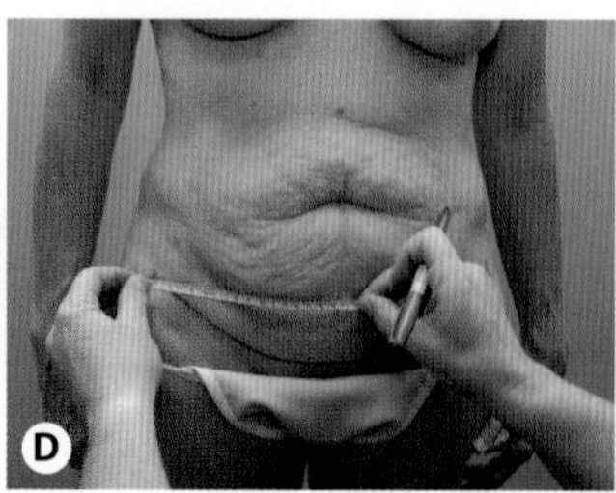

Fig. 7.2 (**A–D**) With the patient strongly lifting the abdominal soft tissue in a smooth even manner, the lower transverse midline incision is marked (A). This mark is placed approximately at the level of or slightly superior to the symphysis pubis, which corresponds to the junction of the upper and middle thirds of the hair-bearing mons (**B**). The mark is then extended laterally in a natural skin fold to be placed at a level the surgeon and patient have agreed on (**C**). The lateral height and length of the incision are measured to ensure symmetry (**D**).

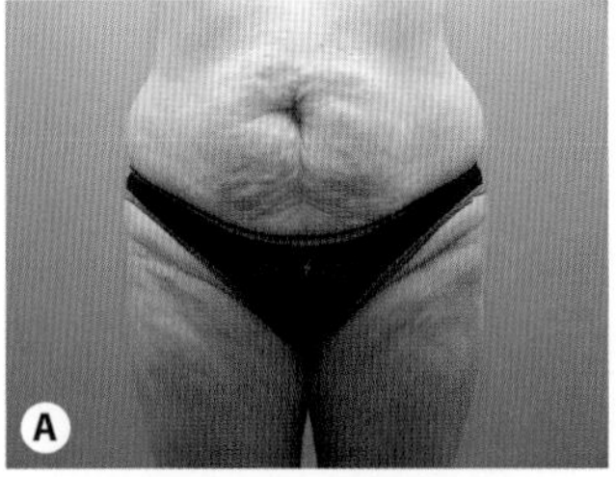
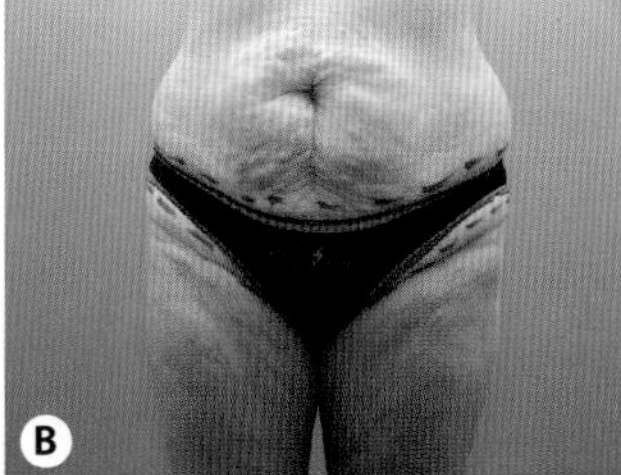
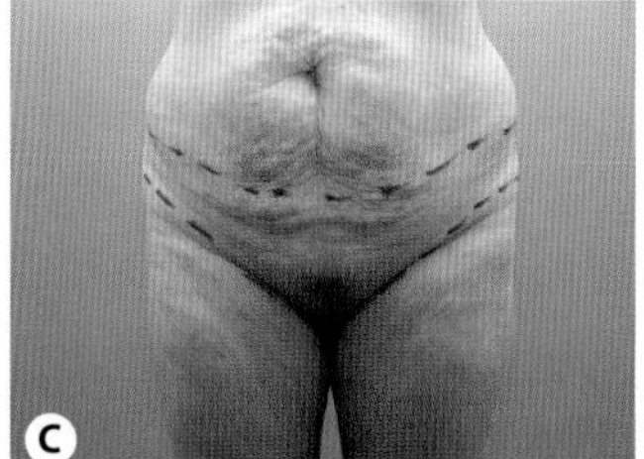
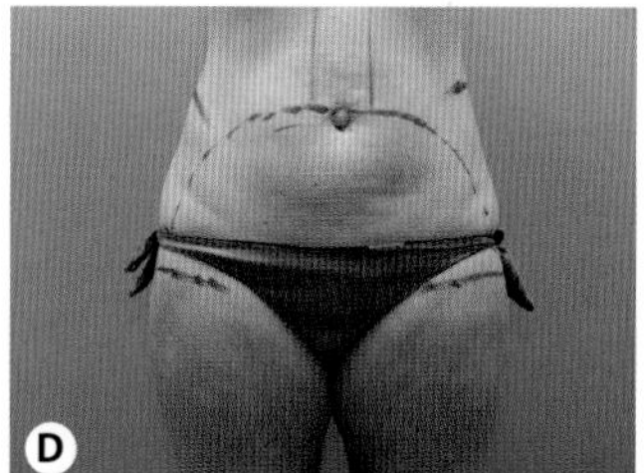
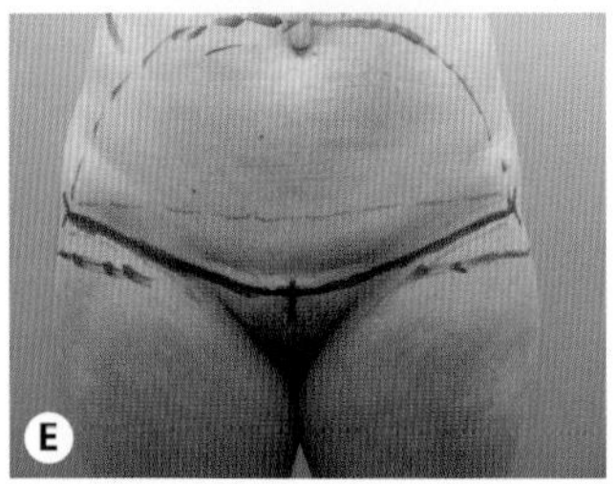

Fig. 7.3 (**A–E**) The patient is often asked to bring in revealing swimwear or lingerie beneath which they would like the abdominoplasty scar to be placed (**Fig. 7.3 A–D**). An outline of the garment is made, allowing the incision to be placed within its borders (**Fig. 7.3 B, C, E**).

proposed incision is then measured to ensure symmetry (**Fig. 7.2 D**).

It is often helpful to ask the patient to bring in their most revealing swimwear or lingerie. This will allow the incision to be placed and concealed within the borders of the garment (**Fig. 7.3 A–E**). The lateral extent of the incision is marked and agreed upon by the patient. This avoids any postoperative concerns about the location and length of the incision.

If the patient has a 'long' waist, if they have only modest abdominal soft-tissue laxity, or if they have previously undergone an abdominoplasty and present for revision, the umbilical defect may not be incorporated within the resection segment and an inverted T closure may be necessary. The lower the initial transverse incision, the more likely an inverted T closure will be needed because of the longer vertical distance to the umbilicus. For patients with greater skin and soft-tissue laxity, the full abdominoplasty incision can be extended to go posterior to the anterior axillary line to address this without creating lateral dog-ears. Doing so results in a technique more appropriately referred to as an extended abdominoplasty (see Chapter 8, Extended Abdominoplasty).

After the lower incision is marked, the proposed upper incision is drawn which estimates the amount of tissue to be resected (**Fig. 7.4 A**). The true extent of tissue resection will be determined intraoperatively. All areas for liposuction are marked at this time. This includes the entire central abdomen, lateral axilla and flanks, hip rolls, and mons (**Fig. 7.4 A–D**).

The patient is brought to the operating room after preoperative markings and photographs are completed. They are placed in the supine position and compression stockings are placed (**Fig. 7.5 A**). The patient is covered with warm blankets to prevent heat loss, and an intravenous line is established (**Fig. 7.5 B**). A warming blanket is used intraoperatively to maintain optimal body temperature (**Fig. 7.5 C**). General anesthesia is administered without the use of nitrous oxide to reduce the risk of intra-abdominal distension. Intravenous antibiotics (Ancef 1 g) and steroids (Decadron 4 mg) are routinely administered unless contraindicated by the patient's medical history.

To minimize bleeding, all incision lines are injected with a solution of lidocaine and epinephrine (**Fig. 7.6 A**). The regions to be liposuctioned are then infiltrated with tumescent solution (**Fig. 7.6 B–E**). Normally the central

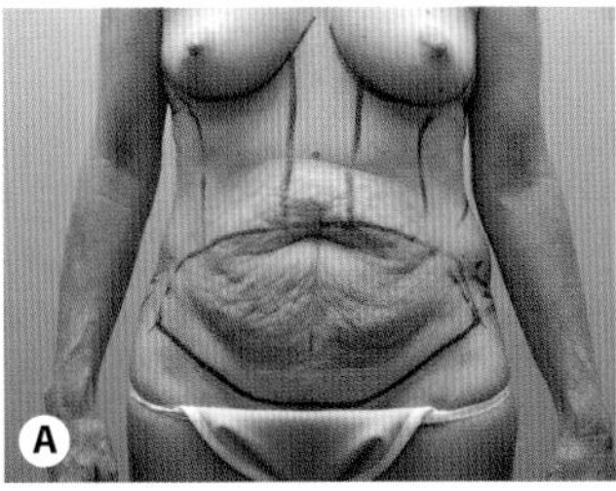
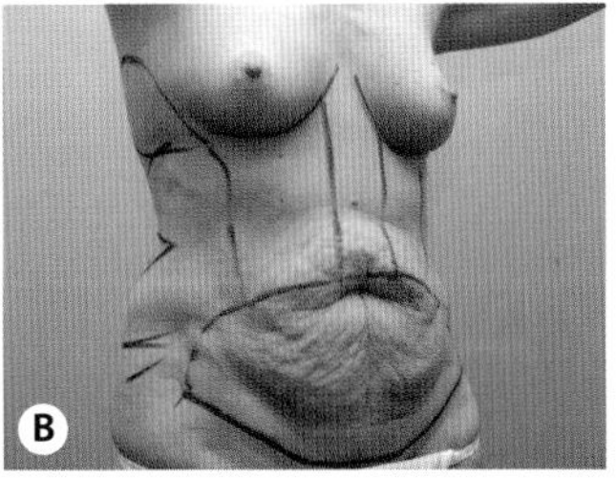
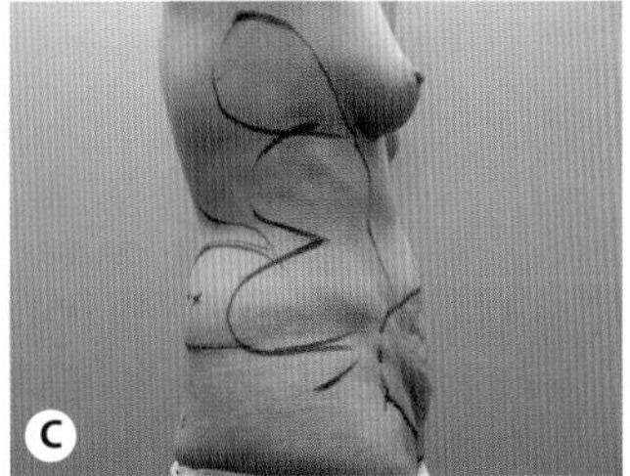
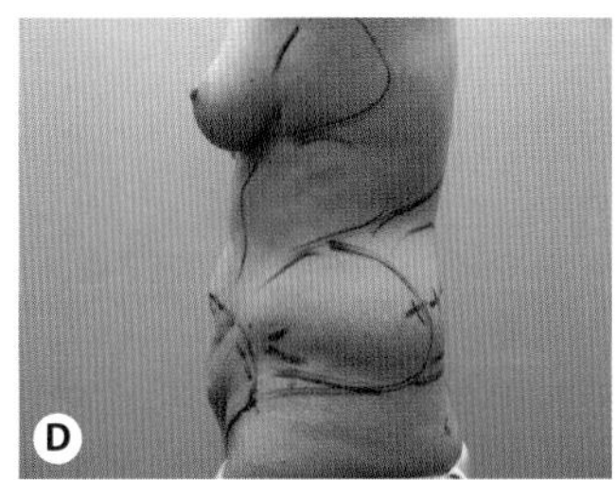

Fig. 7.4 (**A–D**) At this time, the required abdominoplasty marks have been completed. The lower transverse incision has been marked, extending approximately from the left to the right anterosuperior iliac crest. The upper line, which serves as an estimate of the amount of tissue to be resected, is then drawn with the lateral aspects curving strongly cephalad. This is important because significant tissue will be removed laterally, increasing the tension at closure in the lateral portion of the incision and enhancing the shape of the waist (**A, B**). The midline upper abdomen, lateral breast, flanks, and hip rolls are also marked for liposuction, which will be performed concurrently (**A–D**).

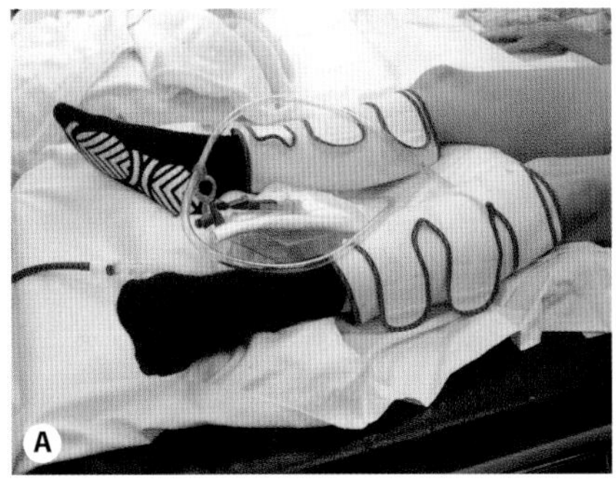
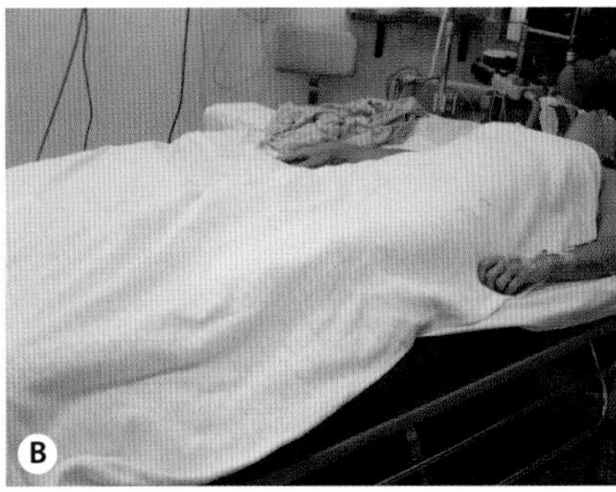
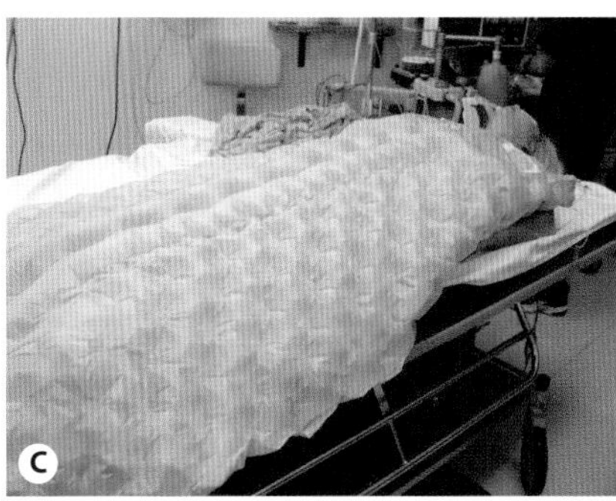

Fig. 7.5 (**A–C**) Sequential compression devices are placed on the patient's legs prior to the induction of anesthesia (**A**). Warm blankets are used to cover the patient immediately upon entering the operating room, and then a forced warmed air heating blanket is utilized to maintain optimum core body temperature (**B, C**).

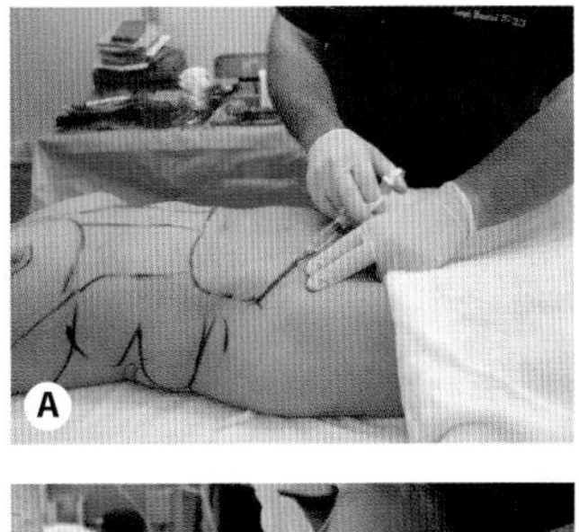
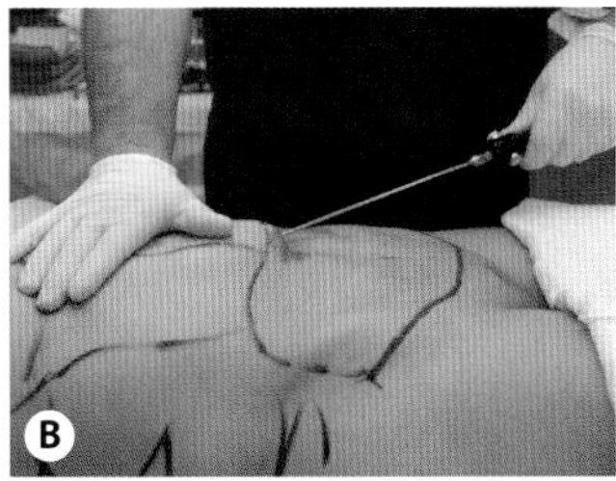
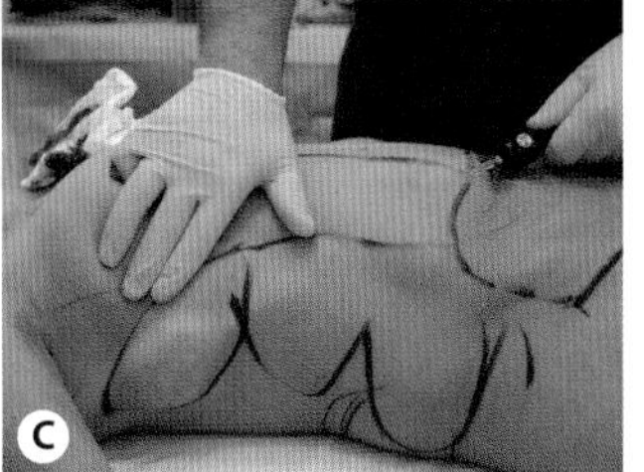
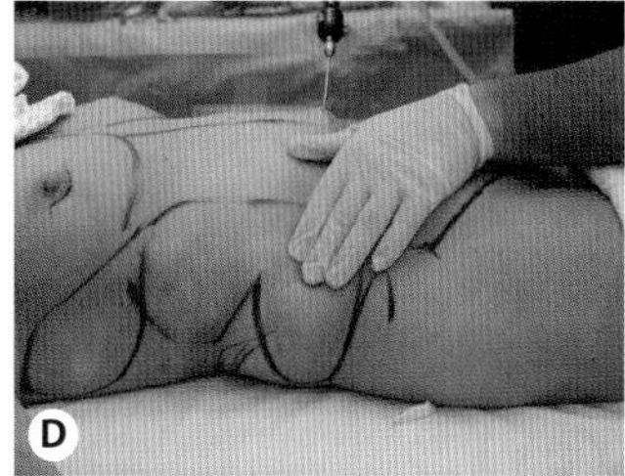
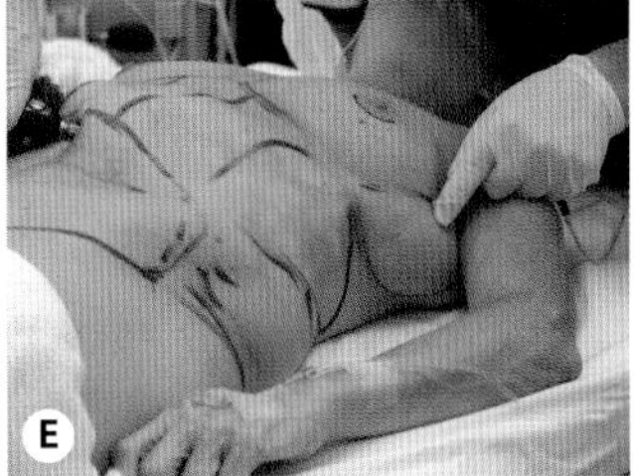
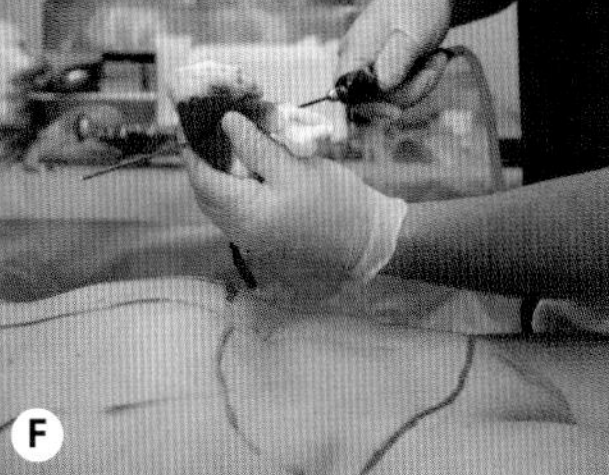

Fig. 7.6 (**A–F**) The lower transverse incision line is injected with dilute lidocaine and epinephrine (**A**). Several entry sites, including the superior portion of the umbilicus, are used to perform tumescent infiltration (**B, C**). The entire midline, upper abdomen, lateral breast, flanks, and hip rolls are infiltrated using the umbilical entry site (**C–E**). The cannula is frequently cleansed with Betadine solution when it is withdrawn and a new entry site is used (**F**). An infiltration entry site is also made within the abdominal skin to be excised to further treat the hip rolls and mons.

abdomen, upper abdomen, lateral abdomen, flanks, hip rolls, and mons are infiltrated. The loose areolar plane between the abdominal wall and the subcutaneous tissue is also infiltrated to facilitate rapid dissection during tissue elevation.

For a full or complete abdominoplasty, it is standard practice to infiltrate between 4 and 6 L of fluid, as this facilitates complete exsanguination of the tissue to be suctioned. Vessel compression and tissue exsanguination prevent stagnation of blood in the abdominoplasty flap. Blood stagnation may result in the formation of vascular microthrombi and the release of inflammatory mediators detrimental to flap viability.

This infiltration thoroughly hydrates the tissue, allows cannulas to be passed with minimal trauma, and compresses

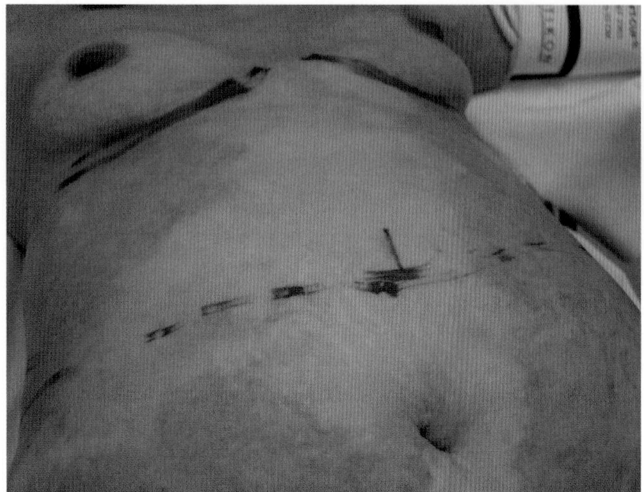

Fig. 7.7 The infiltration is performed prior to prepping and draping, which allows an ideal waiting time of approximately 20 minutes to ensure proper vasoconstriction before performing liposuction.

the vessels, rendering them a smaller target for trauma and thus protecting them. It is important to calculate the total dose of lidocaine and modify the volume of tumescent fluid as needed, prior to infiltration. Large-volume infiltration requires more dilute lidocaine concentration (see Chapter 3, Liposuction in Abdominal Contouring).

Infiltration is performed before full prepping and draping both for efficient use of time as well as to allow sufficient time for vasoconstruction to tale effect. Entry sites are prepared with Betadine and the cannula is frequently wiped with Betadine during the infiltration process (**Fig. 7.6 F**). Fluid is infiltrated until tissue turgor is achieved. Following infiltration, the patient is prepared and draped. This allows sufficient time for the epinephrine in the tumescent fluid to achieve the maximum vasoconstrictive effect (**Fig. 7.7**). The interval between infiltration and liposuction is approximately 20 minutes, which is ideal for achieving excellent vasoconstriction.

Liposuction is performed on all infiltrated areas. Suctioning of the lateral axilla and fullness above the breast is best performed through an axillary entry site (**Fig. 7.8 A, B**). Occasionally an inframammary entry site is used, which provides efficient access to the lateral breast, flank, and upper abdomen (**Fig. 7.8 C**). The umbilical entry site is ideal for access to the central abdomen (**Fig. 7.8 D, E**). In the area of proposed undermining, liposuction is performed on the fat superficial to Scarpa's fascia, because subscarpal fat resection will be performed which will remove the fat deep to Scarpa's fascia throughout the entire area.

Additional entry sites within the marked tissue to be excised can used to treat the flanks, hip rolls, and mons (**Fig. 7.8 E, F**). All liposuction is performed on the areas

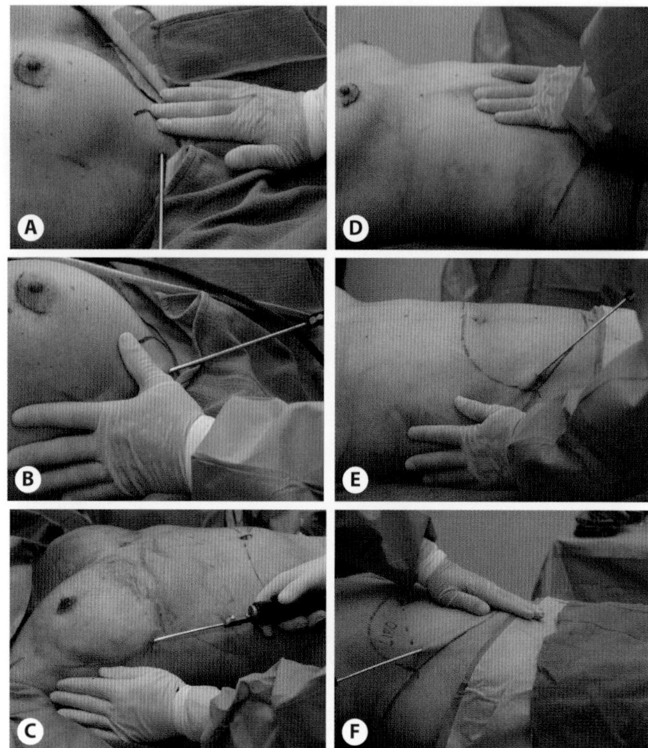

Fig. 7.8 (**A–F**) Liposuction is performed through the entry sites utilized for tumescent infiltration. An entry site in the axilla will allow access to the lateral breast, flank, and upper abdomen (**A, B**). The inframammary entry site can also be used to treat the upper abdomen, lateral breast, and flanks (**C**). Through the umbilical entry site (**D**) the entire midline is suctioned to create a sulcus and enhanced definition of the upper abdomen. The upper abdomen to the level of the inframammary crease is also liposuctioned superficially because all tissue within the undermined area, which often extends to the costal margin, will be treated with subscarpal fat resection (**D**). The hip rolls and mons are thoroughly suctioned using an entry site within the area of tissue to be resected (**E, F**).

outside the central abdominal region where subscarpal fat resection will be performed.

The low transverse incision, previously marked, is made with a number 10 blade into, but not entirely through the dermis (**Fig. 7.9 A**). Electrocautery is then used to complete the incision, sealing the blood vessels within the subdermal plexus (**Fig. 7.9 B**). Electrocautery is also used to deepen the incision through the superficial fascia to reach the deep subcutaneous tissue. The superficial inferior epigastric vessels are identified and controlled (**Fig. 7.9 C, D**). This is important, because these vessels can bleed postoperatively and lead to a hematoma (see Chapter 15, Complications).

A scalpel or electrocautery is used to perform soft-tissue dissection superiorly to the level of the umbilicus. The dissection is beveled through the deep fat to reach the abdominal wall at a point midway between the symphysis and the umbilicus. This is done to improve the final contour and to

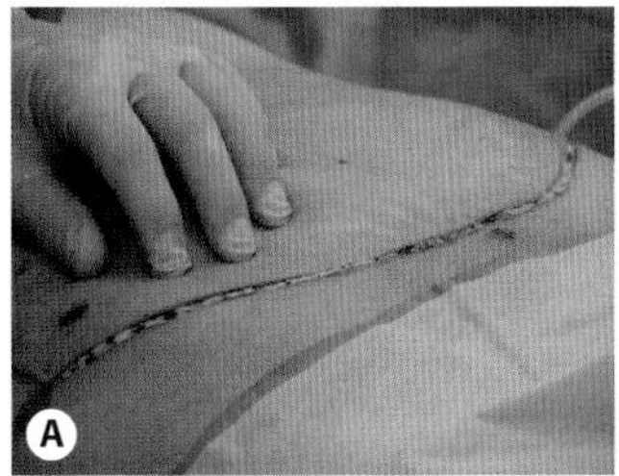

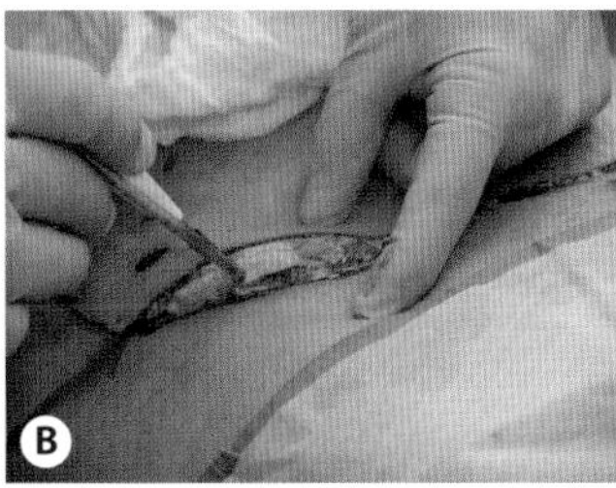

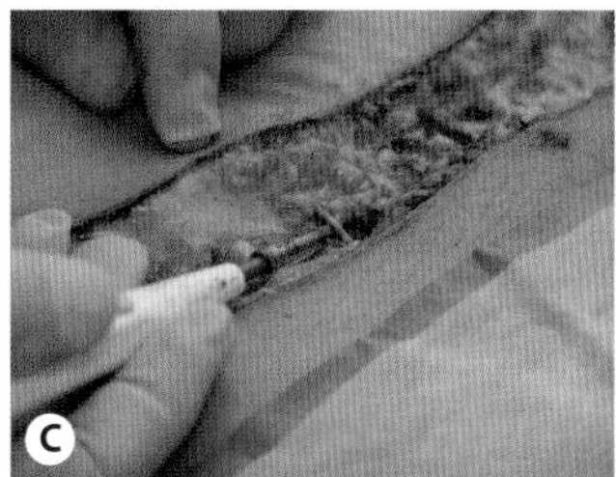

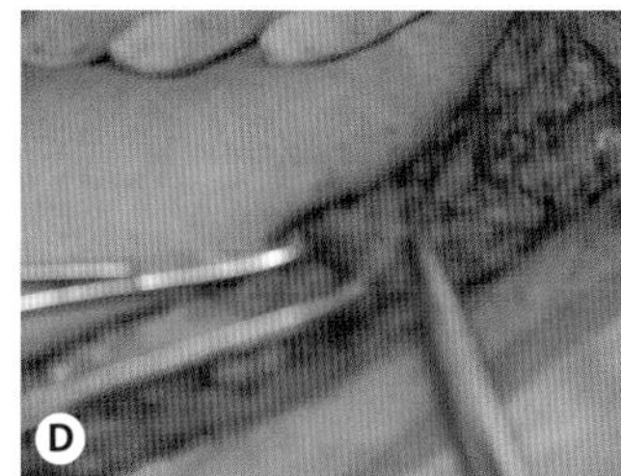

Fig. 7.9 (**A–D**) After liposuction is complete, an incision is made sharply into but not through the dermis of the lower mark (**A**). Electrocautery is then used to deepen the incision through the dermis, controlling the vessels of the subdermal plexus. This allows controlled hemostasis, essentially eliminating incisional bleeding. The superficial inferior epigastric vessels are often easily visualized because of the hydrated nature of the tissue secondary to tumescent infiltration (**C**). These vessels need to be individually controlled, cauterized, or ligated to prevent bleeding, which can result in a postoperative hematoma (**D**).

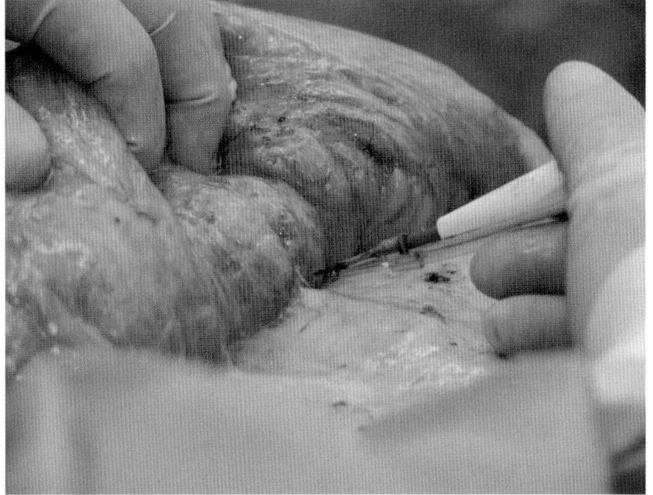

Fig. 7.10 Once the low transverse incision has been made, dissection is performed either sharply or with electrocautery beveling through the deap fat to reach the abdominal wall midway between the symphysis and the umbilicus. Dissection continues to the umbilicus preserving the loose areolar tissue superfical to the abdominal wall. The lower abdominal tissue from the incision line to the umbilicus.

Fig. 7.11 Perforators are identified and controlled. These are particularly prominent and numerous in the periumbilical region.

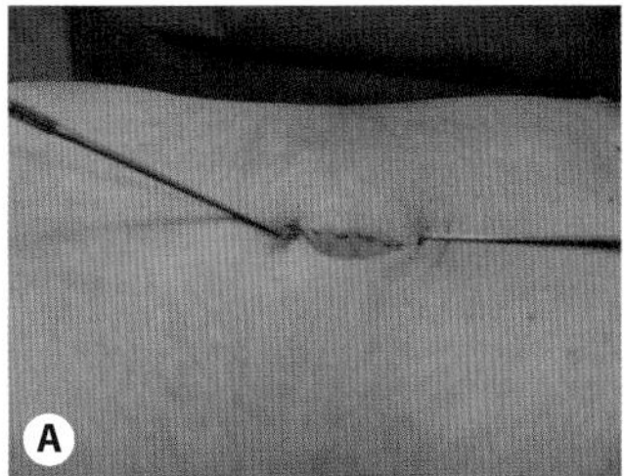

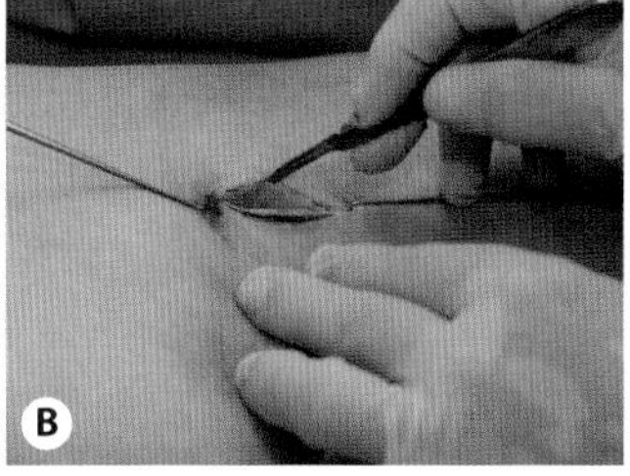

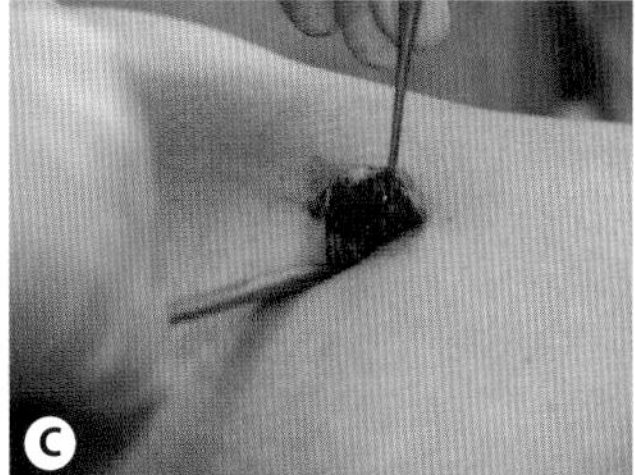

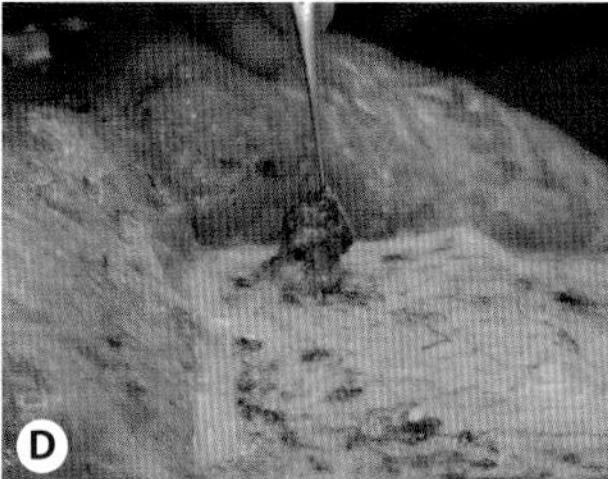

Fig. 7.12 (**A–D**) Once the level of umbilicus is reached, it needs to be carefully released as an important step in creating an aesthetically pleasing result. Two skin hooks are placed at the 12 o'clock and 6 o'clock positions (**A**). A number 11 blade is used in a pushing fashion to incise the umbilicus in a vertical ellipse shape as previously marked (**B**). Metzenbaum scissors are used to carefully dissect the umbilical stalk, leaving attached a small amount of subcutaneous tissue to ensure viability (**C**). Following midline division of the abdominal flap, the umbilical stalk dissection is completed (**D**).

preserve lymphatics which lessens serona formation. (**Fig. 7.10**). Once the level of the umbilicus is reached significant periumbilical perforators are identified and controlled (**Fig. 7.11**). These vessels are the second most likely source for postoperative hematoma and should be properly controlled with either electrocautery or suture ligature. Throughout the course of the dissection, meticulous hemostasis should be maintained to minimize intraoperative blood loss.

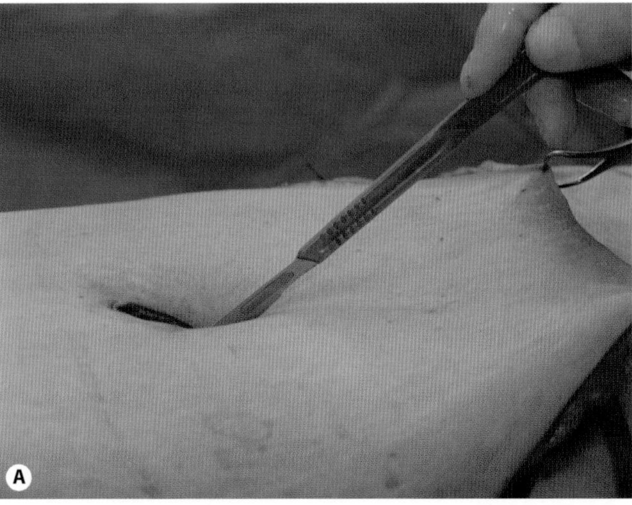

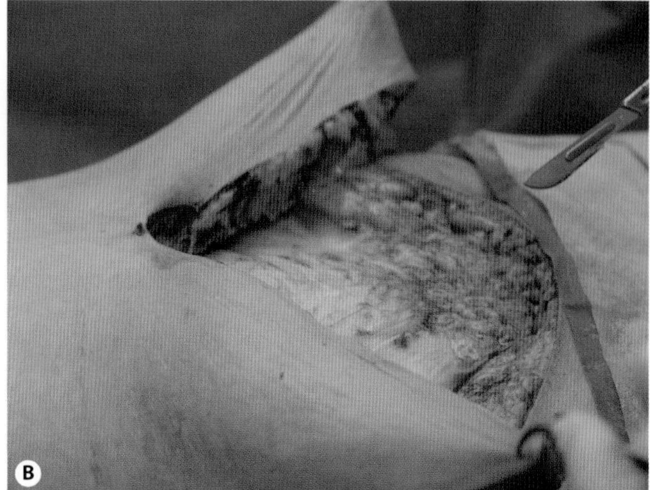

Fig. 7.13 (**A, B**) Once the umbilicus has been incised and dissected free and the lower abdominal flap is split (**A, B**), towel clips are placed at the lower edge of the previous umbilicus location to facilitate further dissection.

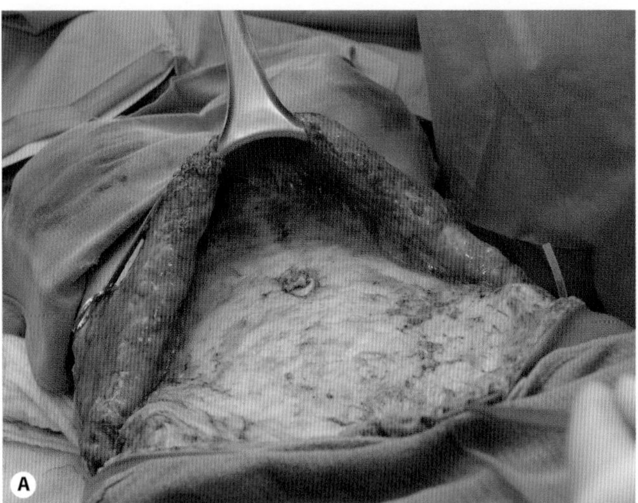

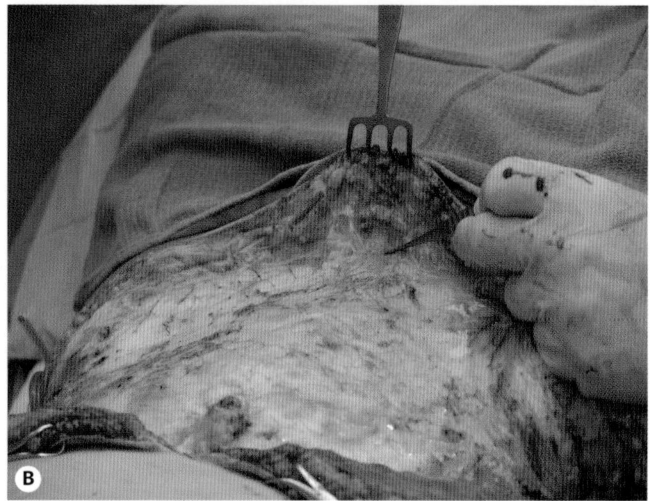

Fig. 7.14 (**A, B**) The dissection continues to the costal margins, using electrocautery to seal all perforating vessels (**A**). Inferior dissection is also performed, elevating the soft tissue to the level of the symphysis pubis (**B**).

The umbilicus is vertically incised and dissected free with scissors (**Fig. 7.12 A–C**). The preferred shape of the umbilical incision is a vertical ellipse. At this point, the inferior flap is split to facilitate subsequent upward dissection (**Fig. 7.13 A, B**). A modest amount of subcutaneous fat is left intact surrounding the umbilical stalk to maintain vascularity (**Fig. 7.12 D**). Dissection continues superiorly to the costal margins and the xiphoid (**Fig. 7.14 A**). Inferior flap elevation is also performed to the level of the pubis symphysis leaving soft tissue attached to the abdominal wall (**Fig. 7.14 B**). At this point the stage is set to perform myofascial plication.

Wide rectus abdominis muscle placation (WRAP) is begun by outlining the medial borders of the rectus abdominis muscle.[13] This defines the diastasis (**Fig. 7.15 A**). The most superior point of the plication marking is the xiphoid process and the most inferior is the pubic symphysis. The lateral line is then marked again from the xiphoid to the pubic symphysis, representing an estimated final line of plication. This estimate is based on the preoperative physical examination and the intraoperative perception of abdominal wall laxity (**Fig. 7.15 B**).

Myofascial plication is performed with a looped number 1 or 0 nylon suture on a tapered needle (**Fig. 7.16 A**). When the suture is first placed at the xiphoid the needle is brought through the existing loop, which secures it without the need to tie a knot (**Fig. 7.16 B**). Plication is performed as either a single line or two lines of closure. In a patient with significant abdominal wall laxity a two-layer closure may be preferable. For patients with moderate abdominal wall

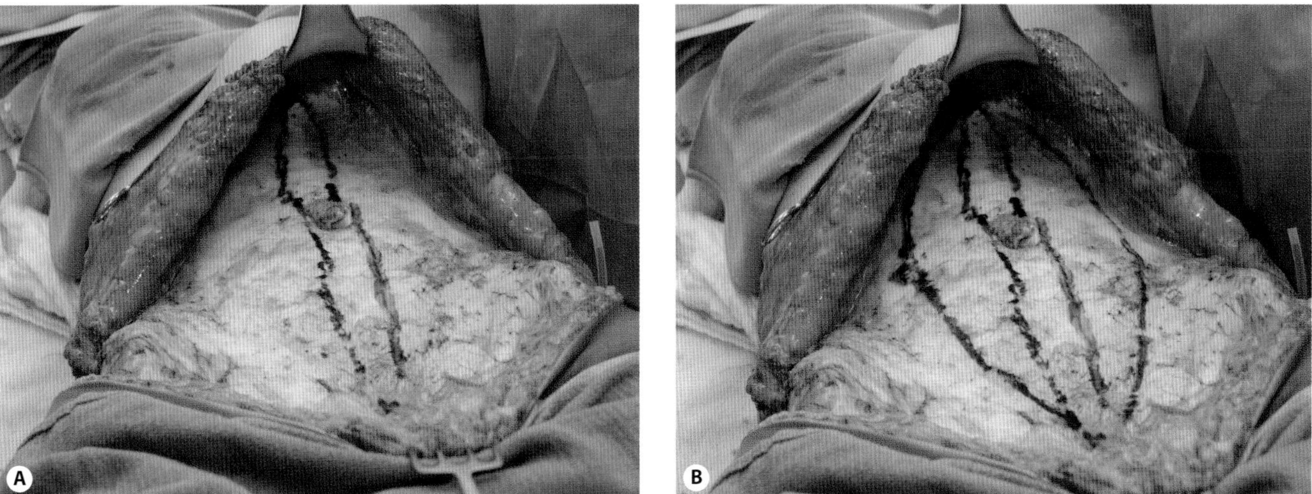

Fig. 7.15 (**A, B**) At this point, markings are made to identify the medial border of the rectus diastasis from the xiphoid to the symphysis pubis (**A**). An additional set of marks are placed laterally as an estimate of the plication to be performed during the second plication layer (**B**).

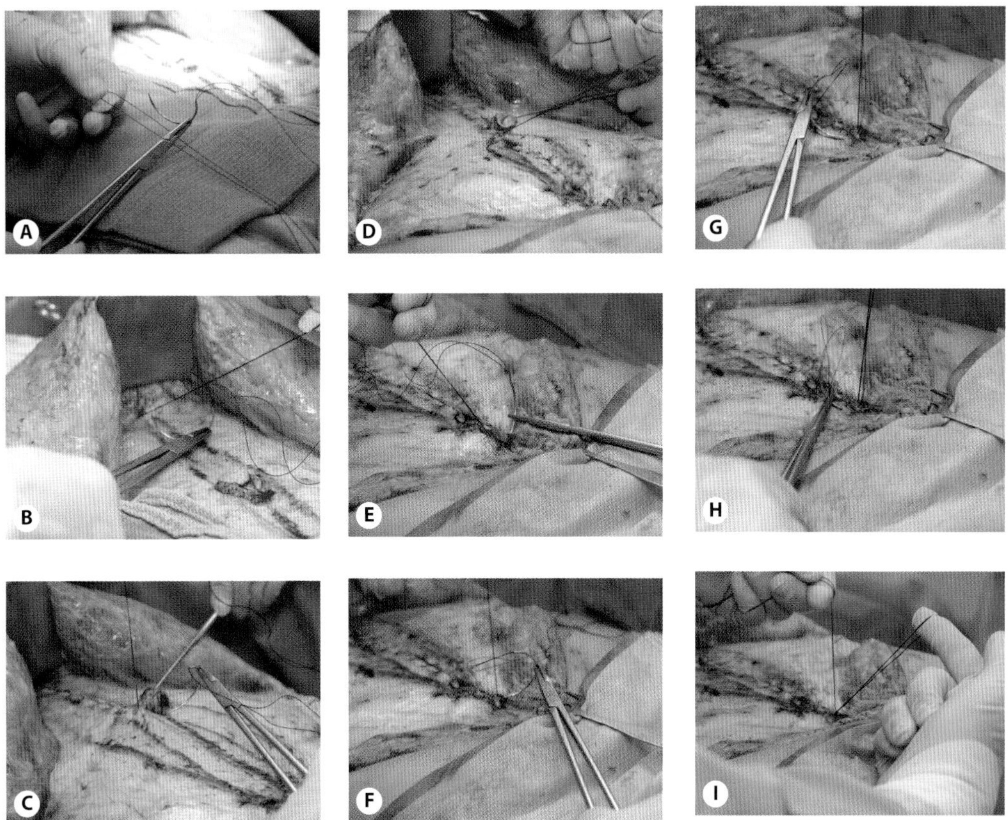

Fig. 7.16 (**A–I**) The abdominal wall plication is performed with a 0 loop nylon suture (**A**). This eliminates the need to tie a knot at the xiphoid. Plication is performed in running fashion down to the level of the umbilicus. At the level of the umbilicus, the suture continues on one edge of the rectus sheath until the inferior edge of the umbilicus is reached. At this point, the plication process is resumed. The plication process should allow sufficient space around the umbilicus to prevent potential ischemia (**B**). The plication continues to the symphysis pubis in a continuous fashion (**C, D**). The knot at the end of the plication suture is buried beneath the edges of the rectus sheath plication (**E**). The suture is brought between these two edges and then held upright (**F**). The needle is then passed through one edge of the rectus sheath and immediately brought back, so that both strands of the suture are deep to the medial edges of the rectus plication. The knot is then tied, which eliminates palpability. This strong muscle plication can be performed as a second layer tailored to the patient's abdominal wall laxity. Patients with significant laxity, especially after massive weight loss, often require the second plication layer (**E–I**).

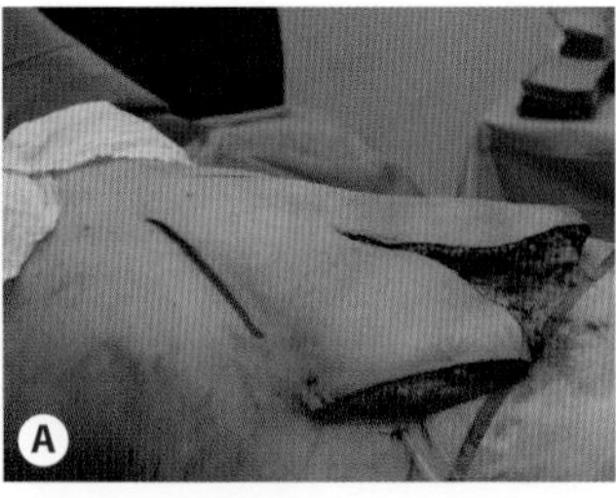

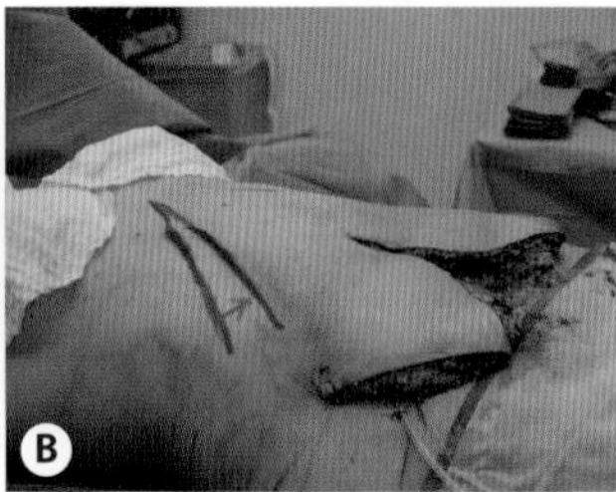

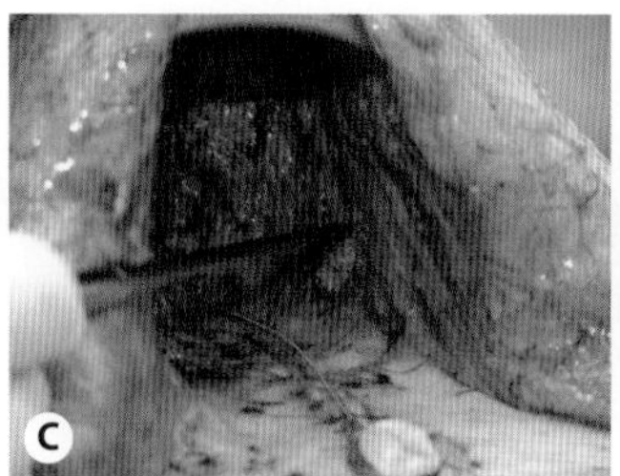

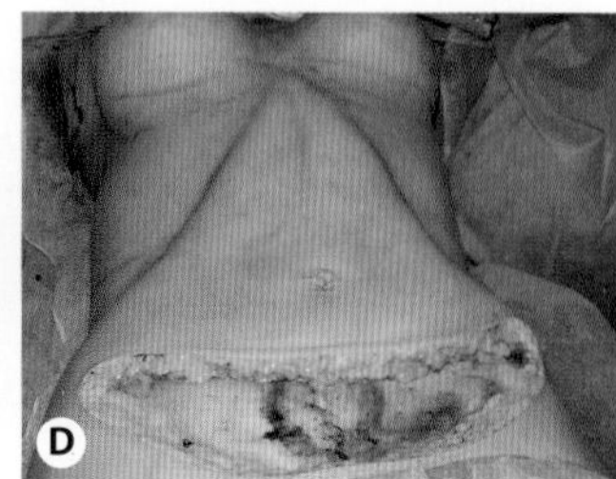

Fig. 7.17 (**A–D**) The continuous undermining that has been performed up to the costal margins has been narrowed toward the midline because of the strong muscle plication (**A, B**). This can create a set of indentations or rolls that need to be addressed. However, additional continuous dissection should not be performed because this will divide important vascular components necessary for flap viability. These indentations can be addressed with discontinuous or blunt undermining.

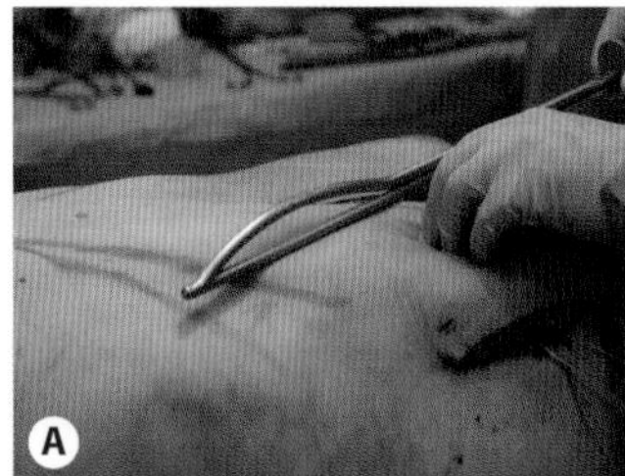

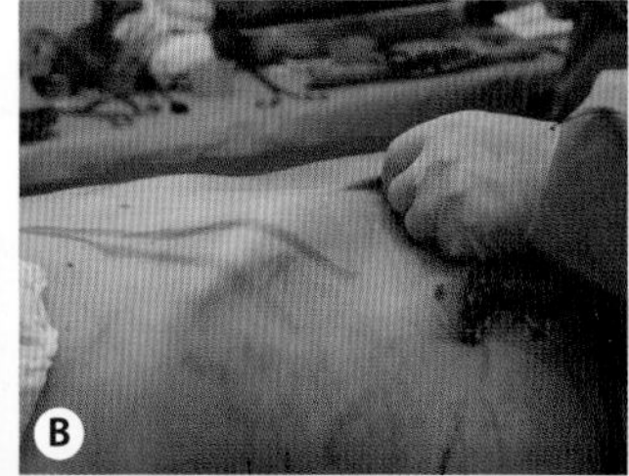

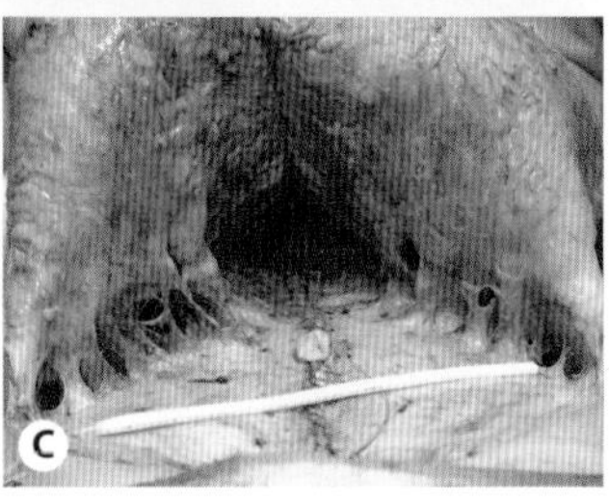

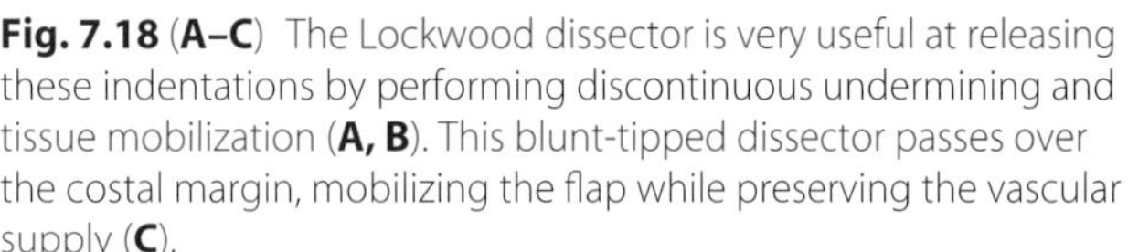

Fig. 7.18 (**A–C**) The Lockwood dissector is very useful at releasing these indentations by performing discontinuous undermining and tissue mobilization (**A, B**). This blunt-tipped dissector passes over the costal margin, mobilizing the flap while preserving the vascular supply (**C**).

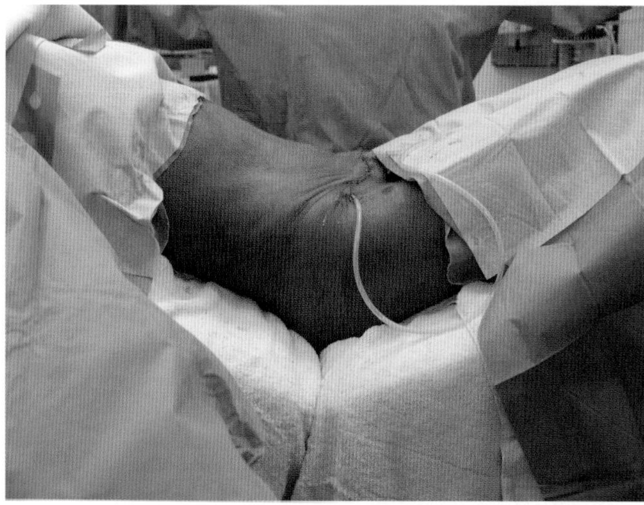

Fig. 7.19 At this point, the patient is placed into a modified jack-knife position prior to skin closure. This will take tension off of the abdominal closure and, in the majority of cases, allow all of the tissue between the low transverse incision and a point superior to the umbilicus to be resected.

laxity a single-line closure is usually sufficient. If the first line of plication has incompletely corrected the abdominal wall laxity, a second line should be performed. The continuous suture courses inferiorly down to the umbilicus. At the upper edge of the umbilicus, the nylon suture continues in a running fashion down one side of the rectus sheath only (**Fig. 7.16 C**). Continuous myofascial plication resumes at the inferior edge of the umbilicus (**Fig. 7.16 D**).

The knot tied at the point of the plication at the level of the pubic symphysis should be buried. This is done by bringing the suture out between the medial edges of the plication and then passing the needle through the opposite rectus sheath deep to superficial and then back superficial to deep, so that all suture strands are between the plication edges (**Fig. 7.16 E–G**).

At this point, a soft-tissue roll medial to the costal margin may be evident which represents the superolateral level of soft-tissue dissection (**Fig. 7.17 A**). This occurs because the level of tissue undermining has been brought medially and inferiorly from the costal margin by the myofascial plication process (**Fig. 7.17 B**). Division of the soft-tissue connection between the abdominal wall and the skin flap in this area is contraindicated, as important vascular connections exist in these pillars that should be respected (**Fig. 7.17 C**). Discontinuous undermining is recommended and is very effective at eliminating the soft-tissue ridge, mobilizing the tissues, and preserving tissue vascularity (**Fig. 7.18 A**). The Lockwood dissector is effective in achieving discontinuous undermining. This dissecting cannula is passed in a direction that parallels the intercostal vessels coursing into the flap (**Fig. 7.18 B**). Discontinuous cannula undermining results in the formation of multiple septa that contain important vascular elements (**Fig. 7.18 C, D**).

Tissue demarcation and resection is performed next. The operating room table is flexed and placed in a modified jack-knife position (**Fig. 7.19**). In the majority of cases the tissue

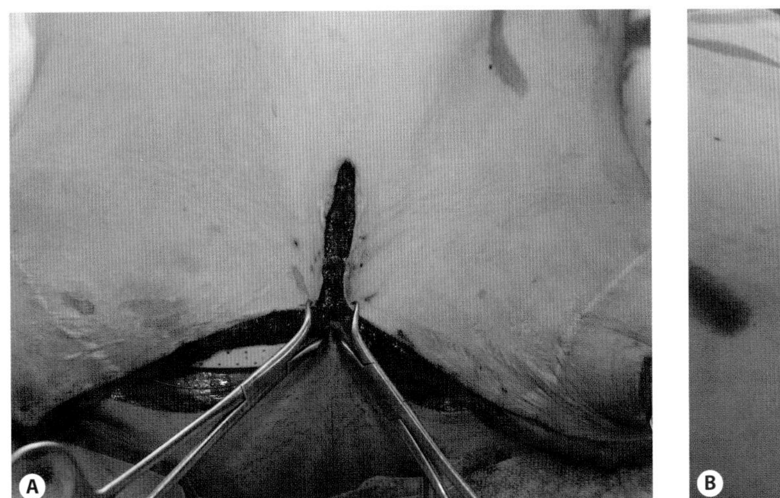
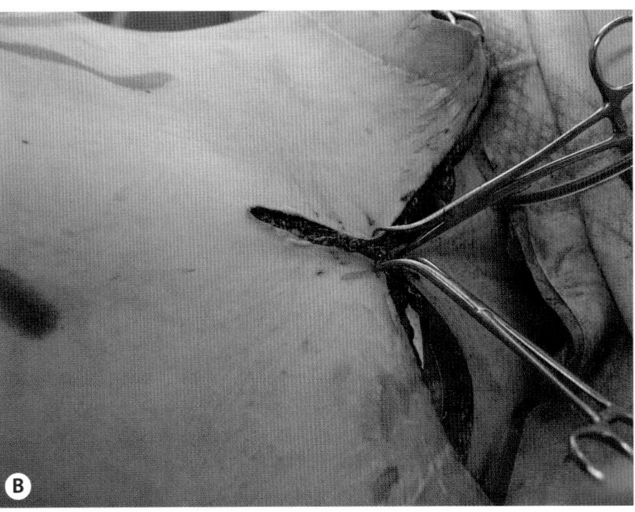

Fig. 7.20(A, B) If the patient has a long waist and only modest abdominal laxity, or if they have previously undergone an abdominoplasty and present for revision, the umbilical defect may not be incorporated within the resection and an inverted T incision closure may be necessary. The lower the initial transverse incision is made, the more likely an inverted T closure will be needed because of the longer vertical distance to the umbilicus present.

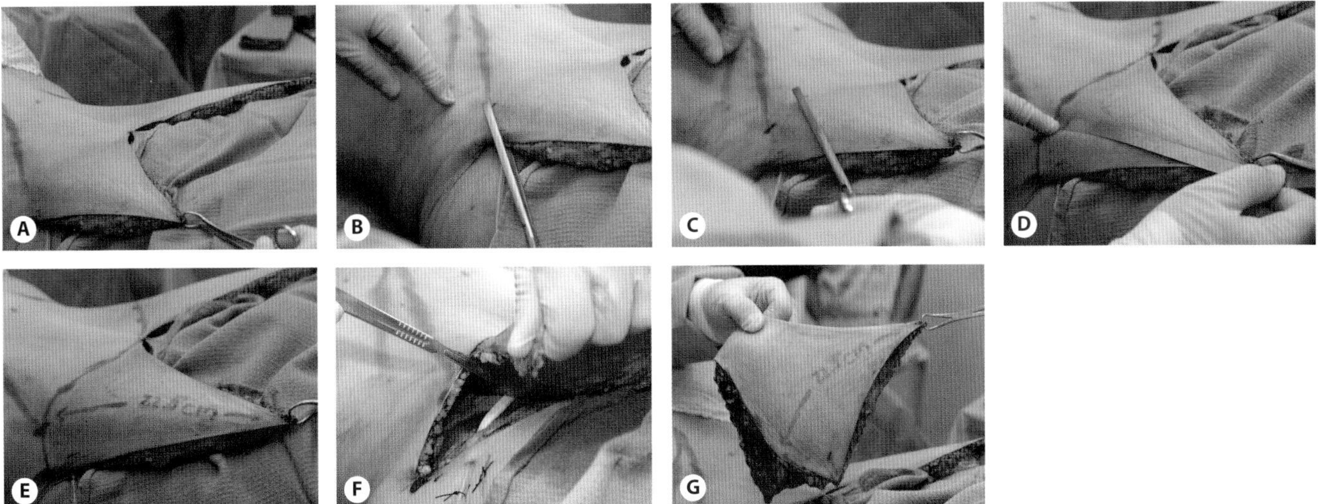

Fig. 7.21 (A–G) Tissue demarcation is done with the patient flexed at the waist in a modest jack-knife position. Towel clips are placed on the tips of the flaps of the divided tissue and a single staple is placed in the midline (**A**). The extent of tissue division in the midline is determined with the demarcator, and additional division of the flap in the midline is performed if necessary, depending on tissue tension. The Pitanguy tissue demarcator is an excellent device. It is used to push the inferior incision edge superiorly while pulling the abdominal flap inferiorly to identify the appropriate amount of tissue to be removed with reasonable tension (**B, C**). Once these points of demarcation are made, the line for resection is then drawn and the amount of tissue to be resected is identified. This should be measured to ensure the left and right areas for resection are identical (**D, E**). A full-thickness resection is then performed using a number 21 scalpel (**F, G**).

to be resected extends superior to the umbilicus. If the tension is too great to achieve this amount of resection safely, a vertical inverted T closure may be necessary (**Fig. 7.20**).

A temporary staple is placed in the midline. Towel clips are placed at the tips of the flaps to be resected and moderate tension is placed on these flaps (**Fig. 7.21 A**). The Pitanguy tissue demarcator is used to determine the appropriate amount of tissue to be resected by pushing the inferior edge of the incision cephalad while simultaneously pulling down on the abdominal tissue flap (**Fig. 7.21 B, C**). Once the resection mark is determined, the two sides are measured and checked for symmetry (**Fig. 7.21 D**). The amount of tissue to be resected should be equivalent on both sides (**Fig. 7.21 E**). The full thickness of the tissue is then resected (**Fig. 7.21 F, G**).

The creation of a new umbilicus is critical for the final aesthetic appearance of the abdominoplasty. A temporary staple closure is performed in the midline and the new location

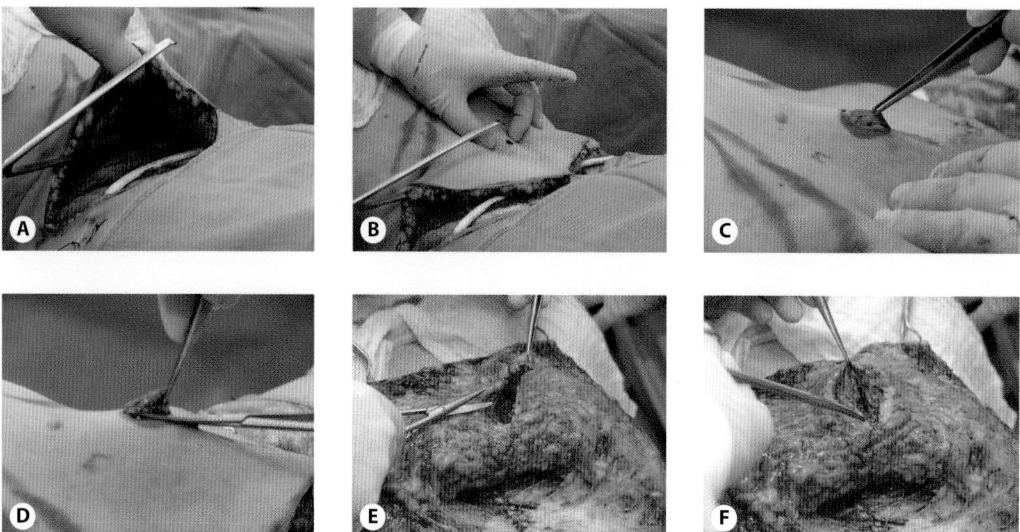

Fig. 7.22 (**A–F**) The single midline staple is left in position to facilitate umbilical location. It must be precisely placed in the midline. The Pitanguy demarcator is used with the inferior blade positioned within the umbilicus and the upper blade, dipped with methylene blue, properly positioned in the midline, with gentle hand pressure pushing the abdominal flap inferiorly (**A, B**). Once the umbilical site is identified, a number 11 scalpel is used in a pushing fashion to excise a vertical ellipse corresponding to the shape of the umbilicus. The skin is removed with a cone of underlying subcutaneous fat (**C, D**). The temporary staple is then released and the flap elevated, and excess tissue is removed from the 3 o'clock to the 9 o'clock positions inferiorly around the perimeter of the umbilical opening, leaving some fullness at the 12 o'clock position to provide additional superior hooding (**E, F**).

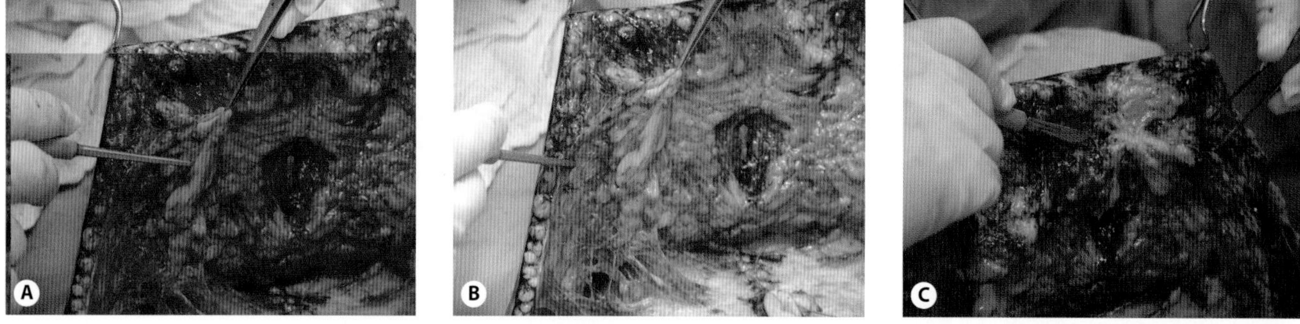

Fig. 7.23 (**A–C**) Subscarpal fat resection is performed next. The subscarpal fat is easiest to delineate from Scarpa's fascia laterally. We recommend sharp dissection using a number 10 scalpel (**A**). The assistant must watch the skin of the abdominal flap to ensure that it is not being tented inwards, which could result in resection through Scarpa's fascia. In the midline, the delineation of the Scarpa's fascia and fat is less distinct (**B**). We recommend a more conservative sharp resection, leaving behind some subscarpal fat for later trimming with scissors (**C**).

for the umbilicus is identified using the Pitanguy demarcator (**Fig. 7.22 A, B**). A vertical ellipse of skin is marked corresponding to the shape of the released umbilicus. The skin is vertically excised along with the subcutaneous tissue beneath the surface surrounding the new umbilical site (**Fig. 7.22 C, D**).The temporary staple closure is released and the flap is elevated, allowing for fat to be removed from the 3 o'clock to the 9 o'clock position, leaving some fat at the 12 o'clock position for superior hooding (**Fig. 7.22 E, F**).

At this point, the stage is set to perform subscarpal fat resection in appropriate patients. Towel clips are placed along the inferior edge of the abdominal soft-tissue flap (**Fig. 7.23 A**). The clips are placed at the same distance from the midline to maintain comparable elevation and tension. This is important to ensure a smooth and even resection. Subscarpal fat is resected throughout the entire area of undermining. Electrocautery or sharp excision can be used. We prefer sharp excision and begin this laterally where the subscarpal fat is very distinct from the overlying Scarpa's fascia (**Fig. 7.23 A**). In the midline, greater fibrous attachment is often present and the distinction between Scarpa's fascia and subscarpal fat is less evident (**Fig. 7.23 C**). Because of this we recommend that the subscarpal fat

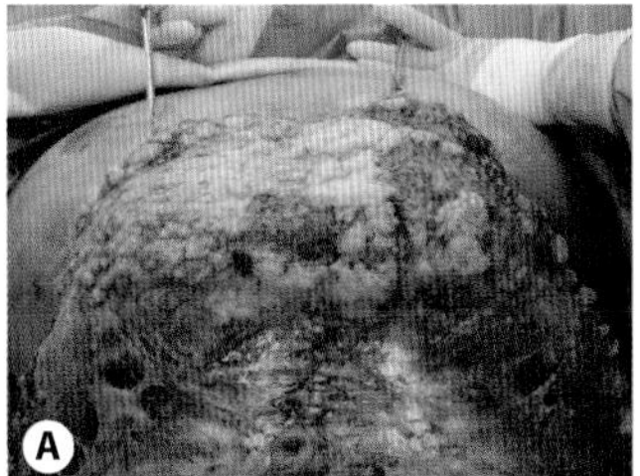

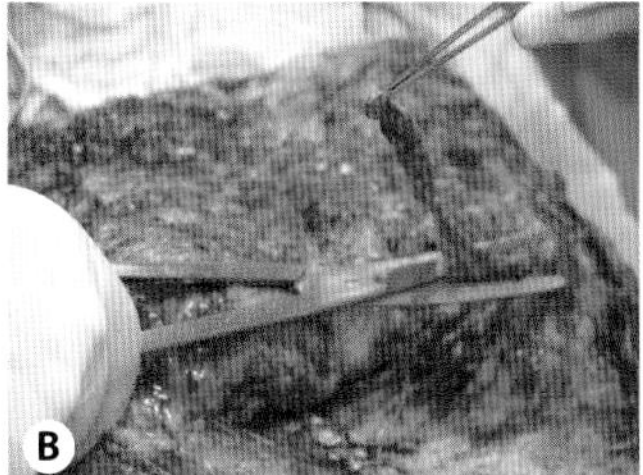

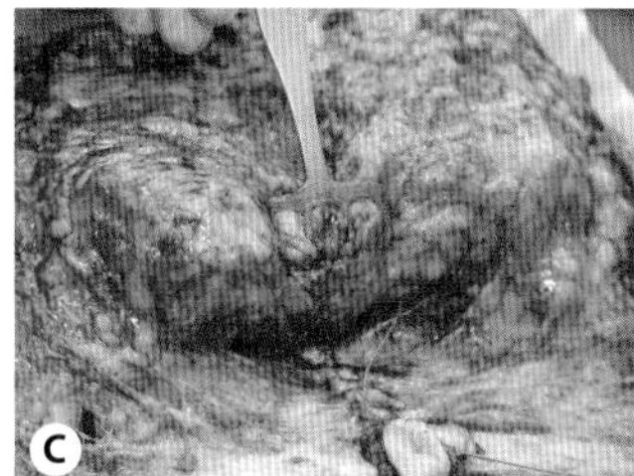

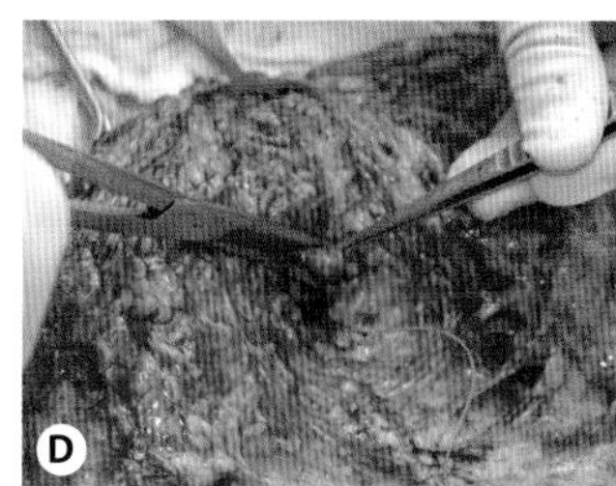

Fig. 7.24 (**A–D**) Because of proper tumescent infiltration, the relatively avascular subscarpal fat is distinctly visible as a bright yellow tissue against the more vascularized red of Scarpa's fascia (**A**). This allows easier identification of the fat and trimming using curved scissors (**B**). The most central and superior aspect of subscarpal fat resection requires additional elevation. We use a Freeman rake, placed perfectly in the midline to elevate the upper portion of the flap (**C**). This will expose the subscarpal fat all the way to the xiphoid, which can be trimmed under direct vision (**D**).

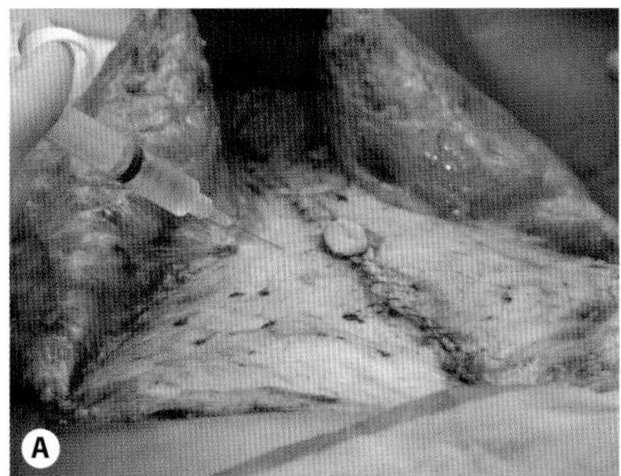

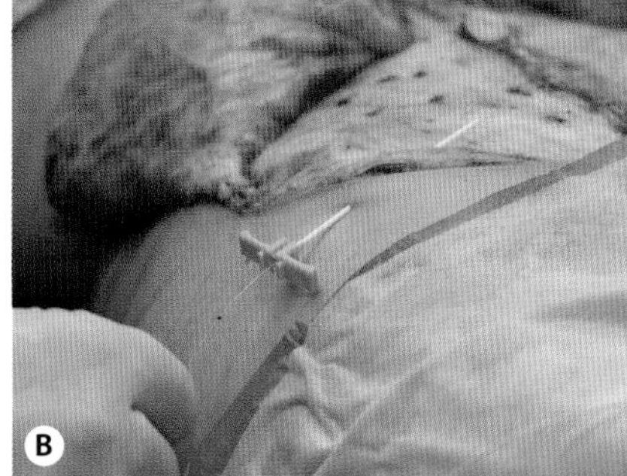

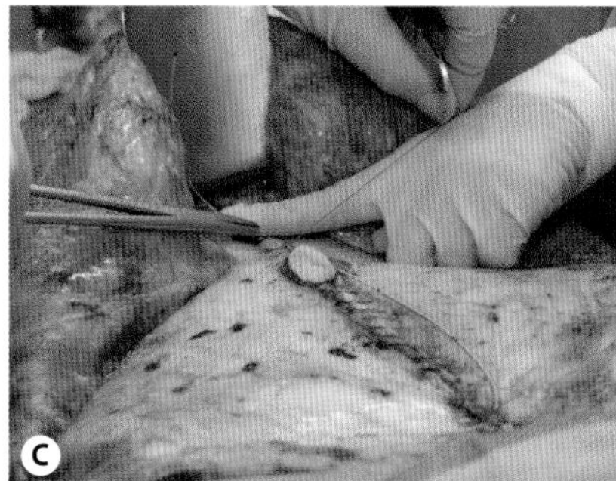

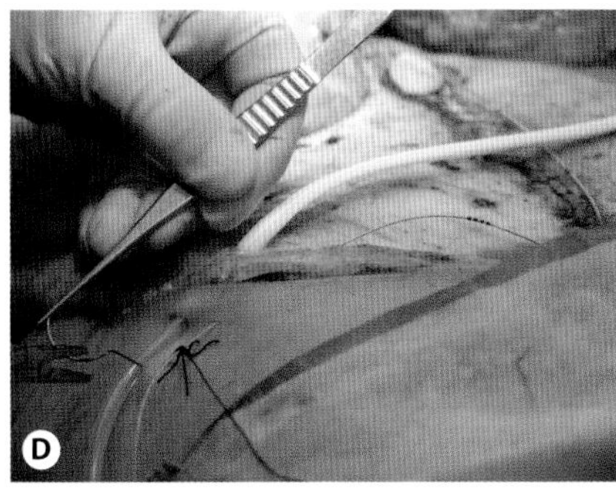

Fig. 7.25 (**A–D**) Marcaine (25 mL 1% plain) is injected into the anterior rectus sheath to aid in postoperative pain management (**A**). A continuous infusing pain pump catheter is placed (**B**), secured with Vicryl sutures along the rectus plication to ensure that the local anesthetic is infused over the strong muscle plication (**C**). Usually a single 7-mm Jackson Pratt drain is used, and both the drain and catheter are secured with silk sutures (**D**).

resection be more conservative in the midline at this point to avoid over-resection. The preservation of Scarpa's fascia is very important to maintain flap viability as well as to allow proper three-layer closure of the transverse incision.

Following sharp resection, residual subscarpal fat is still present in the midline and is a distinct yellow color, easily differentiated from the superficial fat which has better perfusion (**Fig. 7.24 A**). A large curved scissors facilitates final trimming of the residual subscarpal fat (**Fig. 7.24 B**). A Freeman rake is beneficial to facilitate exposure in the xiphoid area (**Fig. 24 C, D**).

Marcaine is injected into the rectus sheath to aid with postoperative pain management (**Fig. 7.25 A**). A continuous infusion pain pump catheter is then placed and secured along the midline (**Fig. 7.25 B, C**). Usually a single 7 mm Jackson Pratt drain is placed. If the patient has undergone significant liposuction or is still significantly overweight, a second drain may be placed. The drain is placed through a stab incision and brought out laterally. The pain pump catheter is inserted and secured in place with suture along the midline to prevent displacement. Both the drain and the catheter are secured with a 2/0 silk suture (**Fig. 7.25 D**). A final inspection for hemostasis is performed prior to closure.

The midline is closed again with a temporary staple. The upper skin margins are strongly advanced bilaterally toward the midline and secured along the way with temporary staples (**Fig. 7.26 A–D**). This creates bilateral advancement flaps which dramatically enhances the final shape and contour of the waist. If redundancy is created in the midline, it will disappear postoperatively. If redundancy is present

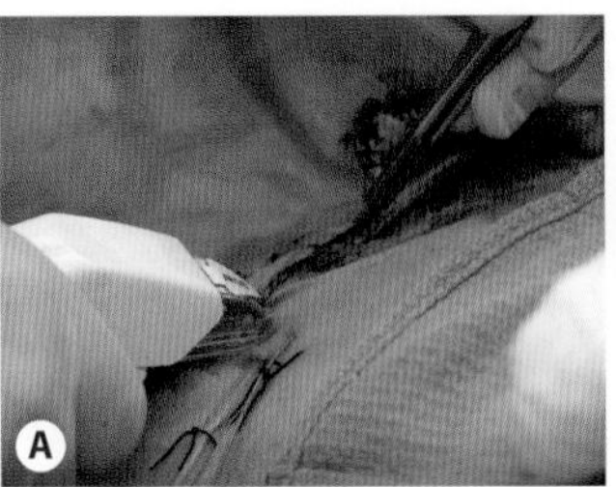
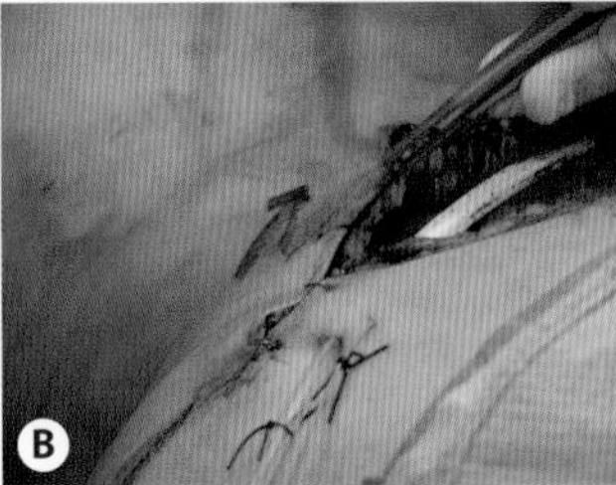
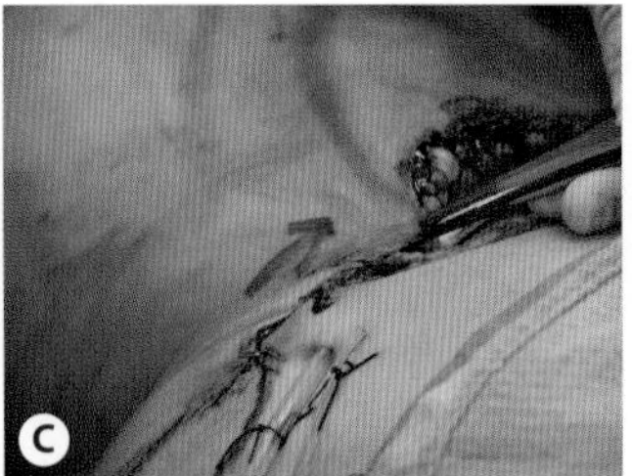
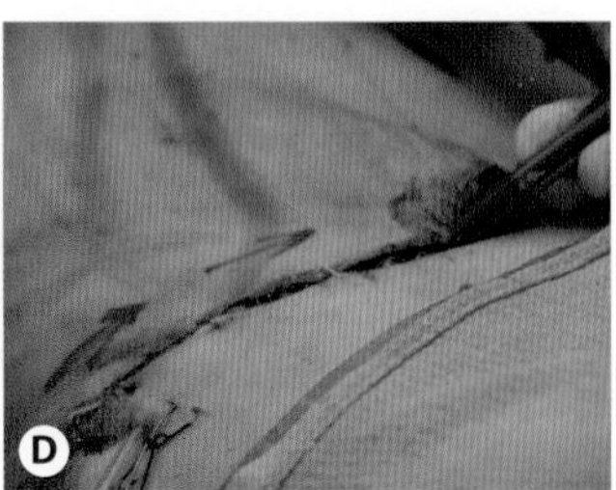

Fig. 7.26 (**A–D**) The abdominoplasty closure is critical to ensure optimal contouring of the hips, waist, and abdomen. A midline staple is placed, and then the upper skin flaps are strongly pulled medially and secured to the lower skin edge with staples (**A**). This effectively creates a bilateral upper abdominal advancement flap (**B, C**). The medial advancement of the upper abdominal tissue provides a dramatic improvement to the waistline and hip rolls and effectively eliminates the lateral dog-ears (**D**).

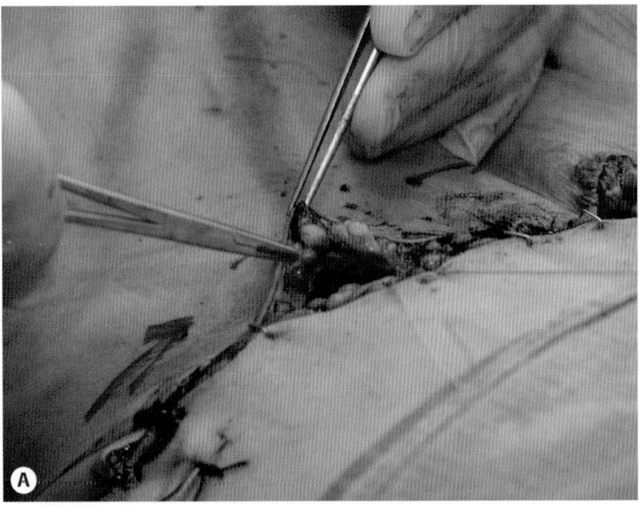
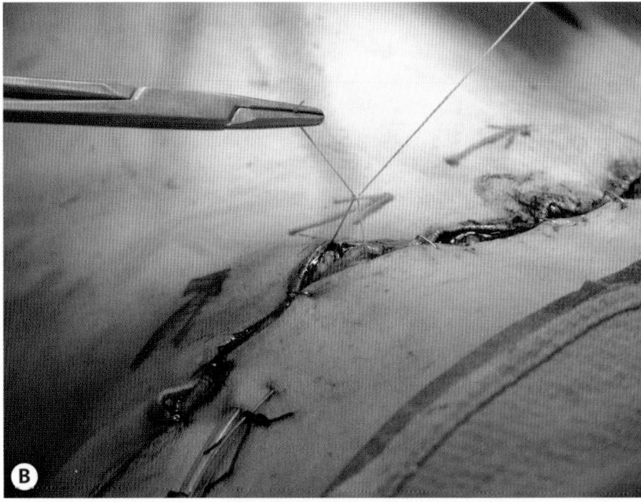

Fig. 7.27 (**A, B**) After a temporary staple closure of the skin, the superficial fascia is closed. Interrupted 1 or 0 Vicryl sutures are used and placed from the upper incision laterally to the lower incision medially, strongly advancing the upper flap. This helps to eliminate lateral dog-ears and achieve dramatic enhancement of the waistline (**A, B**).

laterally at the time of closure, it will probably persist as a dog-ear that will require revision.

A key layer for closure is the superficial fascia (Scarpa's fascia or SFS). This is closed under high tension, which takes the tension off of the skin closure and allows for final skin closure to be performed under minimal tension, which consistently yields a high-quality fine-line scar (**Fig. 7.27 A, B**). Interrupted 0 or 1 Vicryl suture is used for the SFS closure (**Fig. 7.27 A, B**). Again, the superior edge of the SFS is advanced with respect to the lower edge, moving the upper abdominal flap edge toward the midline and enhancing the overall shape, waistline, and contour as well as reducing the incidence of lateral dog-ears.

Final skin closure is performed in a layered fashion with deep dermal 2/0 Vicryl placed every centimeter (**Fig. 7.28**). Each deep dermal suture is used to further advance the upper skin flap medially. The lateral sutures should eliminate any residual small dog-ear present. This second line of

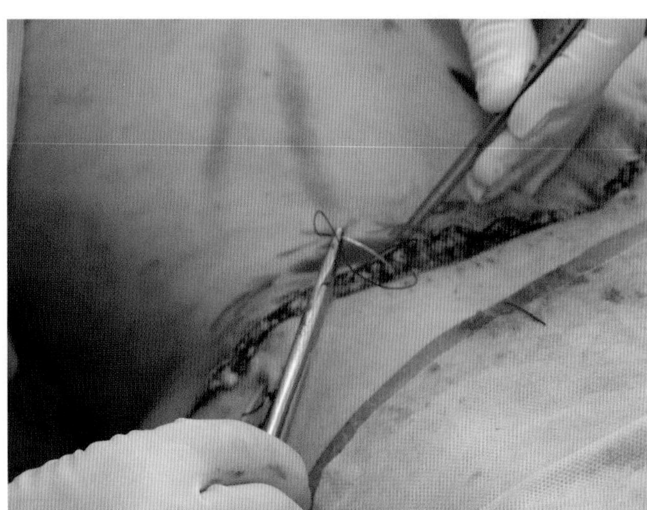

Fig. 7.28 Deep dermal closure is performed with interrupted 2/0 Vicryl sutures spaced approximately 1 cm apart. This is also performed by strongly advancing the upper abdominal skin flap medially, providing a second line of advancement.

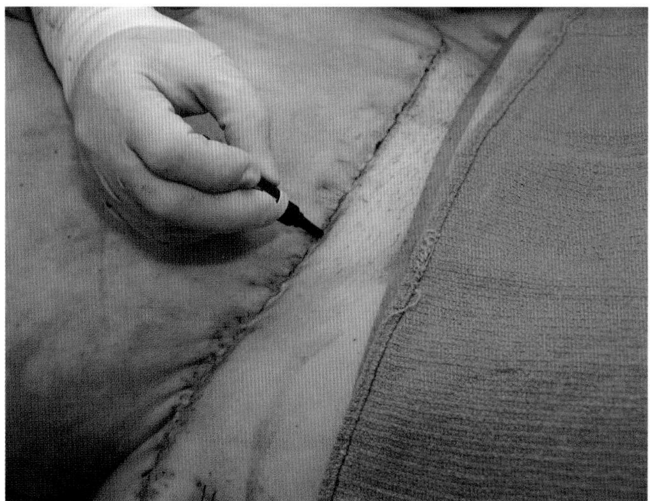

Fig. 7.29 Following the completion of the skin closure with running intradermal 4/0 Monocryl, tissue adhesive is applied, which provides a clean waterproof closure both for the transverse incision and the umbilical closure.

advancement further helps to enhance the shape and contour of the waist.

A continuous intradermal 4/0 Monocryl suture is used for final closure. The umbilicus is also closed with interrupted and running intradermal 4/0 Monocryl. The incisions are all covered with tissue adhesive, which serves as a water impermeable dressing (**Fig. 7.29**).

At the completion of the procedure the vascularity of the abdominal flap is checked by evaluating capillary refill just above the transverse incision in the midline. This is the most poorly perfused area of the flap, so good capillary refill here is a sign of flap viability (**Fig. 7.30**).

Postoperative Care (Box 7.3)

The patient is warmed with a warming blanket and monitored in the recovery room until stable. We find connecting the drain bulbs to high-vacuum wall suction helps quickly reduce the amount of residual tumescent fluid present in the tissues (**Fig. 7.31**). This is important because it promotes tissue adherence immediately and reduces the chance of subsequent seroma formation. Frequent perioperative evaluation of the abdominal soft-tissue perfusion time is important to verify that the abdominal binder is not too tight and to ensure that there are no unwanted folds or creases that could lead to reduced vascular supply to the abdominal skin (**Fig. 7.32**).

We recommend that patients undergoing full abdominoplasty stay overnight in our accredited facility. Doing so

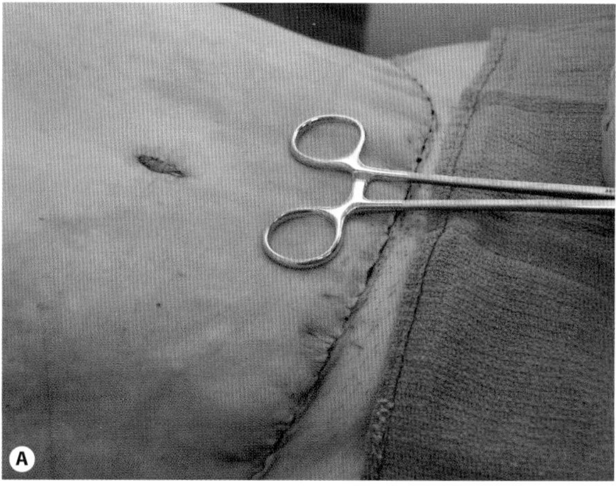

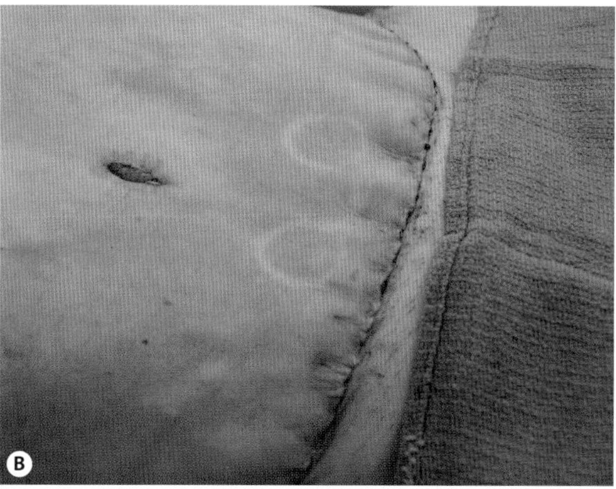

Fig. 7.30 (**A, B**) Although the tissue has been thoroughly liposuctioned superficially, all fat deep to Scarpa's fascia has been resected, and closure has been performed under appropriate tension, excellent perfusion is noted at the completion of the procedure (**A, B**).

Box 7.3 Postoperative instructions for full abdominoplasty

- Maintain a partially flexed position at the waist for the first 1–2 weeks
- Wear the abdominal binder at all times except for showering
- Make sure the binder is maintained low enough on the abdomen to cover the incision and mons
- Verify that there are no significant creases, folds, or the presence of drain tubes underneath the binder
- Avoid smoking or exposure to nicotine-containing products
- Breathe deeply and use the incentive spirometer frequently
- Drink plenty of fluids: 8 oz/hr is the goal
- Move legs frequently while resting and walk regularly
- Drain care as instructed
- Continue to take multivitamin daily. Resume medications as instructed
- No vigorous activity or heavy lifting for 4–6 weeks

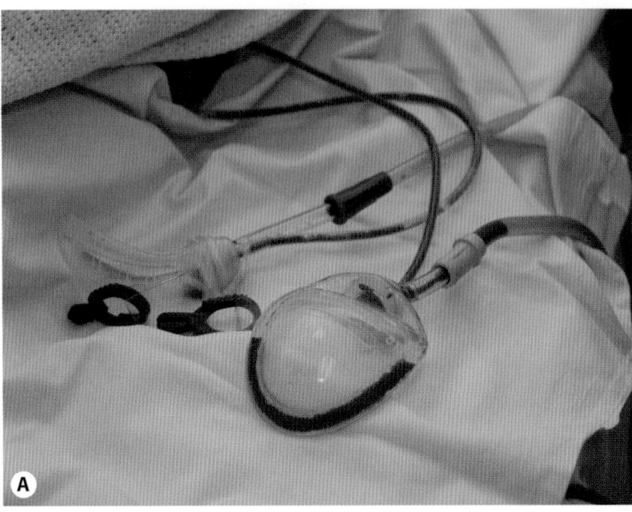

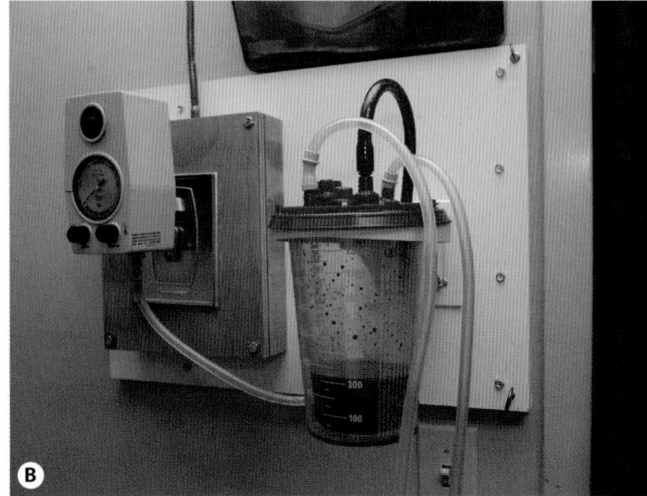

Fig. 7.31 (**A, B**) In the recovery area we find it useful to connect the drains to high-vacuum wall suction. This aids in evacuating residual tumescent fluid and any drainage that has already accumulated.

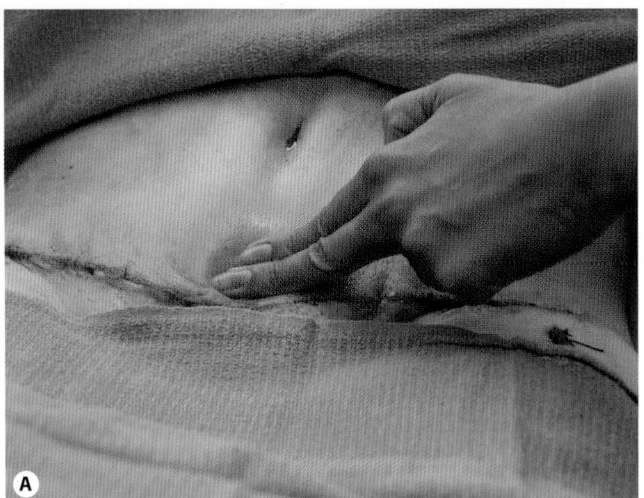

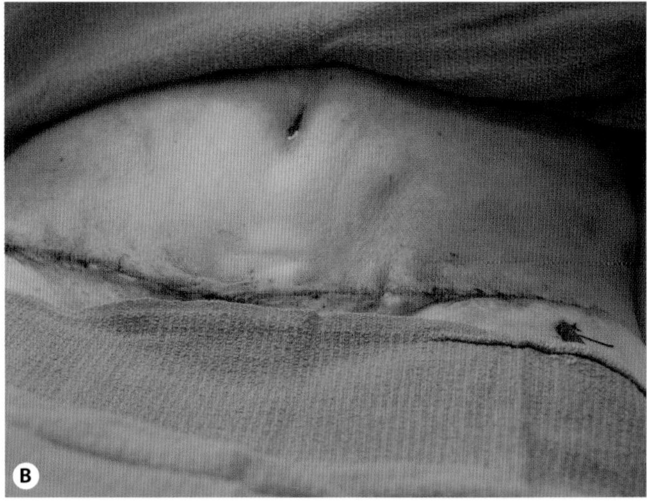

Fig. 7.32 (**A, B**) It is important to verify that perfusion of the abdominal flap has remained excellent. This also allows the opportunity to make sure that the abdominal binder is properly positioned, and that it is not too tight. Making sure that there are no folds in the binder and foam as well as the drain tubing is also important, as these can irritate or damage the underlying skin.

will allow more diligent monitoring of fluid status, as well as better pain management and assurance that the patient is walking periodically and using the incentive spirometer frequently. Most full abdominoplasty patients are kept in our overnight facility cared for by a trained nurse. Some patients wish to go home and then are seen usually the next day or so. We usually see all our body contouring patients the following day, and frequently during the first postoperative week.

On discharge, patients are sent home with oral antibiotics, pain medication, and vitamins, which are started preoperatively. They are instructed to keep their waist slightly flexed and to refrain from heavy lifting or vigorous activity. Frequent movement of the lower extremities while in bed and regular walking is encouraged to help reduce the chance of DVT/PE. Patients are instructed to stay well hydrated by drinking plenty of fluids. Instructions regarding drain care are provided to the patient and their caregiver. The abdominal binder is worn at all times in the immediate postoperative period, except for showering, which is allowed on postoperative day 2. Preoperative and postoperative photographs are shown in **Figs 7.33–7.37**.

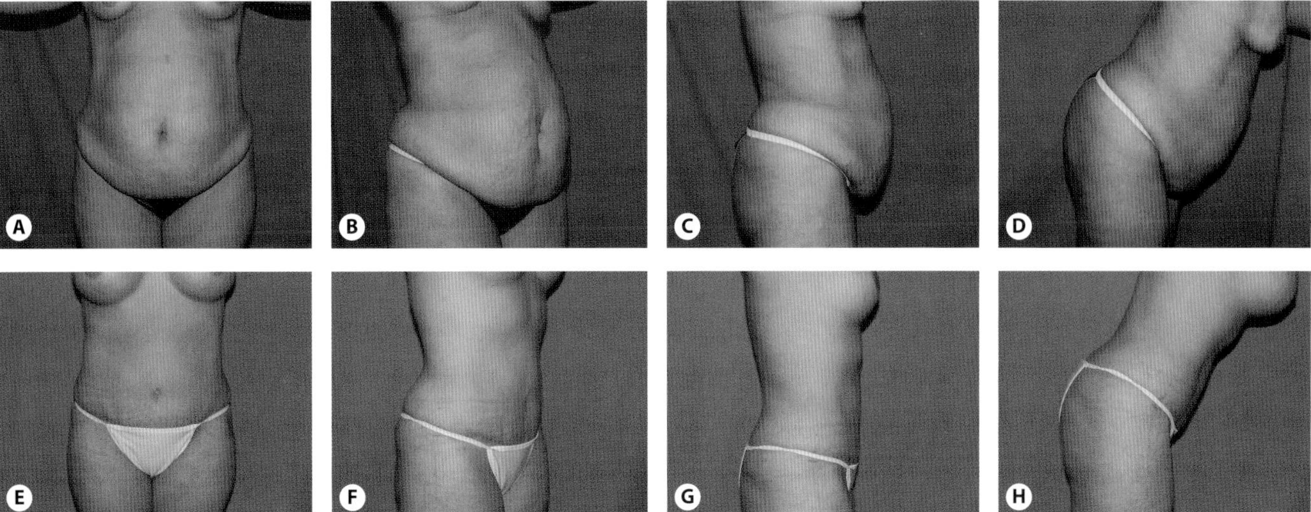

Fig. 7.33 (A–H) A 45-year-old woman. Preoperative photographs demonstrate a moderate amount of abdominal excess adiposity and soft-tissue laxity. There is visible abdominal wall laxity and poor skin quality secondary to striae. She underwent full abdominoplasty with myofascial plication and concurrent liposuction. Postoperative results demonstrate a significant reduction in the amount of abdominal striae, soft-tissue excess, and abdominal wall laxity. Postoperatively, she has much improved silhouette and contour.

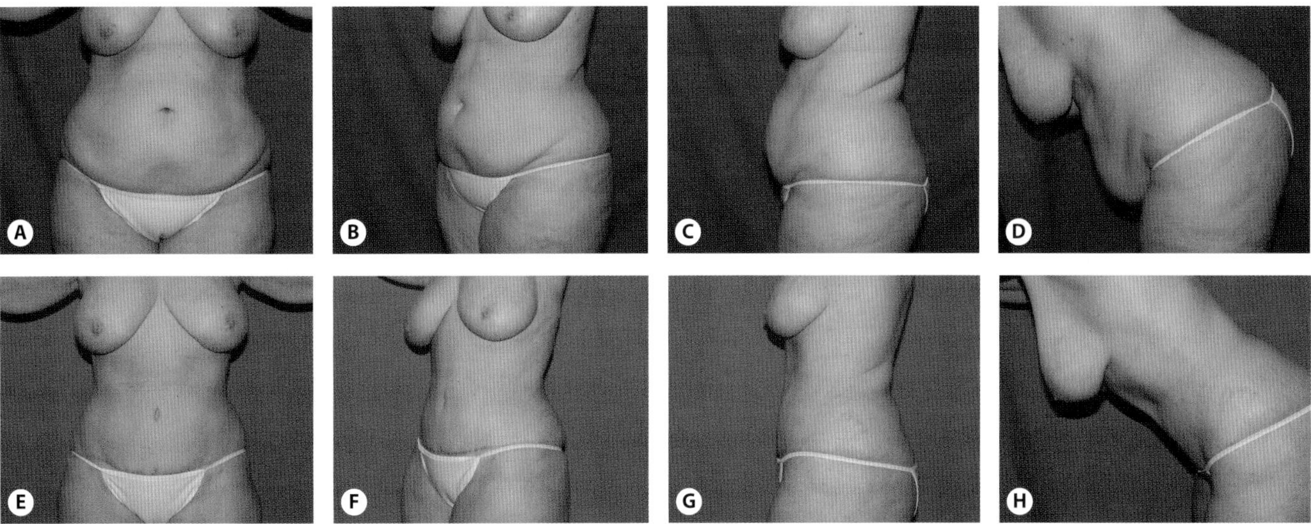

Fig. 7.34 (A–H) A 63-year-old woman. This patient demonstrates relatively good skin quality and body habitus for her age. Preoperatively there was excess adiposity and moderate abdominal wall laxity. She underwent full abdominoplasty with myofascial plication and concurrent liposuction. The postoperative photographs show the usefulness of concurrent liposuction with abdominoplasty to improve the contour of the entire midsection from the costal margins to the pubic symphysis.

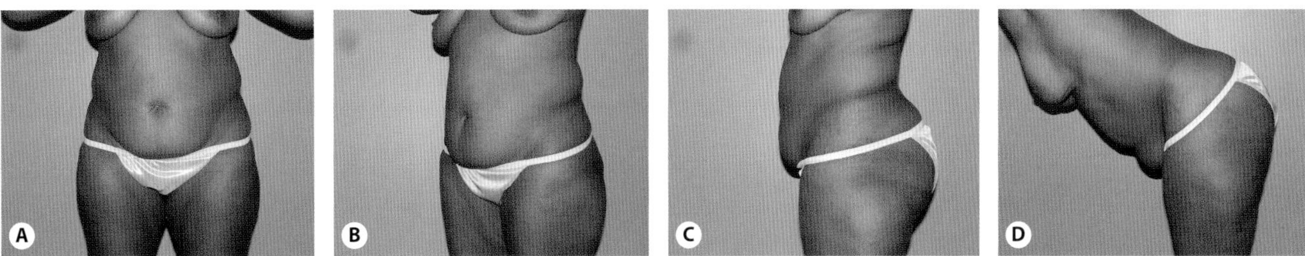

Fig. 7.35 (A–J) A 50-year-old woman. This patient had a moderate to significant amount of excess adiposity circumferentially in the trunk and buttocks area. She underwent a full abdominoplasty with myofascial plication and concurrent liposuction of the abdomen and the middle and lower back. She also desired increased volume and projection of her buttocks. Buttocks augmentation with fat grafting was also performed. Postoperatively, the patient demonstrates significantly improved contour of the abdomen, with improvement of the soft-tissue laxity, thinning of the trunk, and tightening of the abdominal wall.

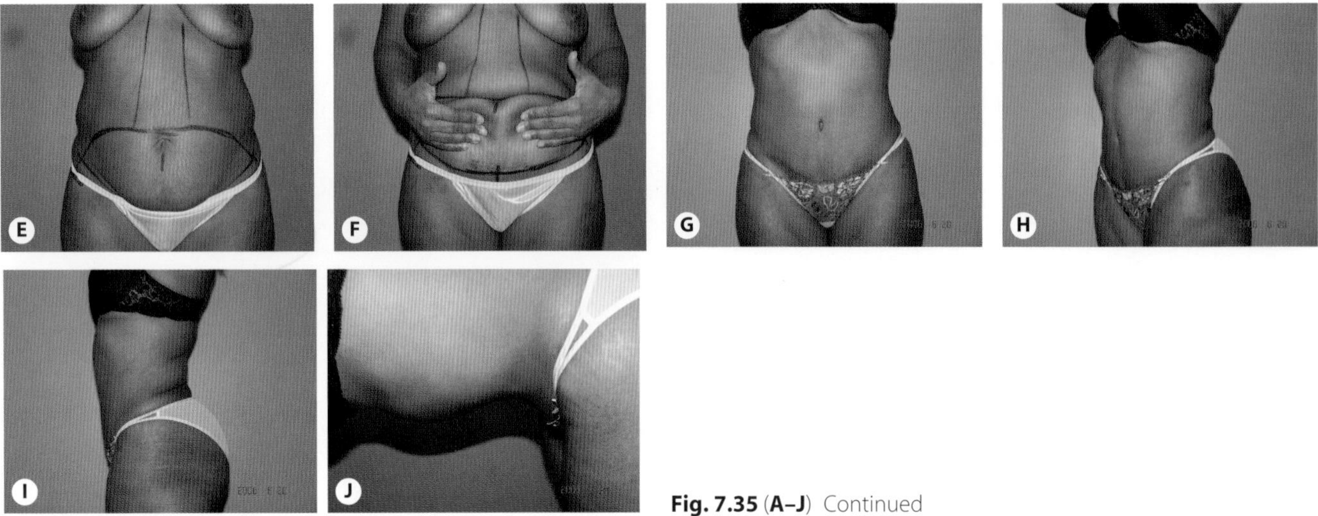

Fig. 7.35 (A–J) Continued

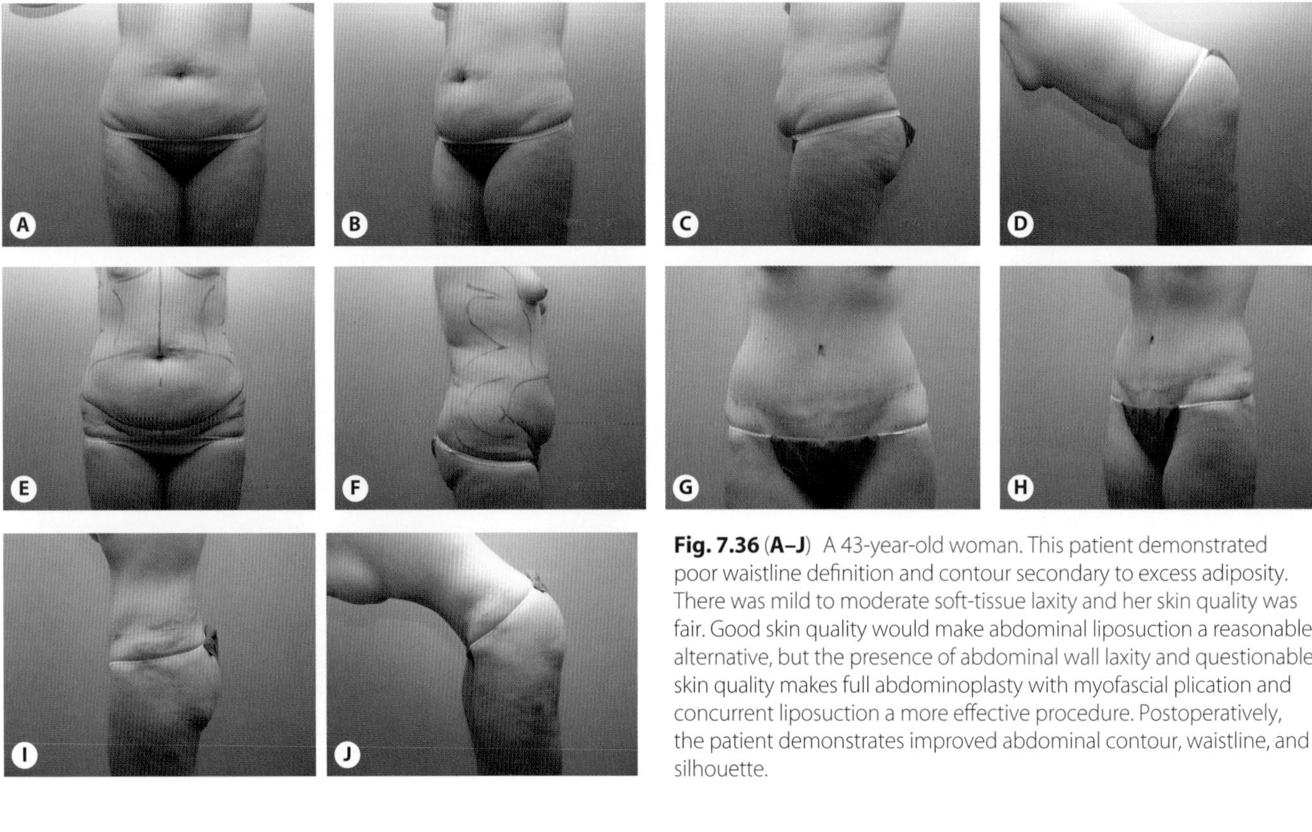

Fig. 7.36 (**A–J**) A 43-year-old woman. This patient demonstrated poor waistline definition and contour secondary to excess adiposity. There was mild to moderate soft-tissue laxity and her skin quality was fair. Good skin quality would make abdominal liposuction a reasonable alternative, but the presence of abdominal wall laxity and questionable skin quality makes full abdominoplasty with myofascial plication and concurrent liposuction a more effective procedure. Postoperatively, the patient demonstrates improved abdominal contour, waistline, and silhouette.

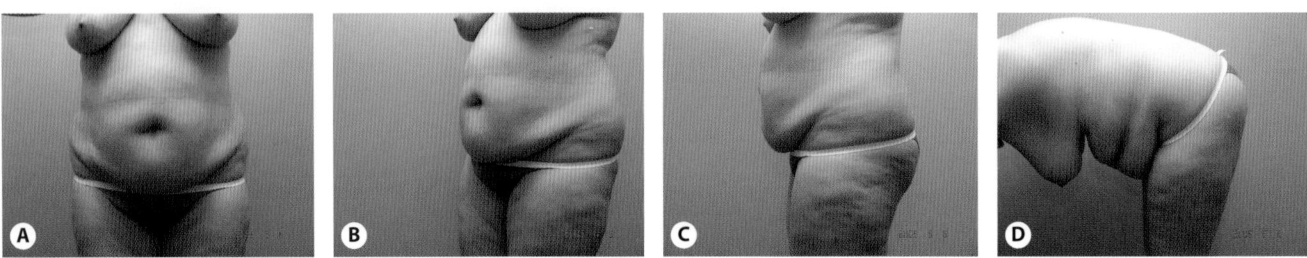

Fig. 7.37 (**A–J**) A 64-year-old woman. This patient had a significant amount of excess adiposity and soft-tissue laxity. She was a reasonable candidate for circumferential abdominoplasty, but her main concern was her abdominal contour. She underwent full abdominoplasty with myofascial plication and concurrent liposuction of the abdomen and lower back. She demonstrates a significant improvement of the abdominal and waistline contour postoperatively.

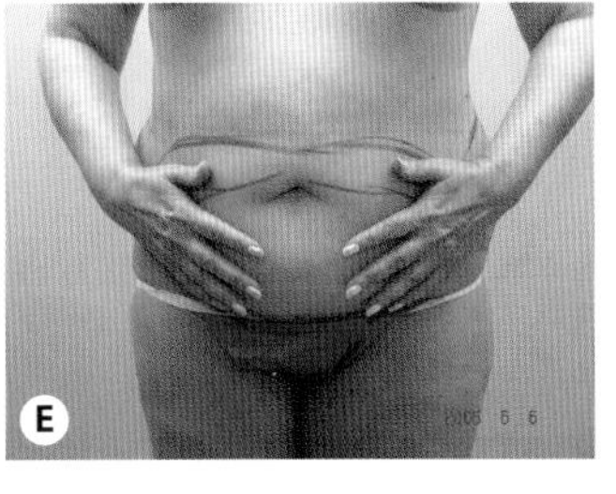
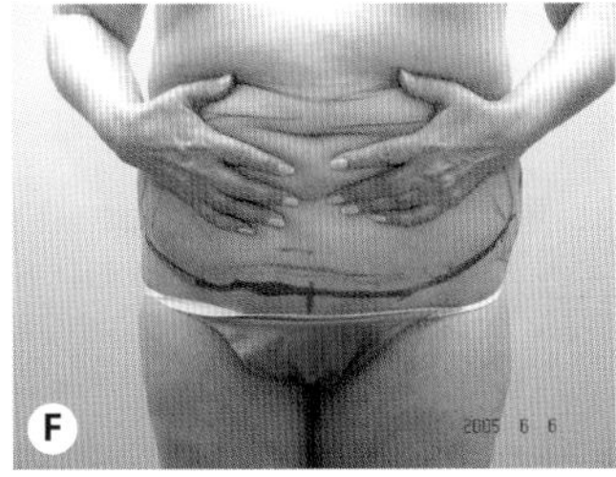
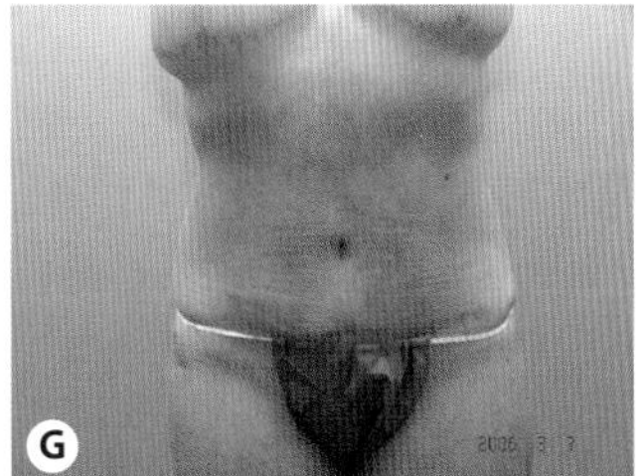
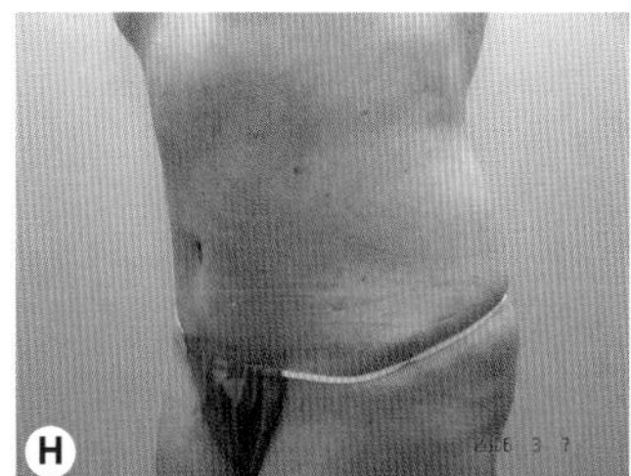
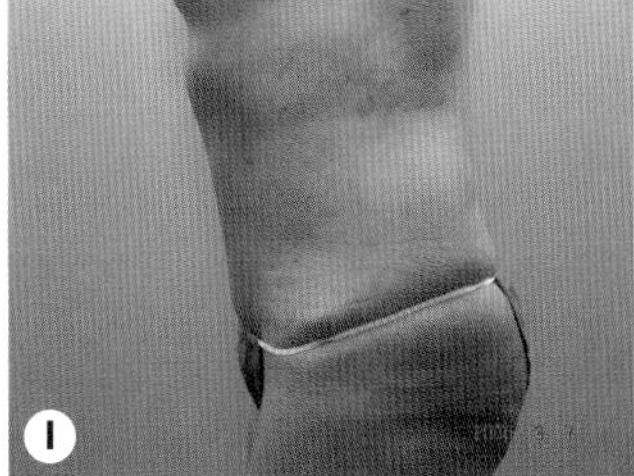
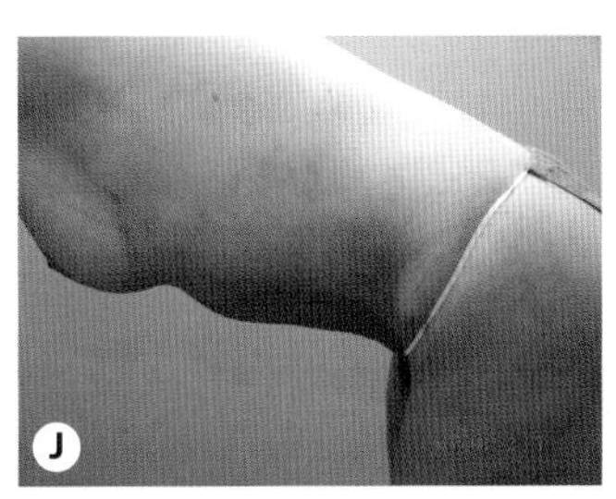

Fig. 7.37 (**A–J**) Continued

Summary

The full or complete abdominoplasty procedure is by far the most commonly performed method of abdominoplasty. This is because the majority of patients presenting for abdominoplasty have significant excess adiposity, skin excess, and rectus diastasis/myofascial laxity. The concurrent use of thorough tumescent liposuction, subscarpal fat resection, and strong myofascial plication allows the surgeon to achieve excellent results. Thinning, tightening, and flattening are laudable goals which can be consistently achieved using these techniques.

Clinical Caveats: Full abdominoplasty

- There are a variety of surgical options available for patients requesting abdominoplasty or abdominal contouring. Each procedure should be tailored according to the goals of the patient and the best aesthetic result possible
- Preoperative instructions/requirements must be methodically followed to maximize safety
- Preoperative markings and photographs are invaluable to achieve the best possible results
- Concurrent liposuction of the abdominal soft-tissue apron and the surrounding area is of great value, especially for the patient with incomplete weight loss or those who have moderate to significant excess adiposity
- It is often better to close the umbilicus defect and have a small inverted 'T' inferiorly in the midline if there is insufficient laxity to allow the location of the umbilicus to be included in the resection. Preoperative discussion with the patient about this should be performed
- Myofascial plication is almost always needed and is beneficial in achieving optimal contour in abdominoplasty procedures
- During closure, strong skin flap advancement medially will reduce the incidence of dog-ears
- Subscarpal fat resection can be performed safely if needed
- Injection of bupivacaine under the rectus sheath will help reduce postoperative discomfort, which facilitates deep breathing and reduces the use of postoperative pain medication
- Overnight care in an accredited facility will allow better fluid status management and pain control, and reduce the chance of DVT with the use of pneumatic compression devices and ambulation
- Evaluation on postoperative day 1 and regularly over the first week will allow proper intervention if care issues arise

References

1. Matarasso A, Swift RW, Rankin M. Abdominoplasty and abdominal contour surgery: a national plastic surgery survey. Plast Reconstruct Surg 2006; 117: 1797.
2. Kim J, Stevenson TR. Abdominoplasty, liposuction of the flanks, and obesity: analyzing risk factors for seroma formation. Plast Reconstruct Surg 2006; 117: 77.
3. Vastine VL, Morgan RF, Williams GS, et al. Wound complications of abdominoplasty in obese patients. Ann Plast. Surg 1999; 42: 34.
4. Guyuron B, Raszewski R. Undetected diabetes and the plastic surgeon. Plast Reconstruct Surg 1990; 86: 471.
5. Manassa EH, Hertl CH, Olbrisch RR. Wound healing problems in smokers and nonsmokers after 132 abdominoplasties. Plast Reconstruct Surg 2003; 111: 2082.
6. Hensel JM, Lehman JA Jr., Tantri MP, et al. An outcomes analysis and satisfaction survey of 199 consecutive abdominoplasties. Ann Plast Surg 2001; 46: 357.

7. Krueger JK, Rohrich RJ. Clearing the smoke: the scientific rationale for tobacco abstention with plastic surgery. Plast Reconstruct Surg 2001; 15; 108: 1063.
8. Borman H. Pregnancy in the early period after abdominoplasty. Plast Reconstruct Surg 2002; 109: 396.
9. Blickstein D, Blickstein I. Oral contraception and thrombophilia. Curr Opin Obstet Gynecol 2007; 19: 370.
10. van Vlijmen EF, Brouwer JL, Veeger NJ, et al. Oral contraceptives and the absolute risk of venous thromboembolism in women with single or multiple thrombophilic defects: results from a retrospective family cohort study. Arch Intern Med 2007; 167: 282.
11. Huang GJ, Bajaj AK, Gupta S, et al. Increased intraabdominal pressure in abdominoplasty: delineation of risk factors. Plast Reconstruct Surg 2007; 119: 1319.
12. Al-Basti HB, El-Khatib HA, Taha A, et al. Intraabdominal pressure after full abdominoplasty in obese multiparous patients. Plast Reconstruct Surg 2004; 113: 2145.
13. Toranto IR. Resolution of back pain with the wide abdominal rectus plication abdominoplasty. Plast Reconstruct Surg 1988; 81: 777.

Suggested Reading

Dillerud E. Abdominoplasty combined with suction lipoplasty: A study of complications, revisions, and risk factors in 487 cases. Ann Plast Surg 1990; 25: 333.

El-Khatib HA, Bener A. Abdominal dermolipectomy in an abdomen with pre-existing scars: a different concept. Plast Reconstruct Surg 2004; 114: 992.

Grazer FM. Abdominoplasty. Plast Reconstruct Surg 1973; 51: 617.

Hafezi F, Nouhi A. Safe abdominoplasty with extensive liposuctioning. Ann Plast Surg 2006; 57: 149.

Hester RT Jr., Baird W, Bostwick J III, et al. Abdomiinoplasty combined with other surgical procedures: Safe or sorry? Plast Reconstruct Surg 1989; 83: 997.

Hunstad JP. Advanced concepts in abdominoplasty. Perspect Plast Surg 1998; 12: 13.

Hunstad JP. Body contouring in the obese patient. Clin Plast Surg 1996; 23: 647.

Lee MJ, Mustoe TA. A simplified version to achieve aesthetic results for the umbilicus in abdominoplasty. Plast Reconstruct Surg 2002; 109: 2136.

Lockwood TE. High-lateral-tension abdominoplasty with superficial fascial system suspension. Plast Reconstruct Surg 1995; 96: 60.

Matarasso A. Abdominoplasty: A system of classification and treatment for combined abdominoplasty and suction-assisted lipectomy. Aesthet Plast Surg 1991; 15: 111–121.

Matarasso A. Awareness and avoidance of abdominoplasty complications. Aesthet Surg J 1997; 17: 256.

Matarasso A. The male abdominoplasty. Clin Plast Surg 2004; 31: 555.

Netscher DT, Wigoda P, Spira M, Peltier M. Musculoaponeurotic plication in abdominoplasty: How durable are its effects? Aesthet Plast Surg 1995; 19: 531.

Spiegelman JI, Levine RH. Abdominoplasty: a comparison of outpatient and inpatient procedures shows that it is a safe and effective procedure for outpatients in an office-based surgery clinic. Plast Reconstruct Surg 2006; 118: 517.

CHAPTER **8**

Extended Abdominoplasty

Joseph P. Hunstad and Remus Repta

IN THIS CHAPTER

KEY POINTS

The extended abdominoplasty procedure is ideal for patients with significant laxity and excess adiposity of the abdomen and flanks. These patients have substantially more tissue redundancy and excess adiposity than are seen in the full abdominoplasty patient. The extent of the soft-tissue laxity may not extend circumferentially to merit a circumferential abdominoplasty, or the patient may simply not wish to have the additional posterior component performed. Excess adiposity posteriorly without significant soft-tissue laxity is amenable to liposuction and may not require soft-tissue resection. The extended abdominoplasty may involve all of the components of a full abdominoplasty. The transverse incision of an extended abdominoplasty is longer than that of the full abdominoplasty, usually extending up to or beyond the midaxillary line.

Introduction

The majority of patients who present for abdominoplasty are well suited for full abdominoplasty. The amount of excess adiposity and soft-tissue laxity in most abdominal contouring patients requires anterior resection with a transverse scar that often spans from one anterior superior iliac spine to the other, in order to avoid lateral dog-ears. A smaller number of patients present with smaller, more localized laxity amenable to mini abdominoplasty (see Chapter 5, Mini Abdominoplasty). At the other end of the spectrum, patients with substantial weight loss are best treated with circumferential abdominoplasty (see Chapter 9, Circumferential Abdominoplasty). The extended abdominoplasty procedure therefore occupies a unique niche between full abdominoplasty and circumferential abdominoplasty.

Patients who undergo an extended abdominoplasty have more soft-tissue laxity than a full abdominoplasty incision can correct without resulting in prominent lateral dog-ears. Conversely, a circumferential abdominoplasty may not deliver much added benefit. The amount of soft-tissue laxity and ptosis in the posterior trunk and buttocks may be appreciably less, and the aesthetic benefit to the posterior area from the posterior component of the circumferential

Box 8.1 Relative contraindications for extended abdominoplasty

- Smoking
- Diabetes mellitus
- Malnutrition
- Various wound-healing disorders
- Bowel/bladder dysfunction
- Immunodeficiency
- Medications that inhibit blood coagulation
- A significant history of pulmonary or deep vein thrombosis
- Lower extremity lymphedema/venous insufficiency
- Significant medical problems including COPD/pulmonary issues, renal insufficiency, anemia, and other systemic issues that may make abdominal tightening surgery dangerous

Note: Age alone should not be a contraindication to abdominoplasty procedures if the patient is in good health. Patients who have a history of chronic pain should also be approached cautiously, as postoperative care may be significantly affected.

Box 8.2 Preoperative recommendations for extended abdominoplasty

- Smoking cessation/avoidance of nicotine exposure for 4–6 weeks prior to surgery
- Multivitamin daily
- Stop aspirin/other blood thinning products with primary care doctor's permission
- Abstain from all dietary/herbal supplements not approved by the surgeon
- Basic laboratory work should be tailored to each patient. It may include CBC, Chem. 7, Factor V Leiden, and PT/PTT/INR
- Medical clearance if needed
- Wearing abdominal binder for 2 weeks before surgery is encouraged
- Shower with a gentle antimicrobial soap the night before and day of surgery

abdominoplasty may be negligible. Lastly, there are occasional patients who cannot accept a posterior incision or scar. Their reasons may be varied, but the point is that they wish for maximum correction of their abdominal soft-tissue laxity without having to undergo a circumferential abdominoplasty.

Patient Selection (Box 8.1)

Indications for an extended abdominoplasty include patients who are overweight or modestly obese, and those who have had significant weight fluctuations and or weight loss. These patients are concerned about the fullness of the central abdomen, as well as the fullness and laxity of the tissues in the flank area. The amount of laxity makes resection of the appropriate amount of soft tissue difficult using a full abdominoplasty incision without creating lateral dog-ears. Any excess adiposity in the posterior trunk can be treated with concurrent liposuction if the quality of the skin and the soft-tissue laxity are appropriate.

Preoperative Considerations (Box 8.2)

The preoperative considerations for extended abdominoplasty are the same as those for full or circumferential abdominoplasty. A focused history and physical examination should be performed. Any existing abdominal scars should be noted and discussed, as these may require modification of the abdominoplasty design in order to avoid complications (see Chapter 14, Management of Pre-Existing Abdominal Scars). Preoperative laboratory analysis may include a complete blood count, a basic metabolic panel, and a coagulation profile, but the precise studies should be tailored to suit the needs of the patient based on their medical history.

As with all abdominoplasty procedures, the most significant complication that can occur is DVT/PE and death. Because myofascial plication may result in increased intra-abdominal pressure and a compensatory reduction in venous return from the lower extremities, we require patients to wear an abdominal binder for 2 weeks preoperatively.[1,2] This serves two goals, including allowing the patient to get accustomed to wearing a binder, which they will have to do postoperatively, but – more importantly – preparing the patient's body for the increased intra-abdominal pressure associated with myofascial implications, which can have a negative effect on venous return and pulmonary function.

Exposure to tobacco or any other nicotine products should be avoided for 6 weeks preoperatively and several weeks postoperatively in order to reduce the deleterious effects of nicotine and other smoking byproducts on the healing process.[3,4] Similarly, we recommend that patients cease the use of birth control pills several weeks preoperatively in an attempt reduce the incidence of DVT/PE associated with these medications.[5] Patients are provided with a vitamin supplement pack preoperatively to make sure that the body's healing ability is optimized.

Operative Approach

The operative approach for extended abdominoplasty is almost identical to that for full abdominoplasty, which is discussed in great detail in Chapter 7. The same sequence of preoperative photographs and markings is used. The obvious difference is the longer transverse incision used for extended abdominoplasty (**Fig. 8.1**). Because of this, it may be necessary to have the assistant partially lift or roll the flank area when closure is performed. The entire case is performed with the patient supine unless liposuction of the back area is planned, in which case the procedure is performed prone first and then the patient is repositioned supine for the abdominoplasty component. Small areas of the flank may be liposuctioned while the patient is in the supine position.

In addition to a longer transverse scar, the amount of concurrent liposuction needed is often greater than with a full abdominoplasty. Frequently, liposuction of the lateral chest, flanks, and hips is performed concurrently with the extended abdominoplasty (**Fig. 8.1**).

A

D

B

E

C

F

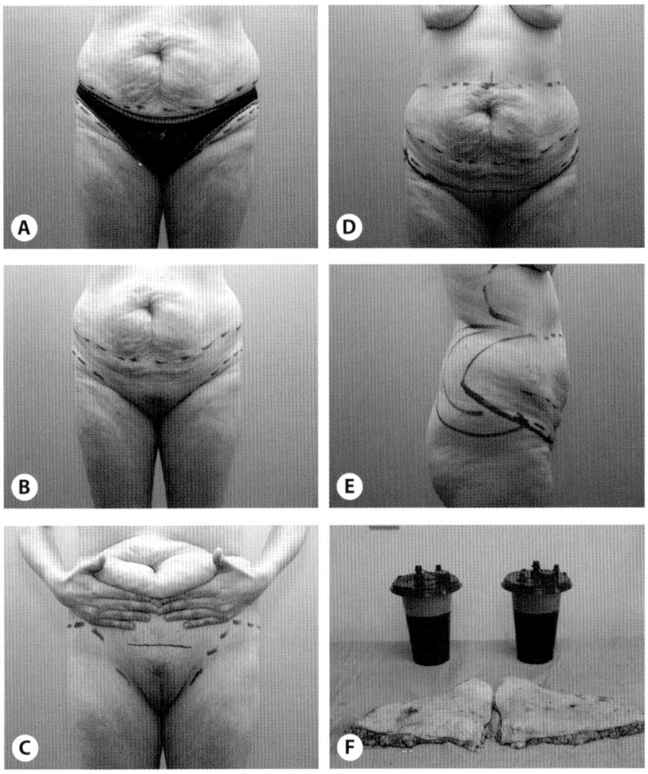

Fig. 8.1 **(A)** Patients with a strong desire to conceal the extended abdominoplasty scar are requested to wear revealing undergarments or swimwear. The borders of these garments can be marked ensuring that the final incision will be hidden. **(B)** After the markings of the swimwear are made, the proposed incision line can then be drawn. **(C)** We request our patients strongly lift their abdominal soft-tissue superiorly and then the initial transverse mark is made at the level of the symphysis pubis. **(D)** The incision line is then extended in a natural fold latterly to encompass the area for resection which is by definition greater than that of a full abdominoplasty. **(E)** The lateral extent of the incision is dependent upon the amount of soft-tissue laxity. In this case, the laxity extended to the posterior axillary line. The areas for liposuction are marked as well. Concurrent liposuction greatly enhances the final result by contouring adjacent areas, particularly the hip rolls and flanks, achieving a more harmonious contour. **(F)** The abdominoplasty resection is noted as well as the liposuction aspirate.

Postoperative Care (Box 8.3)

The postoperative care for a patient undergoing an extended abdominoplasty is identical to that for a full abdominoplasty and is covered in great detail in Chapter 7. Because of the larger extent of undermining and liposuction, the use of additional drains may be beneficial to prevent postoperative seroma. As there is a theoretical increase in the potential incidence of seroma following extended abdominoplasty, the proper use of an abdominal binder postoperatively is especially important. Before and after photographs are shown in **Figs 8.2–8.51**.

Box 8.3 Postoperative instructions for extended abdominoplasty

- Maintain a partially flexed position at the waist for the first 1–2 weeks
- Wear the abdominal binder at all times except for showering
- Make sure the abdominal binder is maintained low enough on the abdomen
- Verify that there are no significant creases, folds, or drain tubes underneath the binder. The drain should exit inferiorly from beneath the binder. Having the drain exit superiorly can result in the drain tubing pressing on the abdominal skin, and could result in ischemia
- Avoid smoking or exposure to nicotine-containing products
- Breathe deeply and use the incentive spirometer frequently
- Drink plenty of fluids: 8 oz/h is the goal
- Move legs frequently while resting, and walk regularly
- Drain care as instructed
- Continue to take multivitamin daily. Resume medications as instructed
- No vigorous activity or heavy lifting for 4–6 weeks

Figs 8.2–8.51 Extended abdominoplasty before and after images

Figs 8.2–8.13

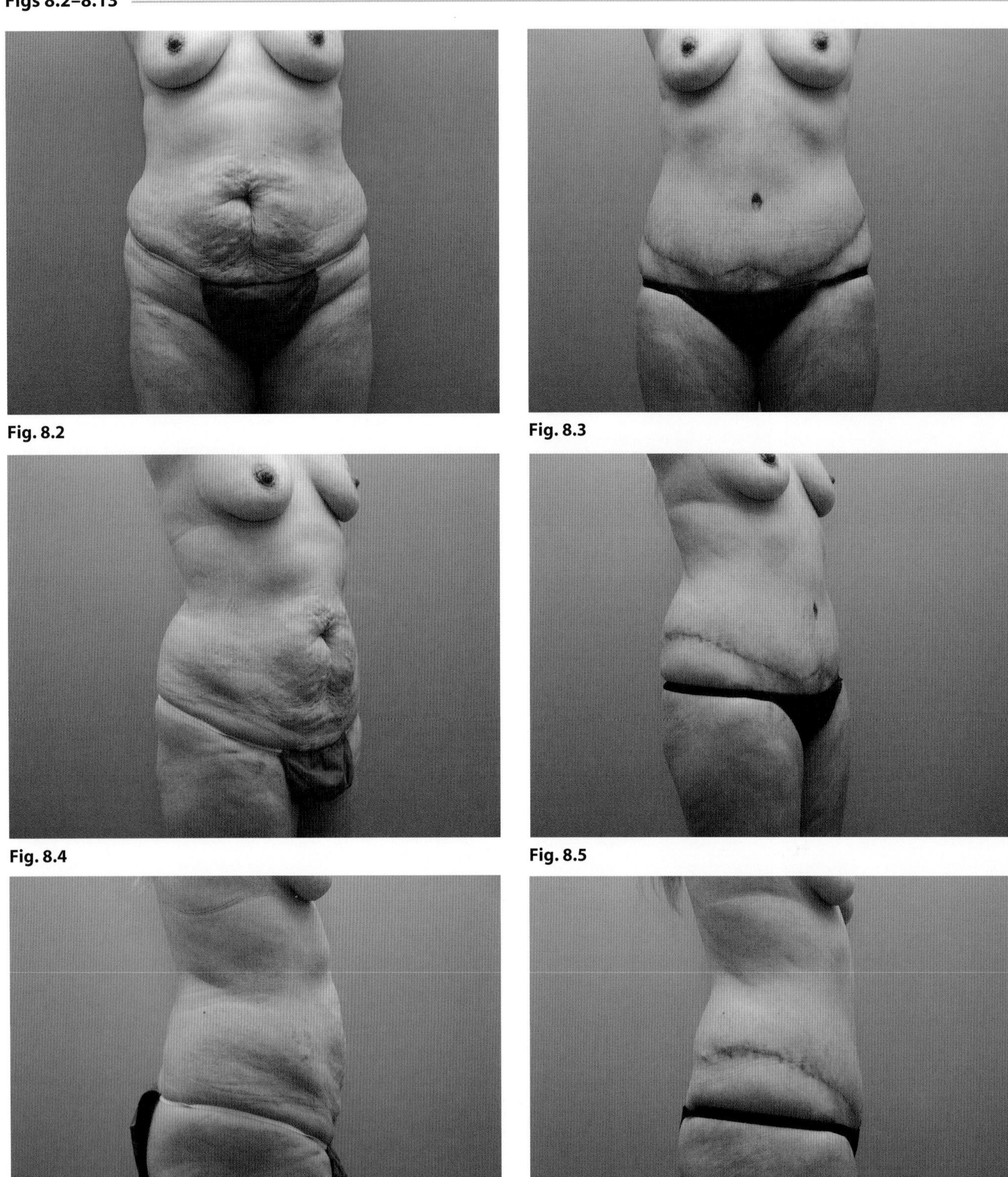

Fig. 8.2

Fig. 8.3

Fig. 8.4

Fig. 8.5

Fig. 8.6

Fig. 8.7

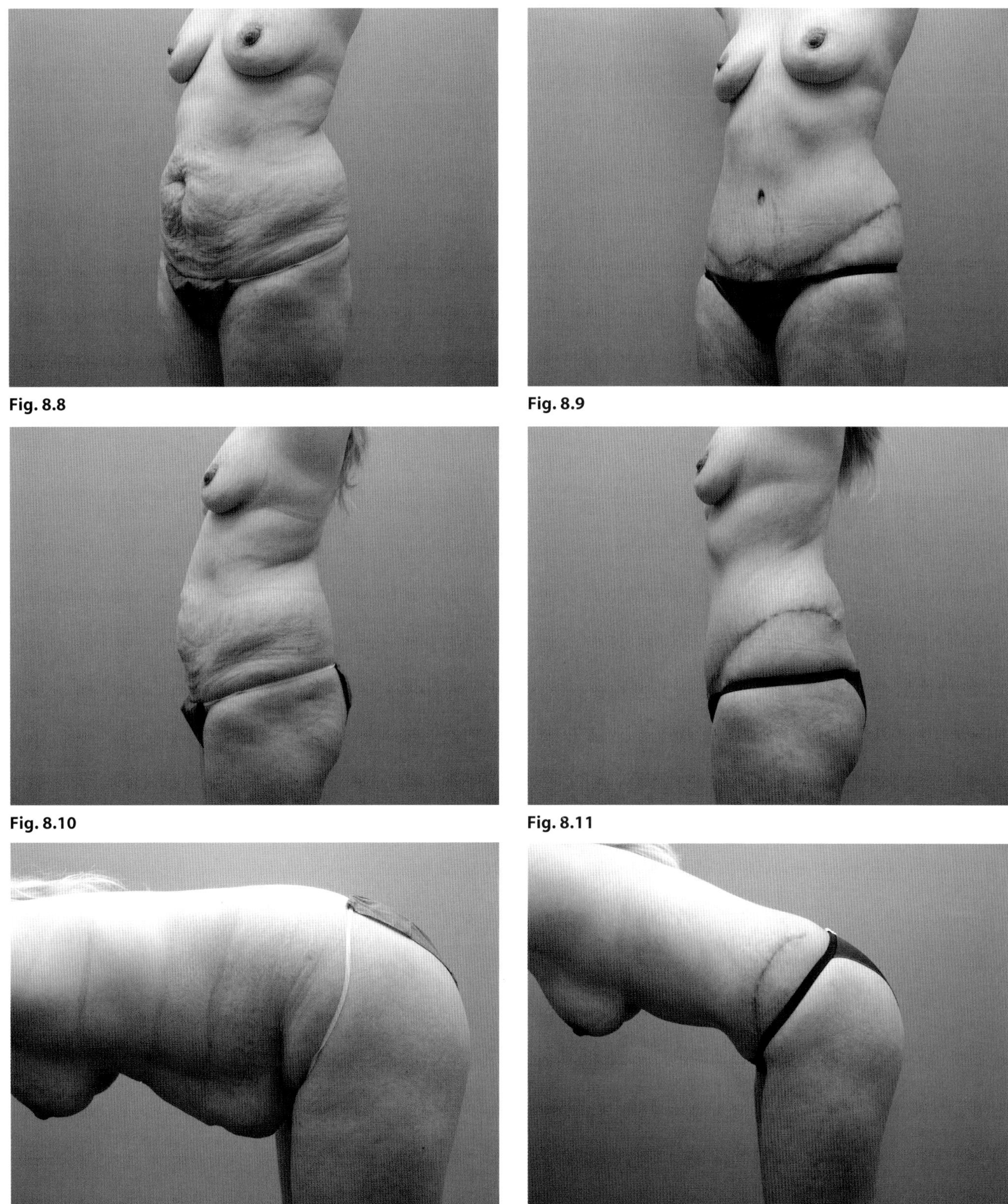

Fig. 8.8

Fig. 8.9

Fig. 8.10

Fig. 8.11

Fig. 8.12

Fig. 8.13

Fig. 8.2–8.13 This 31-year-old multiparous woman presented with concerns with abdominal and hip laxity, excess adiposity, and abdominal fullness. She was very concerned about the laxity and fullness of her hips. She underwent an extended abdominoplasty with concurrent liposuction of the abdomen, mons, and hip rolls. Significant contour improvement was achieved, with thinning, tightening, and flattening of the abdomen and a greatly enhanced silhouette. The diver's view shows the benefit of strong myofascial plication.

Figs 8.14–8.25

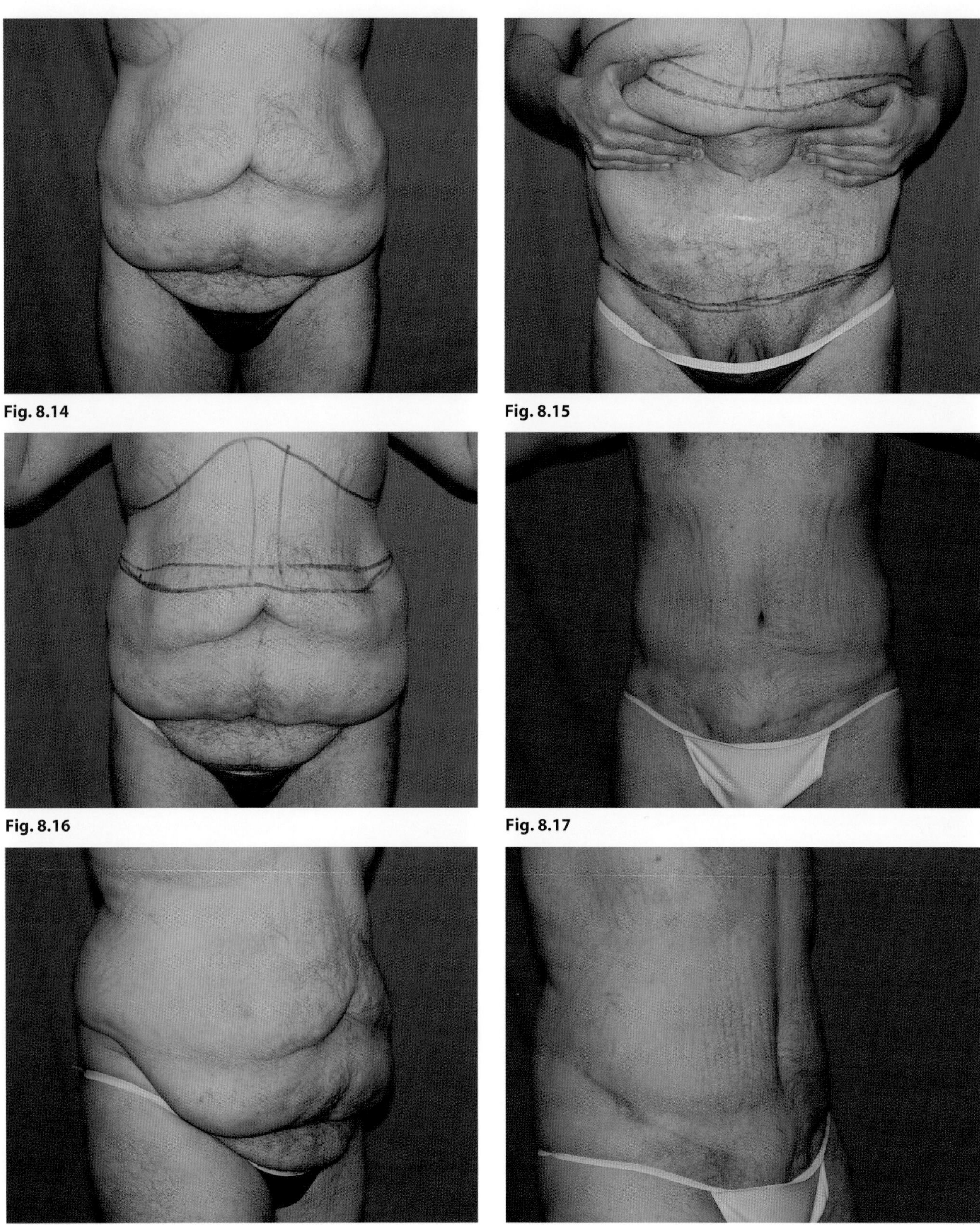

Fig. 8.14

Fig. 8.15

Fig. 8.16

Fig. 8.17

Fig. 8.18

Fig. 8.19

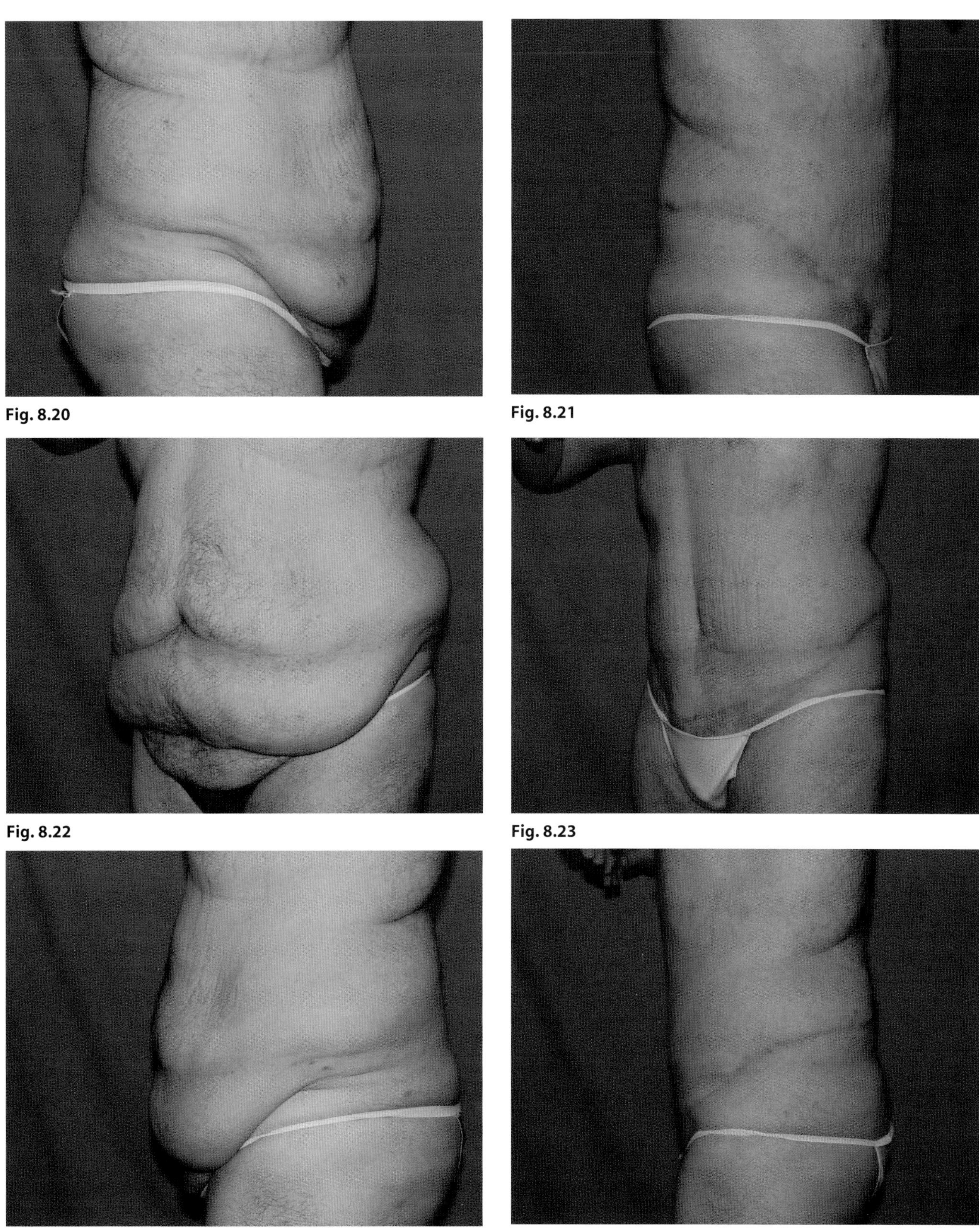

Fig. 8.20

Fig. 8.21

Fig. 8.22

Fig. 8.23

Fig. 8.24

Fig. 8.25

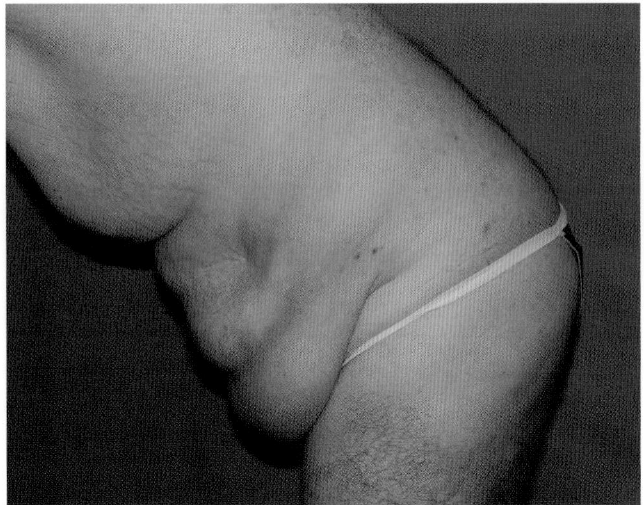

Fig. 8.26

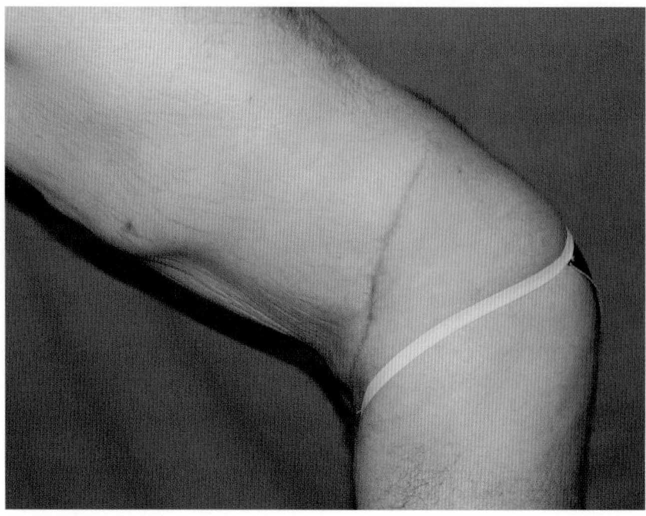

Fig. 8.27

Fig. 8.14–8.27 This 35–year-old man lost 40 kg with diet and exercise. He presented with marked laxity and redundancy of the abdomen and hips. The large abdominal soft-tissue apron bothered him a great deal. He underwent an extended abdominoplasty with thorough liposuction of the abdomen, pubic area, and hip rolls, which dramatically enhanced his overall contour. He was pleased with his enhanced shape, improved umbilical appearance, and flat abdomen.

Figs 8.28–8.30

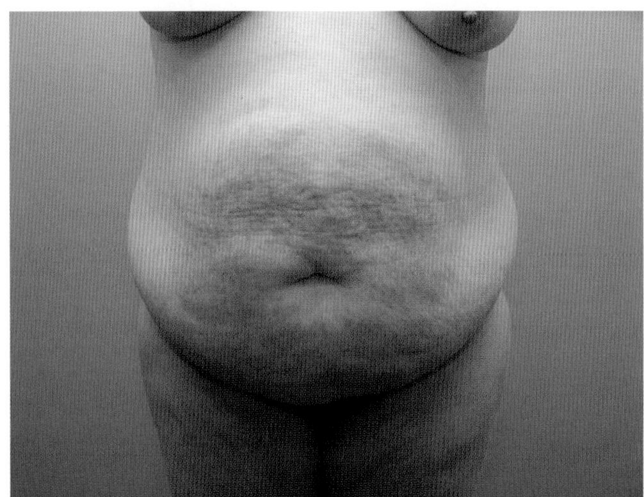

Fig. 8.28

Fig. 8.29

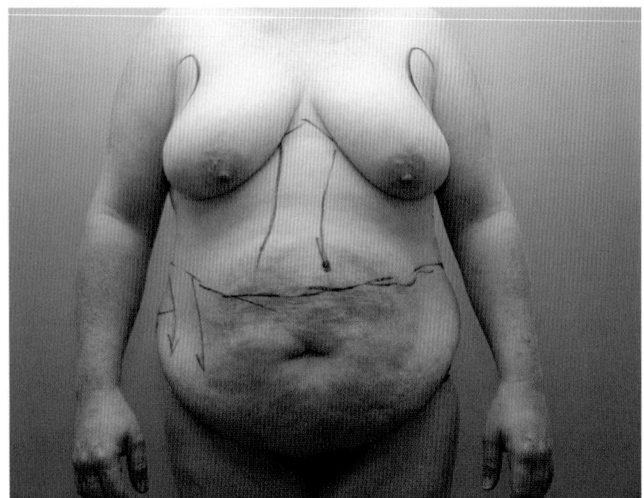

Fig. 8.30

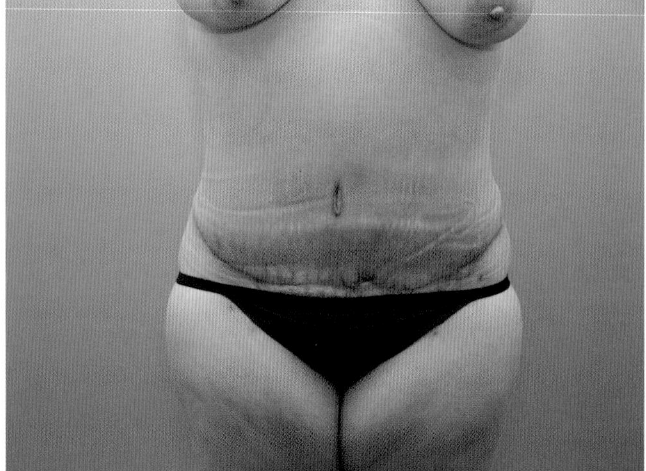

Fig. 8.31

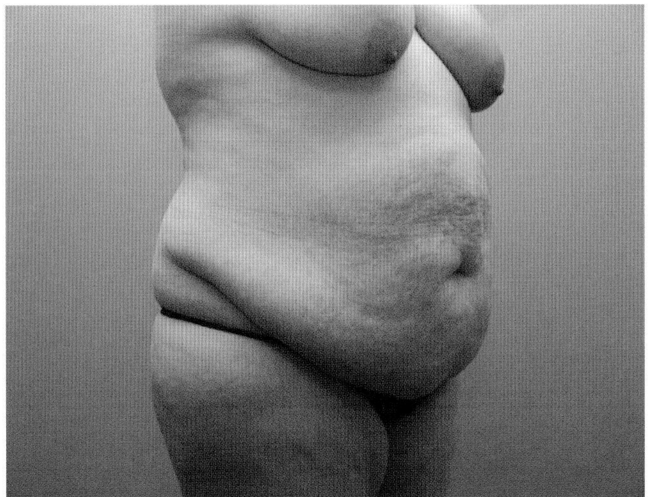

Fig. 8.32

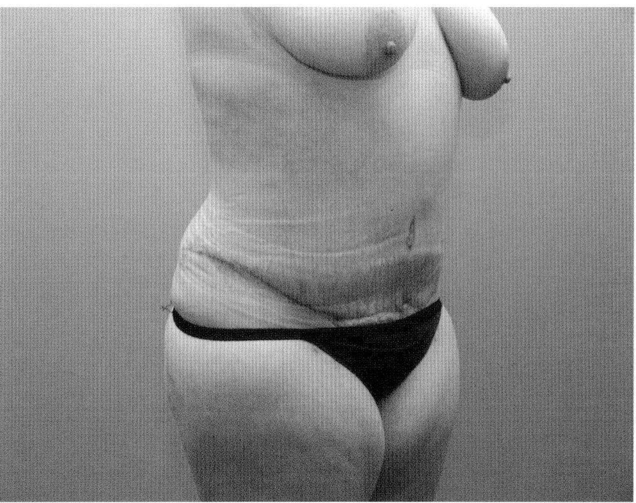

Fig. 8.33

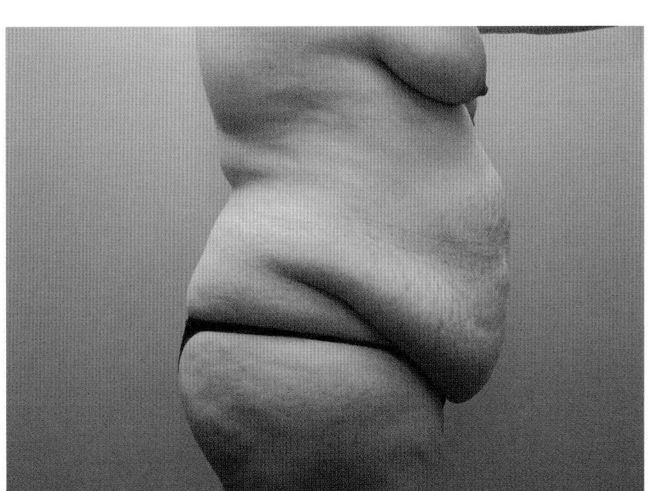

Fig. 8.34

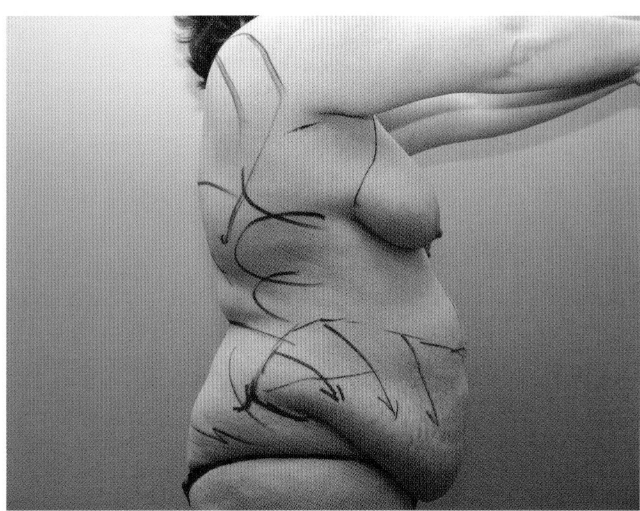

Fig. 8.35

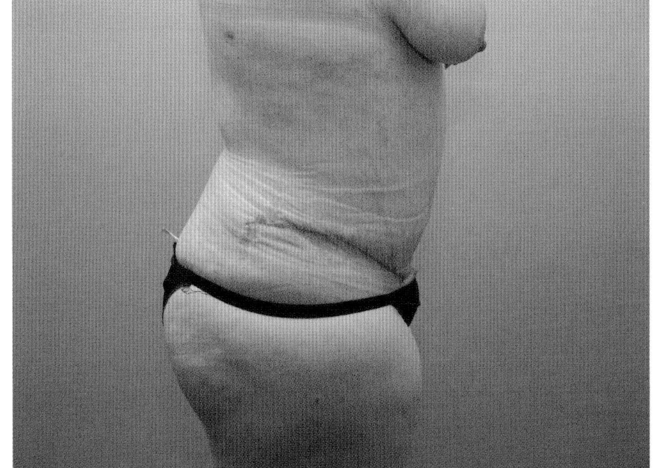

Fig. 8.36

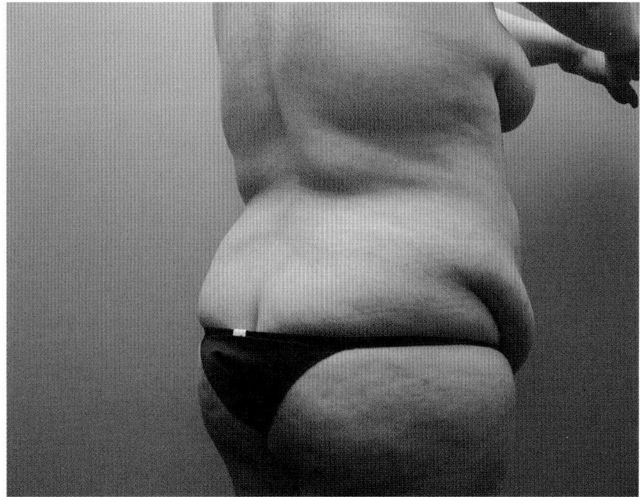

Fig. 8.37

Figs 8.38–8.49

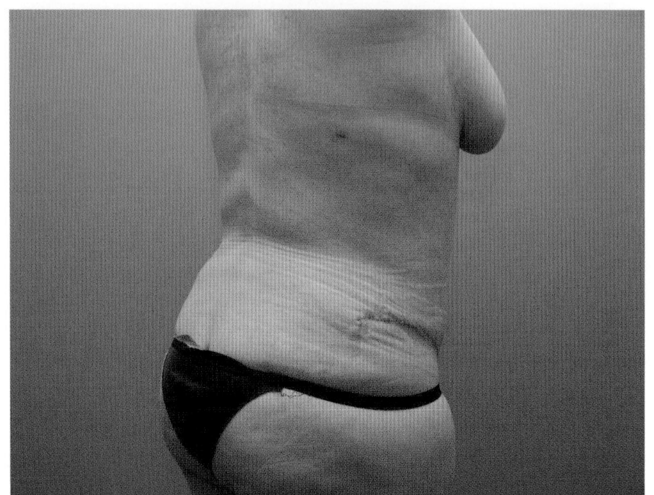
Fig. 8.38

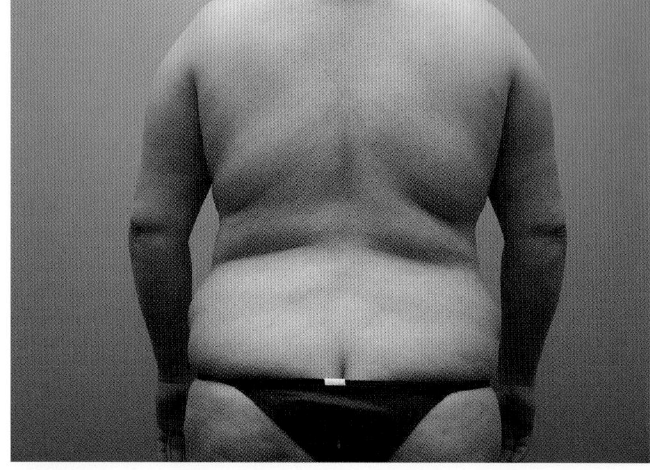
Fig. 8.39

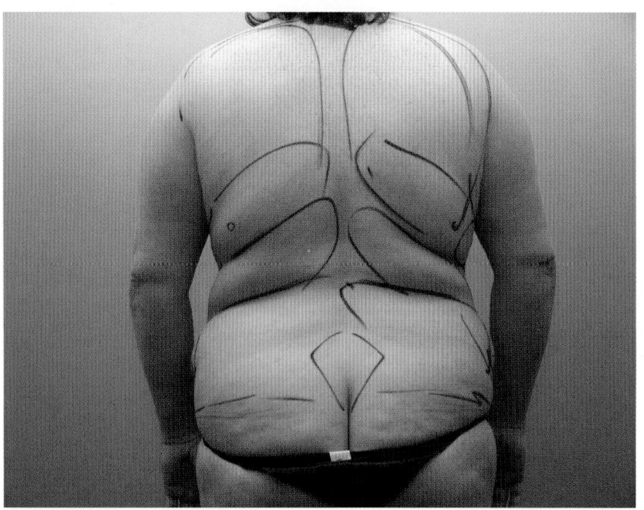
Fig. 8.40

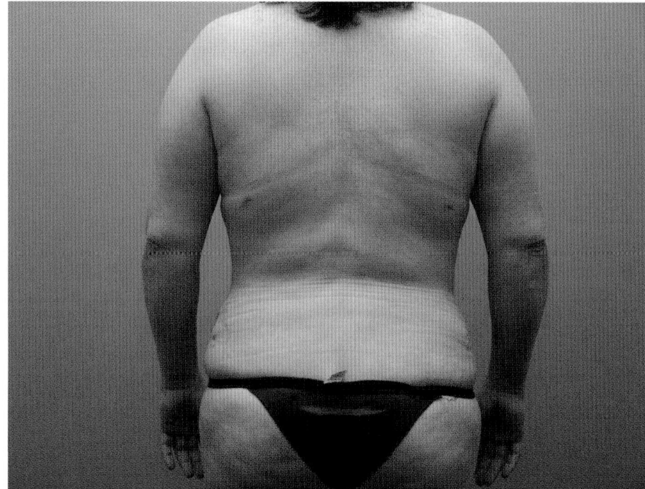
Fig. 8.41

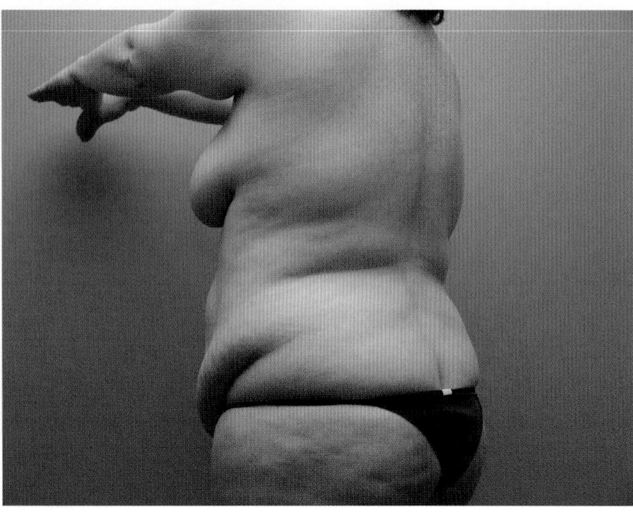
Fig. 8.42

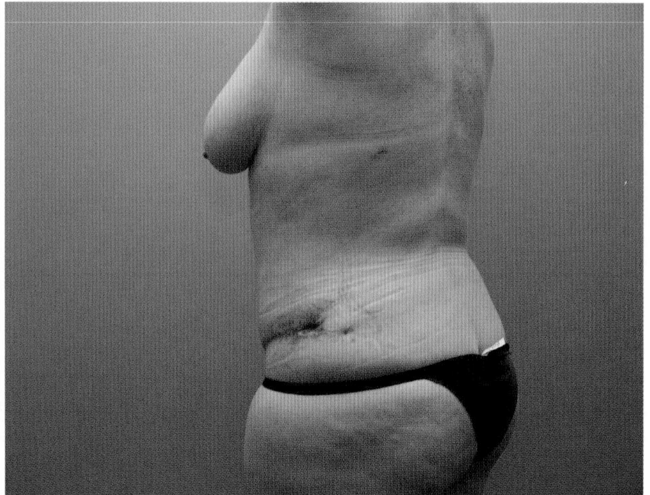
Fig. 8.43

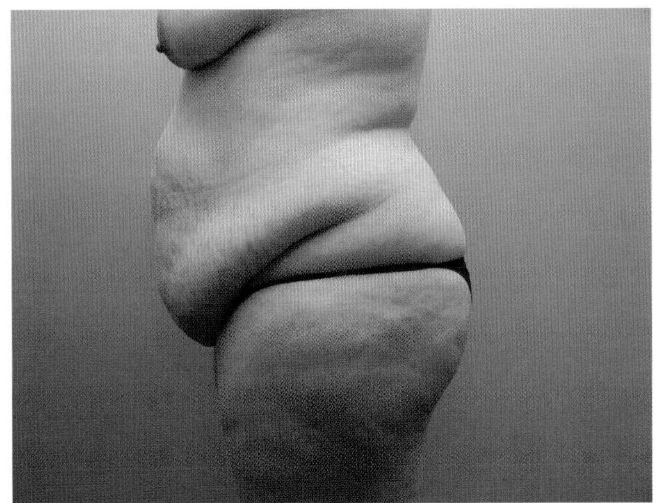
Fig. 8.44

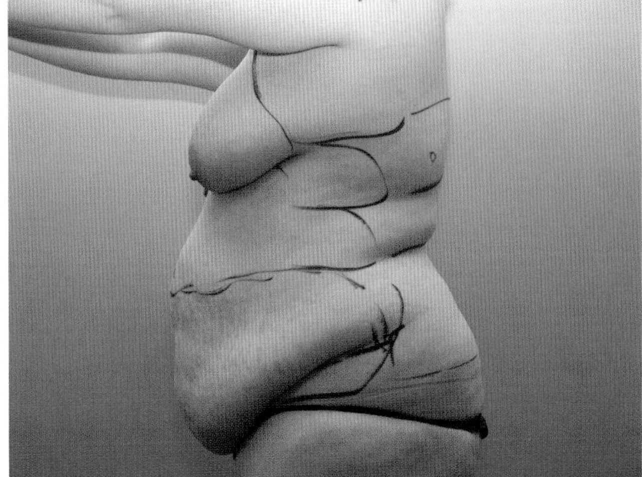
Fig. 8.45

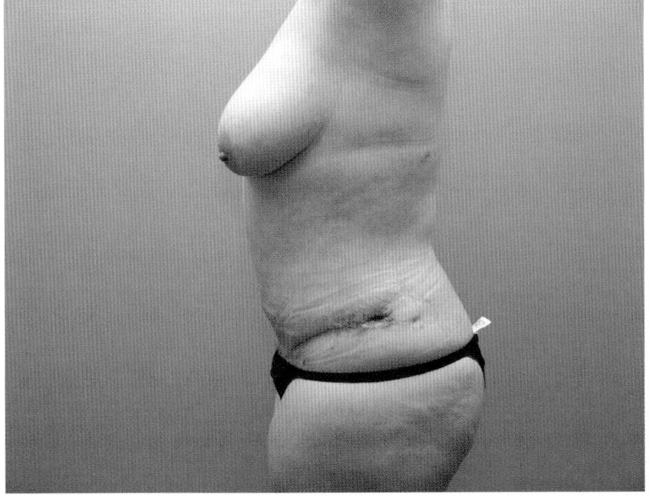
Fig. 8.46

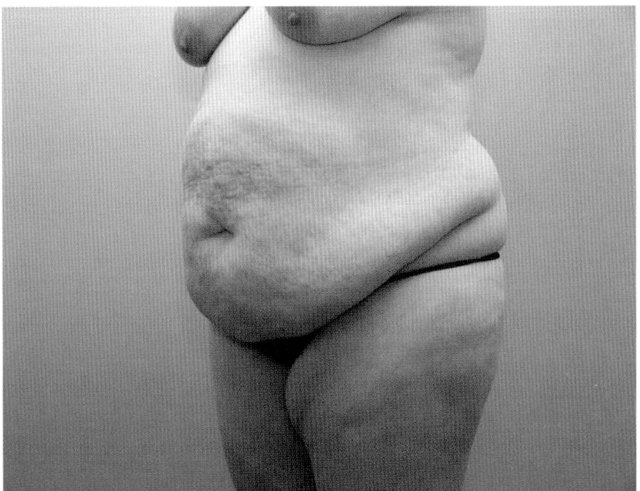
Fig. 8.47

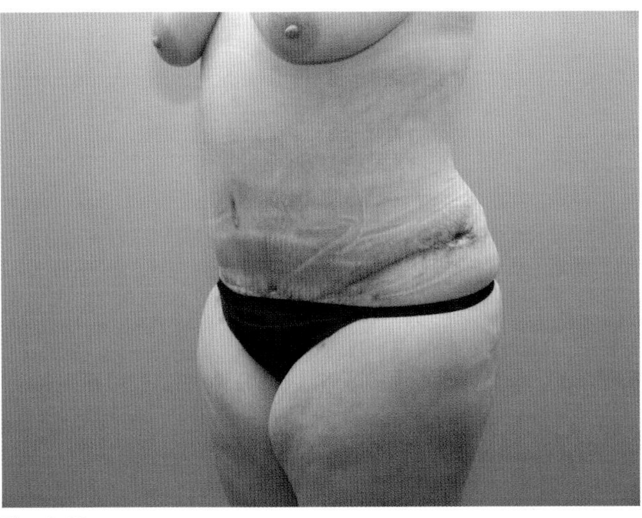
Fig. 8.48

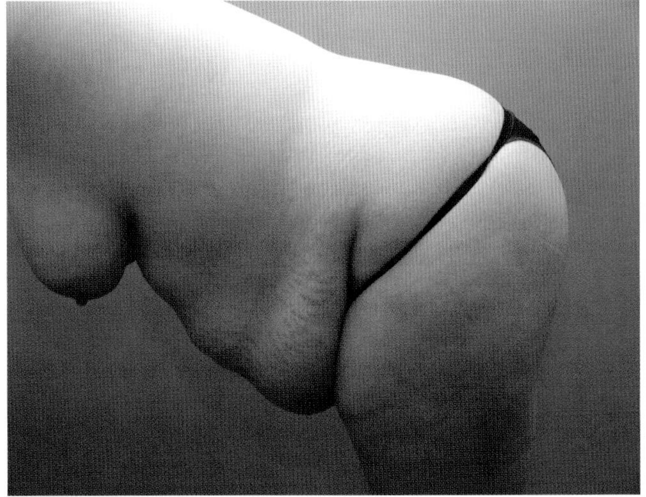
Fig. 8.49

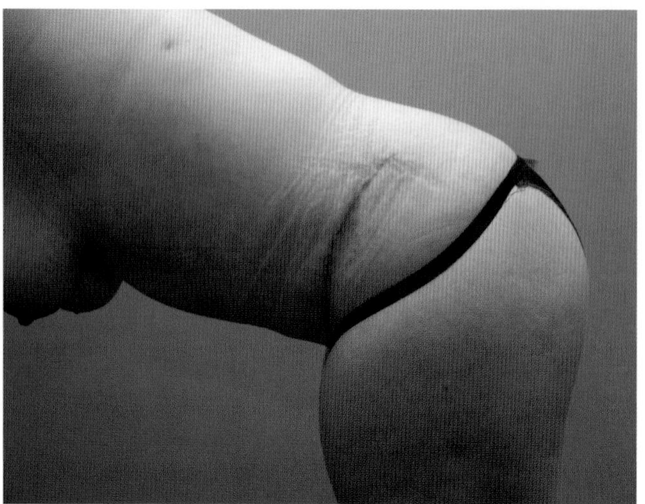

Fig. 8.50

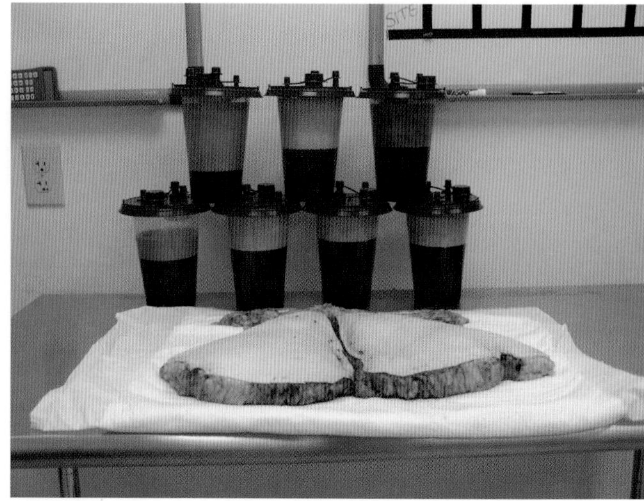

Fig. 8.51

Fig. 8.28–8.50 This 38-year-old woman presented for consultation weighing 86 kg with a height of 5′3″. She had a BMI of 39, was relatively healthy with a stable weight, and was not on any medications. She underwent an extended abdominoplasty with full liposuction of the abdomen, back, and mons. During surgery, the skin and fat resected weighed 4244 g and the volume of fat liposuctioned was 5.5 L. She experienced a dramatic improvement in overall shape and contour. Her posture improved following removal of the pannus and excess adiposity. The large redundant back rolls and folds were eliminated by thorough liposuction. The abdominoplasty resection and the total liposuction aspirate are shown in **Fig. 8.51**.

Conclusion/Brief Summary

The extended abdominoplasty procedure is ideal for treating patients who have excess adiposity and soft-tissue laxity greater than would be properly cared for with a full abdominoplasty. Extending the transverse incision laterally up to and beyond the midaxillary line allows proper resection of soft-tissue laxity without creating lateral dog-ears. The longer incision does little to increase patient morbidity, but provides for a much better overall result as well as increased patient satisfaction. Choosing to perform an extended as opposed to a full abdominoplasty reduces the need for future revisions and touch-ups for this selected group of patients.

Clinical Caveats: Extended Abdominoplasty

- A variety of surgical options are available for patients requesting abdominoplasty or abdominal contouring. Each procedure should be tailored based on the goals of the patient and the best aesthetic result possible
- The extended abdominoplasty is best indicated for patients with significant abdominal and flank laxity but not sufficient to warrant a circumferential abdominoplasty, or for patients who do not wish to have a posterior scar
- Preoperative instructions/requirements must be methodically followed to maximize safety
- Preoperative markings and photographs are invaluable to achieve the best possible results
- Concurrent liposuction of the abdominal soft-tissue apron and the surrounding area, particularly the rolls, is of great value, especially for the patient with incomplete weight loss or those who have moderate to significant excess adiposity
- It is often better to close the umbilical defect and have a small inverted 'T' inferiorly in the midline if there is insufficient laxity to allow the umbilicus location to be included in the resection. Preoperative discussion with the patient about this possibility is recommended. However, this is rarely necessary with patients who need an extended abdominoplasty
- Myofascial plication is almost always indicated and beneficial in achieving optimal contour in abdominoplasty procedures
- During closure, strong advancement medially of the upper skin edges bilaterally will reduce or eliminate the incidence of dog-ears and enhance the final shape of the waist
- Subscarpal fat resection can be performed safely as indicated
- Injection of bupivacaine into the rectus sheath will help reduce postoperative discomfort. This facilitates deep breathing and reduces pain medication use postoperatively
- Overnight care in an accredited facility will allow better fluid status management and pain control, and reduce the chance of DVT through the use of pneumatic compression devices and ambulation
- Evaluation postoperative day 1 and regularly over the first week will allow proper intervention if postoperative care issues arise

References

1. Huang GJ, Bajaj AK, Gupta S, et al. Increased intraabdominal pressure in abdominoplasty: delineation of risk factors. Plast Reconstruct Surg 2007; 119: 1319.
2. Al-Basti HB, El-Khatib HA, Taha A, et al. Intraabdominal pressure after full abdominoplasty in obese multiparous patients. Plast Reconstruct Surg 2004; 113: 2145.
3. Manassa EH, Hertl CH, Olbrisch RR. Wound healing problems in smokers and non-smokers after 132 abdominoplasties. Plast Reconstruct Surg 2003; 111: 2082.
4. Krueger JK, Rohrich RJ. Clearing the smoke: the scientific rationale for tobacco abstention with plastic surgery. Plast Reconstruct Surg 2001; 108: 1063.
5. Blickstein D, Blickstein I. Oral contraception and thrombophilia. Curr Opin Obstet Gynecol 2007; 19: 370.

Suggested Reading

Cardenas-Camarena L, Gonzales LE. Large-volume liposuction and extensive abdominoplasty: A feasible alternative for improving body shape. Plast Reconstruct Surg 1998; 102: 1698.

Dillerud E. Abdominoplasty combined with suction lipoplasty: A study of complications, revisions, and risk factors in 487 cases. Ann Plast Surg 1990; 25: 333.

Grazer FM, Goldwyn RM. Abdominoplasty assessed by survey, with emphasis on complications. Plast Reconstruct Surg 1977; 59: 513.

Grazer FM. Abdominoplasty. Plast Reconstruct Surg 1973; 51: 617.

Hafezi F, Nouhi A. Safe abdominoplasty with extensive liposuctioning. Ann Plast Surg 2006; 57: 149.

Hester RT Jr., Baird W, Bostwick J III, et al. Abdominoplasty combined with other surgical procedures: Safe or sorry? Plast Reconstruct Surg 1989; 83: 997.

Hunstad JP. Advanced concepts in abdominoplasty. Perspect Plast Surg 1998; 12: 13.

Hunstad JP. Body contouring in the obese patient. Clin Plast Surg 1996; 23: 647.

Lee MJ, Mustoe TA. A simplified version to achieve aesthetic results for the umbilicus in abdominoplasty. Plast Reconstruct Surg 2002; 109: 2136.

Lockwood TE. High-lateral-tension abdominoplasty with superficial fascial system suspension. Plast Reconstruct Surg 1995; 96: 60.

Matarasso A. Abdominoplasty: A system of classification and treatment for combined abdominoplasty and suction-assisted lipectomy. Aesthet Plast Surg 1991; 15: 111–121.

Matarasso A. Awareness and avoidance of abdominoplasty complications. Aesthet Surg J 1997; 17: 256.

Matarasso A, Swift RW, Rankin M. Abdominoplasty and abdominal contour surgery: a national plastic surgery survey. Plast Reconstruct Surg 2006; 117: 1797.

Matarasso A. The male abdominoplasty. Clin Plast Surg 2004; 31: 555.

Netscher DT, Wigoda P, Spira M, Peltier M. Musculoaponeurotic plication in abdominoplasty: How durable are its effects? Aesthet Plast Surg 1995; 19: 531.

Kim J, Stevenson TR. Abdominoplasty, liposuction of the flanks, and obesity: analyzing risk factors for seroma formation. Plast Reconstruct Surg 2006; 117: 77.

Pitanguy I. Abdominal lipectomy. Clin Plast Surg 1975; 2: 401.

Spiegelman JI, Levine RH. Abdominoplasty: a comparison of outpatient and inpatient procedures shows that it is a safe and effective procedure for outpatients in an office-based surgery clinic. Plast Reconstruct Surg 2006; 118: 517.

Teimourian B, Gotkin RH. Contouring of the midtrunk in overweight patients. Aesthet Plast Surg 1989; 13: 145.

Vastine VL, Morgan RF, Williams GS, et al. Wounds complications of abdominoplasty in obese patients. Ann Plast Surg 1999; 42: 34.

9

CHAPTER 9

Circumferential Abdominoplasty

Joseph P. Hunstad and Remus Repta

IN THIS CHAPTER

KEY POINTS

Circumferential abdominoplasty is an ideal procedure for patients who have experienced massive weight loss and who have circumferential tissue laxity of the trunk. This procedure requires the patient to be repositioned during the case. It is performed with the patient prone initially and then in the supine position. This is more efficient than the three-position technique using the left and right lateral decubitus positions followed by the supine position. It can achieve greater symmetry, particularly of the buttocks, because both sides are treated simultaneously. Circumferential abdominoplasty allows for complete correction of buttock ptosis, lateral and anterior thigh laxity, abdominal tissue redundancy, and mons ptosis. It also allows for concurrent strong myofascial plication, which further improves abdominal contour. Circumferential abdominoplasty can be combined with autologous buttock augmentation, vertical abdominal tissue resection, mons reduction, or any number of other ancillary procedures (see Chapter 13, Ancillary Procedures).

Introduction

Circumferential abdominoplasty, also referred to as a body lift, is the most powerful form of midbody or trunk contouring. It differs from belt lipectomy in its concurrent use of thorough tumescent liposuction, strong myofascial plication, and often subscarpal fat resection. In addition, the resection is usually centered lower on the trunk, with a final scar placement that is more caudal than in belt lipectomy.[1,2] The combination of circumferential soft-tissue resection and myofascial plication achieves a profound improvement in body shape and contour for patients with soft-tissue redundancy, abdominal wall laxity, and buttock ptosis. This procedure allows maximal soft-tissue resection without the need to modify the resection pattern to prevent dog-ears.

Patient Selection (Box 9.1)

Patient selection criteria for circumferential abdominoplasty include the same criteria as for full abdominoplasty plus the addition of buttock ptosis, lateral and posterior thigh laxity, and patient acceptance of a circumferential incision. Patients will often demonstrate their desire for circumferential abdominoplasty by pulling their thigh and buttock skin upwards, demonstrating correction of anterior and lateral thigh soft-tissue laxity as well as correction of buttock shape and ptosis (**Fig. 9.1**).

Box 9.1 Relative contraindications for circumferential abdominoplasty

The relative contraindications are similar to those for full abdominoplasty. Because the circumferential abdominoplasty is a more extensive operation, the importance of minimizing these potential sources of complications should be emphasized.

- Smoking
- Diabetes mellitus
- Malnutrition
- Various wound healing disorders
- Bowel/bladder dysfunction
- Immunodeficiency
- Medications that inhibit blood coagulation
- A significant history of pulmonary or deep vein thrombosis
- Lower extremity lymphedema/venous insufficiency
- Significant medical problems, including COPD/pulmonary issues, renal insufficiency, anemia, and other systemic issues that may make abdominal tightening surgery dangerous

Note: Age alone should not be a contraindication to abdominoplasty procedures if the patient is in good health. Patients who have a history of chronic pain should also be approached cautiously, as postoperative care may be significantly affected.

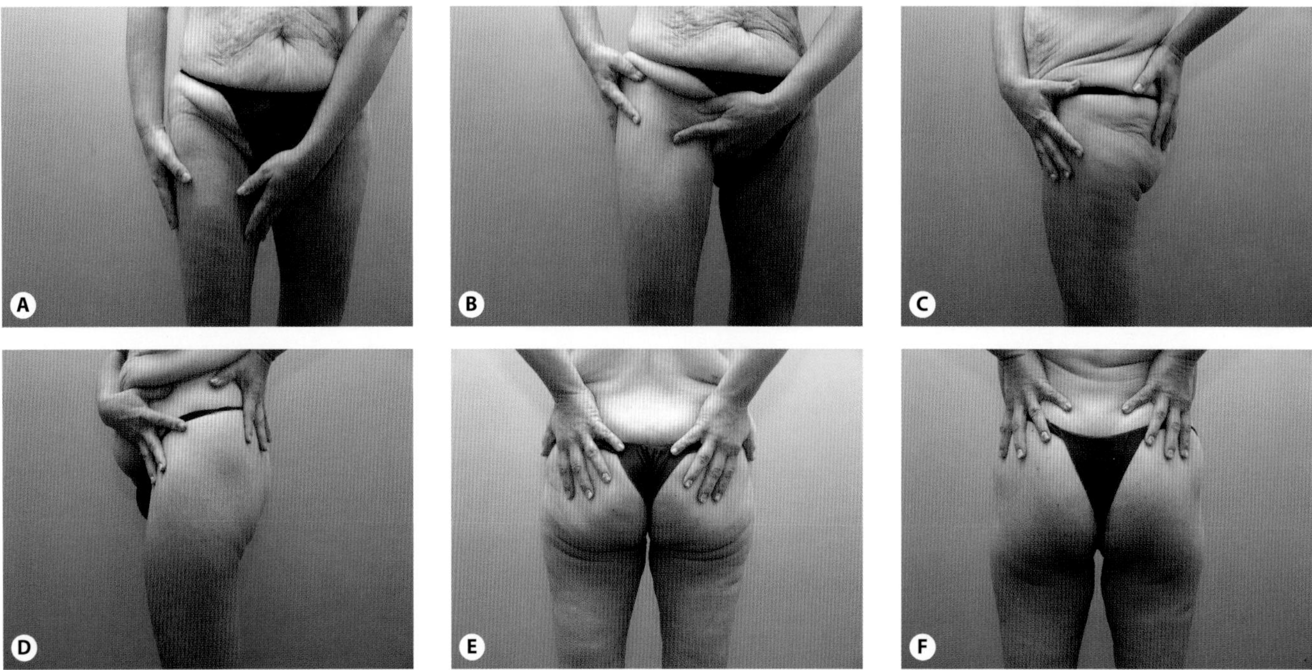

Fig. 9.1 Patients presenting for circumferential abdominoplasty usually demonstrate their desired goal by pulling up on the lax soft tissue of the thighs, hips, buttocks, and abdomen.

Preoperative History and Considerations (Box 9.2)

The patient's general health status is important and should be evaluated. Patients who have experienced massive weight loss, particularly following gastric bypass, may be at risk for healing issues related to malnutrition or other metabolic abnormalities.[3] Complete weight loss is classified as massive weight loss where the patient's residual deformity is essentially that of skin redundancy without excess adiposity, i.e. weight loss of usually more than 100 lb. Basic laboratory tests may include full blood count and a basic metabolic panel, as well as total protein and albumin. If these are within normal parameters then normal wound healing can be expected. If they are not, nutritional correction is needed preoperatively to avoid healing problems. Additional preoperative laboratory analysis is dependent on the facility at which the procedure is to be performed, surgeon and anesthesiologist preference, and any existing health issues the patient may have. For a healthy patient taking no pertinent medications, basic preoperative laboratory analysis should be considered and may include CBC, Chem 7, pregnancy test, and a standard coagulation profile (PT/PTT/INR).

Existing abdominal scars should be diligently taken into account, as these can have a significant impact on the safety and final aesthetic result of the abdominoplasty (see Chapter 14, Management of Pre-Existing Abdominal Scars).[4] Because smoking can have significant negative effects on healing, patients are asked to refrain from smoking or from exposure to tobacco products for 6 weeks preoperatively.[5,6] As most circumferential abdominoplasty patients undergo myofascial plication as part of the procedure, any existing history of pulmonary, bowel, or bladder dysfunction should be considered a relative contraindication, as this can result in worsening of these existing conditions postoperatively.

Box 9.2 Preoperative recommendations for circumferential abdominoplasty

- Smoking cessation/avoidance of nicotine exposure for 6 weeks prior to surgery
- Multivitamin daily
- Stop aspirin/other blood thinning products with primary care doctor's permission
- Abstain from all dietary/herbal supplements not approved by the surgeon
- Basic laboratory work should be tailored to each patient. It may include CBC, Chem 7, Factor V Liden and PT/PTT/INR. Nutritional values, including albumin, may be warranted especially in gastric bypass patients
- Medical clearance if needed
- Wearing abdominal binder for 2 weeks before surgery
- Shower with a gentle antimicrobial soap the night before and day of surgery

Thromboembolism (DVT/PE) is the most serious and worrisome complication of abdominoplasty and other body

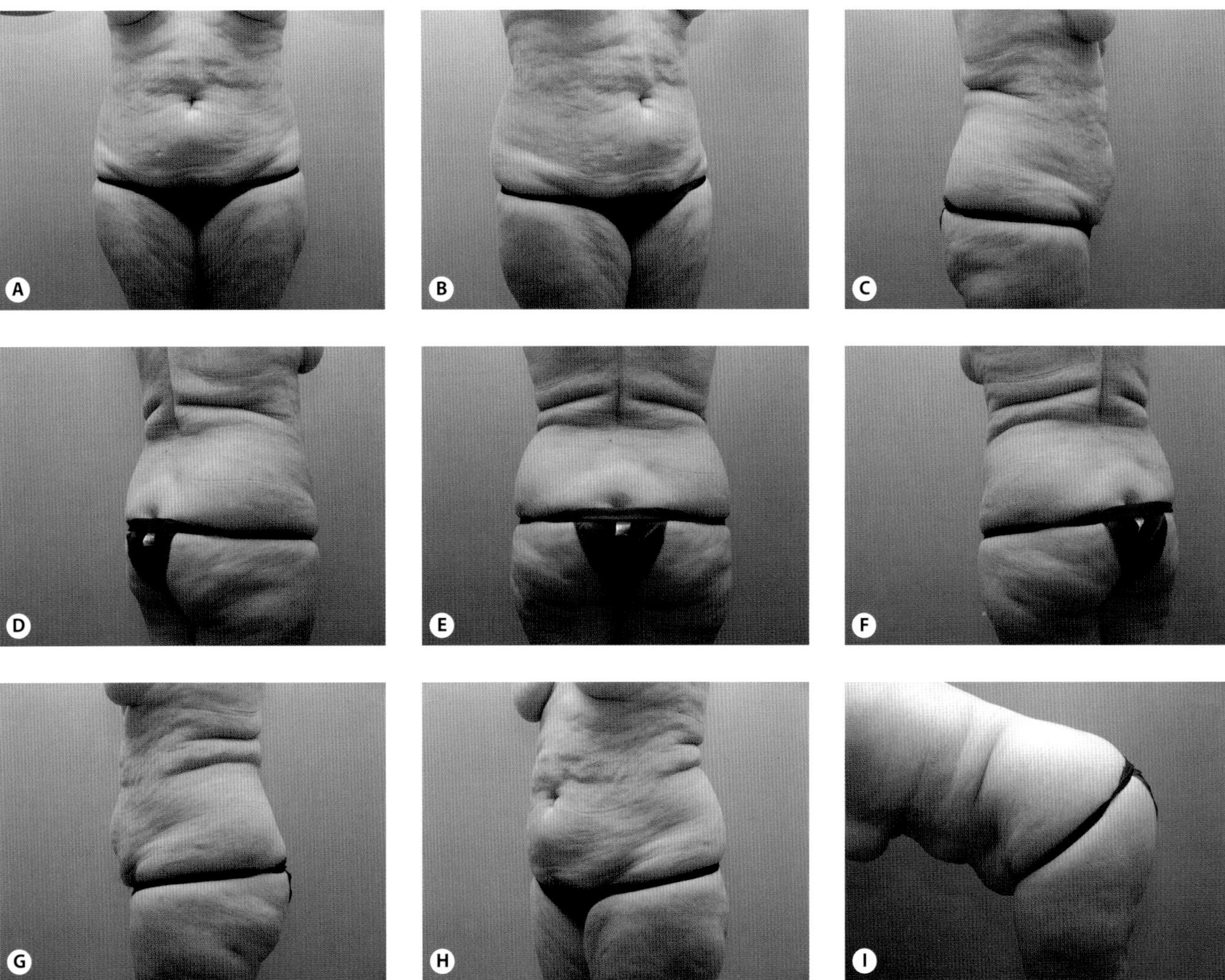

Fig. 9.2 Circumferential abdominoplasty pictures are taken in nine cardinal views. The patient should be relaxed to eliminate tightening of the abdomen and rectus muscles, which allows accurate evaluation of contour and shape. All photographs should include the area from the costal margins to the mid-thigh, because some thigh elevation will occur with this procedure **(A)**. **Figures 9.2B and 9.2H** are left and right oblique views demonstrating the waist, the extent of abdominal laxity, and the anterior thighs and hips. **Figures 9.2C and 9.2G** are left and right lateral views, which further demonstrate the abdominal contour. (**D–F**) Right and left posterior oblique views and the posterior view. These views are helpful in evaluating the buttocks and hip rolls. (**I**) The diver's view, which shows the true degree of abdominal laxity.

contouring procedures: a personal or family history of DVT/PE puts the patient at an elevated risk for similar problems. Appropriate referral and hematologic workup should be obtained prior to the abdominal contouring procedure. There is evidence that hormone replacement therapy and birth control medications can also increase the risk of PE/DVT, and so we discuss this issue with patients and, if feasible, the medications are stopped for several week prior to surgery.[7,8] The appropriate use of lower extremity compression devices, proper intraoperative positioning, perioperative prophylactic medication, and early postoperative ambulation can help reduce the chance of DVT/PE developing.[9,10]

Operative Approach

Preoperative photographs are obtained in the nine cardinal positions: anterior, left and right anterior oblique, left and right lateral, left and right posterior oblique, posterior, and diver's view (**Fig. 9.2**).

The markings for circumferential abdominoplasty begin with the patient strongly lifting the redundant abdominal soft tissue vertically in a cephalad direction. Doing so replicates the tension forces on the final scar that will exist after closure of the incision. With the patient lifting up, the central part of the transverse incision is marked at the level of the pubic symphysis (**Fig. 9.3**). The proposed final incision is then marked in a natural skin fold coursing laterally towards the anterior superior iliac crest (**Fig. 9.4**). The incision continues laterally and posteriorly, ending at the superior level of the buttocks. By reviewing the marking with the patient in a full-length mirror preoperatively, they can help decide on the final position of the incision. Wearing revealing undergarments or the bottom half of a two-piece swimsuit can also help determine the optimum position of the final scar (**Fig. 9.5**).

Once the final position of the scar has been determined, the amount of skin to be resected is identified and marked. This decision process should begin in the mid-axillary line. Using bimanual palpation, the excess tissue to be resected is grasped. Patients will often try and help by leaning toward the surgeon during this process. This should be avoided, as it will result in an overestimation, and to make sure that this does not occur, the patient is asked to place their opposite hand against the wall and lean slightly away from the surgeon (**Fig. 9.6**). This will help prevent over-resection, which is most likely to occur in the midaxillary line! Once they are leaning slightly away from the surgeon, the markings are made. The lower marking is then extended anteriorly to join with the previously marked transverse incision (**Fig. 9.7**).

The average amount of tissue to be resected in the midaxillary line is between 17 and 21 cm. In the most significant case of massive weight loss and tissue laxity, a vertical width of 42 cm has been resected in the midaxillary line! (**Fig. 9.8**). This measurement is repeated on the opposite side to ensure symmetry (**Fig. 9.9**). These are the most critical preoperative markings.

With the patient facing away from the surgeon, bimanual palpation continues at multiple points from the midaxillary

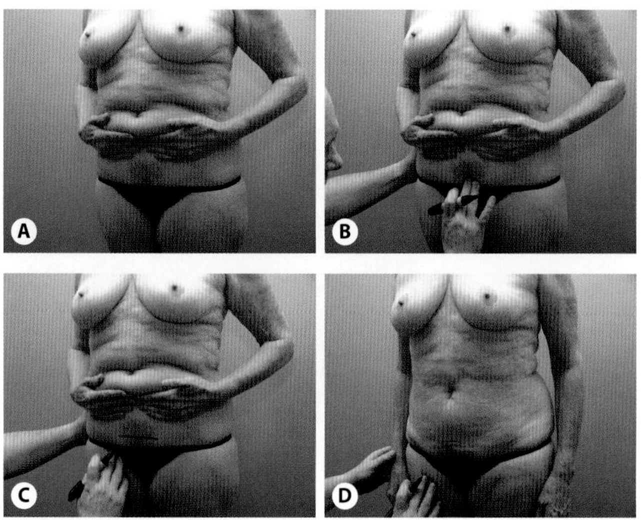

Fig. 9.3 With the patient strongly lifting the abdominal soft tissue in a smooth even manner, the lower transverse midline incision is marked (**A–D**). This mark is placed approximately at the level of or slightly superior to the symphysis pubis, which corresponds to the junction of the upper and middle third of the hair bearing mons (**C**).

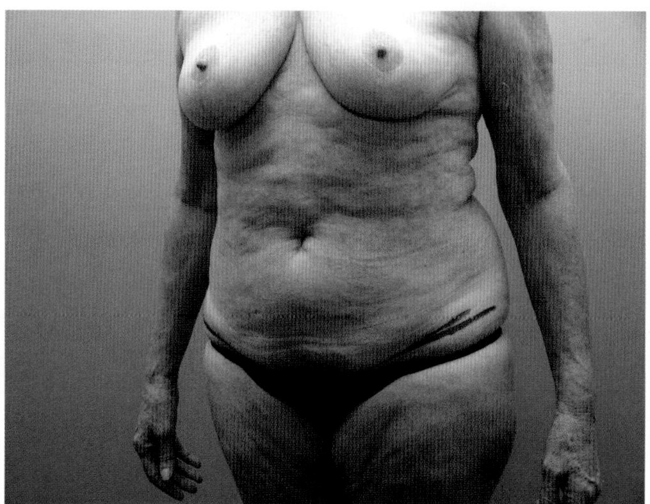

Fig. 9.4 This initial transverse mark is then extended laterally in a natural skin fold to be placed at a level the surgeon and patient have agreed on. The lateral height and extent of the incision are measured on each side to ensure symmetry.

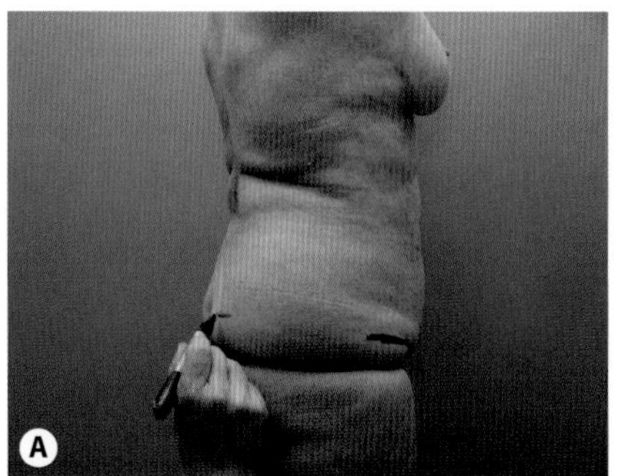

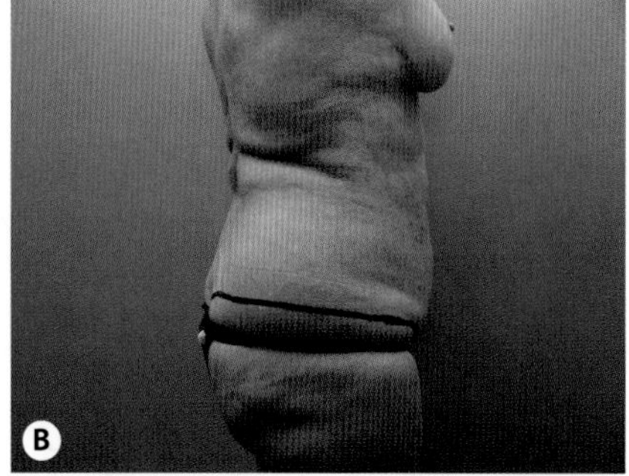

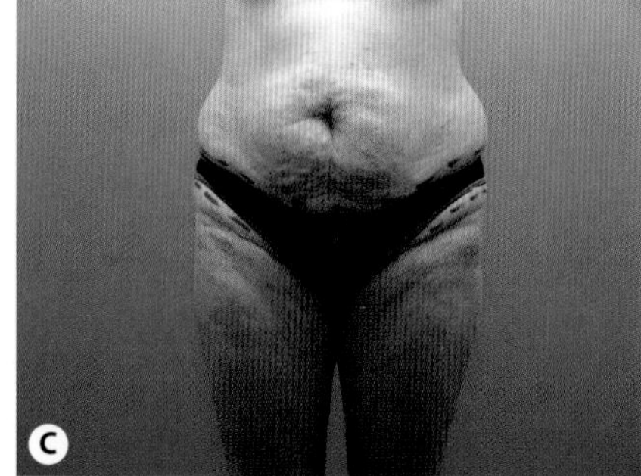

Fig. 9.5 The anterior mark is continued and connected laterally and posteriorly to the superior level of the buttocks (**A, B**). Having the patient wear a revealing undergarment or their swimsuit of choice and reviewing the marks with the patient will help further ensure the proper placement and concealment of the final scar (**C**).

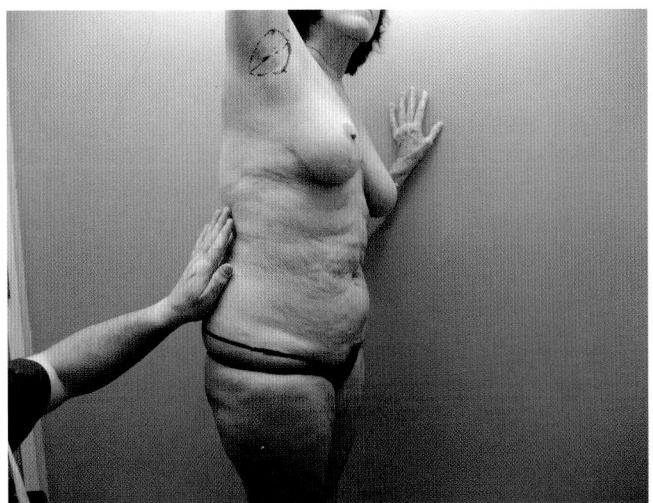

Fig. 9.6 The patient is asked to lean slightly away from the surgeon when the lateral estimate of tissue resection is made. This helps ensure that the amount of resection is not overestimated.

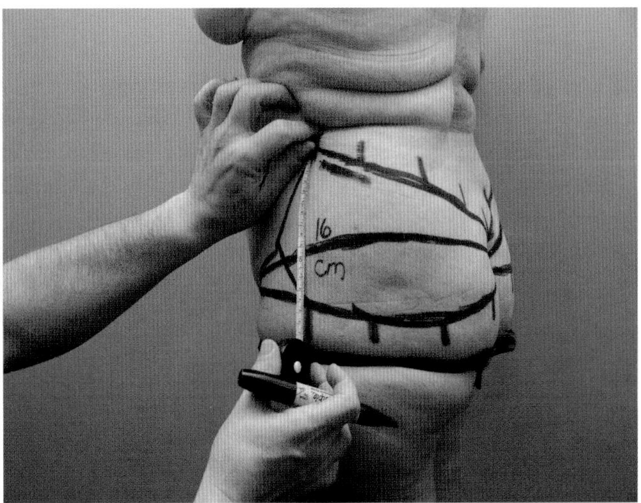

Fig. 9.9 Measurement of the resection amount in the left midaxillary line.

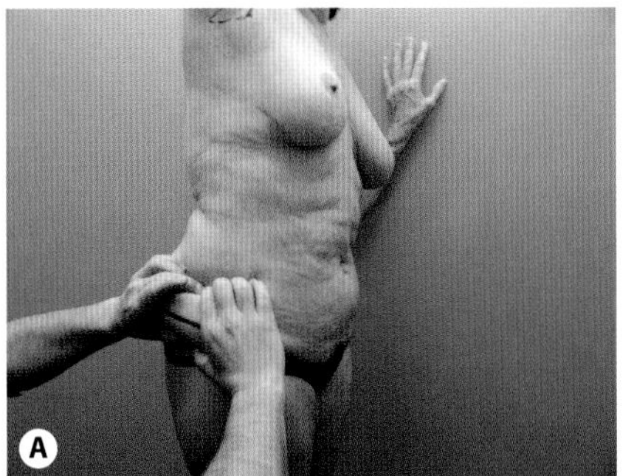

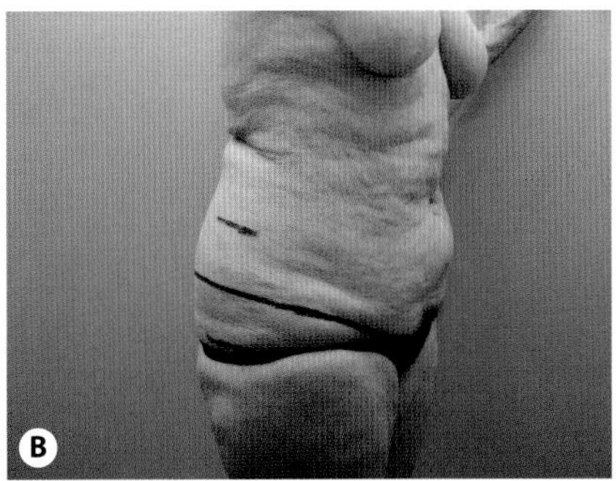

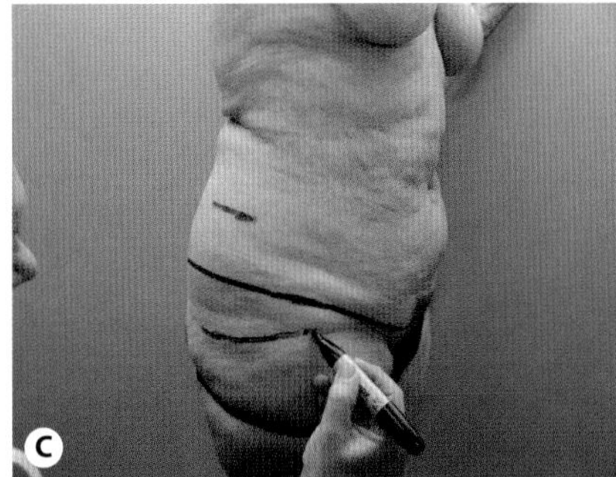

Fig. 9.7 Bimanual estimation is performed and marked along the planned final scar placement (**A, B**). The lower mark of this estimate is continued anteriorly to join the initial transverse abdominoplasty mark (**C**).

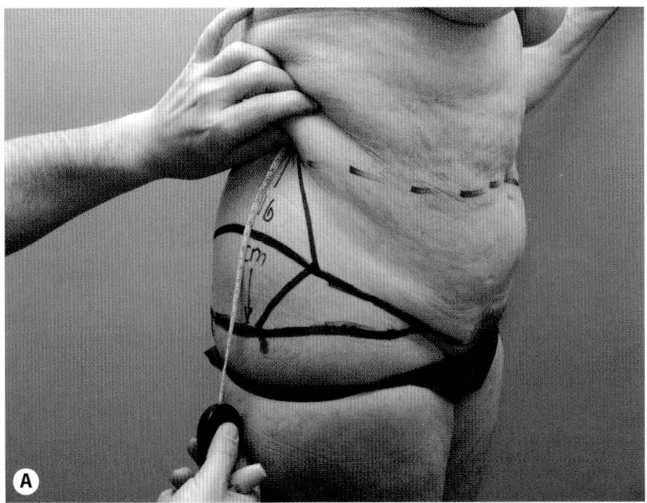

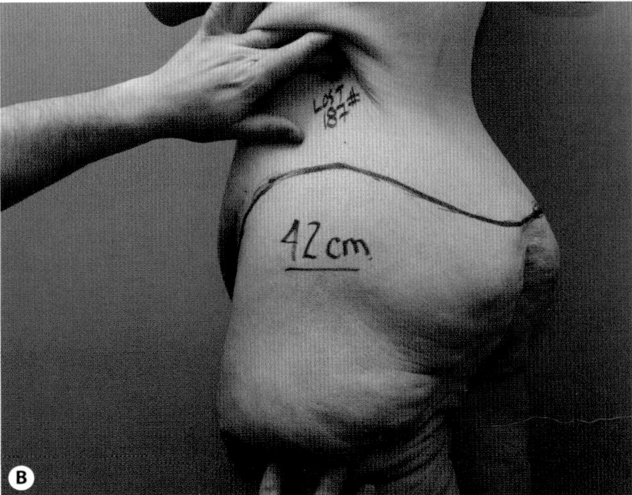

Fig. 9.8 A and B Measurement of the amount of resection in the right midaxillary line. The average amount is usually 17–21 cm, but in some massive weight loss patients with significant laxity this has been as much as 42 cm.

line to the posterior midline to estimate the amount of soft tissue to be resected (**Fig. 9.10**). Because of the strong adherence in the posterior midline, the amount of resection at this point is minimal and care must be taken not to overestimate this amount, as excessively tight closure in this area can lead to wound healing complications. It should be remembered that the posterior midline is the most frequent site for wound healing complications. The estimate of soft-tissue resection is done bilaterally and side-to-side comparison is performed to ensure symmetry.

The lower incision at the midaxillary line is carefully extended anteriorly to intersect with the initially drawn lower abdominal incision just lateral to the mons (**Fig. 9.11**). The upper incision line is extended anteriorly to the area superior to the umbilicus (**Fig. 9.12**). This upper mark serves only as an estimate, and the final resection line will

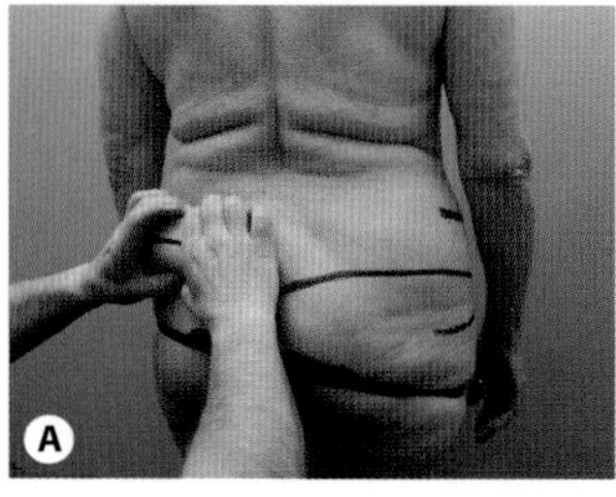

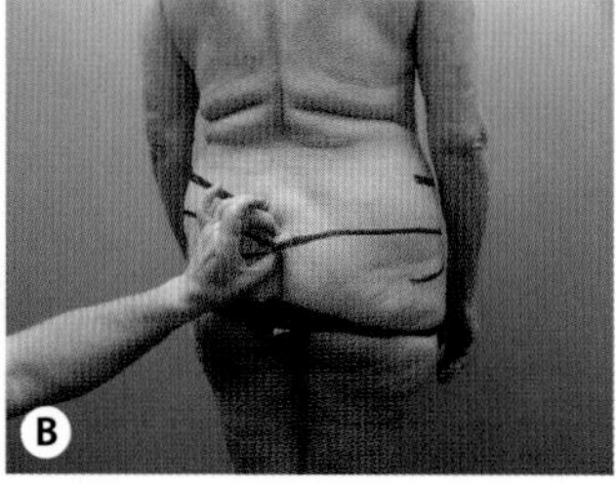

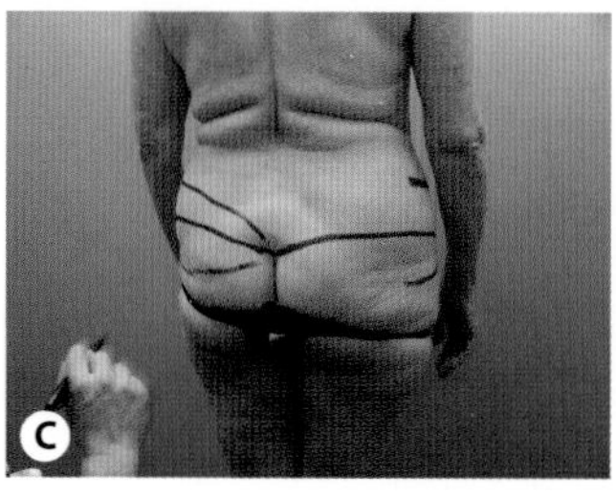

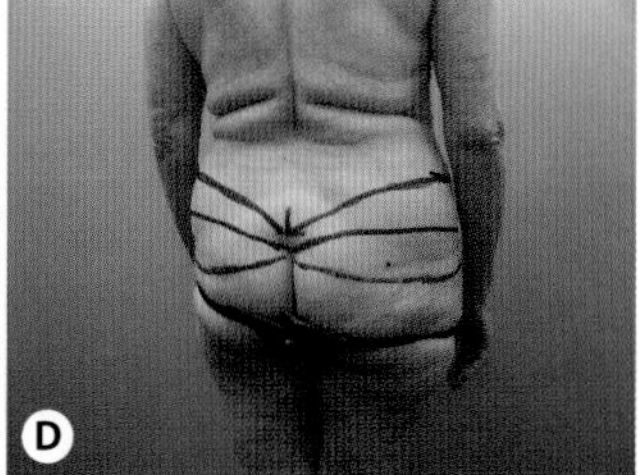

Fig. 9.10 Bimanual estimation and marking of the amount of soft-tissue resection posteriorly (**A–C**). Only a small amount of resection is usually needed centrally above the intergluteal crease (**B**).

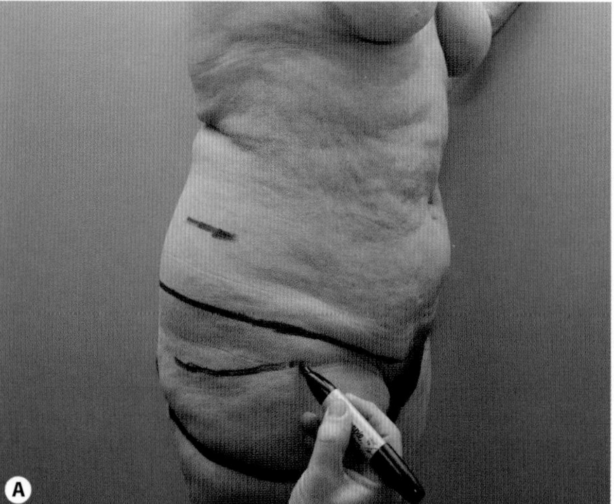

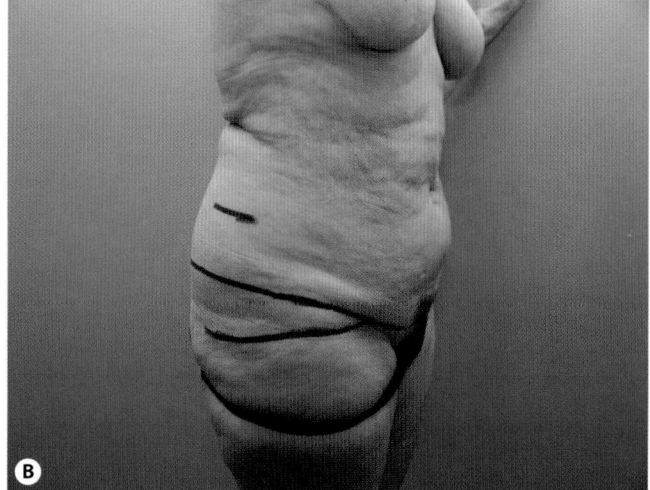

Fig. 9.11 The lower posterior incision mark is continued to the midaxillary line based on bimanual estimation, and then tapered naturally into the anterior transverse marking.

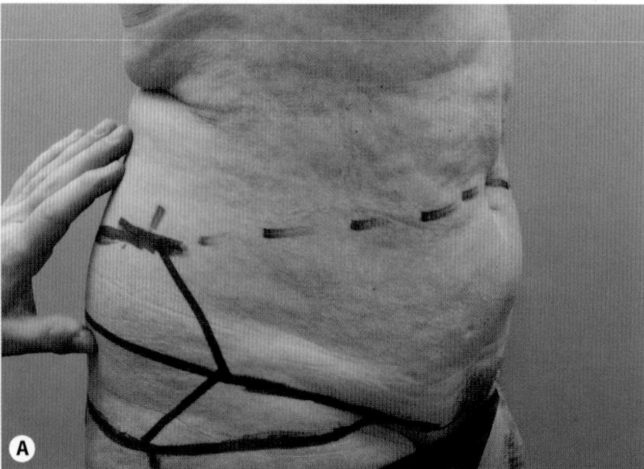

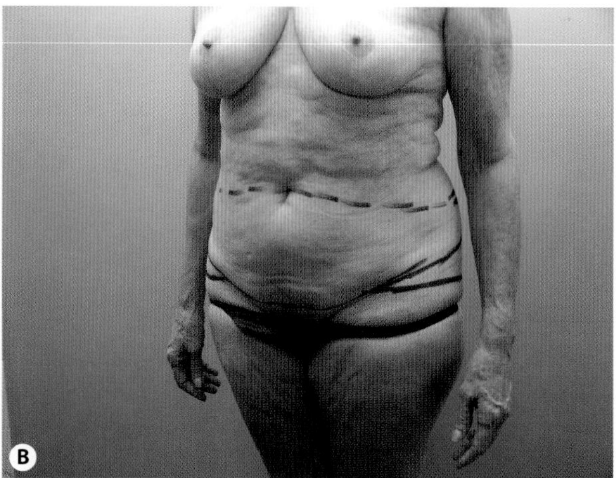

Fig. 9.12 The upper posterior incision mark is continued toward the supraumbilical area as a dashed line, indicating that this is a general estimate of the amount of tissue resection anteriorly.

be determined intraoperatively using a tissue demarcator. A dotted line is usually drawn to signify that this is only an estimate. At this point, a temporary 'V' closure marking is made with the base at the midaxillary line and the point anteriorly at approximately the anterior axillary line (**Fig. 9.13**). Realignment marks are placed bilaterally to facilitate closure (**Fig. 9.14**).

For patients with significant weight loss who have buttock laxity and inadequate buttock volume, autologous buttock augmentation is a wonderful solution and can be easily performed during a circumferential abdominoplasty. In this case, the drawings are similar, as if all of the posterior tissue were to be resected, reducing the amount appropriately to take into account the added tissue from the autologous augmentation. The tissue for augmentation is marked in the area of proposed resection (**Fig. 9.15**). Either this tissue is left in its native position, sewn inferiorly over the gluteus, treated with purse-string sutures to augment projection, or the lateral aspect is elevated and rotated inferiorly. We prefer the method of purse-string gluteoplasty because of its reliability, simplicity, and excellent results. The lowest risk of complication occurs when the tissue is left in its normal location without elevation and rotation. Additional details for autologous buttock augmentation are described in Chapter 13, Ancillary Procedures.

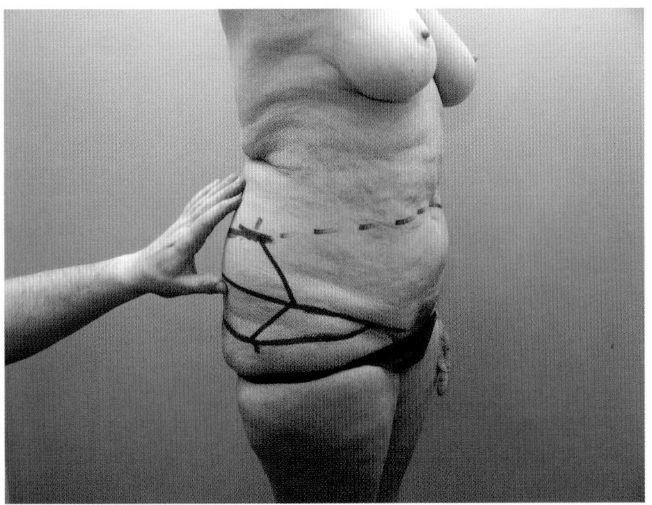

Fig. 9.13 A 'V' closure marking is placed in the midaxillary line bilaterally, or in the general area where access to the patient will be obscured in the prone position. The apex of the 'V' is along the intended final scar placement marked initially and the base of the 'V' posteriorly.

Patients who have a tremendous amount of abdominal soft-tissue laxity, as seen after massive weight loss, usually have laxity in the vertical as well as in the transverse dimension. It is therefore important to discuss with these patients the possibility of also reducing the transverse laxity via an anterior vertical resection. The pros and cons of doing so must be communicated to the patient, as an improved contour can be achieved in this manner. The drawback of vertical resection is the extra scar, which cannot be concealed by a two-piece swimsuit. Often, patients who have achieved massive weight loss would like better overall contour and reduction of the excess soft-tissue laxity, and have no intention of wearing a two-piece swimsuit or revealing clothing. For patients who already have an anterior midline scar from previous abdominal surgery, a vertical resection during circumferential abdominoplasty is an easy decision to make. The amount of the anterior vertical wedge soft-tissue resection is estimated and marked at this time through bimanual estimation. The final amount of resection should be verified intraoperatively after the anterior transverse resection has been performed. The base of this vertical resection should curve medially and end at the transverse resection in the form of an incomplete ellipse (**Fig. 9.16**).

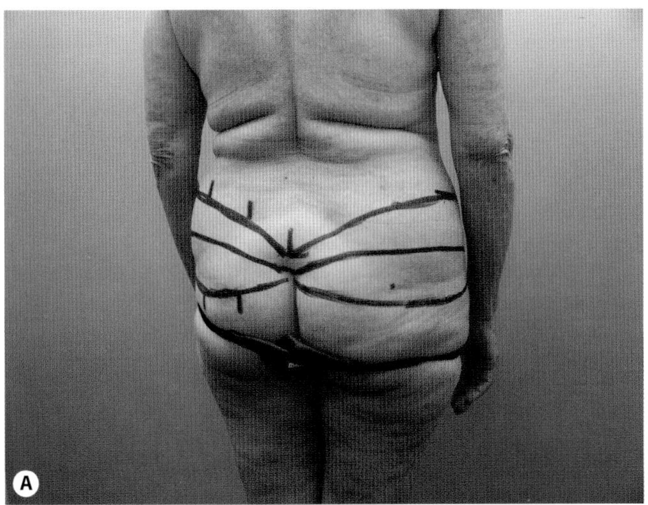

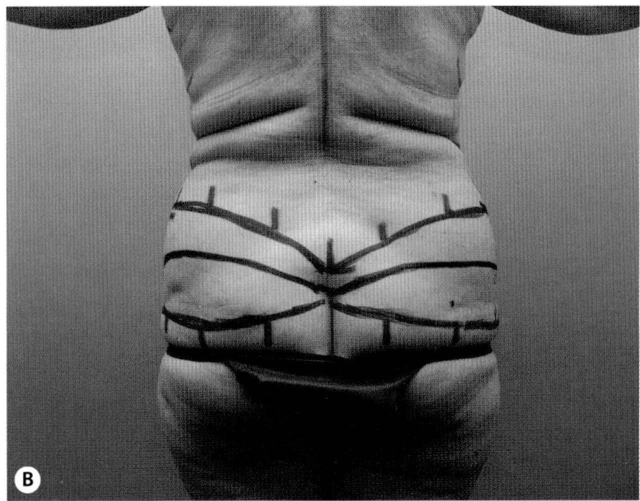

Fig. 9.14 Realignment marks are placed posteriorly to facilitate closure. The posterior component of the circumferential abdominoplasty is less forgiving of asymmetric tissue advancement, largely because of the presence of the intergluteal crease.

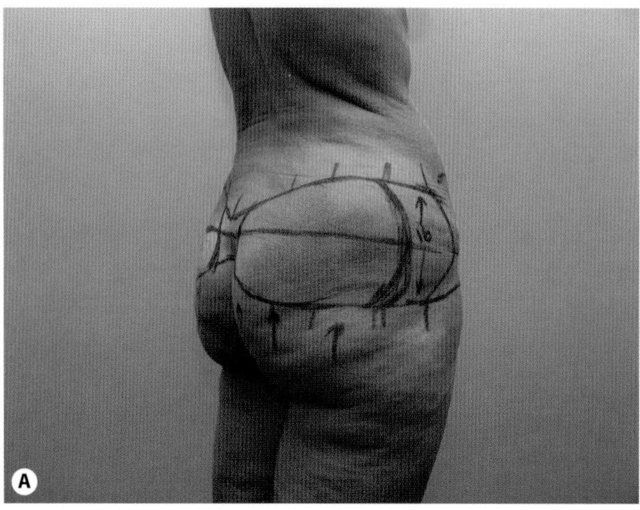

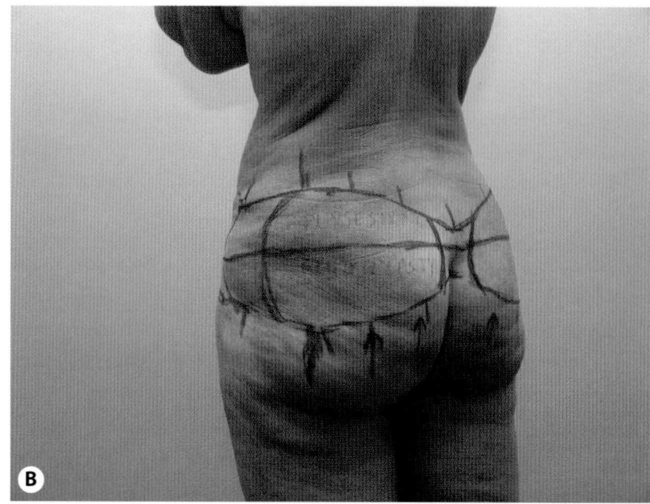

Fig. 9.15 For patients who are also undergoing autologous buttock augmentation the appropriate markings can be made at this time. This patient will be undergoing a purse-string gluteoplasty augmentation. The central mounds are delineated within the confines of the tissue that would usually be resected. Some modification of the amount of resected soft tissue posteriorly may be necessary to allow acceptable tension over the tissue used in the buttock augmentation.

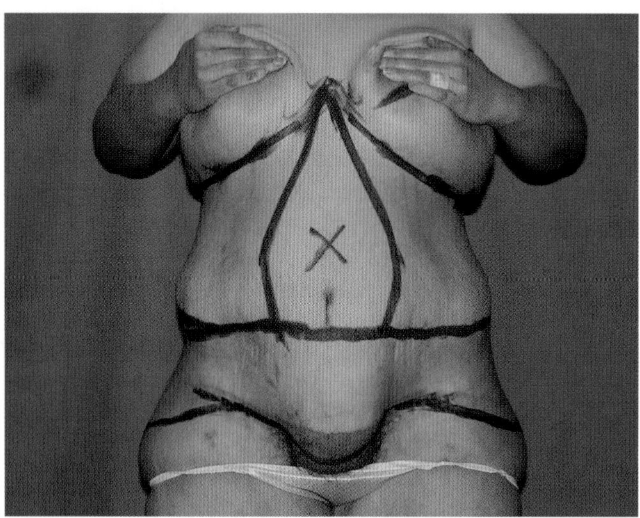

Fig. 9.16 Patients with significant transverse abdominal soft-tissue laxity may benefit from the addition of an anterior vertical ellipse resection. It is important to note that the base of the wedge should be designed to *taper inwards* toward the midline as it approaches the upper transverse incision of the abdominoplasty. Failing to do so by excising excess abdominal tissue in the form of an inverted V, will result in excess soft-tissue resection at the incision line at the position of the inverted T.

The markings are rechecked, ensuring symmetry and the ability to safely reapproximate the two sides. Markings for concurrent liposuction are carefully made throughout the entire upper abdomen, axilla, flanks, hips, and mons, and all preoperative markings are again reviewed. An additional set of preoperative photographs should be taken showing the surgical markings. These photographs are critical when evaluating the postoperative results (**Fig. 9.17**).

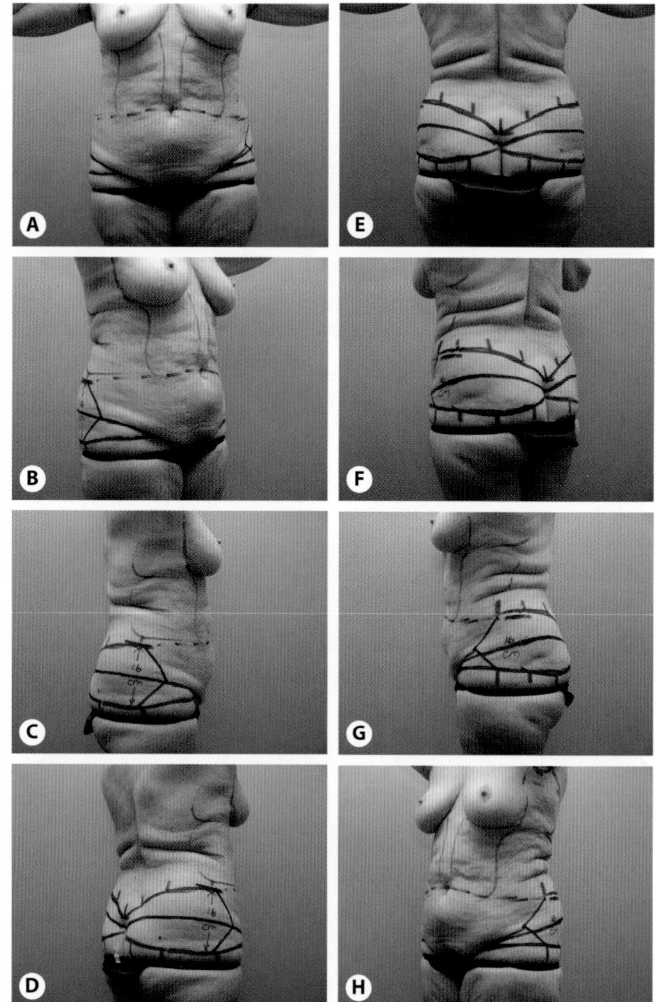

Fig. 9.17 At this time, the areas that will undergo liposuction are identified and marked and a complete set of photographs are taken that demonstrate the markings and the operative plan.

The patient is brought to the operating room, an intravenous line is established, and sequential compression devices are placed on the lower extremities and activated. General anesthesia is induced, a Foley catheter is placed, and intravenous antibiotics and steroids are administered (Ancef 1 g and Decadron 4 mg) (**Fig. 9.18**). If concurrent abdominal liposuction is planned, all areas to be suctioned are then infiltrated with tumescent fluid. Detailed information on infiltration and liposuction is given in Chapter 3, Liposuction in Abdominal Contouring. A thorough all-layer tumescent infiltration (superficial, intermediate, and prefascial) is performed. The incision lines are also infiltrated in the immediate subdermal layer to provide vasoconstriction at the incision line (**Fig. 9.19**). If abdominal liposuction is not planned, the incision line and periumbilical areas only are infiltrated with dilute mixture of lidocaine and epinephrine. The patient is carefully turned prone, properly padded, and a perforating towel clip is used to recheck the incision lines bilaterally to verify that resection and closure can be performed without undue tension (**Fig. 9.20**). The posterior surgical site is then infiltrated. This may include tumescent infiltration if liposuction is anticipated, or incision line-only infiltration if liposuction is not planned (**Fig. 9.21**). If autologous buttock augmentation is planned, the skin to be removed from the central mound is infiltrated subdermally to minimize bleeding.

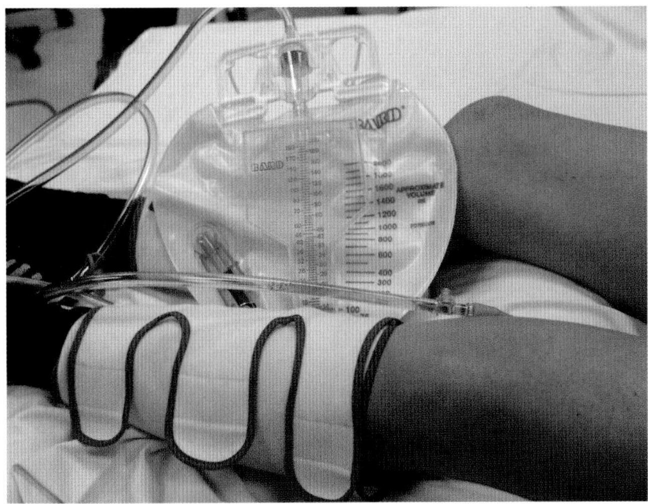

Fig. 9.18 Sequential compression devices are placed on the lower extremities once the patient arrives in the operating room. A Foley catheter is inserted after general anesthesia is started.

Prepping and draping are performed in standard fashion. Care is taken to ensure that the preparation extends below the infragluteal crease so as to visualize the entire buttocks up to the level of the mid-back. Methylene blue tattoo points are placed at each alignment mark, distinguishing successive marks with either one or two tattoo dots (**Fig. 9.22**). If the markings are lost during the procedure, these tattoo points remain and are critical for correct tissue realignment during closure.

The incision is made into but not through the dermis using a number 10 blade. Electrocautery is used to complete the

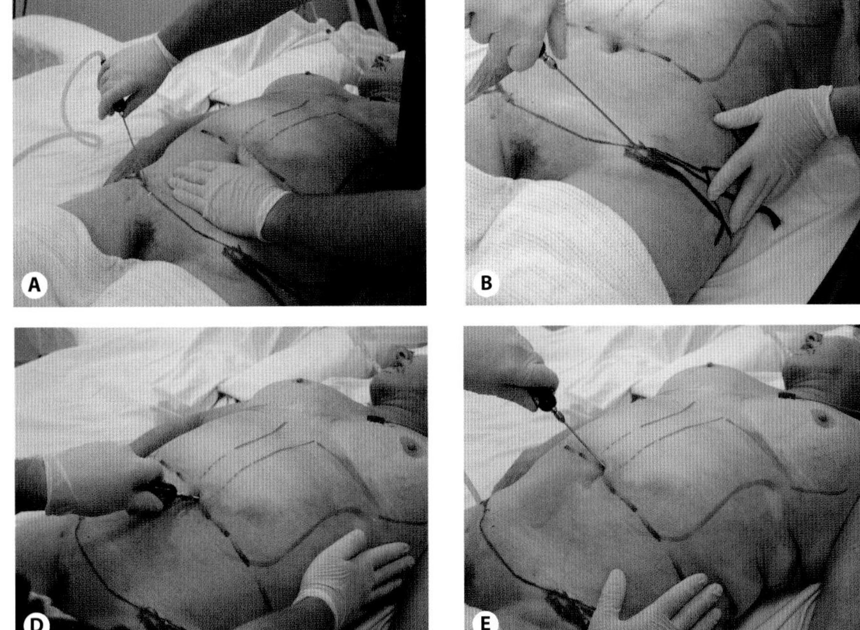

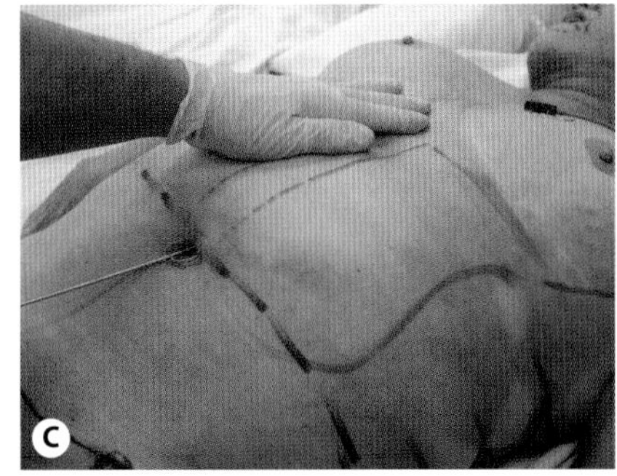

Fig. 9.19 With the patient in the supine position tumescent infiltration is performed in all of the areas to be liposuctioned. If liposuction is not planned, the incision lines and the periumbilical area are infiltrated for intraoperative hemostasis.

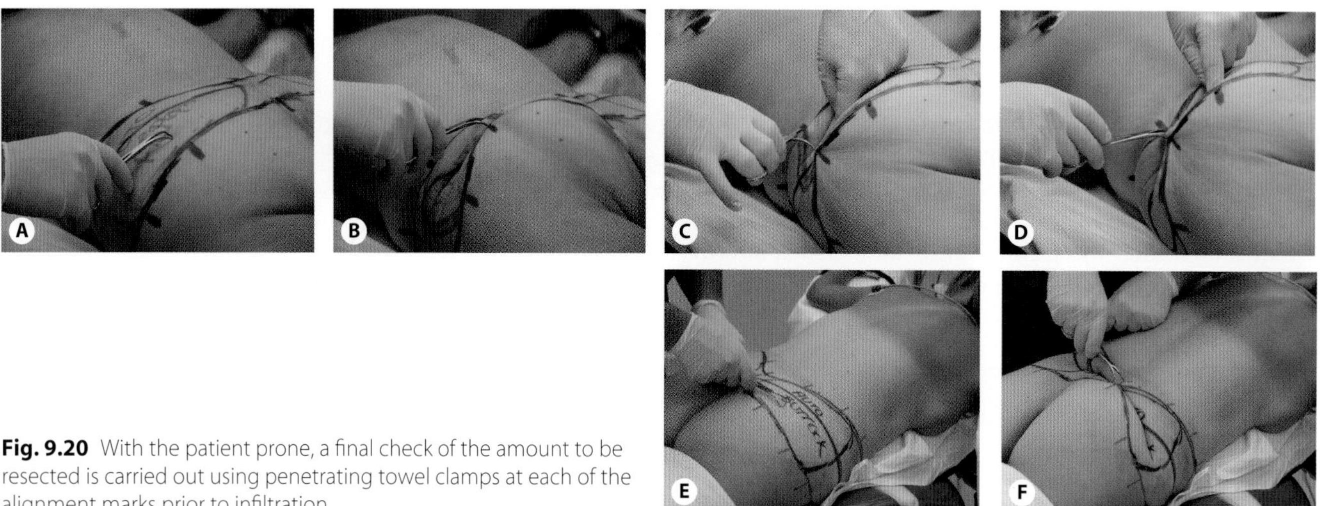

Fig. 9.20 With the patient prone, a final check of the amount to be resected is carried out using penetrating towel clamps at each of the alignment marks prior to infiltration.

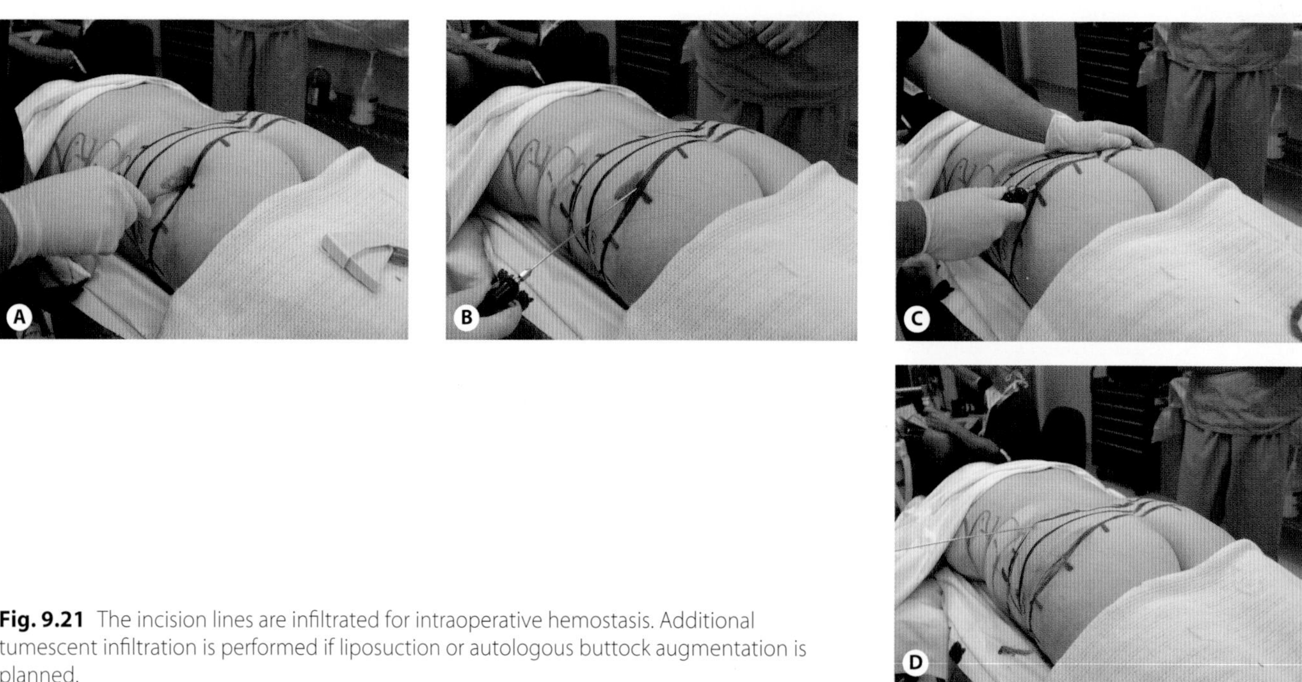

Fig. 9.21 The incision lines are infiltrated for intraoperative hemostasis. Additional tumescent infiltration is performed if liposuction or autologous buttock augmentation is planned.

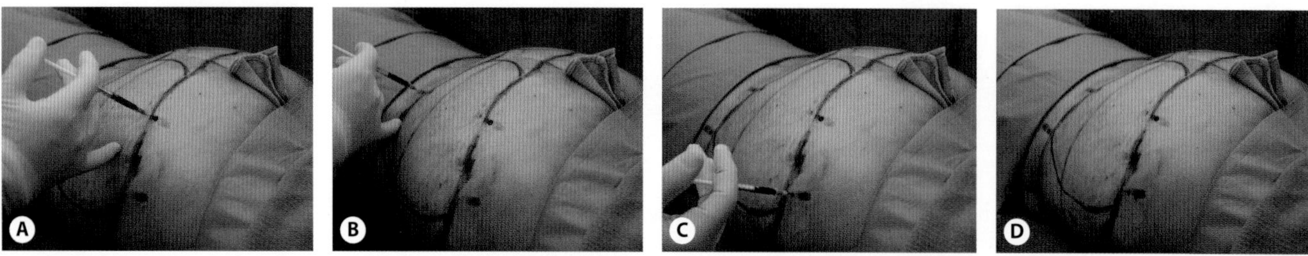

Fig. 9.22 After standard prepping and draping methylene blue is used to tattoo the vertical realignment marks. Successive realignment marks are differentiated with one or two tattoo dots. These tattoos ensure proper alignment of the two sides even if the marks wear off during surgery.

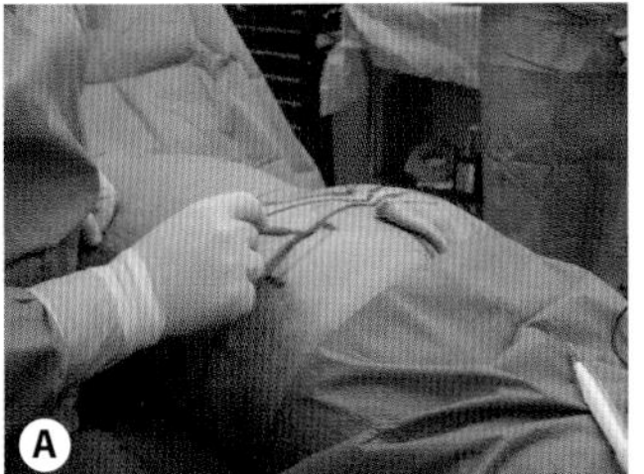
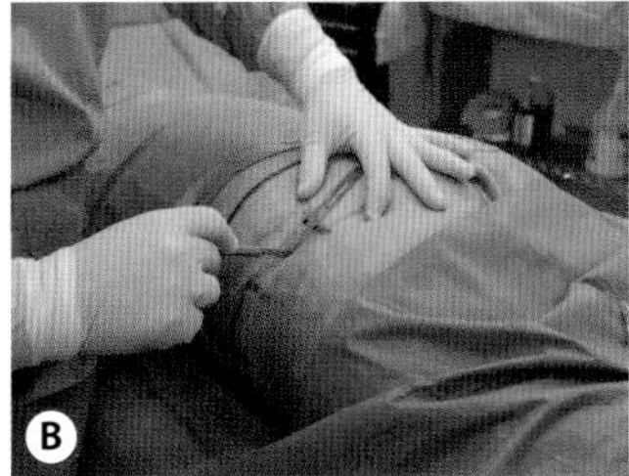
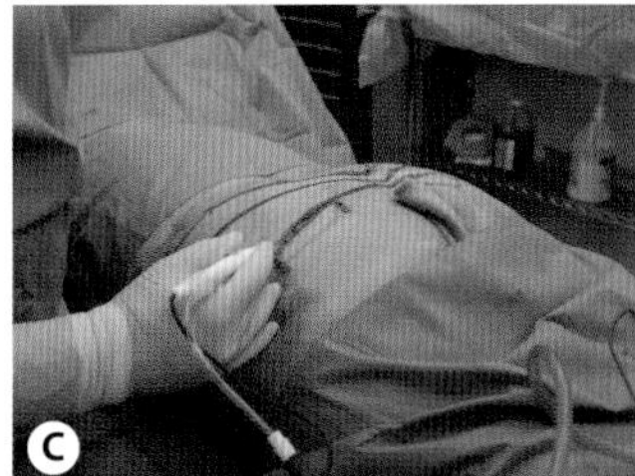
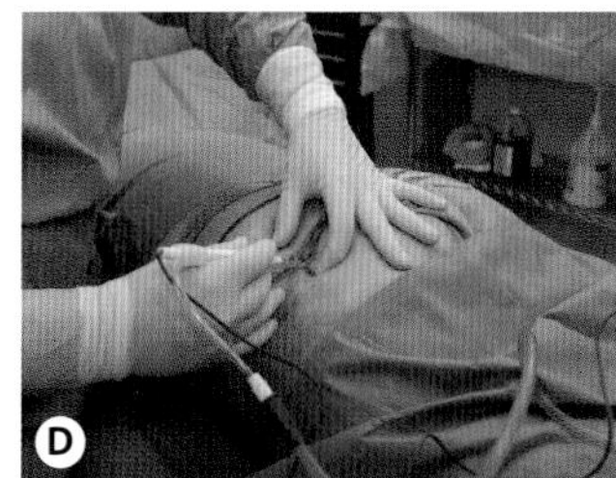

Fig. 9.23 A number 10 blade is used to make the initial incision into but not completely through the dermis. Completion of the skin incision and subsequent dissection with electrocautery helps minimize blood loss.

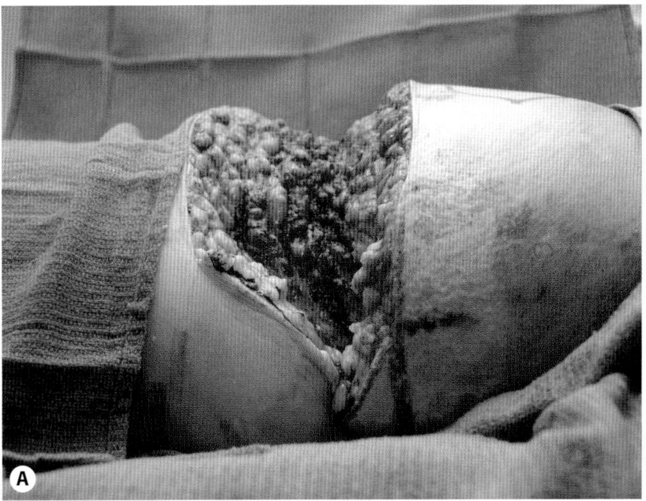
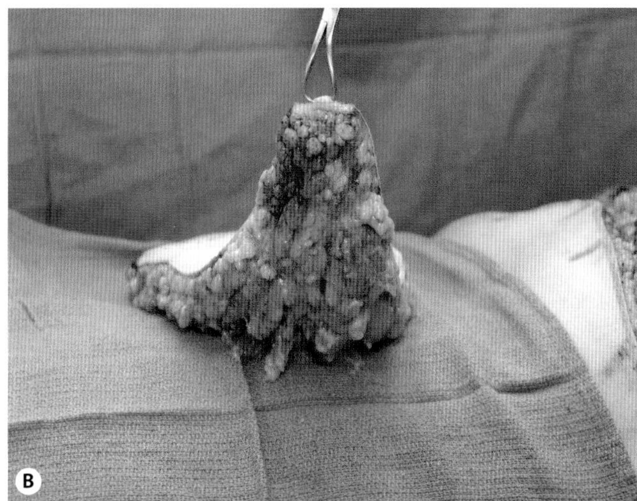

Fig. 9.24 Resection of the posterior tissue should be performed with a gentle inward bevel from both sides, which minimizes dead space once the incision is closed.

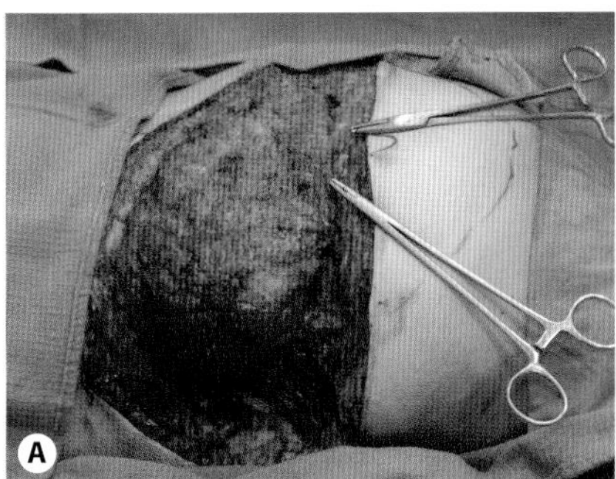
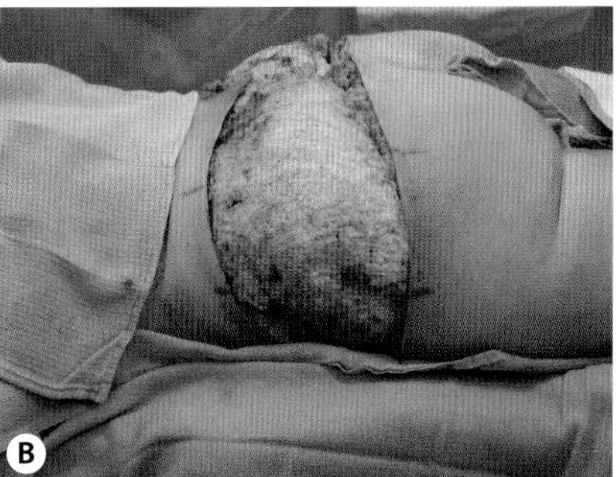
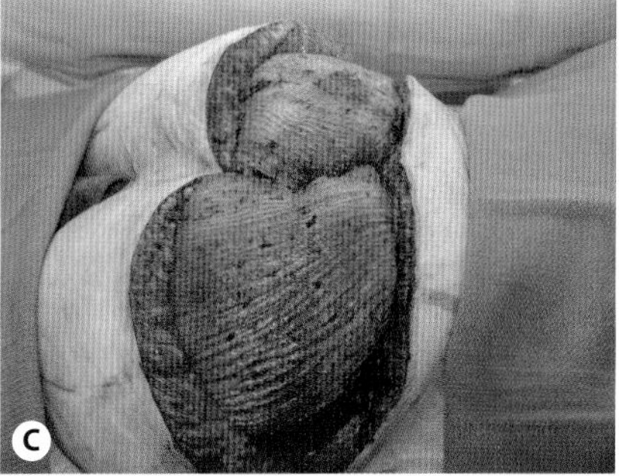

Fig. 9.25 If autologous buttock augmentation is performed, the dissection is carried straight down to the underlying gluteal fascia and the skin overlying the central mound (if a purse-string gluteoplasty is used) is either de-epithelialized or removed.

incision and for all subsequent dissection (**Fig. 9.23**). The inferior incision should be made first, with superior undermining and demarcation to determine the appropriate amount of resection. This will prevent over-resection and excessive tension on the incision line. As experience is gained, however, both incision lines can be made concurrently, with the intervening tissue resected and closure performed with appropriate tension. If there is excessive tension on closure, inferior undermining and, if necessary, superior undermining, will enhance tissue mobilization and reduce tension on the incision line. It will, however, create a larger undesirable area of dead space that will require prolonged drainage and may be associated with an increased risk of seroma formation.

The proper method of tissue dissection is to bevel inwards, down to the muscle fascia at the level of the final incision line. This should be done for both the inferior and superior incisions, creating a 'V'-shaped resection. This will allow closure without undermining, which minimizes the risk of seroma formation (**Fig. 9.24**). If autologous buttock augmentation is performed, the skin of the intervening tissue is either removed or de-epithelialized (**Fig. 9.25**). The soft tissue of the lower buttocks may undermined if necessary, but only down to the level of the infragluteal crease and then lifted over the autologous tissue for closure (see Chapter 13, Ancillary Procedures.

Laterally, the resection ends at a point in the anterior axillary line. A temporary 'V' resection is carried out based in the midaxillary line, full thickness to the muscle fascia and ending at a point in the anterior axillary line (**Fig. 9.26**). Perfect hemostasis is achieved with electrocautery to minimize the risk of postoperative hematoma. A temporary closure is then performed bilaterally from the midaxillary line to the anterior axillary line, closing the temporary 'V' with number 0 Prolene (**Fig. 9.27**).

Fig. 9.26 The resection is carried out to the previously marked 'V', which usually corresponds to the mid or anterior axillary line and the lateral extent of access to the patient.

A drain is then draped across the midline and the tubing is coiled and placed deep to the temporary 'V closure (**Fig. 9.28**). The tattooed alignment marks can be brought together temporarily with towel clips or staples prior to suturing. The superficial fascia (SFS) is closed with number 1 or 0 Vicryl (**Fig. 9.29**). Sutures are placed every 1–2 cm, depending on tissue tension. The skin is reapproximated with deep dermal 2/0 Vicryl sutures placed approximately every centimeter (**Fig. 9.30**). Final closure is achieved with intradermal 4/0 Monocryl. The incision is then coated with tissue adhesive as a water-impermeable dressing (**Fig. 9.31**). The patient is then carefully repositioned into the supine position for the anterior portion of the case.

The patient is then reprepped and draped. Adequate padding is assured, and a heated air blanket is placed on the lower extremities. Thorough abdominal liposuction is performed on patients who have excess adiposity and who

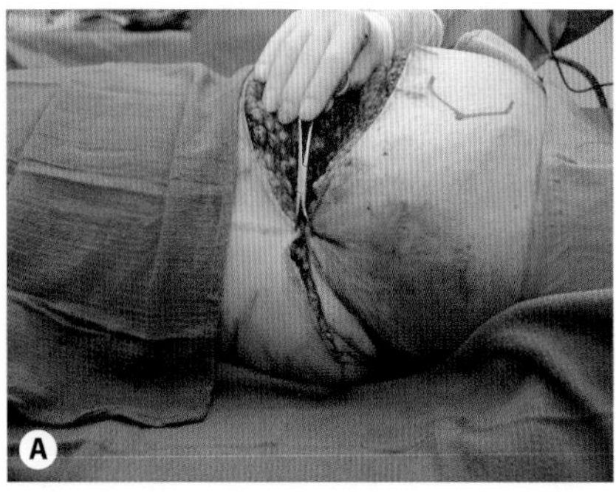

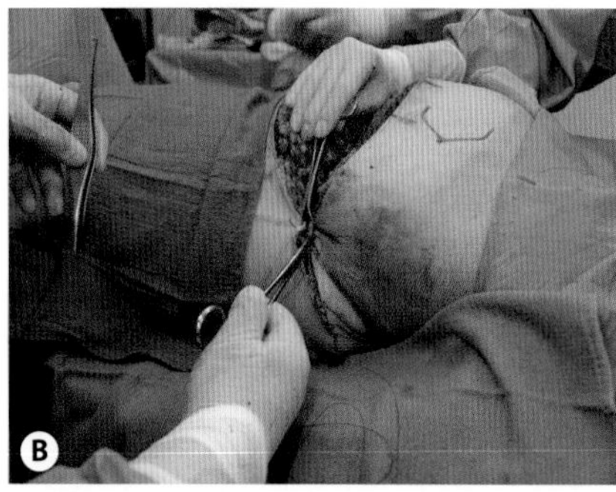

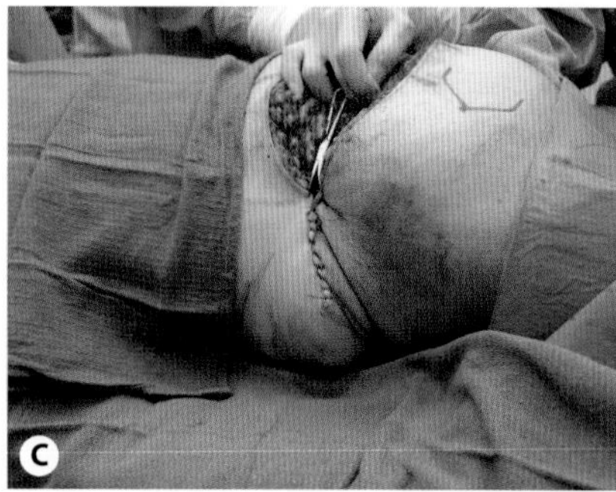

Fig. 9.27 The termination of the posterior resection at the 'V' marking allows temporary closure with size 0 Prolene. This simply facilitates temporary skin closure to allow repositioning of the patient in the supine position and continuation of the procedure.

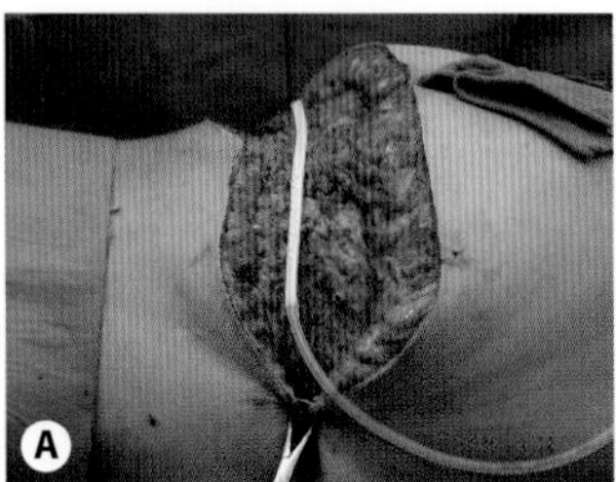

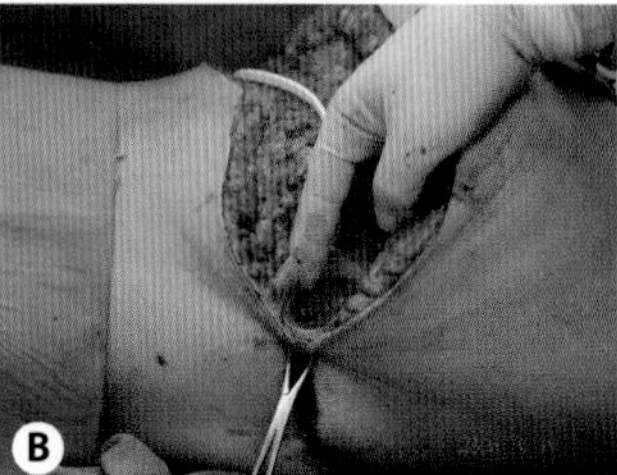

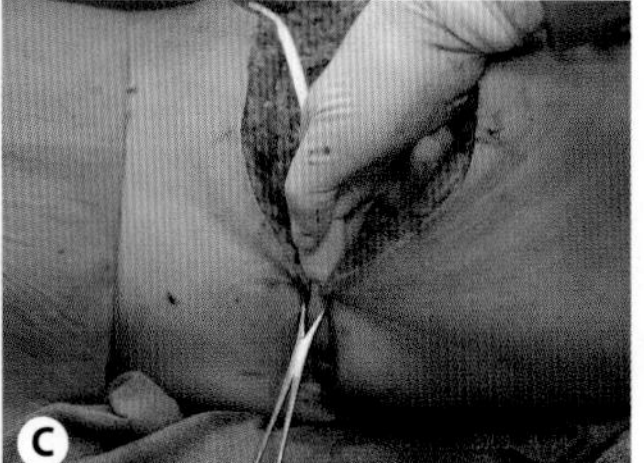

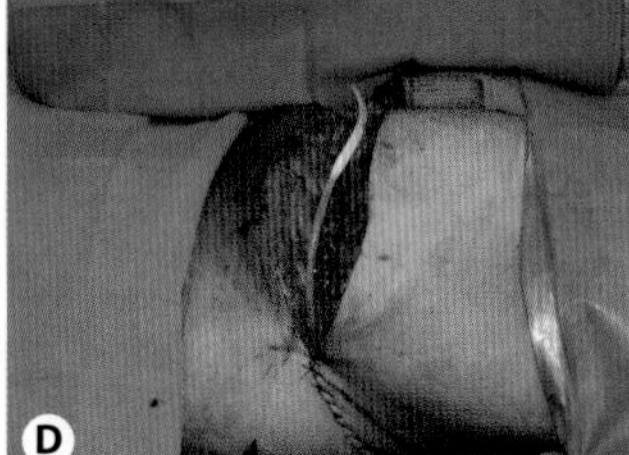

Fig. 9.28 Prior to closure of the posterior portion of the case, a drain is draped across the superior portion of the surgical site and the tubing is coiled and placed deep to the temporary 'V' closure.

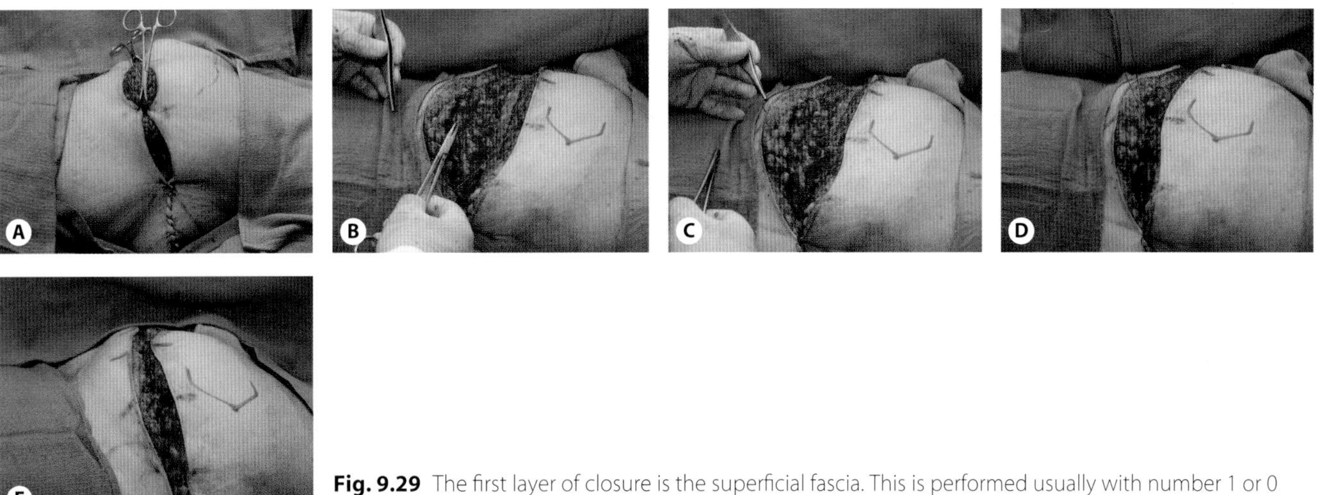

Fig. 9.29 The first layer of closure is the superficial fascia. This is performed usually with number 1 or 0 Vicryl.

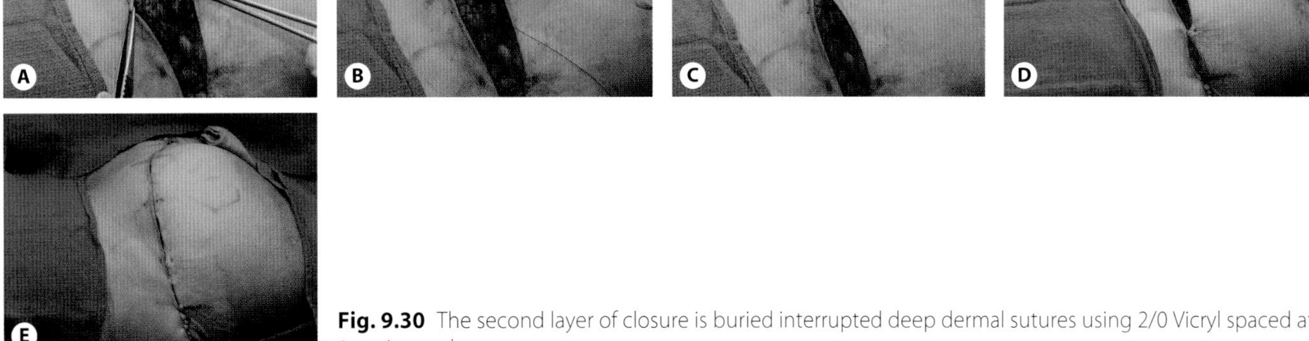

Fig. 9.30 The second layer of closure is buried interrupted deep dermal sutures using 2/0 Vicryl spaced at 1 cm intervals.

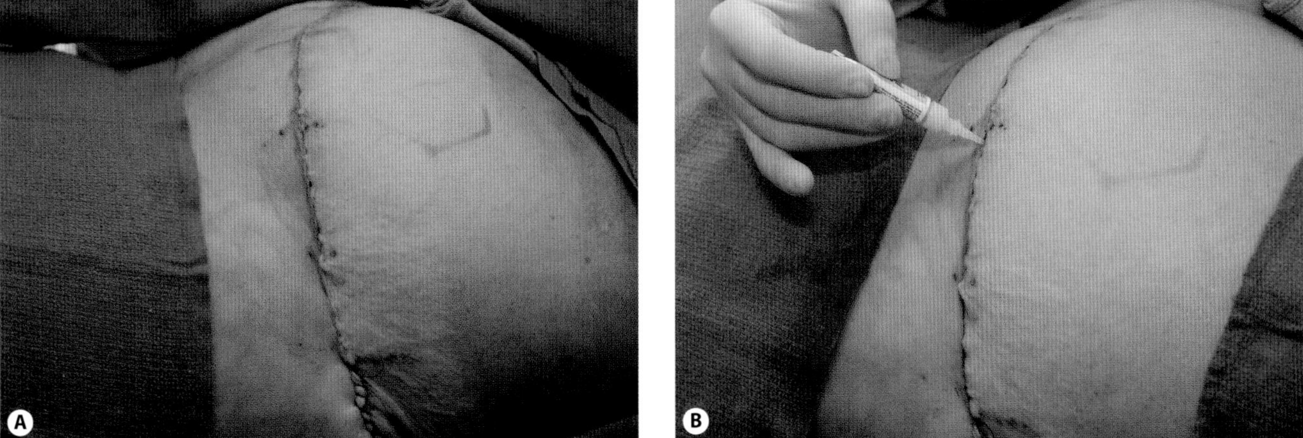

Fig. 9.31 Formal closure is achieved with running intradermal 4/0 Monocryl sutures followed by the application of tissue adhesive as a water-impermeable dressing.

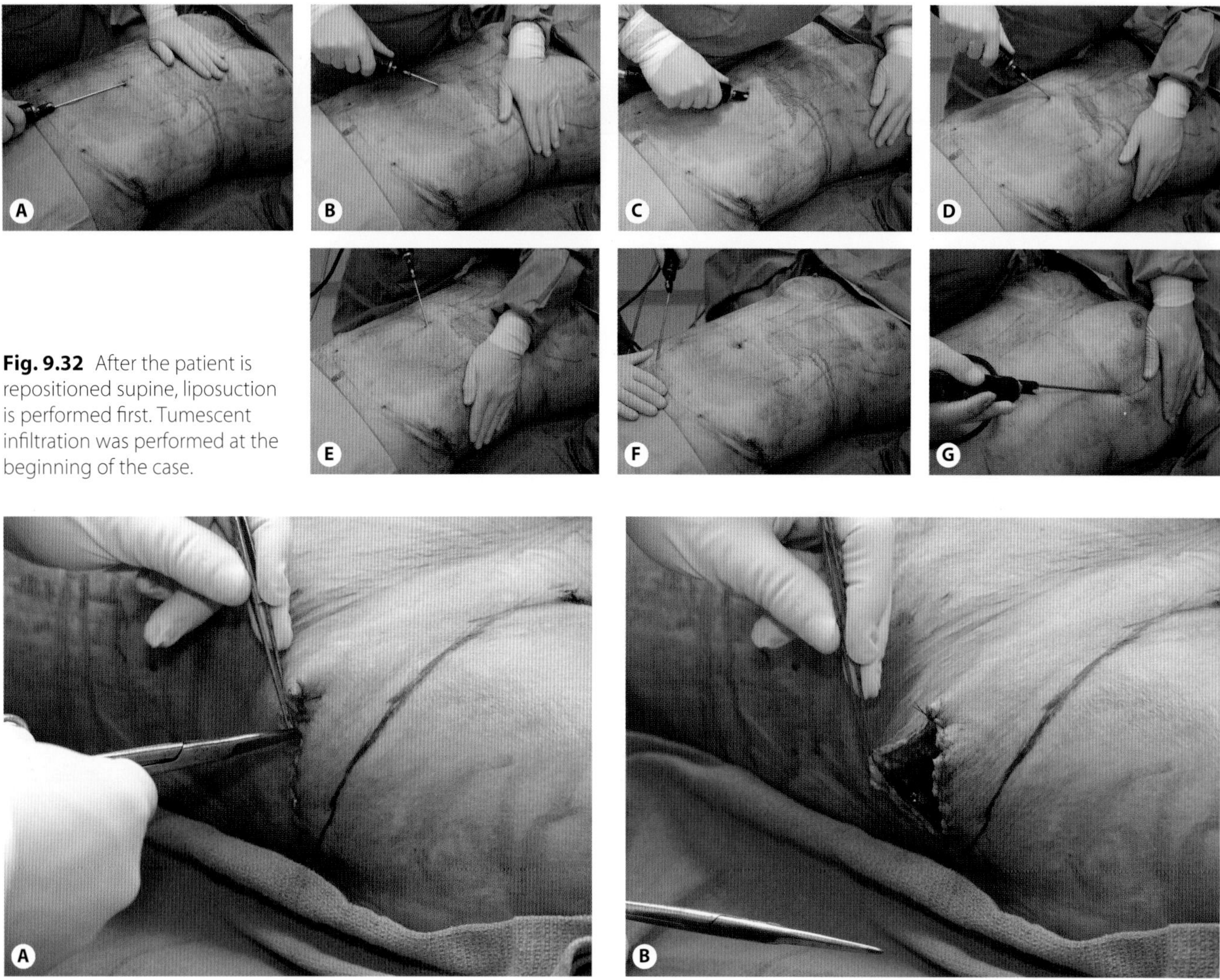

Fig. 9.32 After the patient is repositioned supine, liposuction is performed first. Tumescent infiltration was performed at the beginning of the case.

Fig. 9.33 The Prolene sutures used to temporarily close the 'V' are removed after liposuction is complete.

were infiltrated with tumescent fluid at the beginning of the case (**Fig. 9.32**). Liposuction is carried out in all layers except in the central abdomen, where it is performed in the layer superficial to Scarpa's fascia. This is because the tissue deep to this layer will usually be excised during resection of the subscarpal fat. In patients with complete weight loss who have minimal excess adiposity, liposuction is omitted.

The temporary lateral Prolene sutures are removed (**Fig. 9.33**). The remaining inferior incision is completed from one midaxillary line to the other. The incision is made partway into the dermis, and then the electrocautery is used to complete the incision and continue the dissection down to the abdominal wall (**Fig. 9.34**). The coiled drain is brought out below the incision on the left side and secured with a silk suture (**Fig. 9.35**). The superficial inferior epigastric vessels should be identified and carefully controlled with either electrocautery or a ligature (**Fig. 9.36**).

Dissection is then performed with electrocautery to the level of the umbilicus. The loose areolar tissue is protected to facilitate subsequent tissue adherence and reduce seroma formation (**Fig. 9.37**). Large periumbilical perforators are frequently encountered that must be carefully controlled to prevent rectus sheath hematoma (**Fig. 9.38**). These vessels can be impressive in caliber, especially in the massive weight loss patient. It is frequently noted that vascular hypertrophy with weight gain is maintained even after massive weight loss has occurred.

The umbilicus is incised vertically and scissor dissection is performed down to the abdominal wall, leaving some subcutaneous fat on the umbilical stalk to maintain vascularity (**Fig. 9.39**). The abdominal flap is split, anticipating its complete removal (**Fig. 9.40**).

Dissection continues superiorly to the level of the costal margin. The medial borders of the rectus sheath are marked

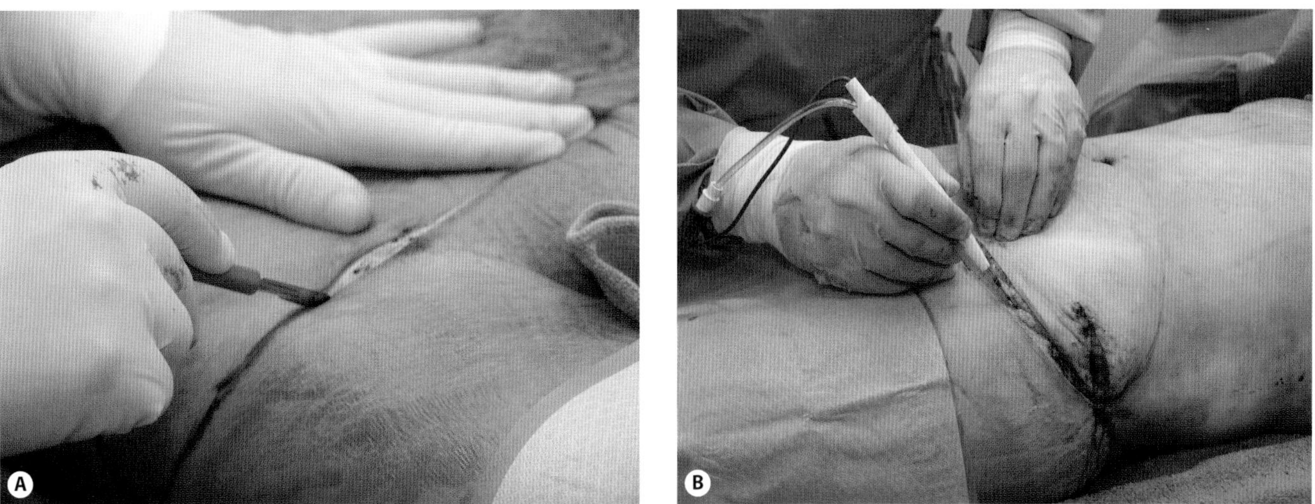

Fig. 9.34 The anterior transverse mark which connects at each 'V' closure is incised. A number 10 scalpel is used to make the incision into but not completely through the dermis. The electrocautery is used to complete the skin incision and begin the dissection.

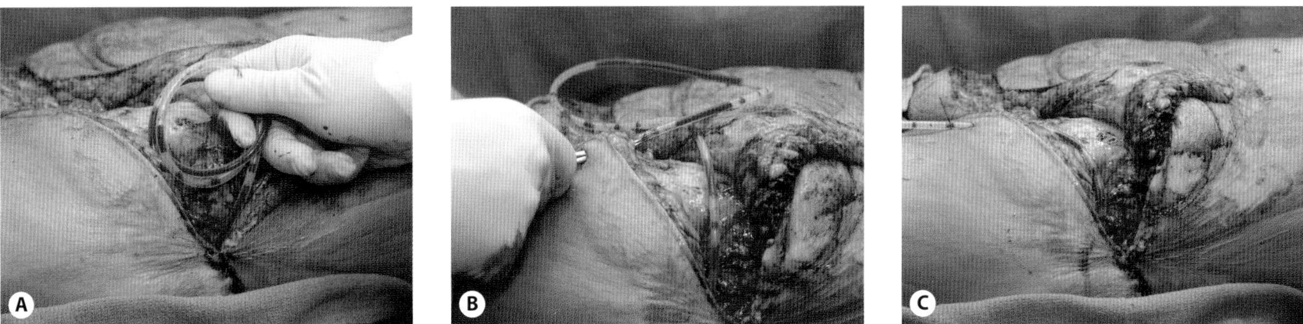

Fig. 9.35 At this time, the coiled tubing from the posterior drain is brought out, placed through a skin puncture inferior to the lateral portion of the transverse incision, and secured with silk sutures.

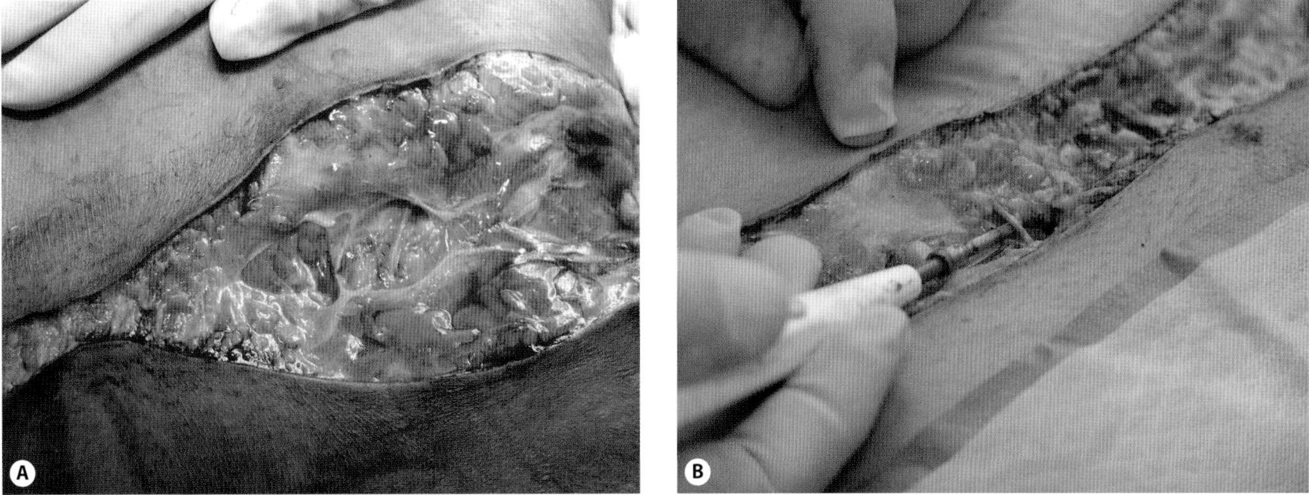

Fig. 9.36 During the initial anterior dissection an attempt should be made to identify and control the superficial inferior epigastric vessels with either electrocautery or ligature.

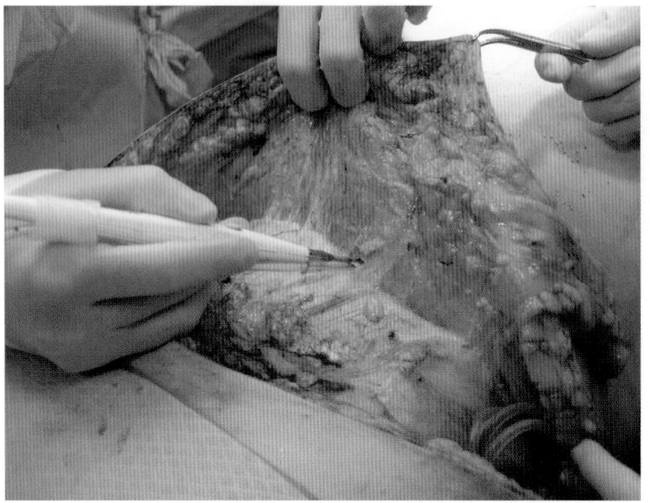

Fig. 9.37 Dissection of the abdominal soft-tissue apron is performed with electrocautery, taking care to preserve as much of the loose areolar tissue as possible.

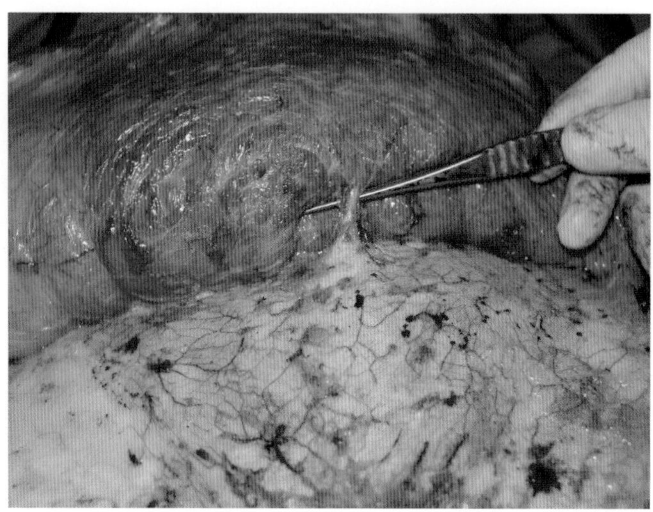

Fig. 9.38 As the dissection progresses care should be taken to properly control perforators, especially in the periumbilical area where they can often have an impressive caliber.

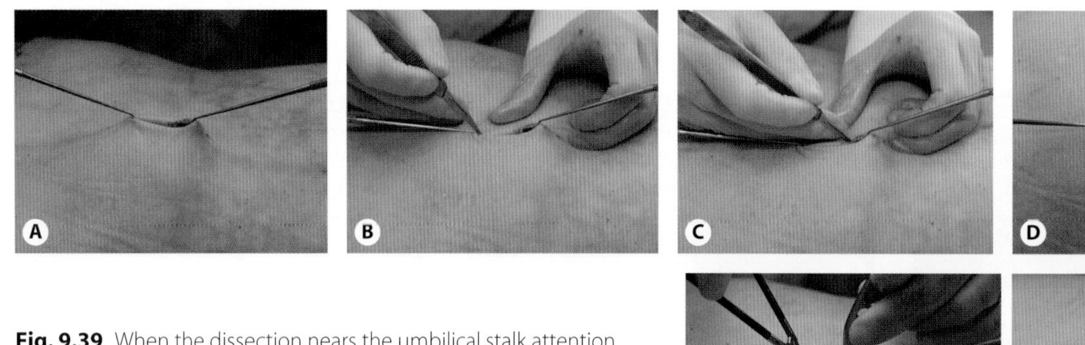

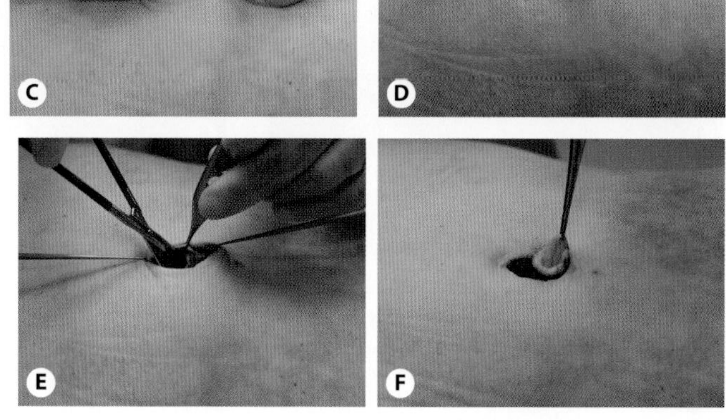

Fig. 9.39 When the dissection nears the umbilical stalk attention is turned to releasing the umbilicus. This is performed by using two single hooks to place the umbilicus under tension vertically. A number 11 blade is used to incise the umbilicus, and then scissors are used to dissect the stalk from the surrounding soft tissue down to the abdominal wall. Care is taken to preserve some fat on the stalk to maintain vascularity.

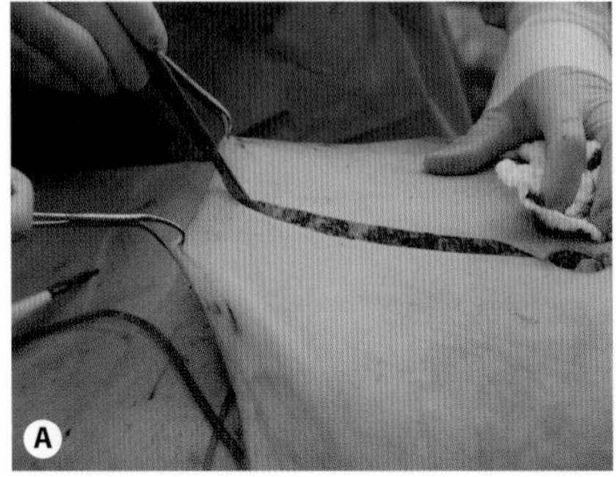

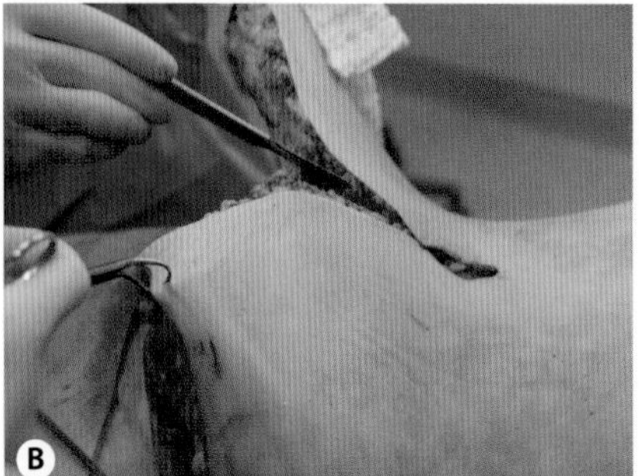

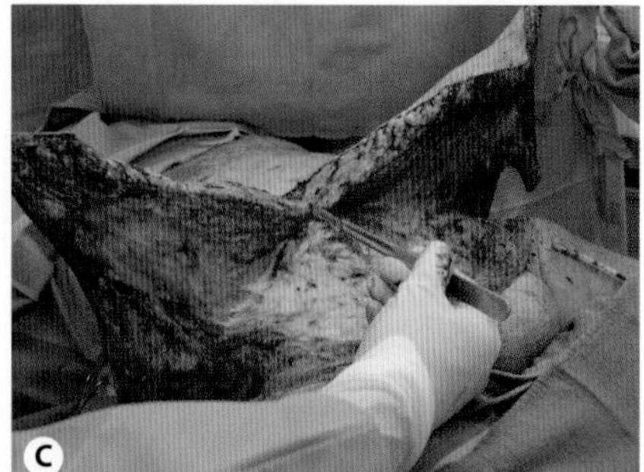

Fig. 9.40 Once the umbilicus is released, the inferior abdominal soft-tissue apron is split in anticipation of its removal, as well as to help visualize the dissection superiorly.

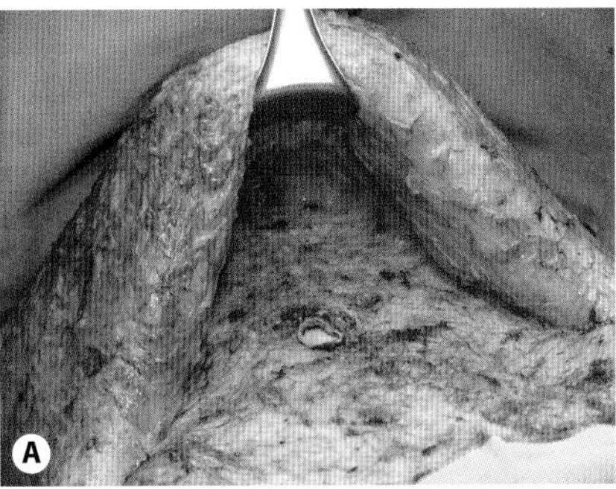
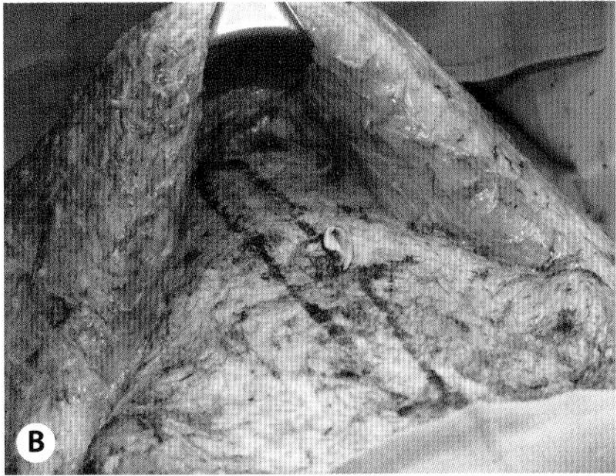
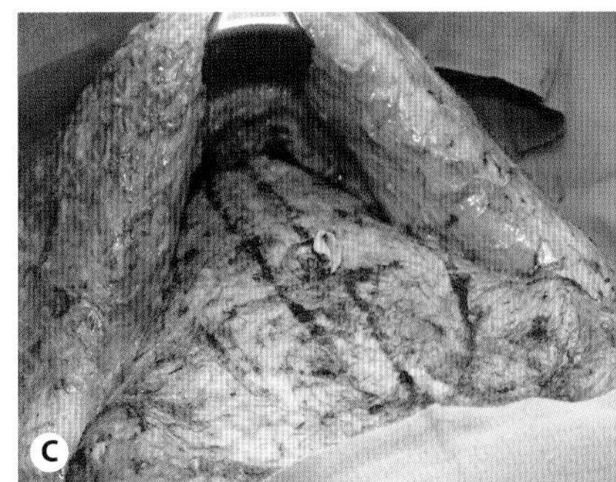

Fig. 9.41 The dissection is performed up to the costal margins and the xiphoid. The medial borders of the diastasis recti as well as the lateralmost extent of the estimated myofascial laxity are marked with methylene blue.

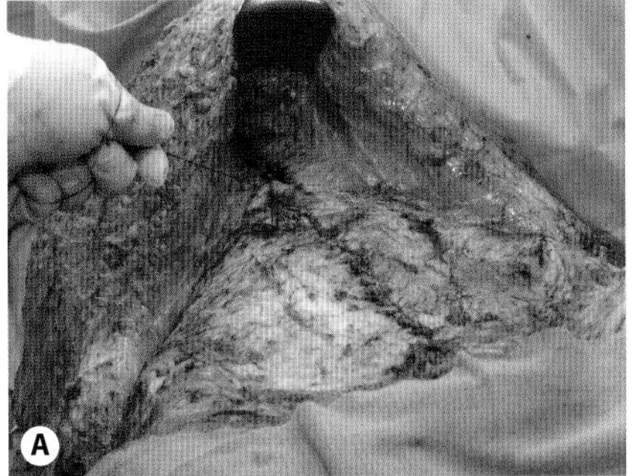
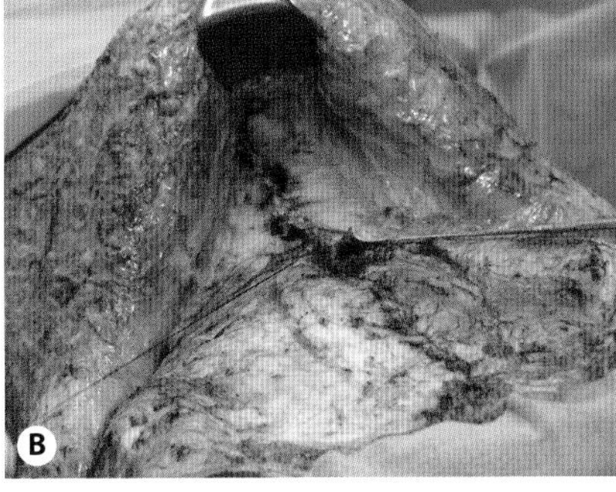
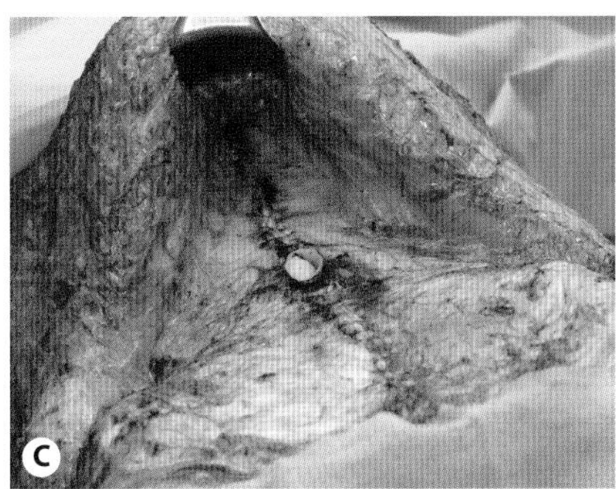

Fig. 9.42 Myofascial plication is performed using number 0 looped nylon. Plication starts at the xiphoid and is performed in a running fashion at the medial borders of the diastasis recti down to the pubic symphysis. The suture is placed on one side of the fascia at the level of the umbilicus, and plication resumes at the marks inferior to it. The benefit of the looped nylon is that a knot at the xiphoid is avoided. At the termination of the plication near the pubic symphysis the suture is tied in a manner that places the knot inside the plication, as described in Chapter 7.

with methylene blue, delineating the diastasis recti. The proposed lateral edge of the rectus sheath plication is also marked with methylene blue (**Fig. 9.41**). The myofascial plication is performed with number 0 looped nylon, avoiding the need to place a knot at the level of the xiphoid. The suture is run from the xiphoid to just above the umbilicus, at which point it continues along one edge of the rectus sheath. Plication resumes at the inferior edge of the umbilicus down to the level of the pubic symphysis, where the suture is tied in a manner that buries the knot deep to the fascial plication, as described in Chapter 7. A second layer of plication can be performed to further correct residual myofascial laxity if needed (**Fig. 9.42**).

Marcaine 0.5% is injected into the rectus sheath bilaterally to aid in postoperative pain control (**Fig. 9.43**). A local anesthetic pain pump is placed and secured along the myofascial plication in the midline to provide additional pain relief (**Fig. 9.44**). The anterior drain is laid across the lower abdomen and brought out through the skin inferior to the incision on the right side and secured with a silk suture (**Fig. 9.45**).

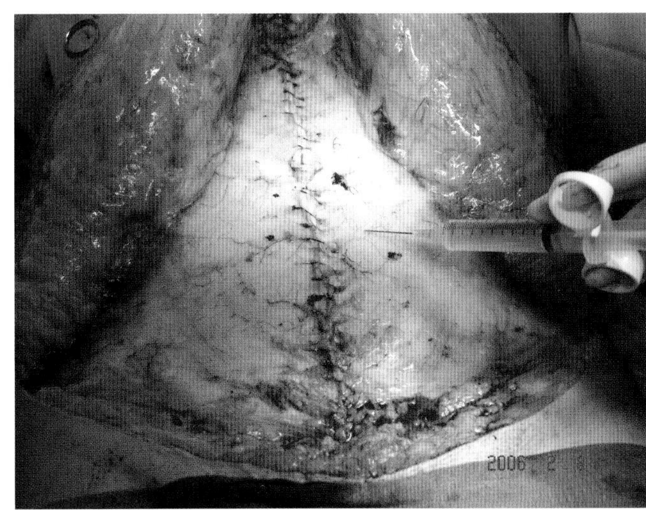

Fig. 9.43 After plication has been performed, 0.5% marcaine is injected under the anterior rectus sheath to help with postoperative pain control.

Tissue demarcation is performed next using the Pitanguy demarcator. The bed can be flexed for this maneuver, but care should be taken not to overestimate the amount of tissue resection (**Fig. 9.46**). Next, the areas for resection are measured to ensure symmetry (**Fig. 9.47**). The excess tissue is resected and a temporary midline staple is placed to facilitate identification of the new umbilical location, which is accomplished using the Pitanguy demarcator. A small

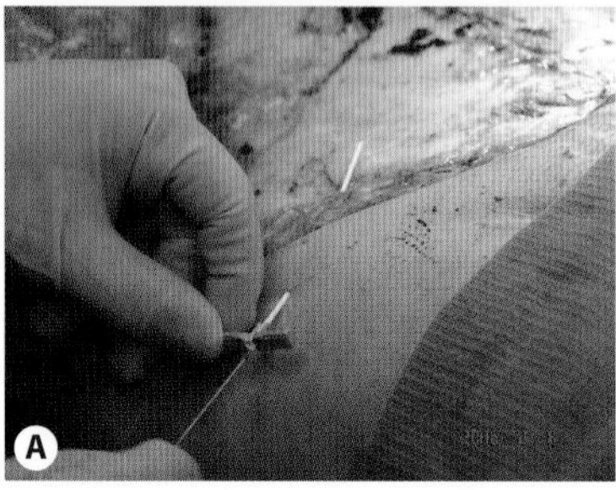

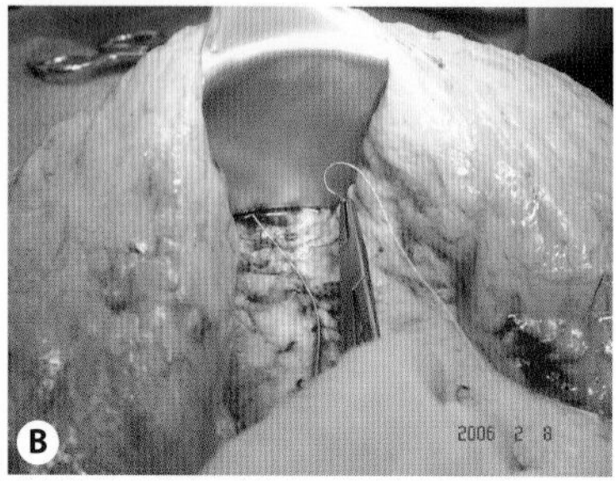

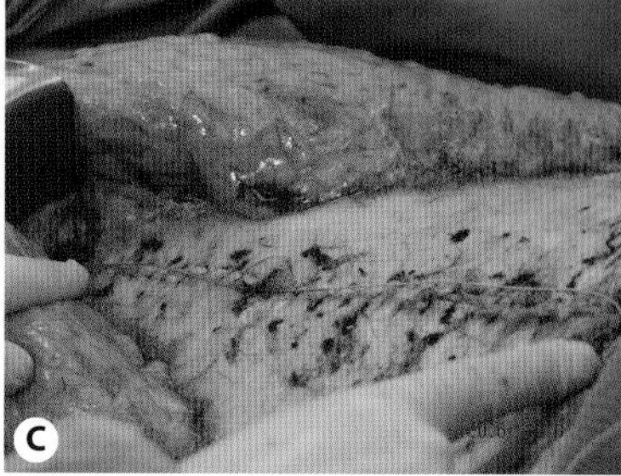

Fig. 9.44 A pain pump catheter is inserted beneath the edge of the lower incision and secured along the myofascial plication in the midline as well as at the skin entry point.

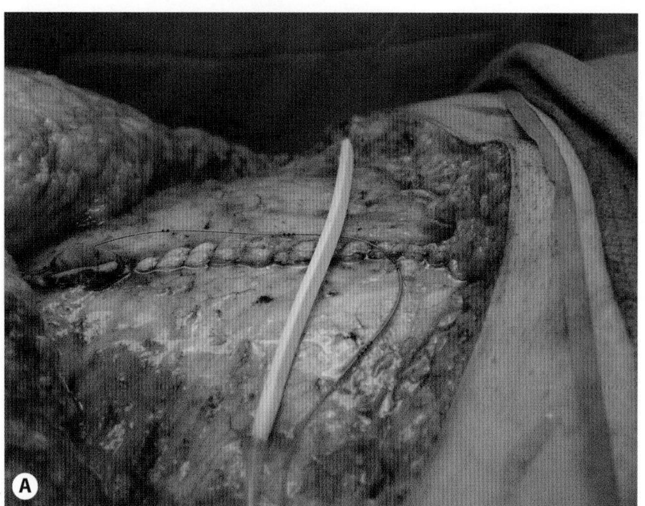

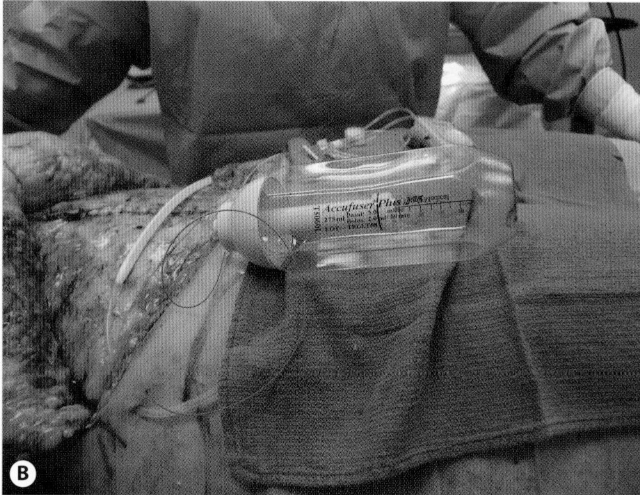

Fig. 9.45 A single drain is usually used. This is draped inferiorly, brought out below the lower incision edge near the pain pump catheter, and secured with silk suture.

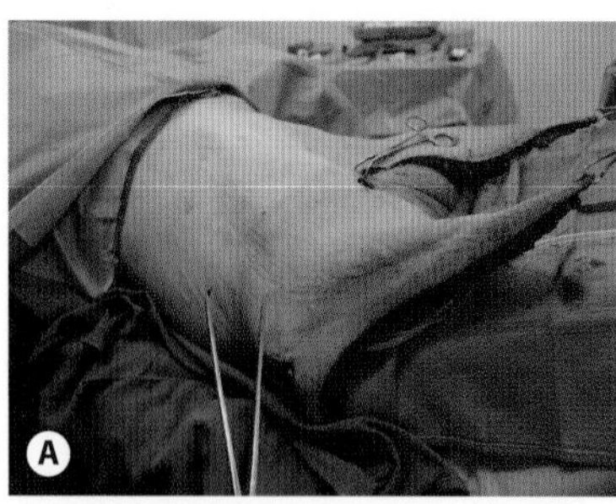

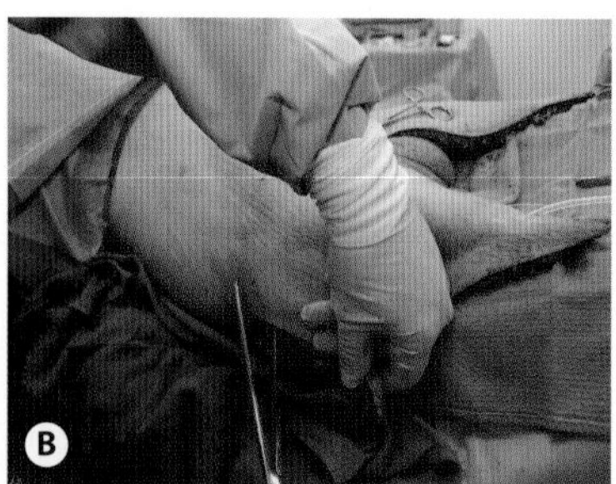

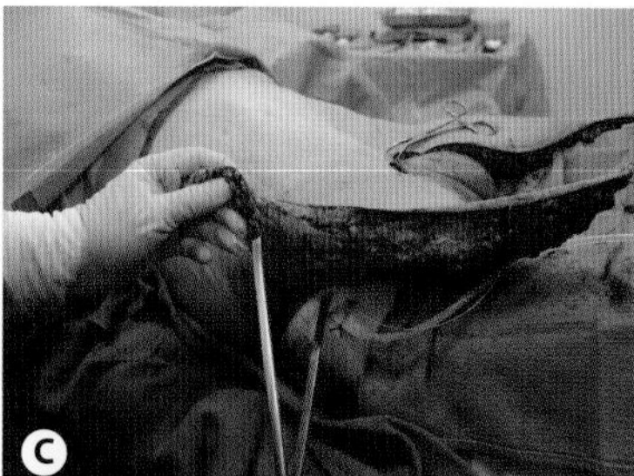

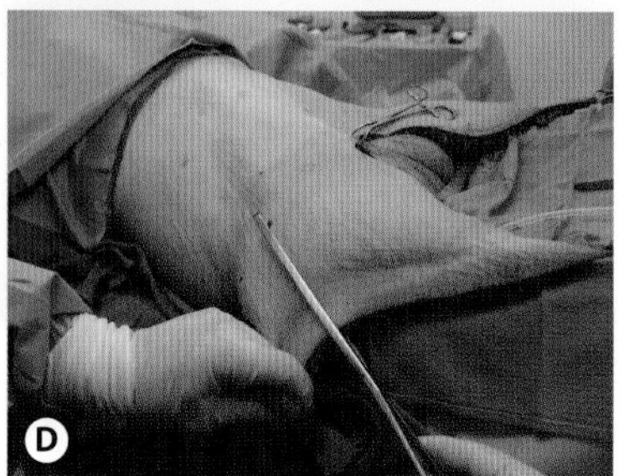

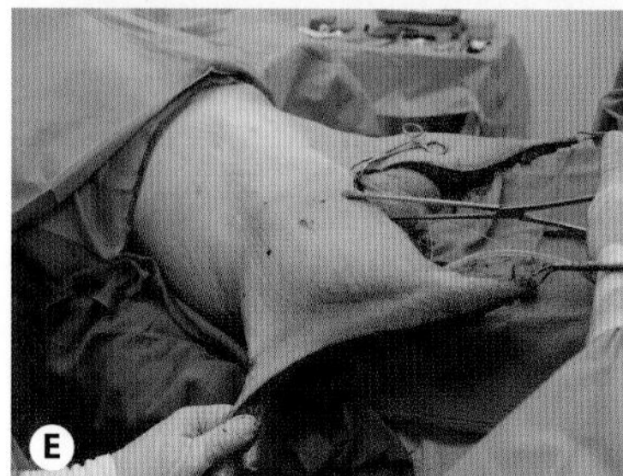

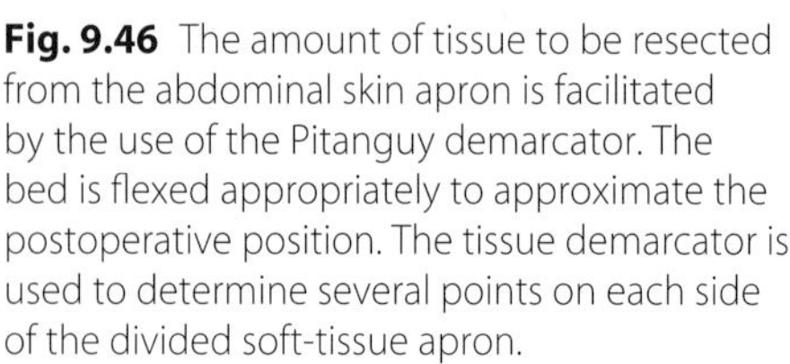

Fig. 9.46 The amount of tissue to be resected from the abdominal skin apron is facilitated by the use of the Pitanguy demarcator. The bed is flexed appropriately to approximate the postoperative position. The tissue demarcator is used to determine several points on each side of the divided soft-tissue apron.

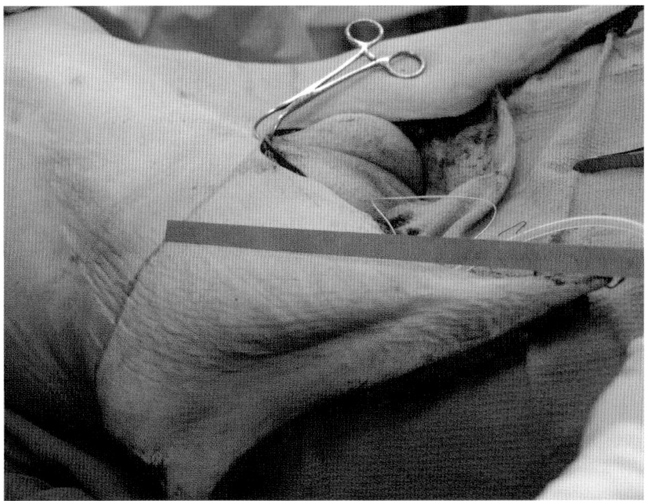

Fig. 9.47 The areas to be resected are measured and compared to ensure symmetry.

vertical ellipse is drawn, excised, and carefully defatted. The umbilicus is sewn into position with interrupted buried and intradermal 4/0 Monocryl. An intracuticular suture for umbilical closure is important to minimize any visible scarring (**Fig. 9.48**). Additional details on the umbilicus are covered in Chapter 12, The Umbilicus in Body Contouring.

The table is flexed appropriately to reduce the tension on the closure site. Final skin closure is performed with interrupted number 1 or 0 Vicryl through the superficial fascia, interrupted deep dermal 2/0 Vicryl, and intradermal 4/0 Monocryl. Tissue adhesive is then applied (**Fig. 9.49**) as a water impermeable dressing.

Perfusion of the abdominal soft-tissue apron is checked at this point by evaluating capillary refill in the most poorly perfused area, which is located in the midline between the umbilicus and the transverse incision (**Fig. 9.50**).

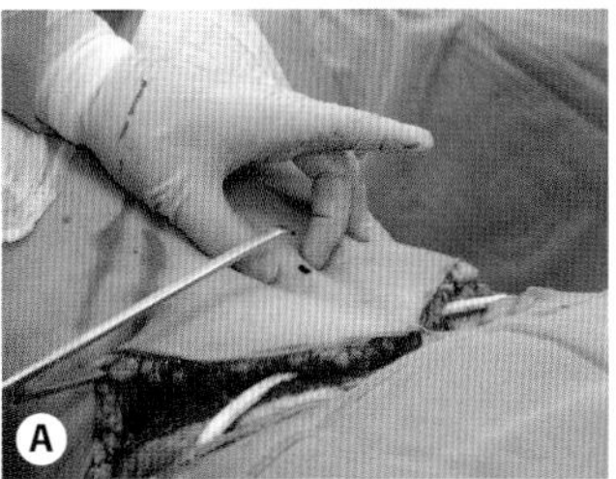

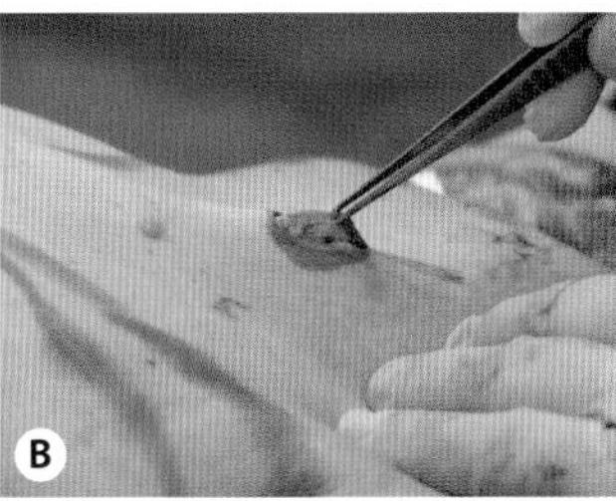

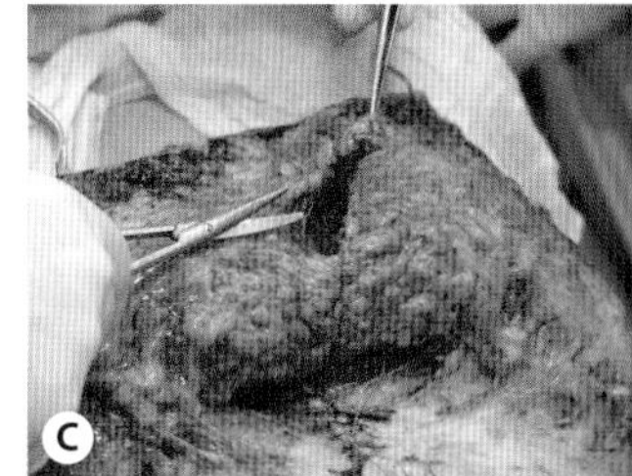

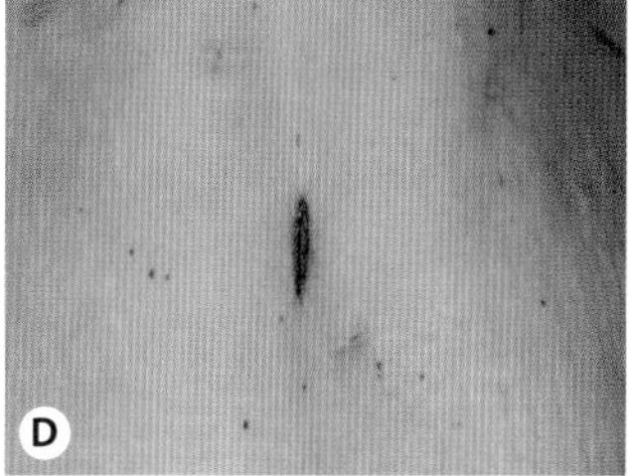

Fig. 9.48 The location of the neoumbilicus is also determined by using the Pitanguy demarcator. Once the location is marked, a small ellipse of skin and soft tissue is excised. The umbilicus is brought into this opening and secured with 4/0 Monocryl in buried interrupted as well as running intradermal sutures.

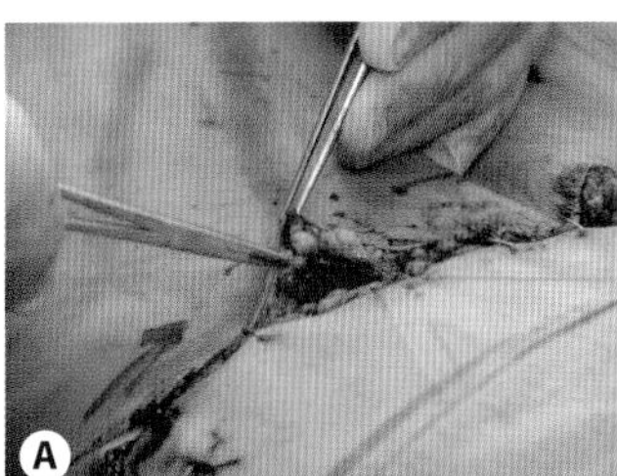

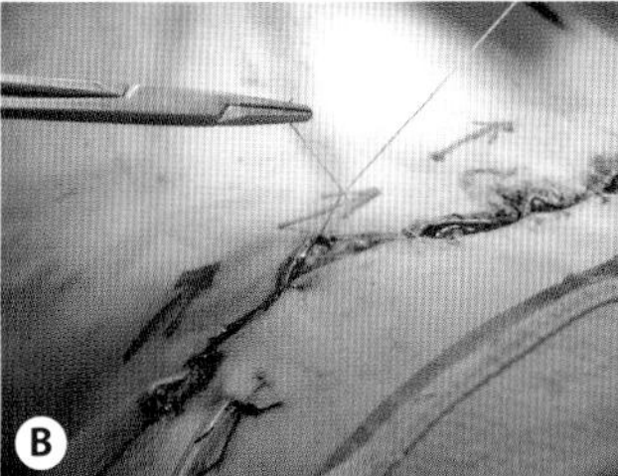

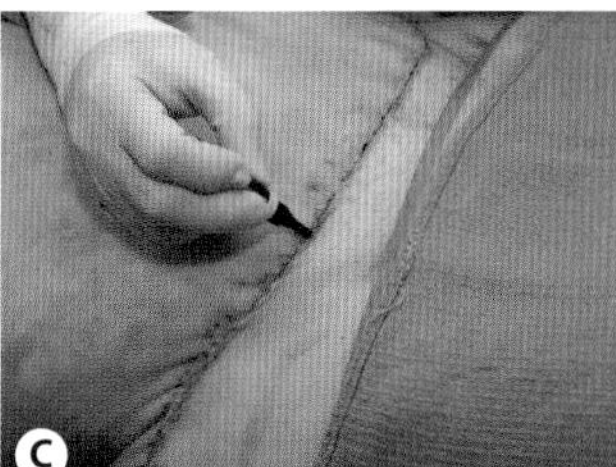

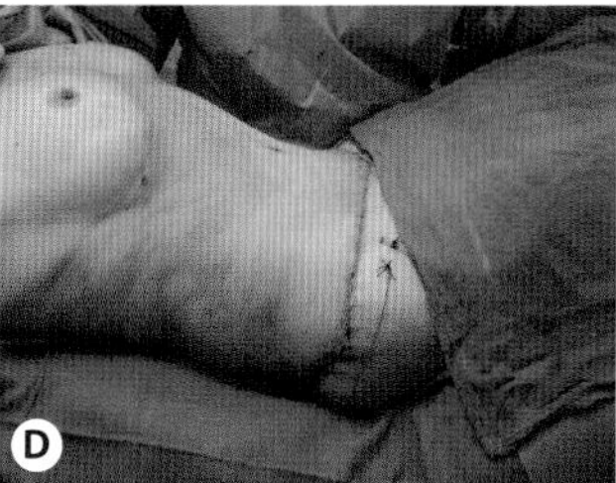

Fig. 9.49 The bed is flexed in a semi-Fowler position to reduce tension and facilitate closure. Closure is achieved with number 1 or 0 Vicryl through the superficial fascia, 2/0 buried deep-dermal Vicryl, and 4/0 running intradermal Monocryl. Tissue adhesive is used as a water-impermeable dressing.

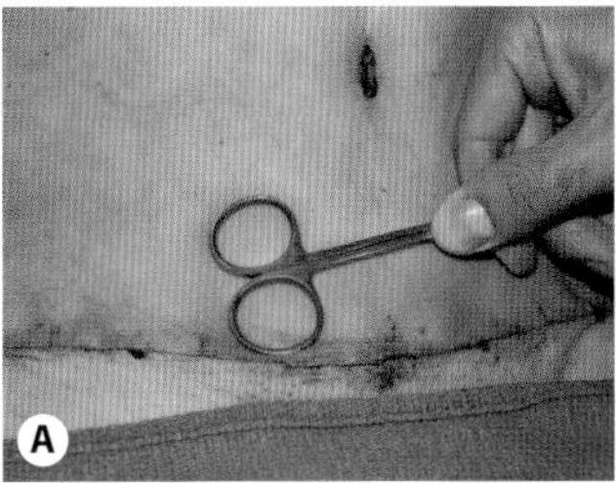

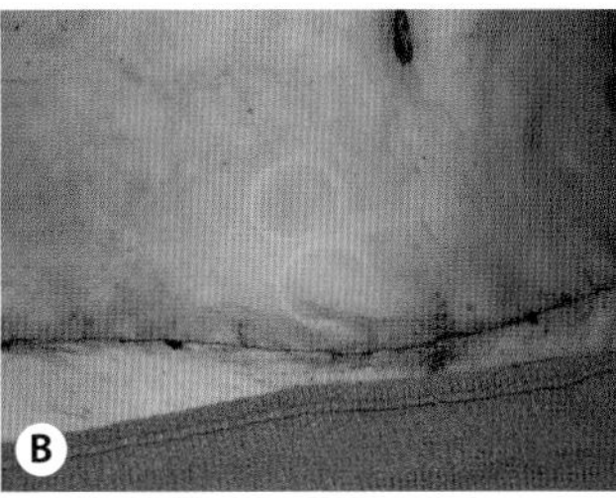

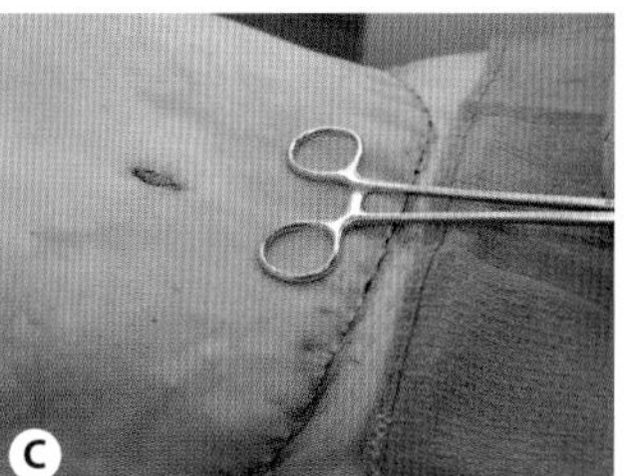

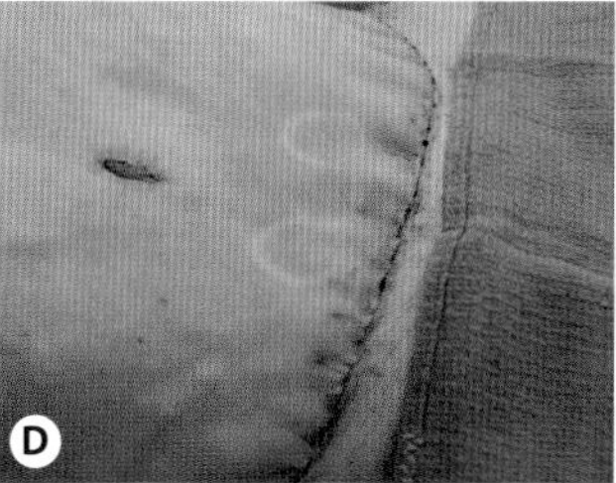

Fig. 9.50 Perfusion of the abdominal soft-tissue apron is checked by evaluating the capillary refill above the incision overlying the suprapubic area. This area is the furthest away from the blood supply and therefore the most poorly perfused.

Postoperative Care (Box 9.3)

The patient is warmed with a warming blanket and monitored in the recovery room until stable. We find that connecting the drain bulbs to high-vacuum wall suction will help rapidly reduce the amount of residual tumescent fluid in the tissues (**Fig. 9.51**), thereby more rapidly re-establishing tissue adherence and significantly reducing the incidence of seroma. Evaluation of abdominal soft-tissue perfusion in the perioperative period is important to verify that the abdominal binder is not too tight and to ensure that there are no unwanted folds or creases that could potentially reduce vascular supply to the skin (**Fig. 9.52**).

Box 9.3 Postoperative instructions for circumferential abdominoplasty

Many of the postoperative instructions for circumferential abdominoplasty are similar to those for full and extended abdominoplasty. Because more of these patients are likely to be massive weight loss patients following gastric bypass, a longer healing time may be needed and the duration of certain restrictions such as activity may need to be modified.

- Maintain a partially flexed position at the waist for the first 1–2 weeks
- Wear the abdominal binder at all times, except for showering
- Make sure the binder is maintained low enough on the abdomen
- Verify that there are no significant creases, folds, or the presence of drain tubes underneath the binder
- Avoid smoking or exposure to nicotine-containing products
- Breathe deeply and use the incentive spirometer frequently
- Drink plenty of fluids: 8 oz/h is the goal
- Move legs frequently while resting, and walk regularly
- Drain care as instructed
- Continue to take multivitamin daily. Resume medications as instructed
- If buttock augmentation has been performed use ample padding when sitting
- No vigorous activity or heavy lifting for 4–6 weeks. Submersion under water, including swimming, is prohibited until proper healing has occurred and all of the drains have been removed

Patients undergoing circumferential abdominoplasty usually benefit from overnight care in a medical facility, which will permit more diligent fluid status monitoring as well as better pain management, and ensure that the patient is walking periodically and using the incentive spirometer frequently. Patients are seen in the office for follow-up shortly after the procedure and a number of times during the first few weeks after surgery.

On discharge, patients are sent home with oral antibiotics, pain medication, and vitamins, which are started preoperatively. They are instructed to keep their waist slightly flexed and to refrain from heavy lifting or vigorous activity. If autologous buttock augmentation has been performed concurrently the patient is instructed to have adequate padding in the gluteal area when sitting. Frequent movement of the lower extremities while in bed and regular walking are encouraged to help reduce the chance of DVT/PE. Patients are instructed to stay well hydrated by drinking plenty of fluids. Instructions regarding drain care are provided to the patient and their caregiver. The abdominal binder is worn at all times in the immediate postoperative period, except for showering, which is allowed on postoperative day 2. Preoperative and postoperative photos are shown in **Figs 9.53–9.59**.

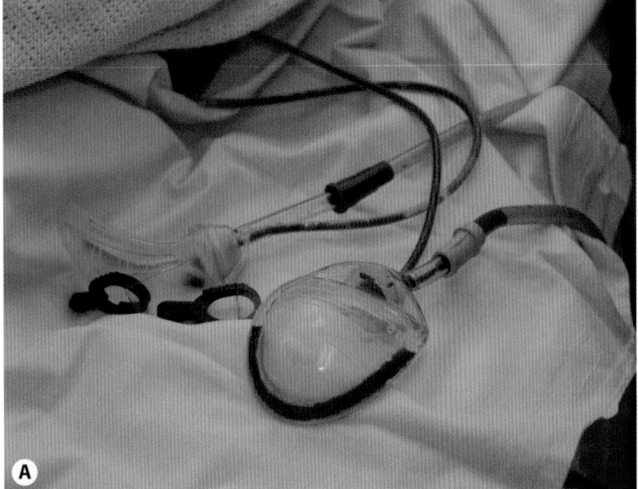

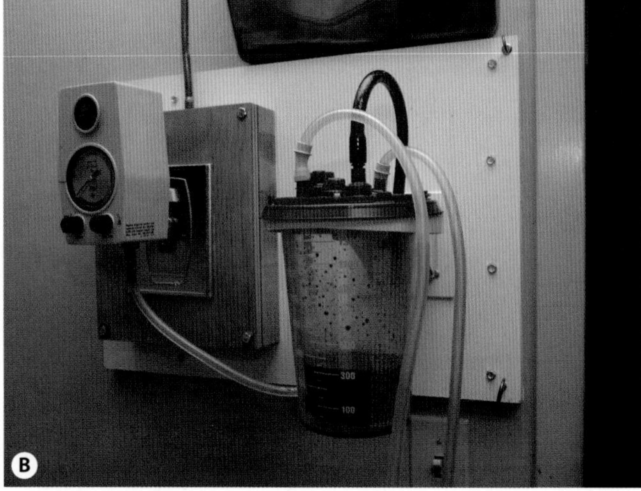

Fig. 9.51 In the postoperative recovery area the drains are connected to vacuum suction to facilitate evacuation of any residual tumescent fluid.

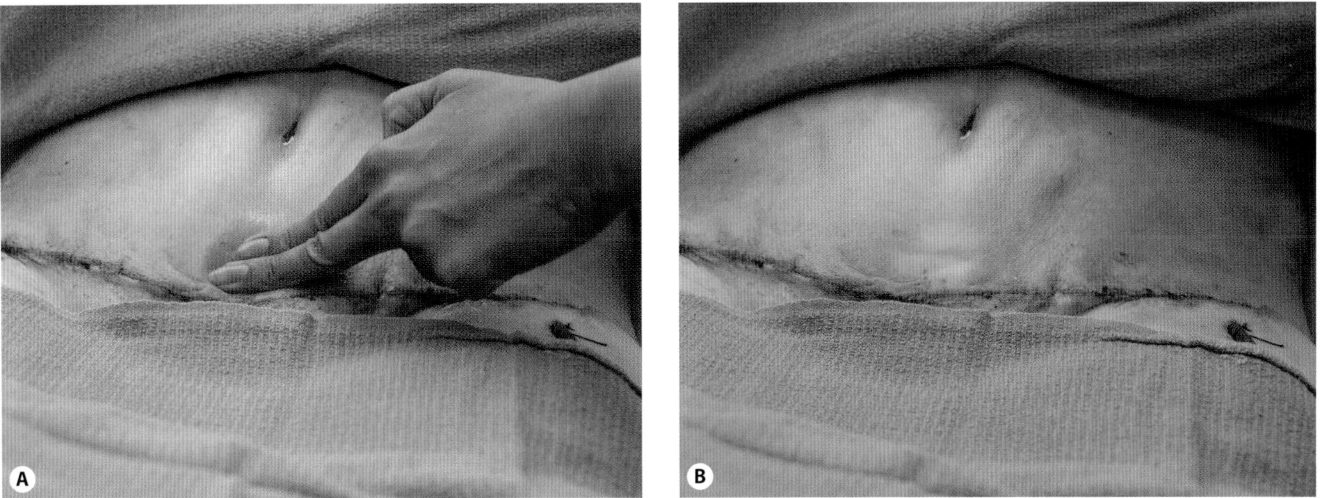

Fig. 9.52 Perfusion of the abdominal soft-tissue is also evaluated in the recovery area. This also serves to verify that the abdominal binder is not too tight, and that there are no unwanted folds or creases in the foam or garment that would negatively affect vascular supply to the skin.

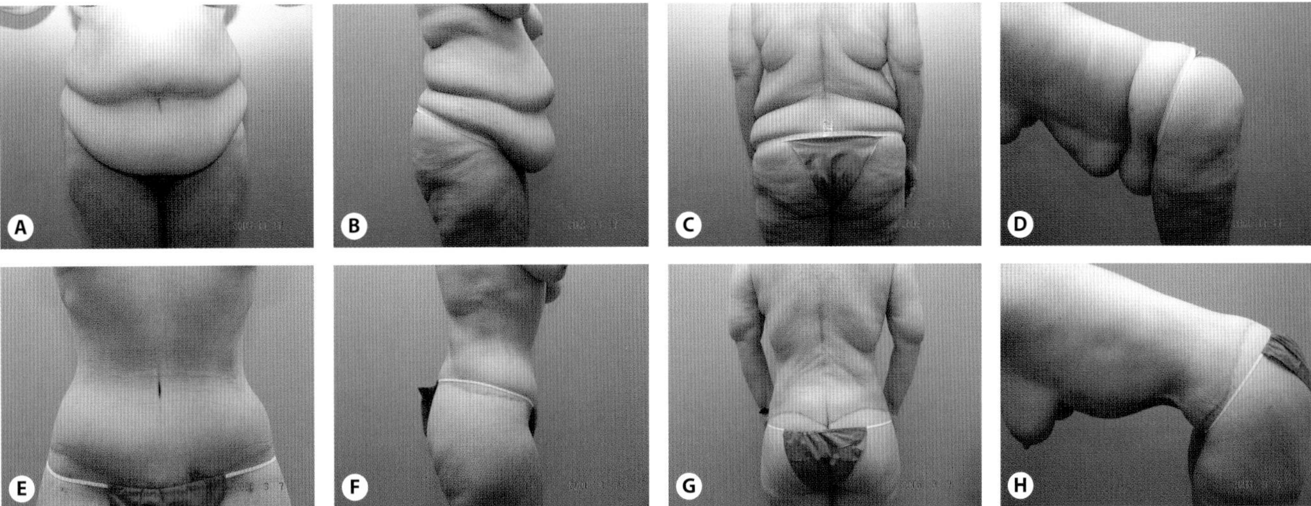

Fig. 9.53 A 55-year-old woman, height 5′2″, weight 167 lb, BMI 30.5. She has excess adiposity circumferentially and significant contour irregularity anteriorly. She underwent circumferential abdominoplasty with myofascial plication and full abdominal liposuction. Her dress size decreased from 10–12 to 4–6.

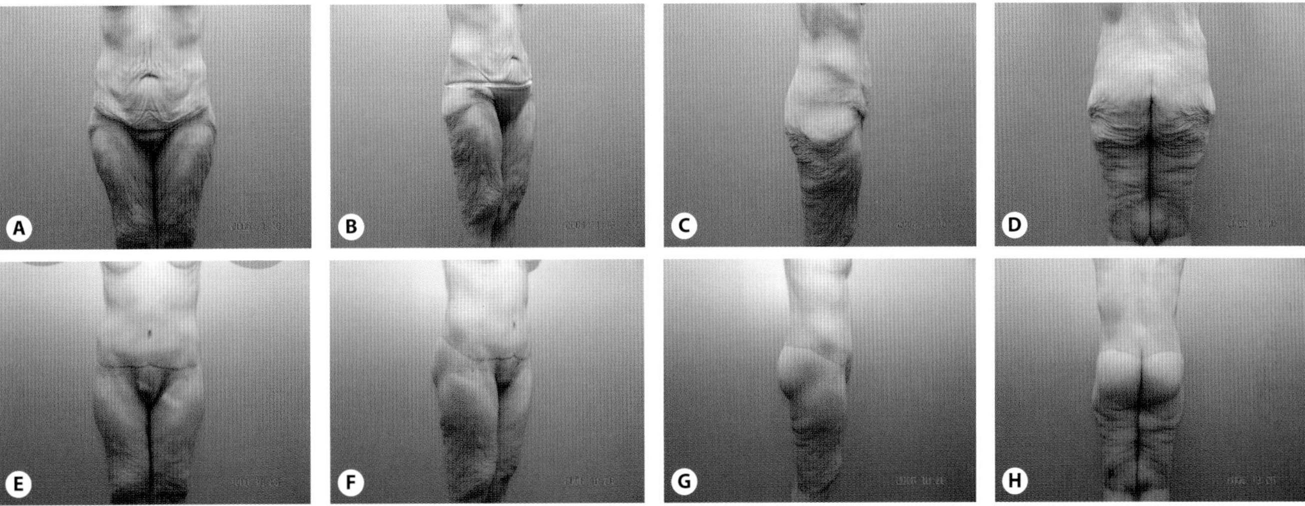

Fig. 9.54 A 54-year-old woman, height 5′1″, 155 lb, BMI 29.3. She has a significant amount of excess skin laxity, with the most significant contour deformity seen in the thighs and lower buttocks. She underwent circumferential abdominoplasty with autologous buttochs augmentation. Excellent correction of the excess soft-tissue laxity is evident, particularly in the hip and thigh area.

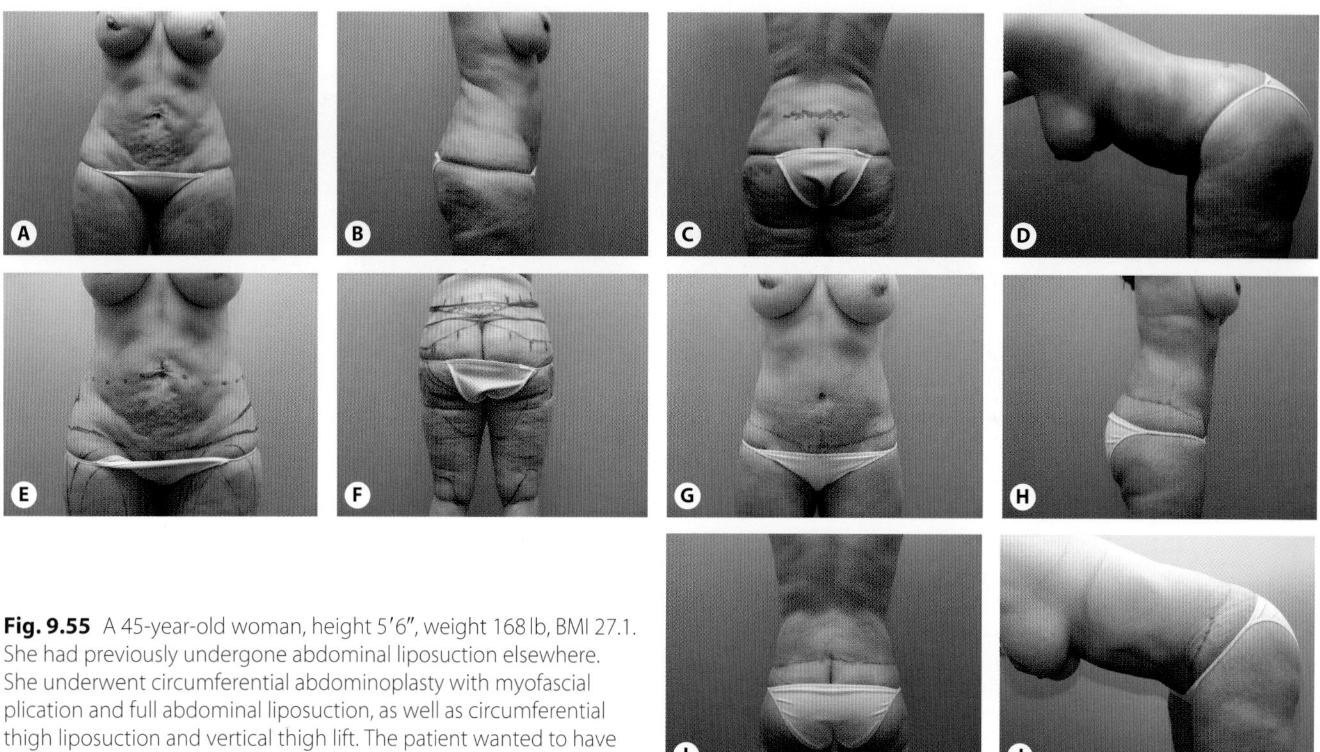

Fig. 9.55 A 45-year-old woman, height 5′6″, weight 168 lb, BMI 27.1. She had previously undergone abdominal liposuction elsewhere. She underwent circumferential abdominoplasty with myofascial plication and full abdominal liposuction, as well as circumferential thigh liposuction and vertical thigh lift. The patient wanted to have her posterior tattoo removed, so the posterior preoperative markings indicate our plan to accomplish this.

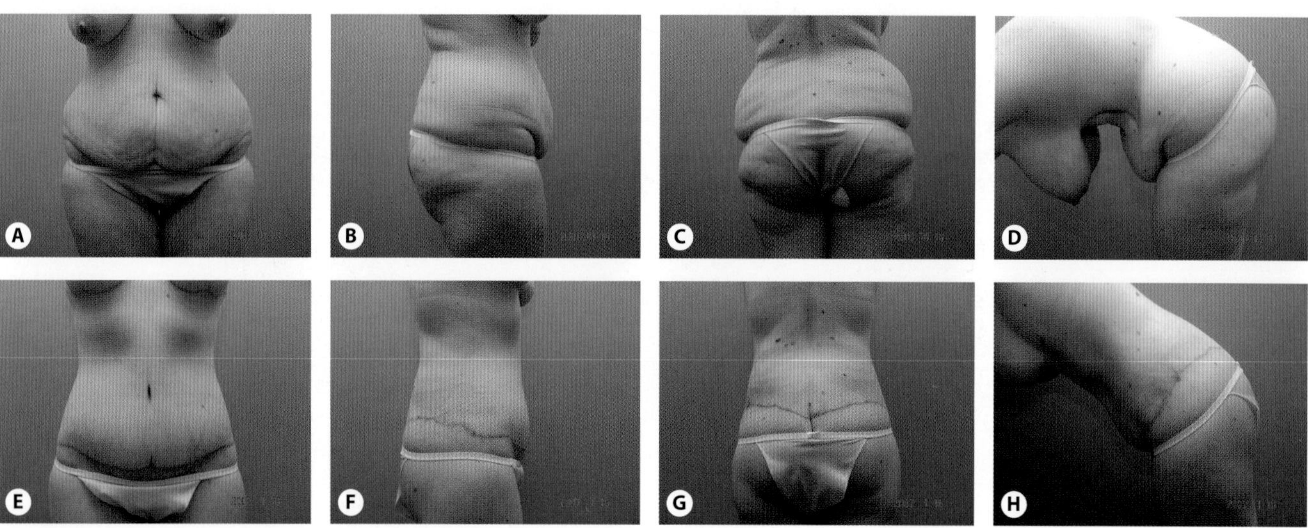

Fig. 9.56 A 36-year-old woman, height 5′5″, weight 153 lb, BMI 25.5. She underwent circumferential abdominoplasty with myofascial plication and full abdominal and concurrent bach liposuction.

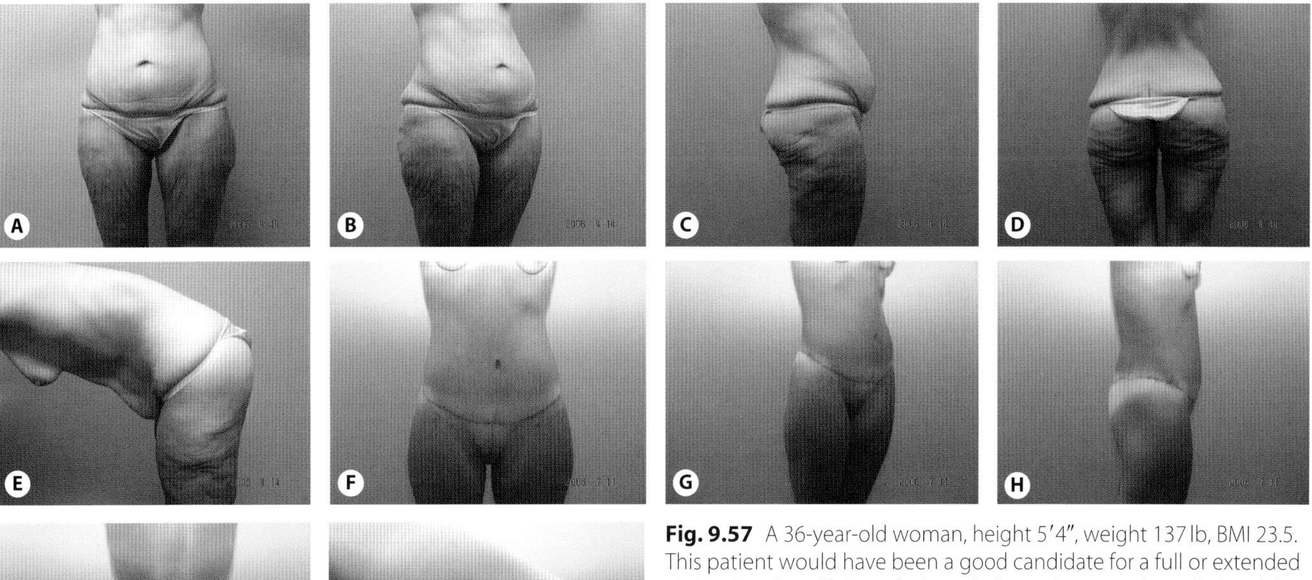

Fig. 9.57 A 36-year-old woman, height 5′4″, weight 137 lb, BMI 23.5. This patient would have been a good candidate for a full or extended abdominoplasty if the soft-tissue laxity and contour irregularity of the hips, thighs, and buttocks were not an issue. She wanted correction of the laxity and contour irregularity of hips, thighs, and buttocks as well, so a circumferential abdominoplasty with myofascial plication but without abdominal liposuction was performed.

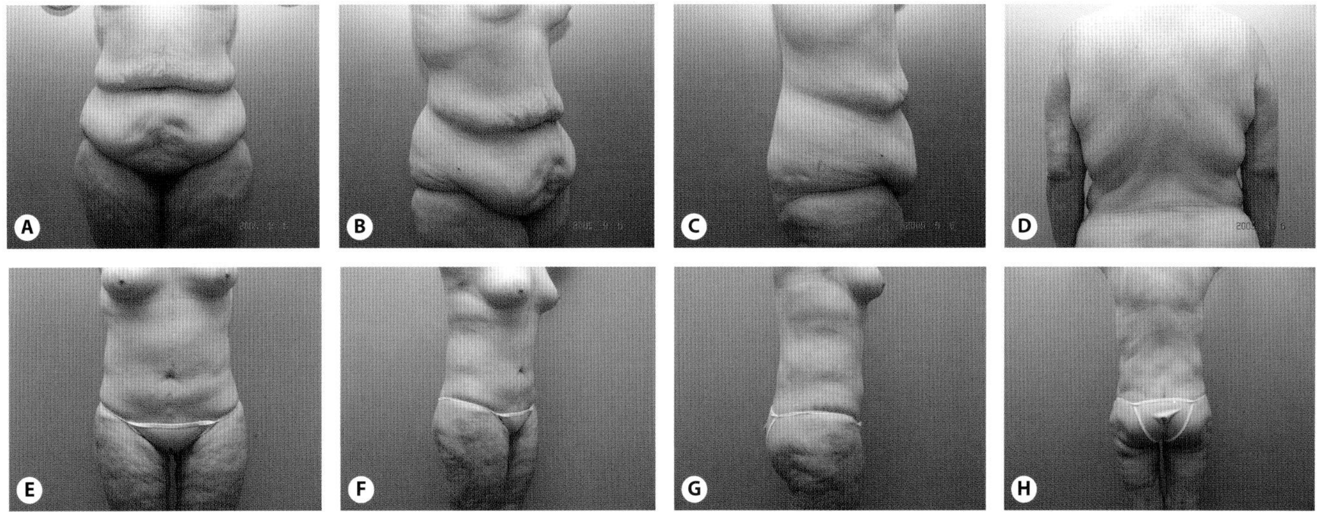

Fig. 9.58 A 35-year-old woman, height 5′4″, weight 185 lb, BMI 31.8. This patient underwent a circumferential abdominoplasty with an anterior vertical soft-tissue resection along with myofascial plication and full abdominal liposuction. She would have been an acceptable candidate for a standard circumferential abdominoplasty without a vertical resection, but the possibility of improved contour with a vertical resection was discussed with her, as well as the pros and cons involved, namely the presence of a vertical scar. She elected to proceed with a vertical resection as well. Postoperatively she has a significantly improved silhouette and contour. The vertical scar is of good quality.

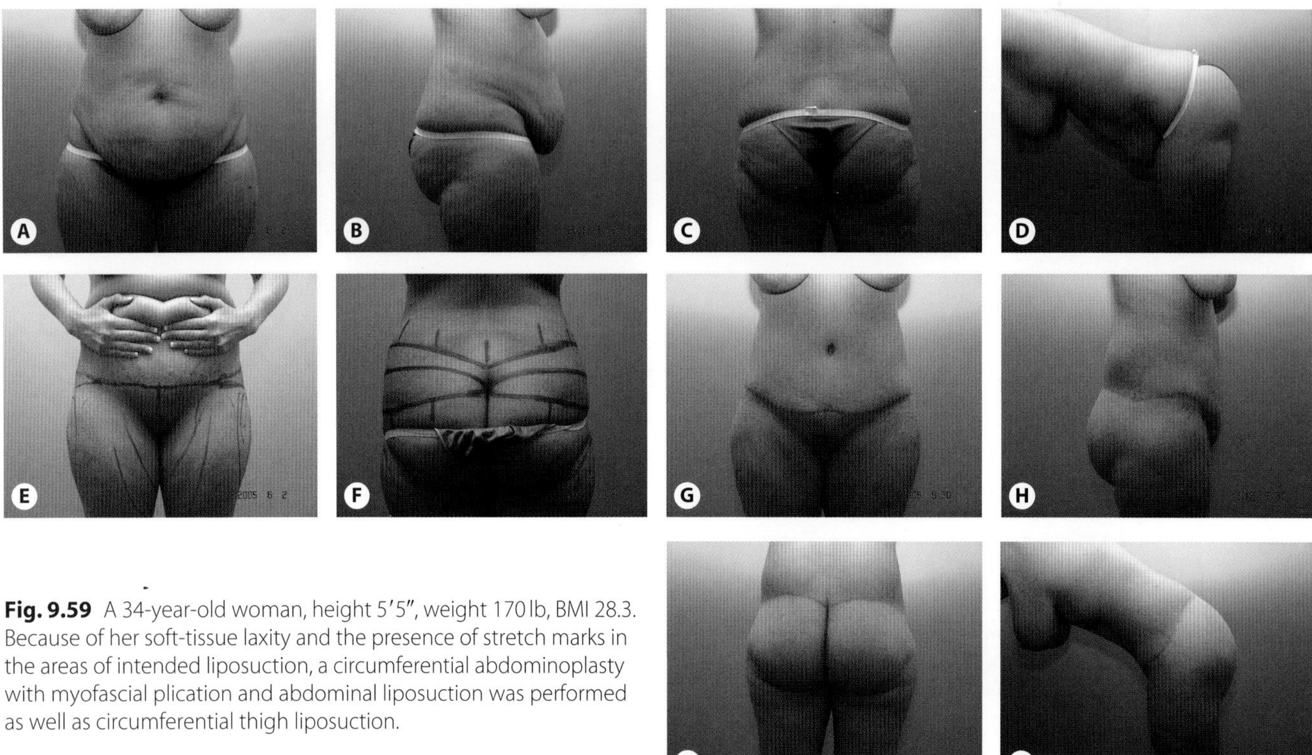

Fig. 9.59 A 34-year-old woman, height 5′5″, weight 170 lb, BMI 28.3. Because of her soft-tissue laxity and the presence of stretch marks in the areas of intended liposuction, a circumferential abdominoplasty with myofascial plication and abdominal liposuction was performed as well as circumferential thigh liposuction.

Summary

Circumferential abdominoplasty is a very powerful procedure for contouring the trunk and buttocks area. It is applicable to a large segment of the body contouring patient population and is the procedure of choice if skin and soft tissue redundancy of the torso is present circumferentially. It combines the benefits and goals of a full abdominoplasty, including thinning, tightening, and flattening the abdominal contour as well as rejuvenation of the buttocks and the anterolateral thighs. Circumferential abdominoplasty patients are consistently some of the happiest and most grateful patients of the body contouring population.

Clinical Caveats: Circumferential abdominoplasty

- Massive weight loss patients are best served by circumferential abdominoplasty with or without a vertical anterior resection to properly address the significant amount of soft tissue laxity
- The procedure must be individualized for each patient. The benefit of autologous buttock augmentation and other ancillary procedures should be considered
- Preoperative instructions/requirements must be methodically followed to maximize safety
- Preoperative markings and photographs are invaluable to achieve the best possible results
- Concurrent liposuction of the abdominal soft-tissue apron is of great value, especially for the patient with incomplete weight loss or those who have moderate to significant excess adiposity
- The vertical resection should end inferiorly with the ends curving medially, similar to an unfinished ellipse as opposed to a triangle
- Subscarpal fat resection can be performed safely if needed
- Injection of bupivacaine under the rectus sheath will help reduce postoperative discomfort, which facilitates deep breathing and reduces postoperatively use of pain medication
- Overnight care in an accredited facility will allow better fluid status management and pain control, and reduce the chance of DVT through the use of pneumatic compression devices and ambulation
- Evaluation postoperative day 1 and regularly over the next week will allow proper intervention if postoperative care issues arise

References

1. Aly AS, Cram AE, Chao M, et al. Belt lipectomy for circumferential truncal excess: the University of Iowa experience. Plast Reconstruct Surg 2003; 111: 398.
2. Hamra ST. Circumferential body lift. Aesthet Surg J 1999; 19: 244.
3. Sebastian JL. Bariatric surgery and work-up of the massive weight loss patient. Clin Plast Surg 2008; 35: 11.
4. El-Khatib HA, Bener A. Abdominal dermolipectomy in an abdomen with pre-existing scars: a different concept. Plast Reconstruct Surg 2004; 114: 992.
5. Manassa EH, Hertl CH, Olbrisch RR. Wound healing problems in smokers and non-smokers after 132 abdominoplasties. Plast Reconstruct Surg 2003; 111: 2082.
6. Krueger JK, Rohrich RJ. Clearing the smoke: the scientific rationale for tobacco abstention with plastic surgery. Plast Reconstruct Surg 2001; 108: 1063.
7. Blickstein D, Blickstein I. Oral contraception and thrombophilia. Curr Opin Obstet Gynecol 2007; 19: 370.
8. van Vlijmen EF, Brouwer JL, Veeger NJ, et al. Oral contraceptives and the absolute risk of venous thromboembolism in women with single or multiple thrombophilic defects: results from a retrospective family cohort study. Arch Intern Med 2007; 167: 282.
9. Davison SP, Venturi ML, Attinger CE, et al. Prevention of venous thromboembolism in the plastic surgery patient. Plast Reconstruct Surg 2004; 114: 43.
10. Broughton G 2nd, Rios JL, Rohrich RJ, Brown SA. Deep venous thrombosis prophylaxis practice and treatment strategies among plastic surgeons: survey results. Plast Reconstruct Surg 2007; 119: 157.

Suggested Reading

Aly AS, Cram AE, Heddens C. Truncal body contouring surgery in the massive weight loss patient. Clin Plast Surg 2004; 31: 611.

Carwell GR. Circumferential torsoplasty. Ann Plast Surg 1997; 38: 213.

Davison SP, Clemens MW. Safety first: precautions for the massive weight loss patient. Clin Plast Surg 2008; 35: 173.

de Jong RH, Grazer FM. Perioperative management of cosmetic liposuction. Plast Reconstruct Surg 2001; 107: 1039.

Gonzalez-Ulloa M. Belt lipectomy. Br J Plast Surg 1961; 13: 179.

Hunstad JP. Advanced abdominoplasty concepts. In: Saleh MS, ed. Perspectives in plastic surgery, Vol. 12. New York: Thieme, 1999; 13–38.

Hunstad JP, Aitken ME. Circumferential body contouring, in body contouring after massive weight loss. St Louis: Quality Medical Publishing, 2006.

Illouz YG. History and current concepts of lipoplasty. Clin Plast Surg 1996; 23: 721.

Iverson RE, Lynch DJ. Practice advisory on liposuction. Plast Reconstruct Surg 2004; 113: 1478.

Klein JA. Tumescent technique for liposuction surgery. Am J Cosmet Surg 1987; 4: 263.

Klein JA. Tumescent technique for regional anesthesia permits lidocaine doses of 35 mg/kg for liposuction. J Dermatol Surg Oncol 1990; 16: 248.

Klein JA. Tumescent technique for local anesthesia improves safety in large volume liposuction. Plast Reconstruct Surg 1993; 92: 1085.

Lockwood TE. Lower body lift with superficial fascial system suspension. Plast Reconstruct Surg 1993; 92: 112.

Lockwood TE. Lower-body lift. Aesthet Surg J 2001; 21: 355.

Pascal JF, Le Louarn C. Remodeling bodylift with high lateral tension. Aesthet Plast Surg 2002; 26: 223.

Pitanguy I. Abdominal lipectomy. Clin Plast Surg 1975; 2: 401.

Rohrich RJ, Broughton G 2nd, Horton B, et al. The key to long-term success in liposuction: a guide for plastic surgeons and patients. Plast Reconstruct Surg 2004; 114.

Rohrich RJ, Raniere J Jr., Beran SJ, Kenkel JM. Patient evaluation and indications for ultrasound-assisted lipoplasty. Clin Plast Surg 1999; 26: 269.

Rohrich RJ, Smith PD, Marcantonio DR, Kenkel JM. The zones of adherence: role in minimizing and preventing contour deformities in liposuction. Plast Reconstruct Surg 2001; 107: 1562–1569.

Teimourian B. Complications associated with suction lipectomy. Clin Plast Surg 1989; 16: 385.

Trott SA, Beran SJ, Rohrich RJ, et al. Safety considerations and fluid resuscitation in liposuction: An analysis of 53 consecutive patients. Plast Reconstruct Surg 1998; 102: 2220.

CHAPTER **10**

Reverse Abdominoplasty

Joseph P. Hunstad, Mauro Deos & Remus Repta

IN THIS CHAPTER

KEY POINTS

Reverse abdominoplasty is an unusual yet useful option for abdominal contouring in patients who have primarily upper abdominal soft-tissue laxity. The advantage of reverse abdominoplasty in these patients is that the resection is in the region of the upper abdominal laxity and fullness, and therefore it is more effective in correcting it. The final scar is ideally hidden within the inframammary fold. In addition, the umbilicus rarely needs to be released and re-inset, as the upward pull generated from the reverse abdominoplasty lifts and rotates the umbilicus and periumbilical soft tissue to their original position. The procedure can be combined with breast augmentation, mastopexy/reduction, or with upper and middle back contouring procedures such as a bra-line back lift (see Chapter 13, Ancillary Procedures).

Introduction

With the exception of endoscopic abdominoplasty, most abdominoplasty procedures involve resection of transverse skin and soft tissue inferiorly and placement of the final scar below or within the bikini or underwear line. Vertical soft-tissue laxity is thus corrected and the final scar is well hidden. Because most patients present with soft-tissue laxity and striae in the lower half of the abdomen, the standard abdominoplasty technique is very effective. Some patients, however, do not fit the classic abdominoplasty body habitus description. These patients may present with mild to significant upper abdominal soft-tissue laxity, relatively little or no lower abdominal laxity, and good lower abdominal skin quality with absence of striae (**Fig. 10.1 A, B**). Upper abdominal tissue resection is more effective at correcting the specific abdominal contour deformity in these patients, and does so by placing the final scar in the inframammary fold, hidden in the inferior border of the bra (**Fig. 10.2**).[1,3] This chapter will review important clinical and operative points of reverse abdominoplasty.

Patient Selection (Box 10.1)

Patients who are good candidates for reverse abdominoplasty have skin laxity or poor skin quality in the upper half of the abdomen, or have a significant amount of soft-tissue redundancy in the upper half of the abdomen that will not be adequately addressed by a full abdominoplasty technique. Poor lower abdominal skin quality

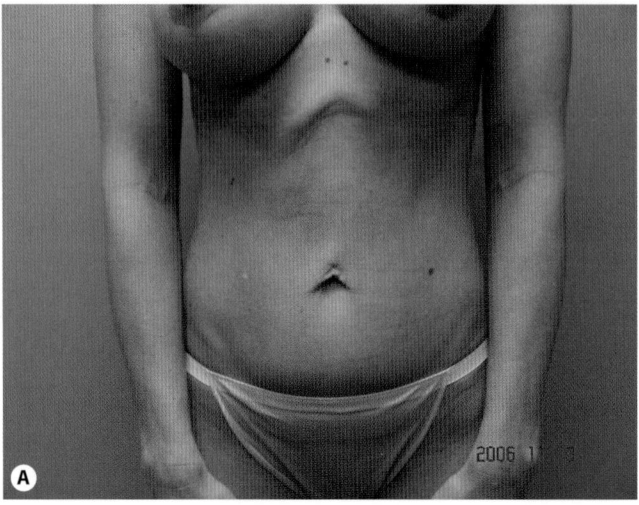

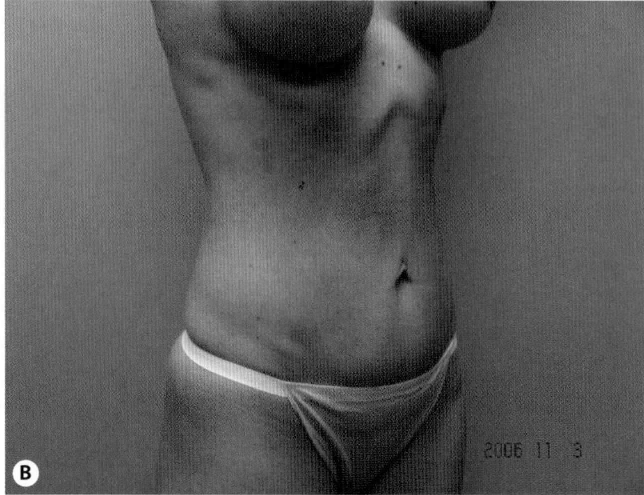

Fig. 10.1 Patients who are candidates for reverse abdominoplasty have upper abdominal skin and soft-tissue laxity that may be insufficiently addressed with standard abdominoplasty procedures. In addition, the ideal candidate has good skin quality without stretch marks, and relatively mild lower abdominal tissue laxity.

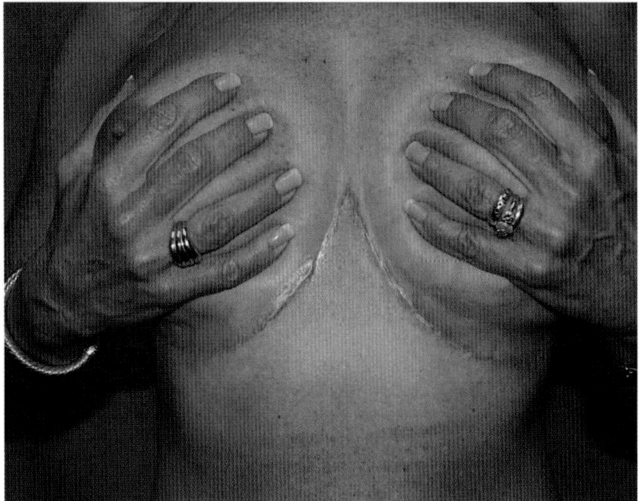

Fig. 10.2 The benefit of reverse abdominoplasty is that the resection is closer to the upper abdominal tissue laxity and hence more capable of correcting the deformity. The final scar can be concealed in the inframammary fold area within the confines of the bra. Concurrent breast procedures, including augmentation, mastopexy, and reduction, can be performed, as the inframammary incision will correspond to the final reverse abdominoplasty scar.

and the presence of striae is a common reason for patients requesting more traditional abdominoplasty procedures. In most patients the striae are located in the lower half of the abdomen, extending superior to or just above the umbilicus. Much less commonly seen are those patients who present with skin and soft-tissue laxity primarily located in the upper half of the abdomen. These patients are ideal candidates for reverse abdominoplasty, bearing in mind that direct excision is the most effective treatment for soft-tissue laxity.

Box 10.1 Relative contraindications for reverse abdominoplasty

The relative contraindications for reverse abdominoplasty are in addition to those that pertain to the standard abdominoplasty patient (see chapters on full, extended, and circumferential abdominoplasty).

- Excess upper abdominal adiposity without significant soft-tissue laxity
- Significant lower or global abdominal soft-tissue laxity
- Previous surgery with low subcostal scars that cannot be excised during the reverse abdominoplasty
- Poor skin quality with extensive lower abdominal striae
- History or concern of hypertrophic/keloid scars in the sternal or parasternal area
- Umbilical shape and position that would benefit from umbilicus release and inset with a standard abdominoplasty

Patients with significant lower as well as upper abdominal skin and soft-tissue laxity are best served by a traditional full abdominoplasty, to be followed in the future by a reverse abdominoplasty only if necessary.[4] The full abdominoplasty is usually sufficient to correct both lower and upper abdominal skin and soft-tissue laxity and excess adiposity. We recommend that the staged procedure, if upper abdominal laxity persists, is performed at least 6 months between procedures.

Additional procedures can also be combined with the reverse abdominoplasty. The most common involve procedures performed with reverse abdominoplasty the breasts and those that allow contouring of the upper and middle back. Various breast procedures, including breast lift with or without augmentation, can be performed in combination with a reverse abdominoplasty, as the two procedures will share a common final transverse scar at or above the level of the inframammary fold. Contouring of the upper and middle back can also be combined with a reverse abdominoplasty in the form of a bra-line back lift (see Chapter 12). This procedure resects the excess soft tissue of the upper and middle back and places the final scar within the confines of the posterior bra line. This allows correction of the soft-tissue laxity of the middle and upper back that cannot be achieved by the posterior component of a circumferential abdominoplasty because of the strong fascial attachments of the midline zone of adherence. The final scar is placed within the bra line, and the lateral extent of the incision in this case is joined with the inframammary scar from the reverse abdominoplasty.

An additional advantage of the reverse abdominoplasty is that the umbilicus usually does not need to be released and re-inset, as the upward pull is directly opposite to the natural downward drift of the aging process.[5] The force and vector created by the reverse abdominoplasty naturally contributes to the rejuvenation of the umbilicus by raising and rotating the umbilicus and periumbilical soft tissue closer to their original position. When a reverse abdominoplasty is performed with complete myofascial plication from the symphysis pubis to the xiphoid, the umbilical stalk can be divided and then reattached in the ideal position following muscle plication.

Preoperative History and Considerations (Box 10.2)

Preoperative evaluation of the reverse abdominoplasty candidate is similar to that for the other abdominoplasty procedures discussed. Fortunately, most candidates are healthy, and are unlikely to be overweight or have a history of massive weight loss. Nevertheless, specific health issues should be addressed as discussed in previous chapters. In particular, smoking, diabetes, pulmonary function, anticoagulation medications, a personal or family history of DVT/PE, and future plans for pregnancy are relative contraindications and must be discussed before proceeding with surgery.

Box 10.2 Preoperative recommendations for reverse abdominoplasty

Most abdominoplasty and abdominal contouring patients benefit from a standard preoperative workup. Fortunately, reverse abdominoplasty patients tend to be middle-aged and fairly health conscious.

- Smoking cessation/avoidance of nicotine exposure for 6 weeks prior to surgery
- Multivitamin daily
- Stop aspirin/other blood thinning products with primary care doctor's permission
- Abstain from all dietary/herbal supplements not approved by the surgeon
- Basic laboratory work should be tailored to each patient. It may include CBC, Chem 7, and PT/PTT/INR. Nutritional values, including albumin, may be warranted, especially for gastric bypass patients
- Medical clearance if needed
- Wearing abdominal binder for 2 weeks before surgery
- Shower with a gentle antimicrobial soap the night before and day of surgery

Operative Approach

Preoperative photographs are taken with the patient in nine cardinal views, as performed for other abdominal contouring procedures, and markings are made with the patient standing. The midline of the abdomen and the inframammary folds are marked bilaterally. The desired final scar placement should be approximately at the level of the inframammary fold. To achieve this, the upper incision should be placed approximately 1–2 cm above the fold, anticipating some descent of the scar postoperatively.

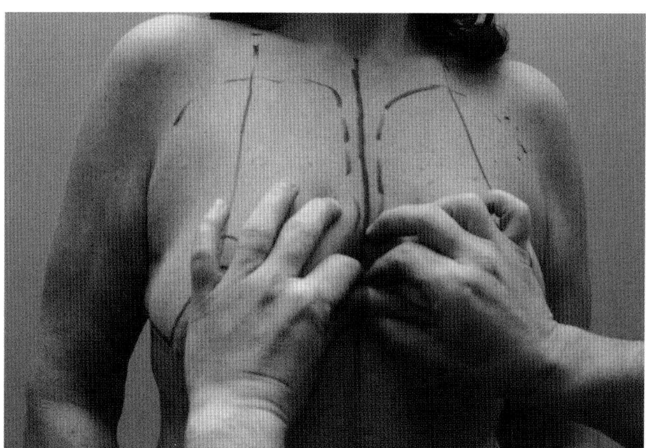

Fig. 10.3 The preoperative marking for reverse abdominoplasty starts with the midline and the inframammary folds bilaterally. Any breast procedure markings can also be performed at this time. The amount to be resected for the reverse abdominoplasty is estimated through bimanual pinch method performed at several points, including the anterior axillary line, the mid-portion of the inframammary line, and the midline. The length of the resection transversely is largely determined by the amount of soft-tissue laxity in order to prevent lateral dog-ear formation.

Using the bimanual pinch method, the amount of soft-tissue resection is estimated (**Fig. 10.3**). This is performed at several points along the incision line, including the anterior axillary point, the mid-portion of the inframammary line, and the midline. The final markings are usually two symmetric ellipses of soft tissue that connect to a narrow area

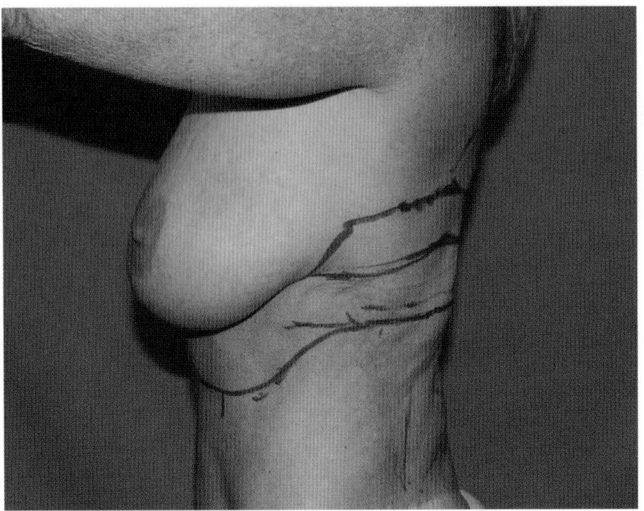

Fig. 10.4 When a bra-line back lift is performed concurrently with reverse abdominoplasty the lateral resection of the reverse abdominoplasty is joined with the bra-line back lift procedure. The resection should be designed to allow final scar placement within the confines of the bra.

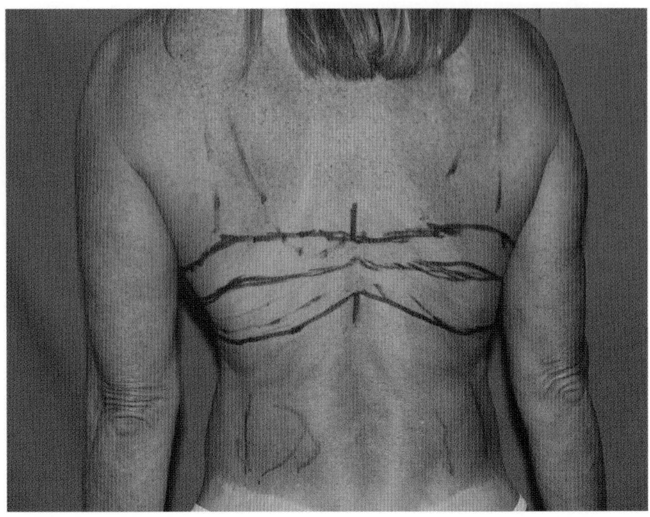

Fig. 10.5 When the reverse abdominoplasty resection is carried beyond the anterior axillary line and/or a bra-line back lift is performed concurrently, it is useful to trace the outline of the bra to make sure that the final scar is kept hidden within the confines of the garment.

of resection in the midline. The actual length of the transverse resection will be determined by the amount of soft-tissue laxity present. The lateral resection is carried out to the extent needed to prevent dog-ears. If a bra-line back lift is performed concurrently with the reverse abdominoplasty, the lateral and posterior resections should be designed to leave the final scar within the bra line (**Fig. 10.4 A, B**). Outlining the border of the bra is helpful (**Fig. 10.5**).

The procedure is performed in the supine position unless a bra-line back lift or other posterior procedure is also planned. If a posterior procedure is planned, it is performed first with the patient in the prone position and the patient is repositioned supine for the reverse abdominoplasty. Standard intraoperative precautions are taken, including lower extremity sequential compression devices, warm air blanket, appropriate padding and positioning, and intravenous antibiotics.

With the patient in the supine position, the incision lines are infiltrated with lidocaine containing epinephrine. If abdominal liposuction is planned, tumescent infiltration is performed prior to prepping and draping to allow sufficient time for vasoconstriction to be achieved. Abdominal liposuction is performed first if it is needed. If concurrent breast procedures are planned, these are usually performed before the reverse abdominoplasty.

The incisions for the reverse abdominoplasty are made with a number 10 scalpel into the dermis. The excess soft-tissue laxity in the upper abdomen outlined preoperatively can be de-epithelialized or resected (**Fig. 10.6**). It is important to note that proper anchoring of the abdominal flap is critical to prevent poor scar formation, as well as descent of the scar below the inframammary fold onto the abdomen. To help ensure this, a segment of de-epithelialized tissue 1 or 2 cm wide along the entire length of the inframammary fold is preserved. This will preserve the inframammary fold architecture and also provide a stronger anchor point for the abdominal flap.

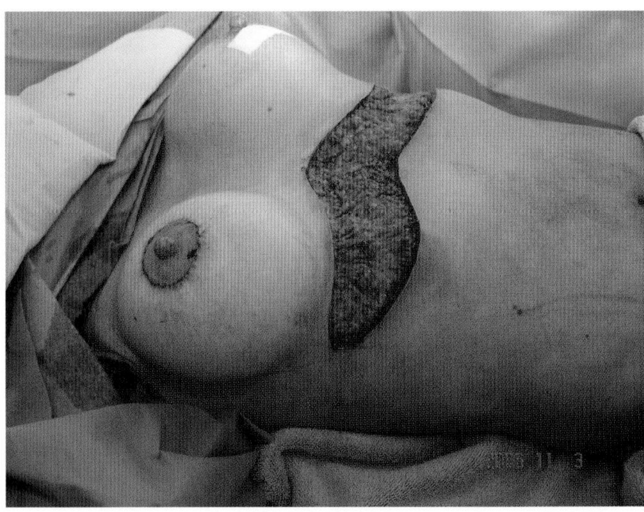

Fig. 10.6 The segment of soft-tissue laxity identified preoperatively can be resected or de-epithelialized. De-epithelialization preserves some additional tissue that can be used to secure the abdominal flap.

Dissection of the abdominal flap is performed in a manner comparable to standard abdominoplasty techniques except in reverse. The intercostal and subcostal vessels should be protected to maintain this important blood supply to the flap. The soft tissues are elevated off the abdominal wall fascia using electrocautery, and dissection is performed to the umbilical stalk, which is usually preserved. More inferior dissection can be performed if visualization permits, but is usually unnecessary. The superficial epigastric and circumflex vessels are preserved with this technique unless an inferior abdominal resection is also performed.

Myofascial plication is performed in similar fashion to other abdominoplasty techniques using a size 1 or 0 looped nylon suture on a tapered needle. Most candidates for reverse abdominoplasty do not have the global myofascial laxity seen in standard abdominoplasty patients. Nevertheless, myofascial plication is performed as needed from the pubic symphysis to the xiphoid. This is the reverse of the normal abdominoplasty xiphoid-to-pubic-symphysis plication. The generous incision at the inframammary fold allows for excellent myofascial visualization to the level of the pubic symphysis without the need for other access incisions. Should one be necessary, however, it can be made at the level of pubic symphysis or in the mons pubis to conceal the scar. During myofascial plication, the umbilical stalk can be left in place or released and reattached for better visualization.

The upper abdominal soft tissue can be resected at the beginning of the procedure by following the preoperative markings, as is the case when de-epithelialization of the segment is performed, or it can be done near the completion of the procedure using demarcation. A Jackson Pratt drain and a pain pump catheter are used routinely. These usually exit through the mons region, but can be brought out at the lateral extent of the inframammary line if necessary.

Incision closure begins with suspension and anchoring of the abdominal flap using number 0 or 1 Vicryl or polydioxanone (PDS). These sutures anchor the superficial fasciae of both the abdominal flap and the upper incision to the underlying dense fibrous structures of the inframammary fold and periosteum or perichondrium at the level of the fold. Using a longer-lasting suture and strong anchoring techniques is beneficial in reverse abdominoplasty, as the abdominal flap is suspended against gravity compared to the standard abdominoplasty techniques. The skin is closed with 2/0 Vicryl interrupted deep-dermal buried sutures placed every centimeter. Final closure is achieved with running intradermal 4/0 Monocryl. Tissue adhesive is used as a water-impermeable dressing.

Box 10.3 Postoperative instructions for reverse abdominoplasty

The postoperative care for reverse abdominoplasty patients is comparable to that for standard abdominoplasty listed below. Additional instructions regarding any concurrent procedures are given as needed. A bra may be worn as usual if any breast work has been performed, but it may be somewhat cumbersome as the abdominal binder and underlying foam is placed up to the inframammary fold.

For patients who have a concurrent bra-line back lift, postoperative positioning will have to be modified as the upper back closure will also be under tension. We have found that patients will find a position of partial waist flexion that balances the tension in both surgical sites.

- Maintain a partially flexed position at the waist for the first 1–2 weeks
- Wear the abdominal binder at all times except for showering
- Make sure the abdominal binder is maintained low enough on the abdomen
- Verify that there are no significant creases, folds, or drain tubes underneath the binder
- Avoid smoking or exposure to nicotine-containing products
- Breathe deeply and use the incentive spirometer frequently
- Drink plenty of fluids: 8 oz/h is the goal
- Move legs frequently while resting, and walk regularly
- Drain care as instructed
- Continue to take multivitamin daily. Resume medications as instructed
- No vigorous activity or heavy lifting for 4–6 weeks

Postoperative Care (Box 10.3)

Postoperative care for the reverse abdominoplasty patient is similar to that for other abdominoplasty procedures. Proper drain care, a well-positioned and well-fitted abdominal binder that is not too tight, avoidance of smoking, and adequate hydration and ambulation are the core postoperative care issues for all abdominal contouring procedures. These patients are requested to stay flexed for 7–10 days to allow proper healing. The reverse abdominoplasty patient may have additional instructions based on the additional procedures that were performed concurrently. A loosely fitted bra is worn immediately, or some time after the procedure if a breast operation was performed concurrently. If a bra-line back lift is performed at the same time, a less aggressively flexed positioned is recommended; however, we find that patients will naturally assume the position that affords the best combination of anterior and posterior tension.

Showering is allowed on postoperative day 2. Restriction from heavy lifting and vigorous activity is preferred for 4 weeks postoperatively. The abdominal binder is worn for 3–4 weeks after surgery, and then the patient switches to a more comfortable compression garment afterwards.

Figure 10.7 A,B demonstrates a patient's desire for abdominal contouring when she strongly lifts her upper abdominal skin giving a significant improvement to the entire abdomen. The preoperative markings for a reverse abdominoplasty place the incision line at the level of the inframammary

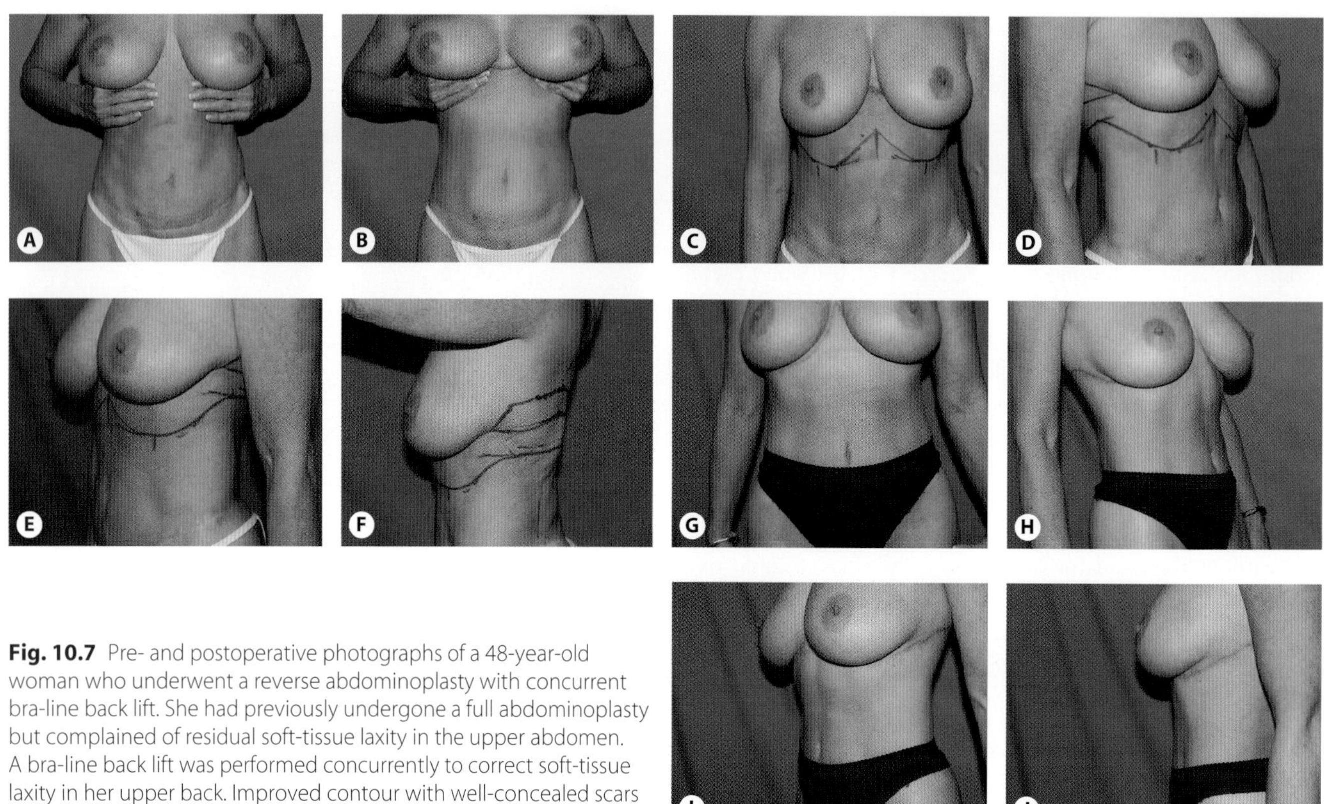

Fig. 10.7 Pre- and postoperative photographs of a 48-year-old woman who underwent a reverse abdominoplasty with concurrent bra-line back lift. She had previously undergone a full abdominoplasty but complained of residual soft-tissue laxity in the upper abdomen. A bra-line back lift was performed concurrently to correct soft-tissue laxity in her upper back. Improved contour with well-concealed scars are noted in the postoperative photographs.

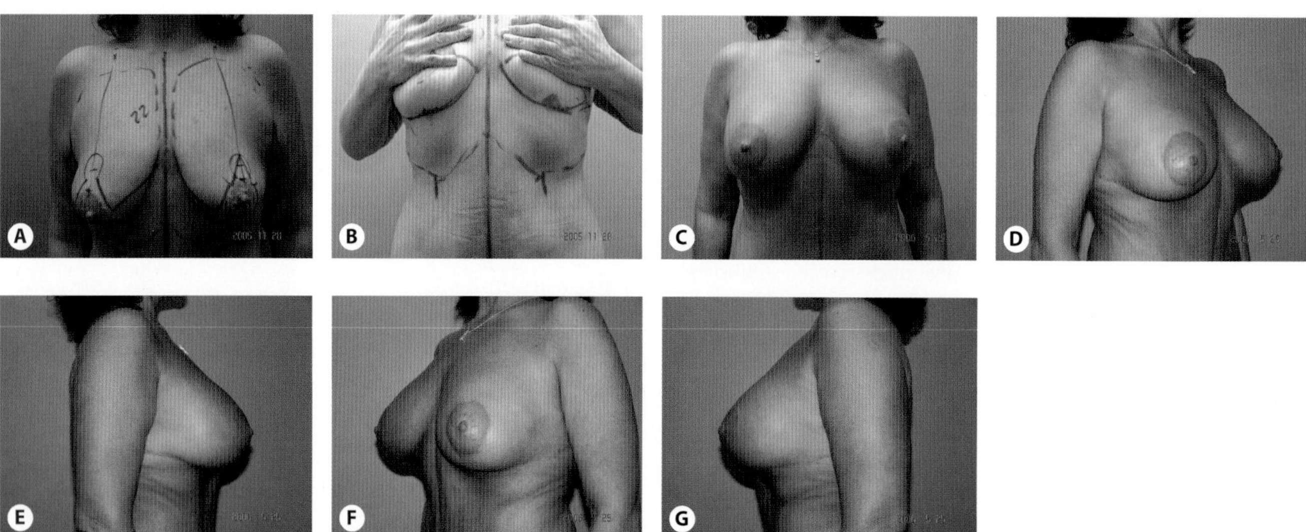

Fig. 10.8 Pre- and postoperative photographs of a 44-year-old woman who underwent a reverse abdominoplasty with concurrent augmentation mastopexy. This patient had previously undergone a circumferential abdominoplasty, and presented for augmentation mastopexy as well as further correction of the soft-tissue laxity in the upper abdomen. The combination of reverse abdominoplasty and augmentation mastopexy resulted in a well-concealed final scar at the inframammary fold. Improved upper abdominal contour as well as improved shape and volume of her breasts are noted.

fold (**Fig. 10.7 C–E**). The excess tissue is determined by bimanual palpation. A reverse abdominoplasty can be performed in combination with a bra-line back lift (**Fig. 10.7 F**). Postoperative results following this procedure reveal a significant improvement to the overall contour of the abdomen and the final incision placed ideally within the inframammary fold (**Fig. 10.7 G–J**).

A reverse abdominoplasty can be performed in combination with a mastopexy as noted in **Fig. 10.8 A–G**. Combining these two procedures requires careful preoperative planning to ensure that the final incision line is placed at the level of the inframammary fold.

Reverse Abdominoplasty with Continuous Progressive Tension Suture

As indicated above, laxity in the upper abdominal region is often difficult to treat. In some cases abdominoplasty may not be indicated, and mini abdominoplasty usually presents unsatisfactory results.

The first description of skin and soft tissue resection in the upper abdomen was by Thorek.[2] However, Rebello and Franco[3] described and systematized the approach in the submammary sulcus for abdominoplasties. Reverse abdominoplasty was practically forgotten for many years following this, because of the perception that this procedure resulted in poor final scarring. Currently, when this procedure is performed using the techniques to be described, reverse abdominoplasty with incisions in the inframammary region can yield very satisfactory results with proper patient selection. The first report on flap fixation to the abdominal wall was by Baroudi and Ferreira[6] to prevent and treat recurrent seroma. Progressive traction of the abdominoplasty flap toward the suprapubic region was described by Harlan and Todd Pollock,[7] who described an abdominoplasty with progressive tension sutures; complication rates were low, as were seroma and ischemia rates, and the suprapubic scars were improved. The technique to be described follows similar principles but with continuous tension sutures, with guidelines to reduce operative time and using premarked suture lines to achieve even, symmetrical lifting and tightening.

Patient Selection

The ideal patient must have skin laxity mainly in the upper portion of the abdomen. There may or may not be muscular diastasis and/or excess fat in the same region. Normally, candidates for mini or full abdominoplasty are not considered for reverse abdominoplasty. Those without a history of hypertrophic keloid scarring should also be considered good candidates. Patients with fair skin tend to heal very well, forming fine line scars in this region. Reverse abdominoplasty can be combined with breast reduction, mastopexy, and augmentation. Patients with a previous mastopexy or breast reduction tend to be good candidates for this procedure, especially if the resulting scar is long and either continuous or almost continuous across the midline. Patients with wide breasts are also good candidates, because wider breasts can hide the incisions more easily. In patients with narrow breasts, this technique is more difficult. If breast augmentation is being performed, this procedure will increase the breast base and improve the results. Breast augmentation can be performed with saline or silicone prostheses, or with the use of a dermal-fat flap made from the excess tissue from the upper part of the reverse abdominoplasty.

Preoperative Markings

Markings are made with the patient standing. One hand pushes the abdominal tissue upwards toward the breast to determine the amount that needs to be resected. The laxity present will determine whether the incision will course across the entire chest from one breast to the other, or whether paired inframammary excisions will suffice. With moderate or significant laxity the incision is usually required to cross the midline. The most lateral mark should be made at the anterior axillary line. The lower line for undermining is usually at the level of the umbilicus, done in a single V-shaped tunnel (**Fig. 10.9**). The amount of rectus abdominis muscle diastasis should be noted, as well as the amount of plication necessary. Myofascial plication should be performed prior to placement of the progressive traction sutures. For patients with limited laxity, undermining can be performed in shape of two narrow tunnels having their superior aspect the width of each breast. These tunnels are joined midway between the breasts and the umbilicus (**Fig. 10.10**). In some cases, undermining to the umbilicus may not be necessary.

Surgical Technique

The areas to be suctioned are infiltrated next using physiologic saline and 1:500 000 epinephrine. Infiltration at the level of the fascia is performed to facilitate subsequent undermining. Liposuction is performed first, treating all areas of excess adiposity to improve contour and shape. Liposuction has proved safe in this procedure, with no vascular compromise. Thin flaps contour better on the abdomen and are lighter than without liposuction. The progressive tension sutures hold a thinner and lighter flap more securely. Liposuction of the entire torso is often performed, beginning posteriorly and laterally and finishing anteriorly.

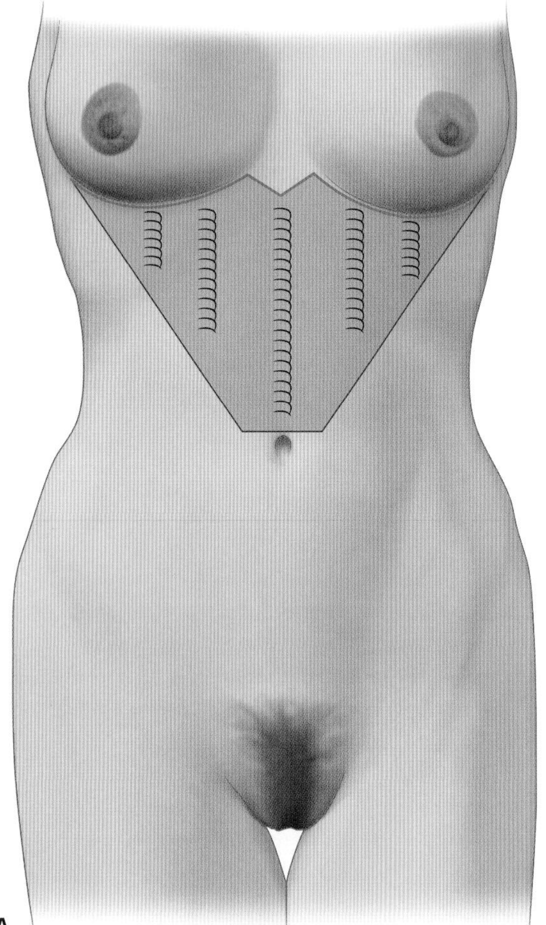

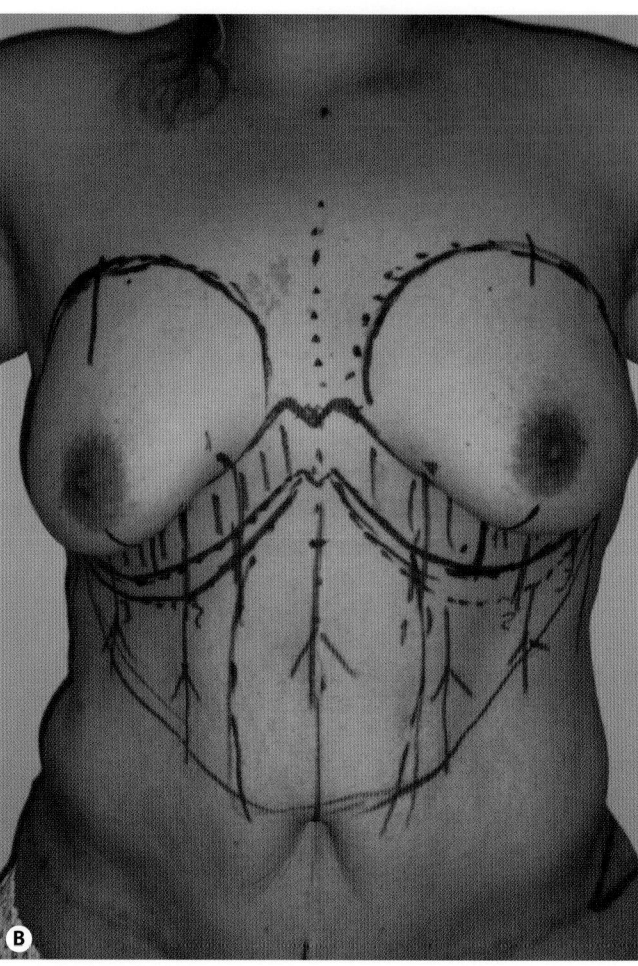

Fig. 10.9 Complete inframammary incision with V-shaped flap and undermining to the level of the umbilicus. Five marked progressive tension suture lines are noted, as well as the excess upper abdominal tissue marked for resection.

The incision is made precisely in the inframammary crease using the preoperative markings. Dissection is performed just superficial to the abdominal wall, and undermining is performed to the level marked preoperatively. Perfect hemostasis is achieved with electrocautery. When undermining is complete, rectus plication is performed using interrupted 2/0 nylon suture and a second layer of continuous 3/0 nylon. When undermining is complete, strong manual elevation of the abdominal skin is performed and markings are made for the anticipated skin resection. Three to five lines of traction sutures are marked, based on skin laxity and the width of lifting. Each suture line should provide superior or cephalic traction to the flap. In wider and heavier flaps, more traction lines (usually five) are placed (**Fig. 10.9**). In narrow work and lighter flaps, three traction lines are usually sufficient. When the incision does not cross the midline, two traction lines are placed within each narrow tunnel (**Fig. 10.10**).

For flap fixation and traction points continuous 2/0 Vicryl on a 4 cm tapered needle is used. The large needle is useful to attach the fascia of the abdominal flap to the underlying abdominal wall fascia. Skin puckers should be avoided. As this continuous suture is being placed, the assistant constantly advances the abdominal tissue cephalad. When the inframammary crease is approached the flap is split in the midline and excess tissue resected symmetrically. Closure at the inframammary fold is performed both deeply to the abdominal wall fascia and to the dermis itself. This provides definition to the inframammary crease. The upper abdominal tension flap is widely fixed to the abdominal wall along the five lines of continuous tension suturing, and there is minimal tension across the incision line. This flap stays in position and does not descend to its original location. Inferior displacement of the breast does not occur.

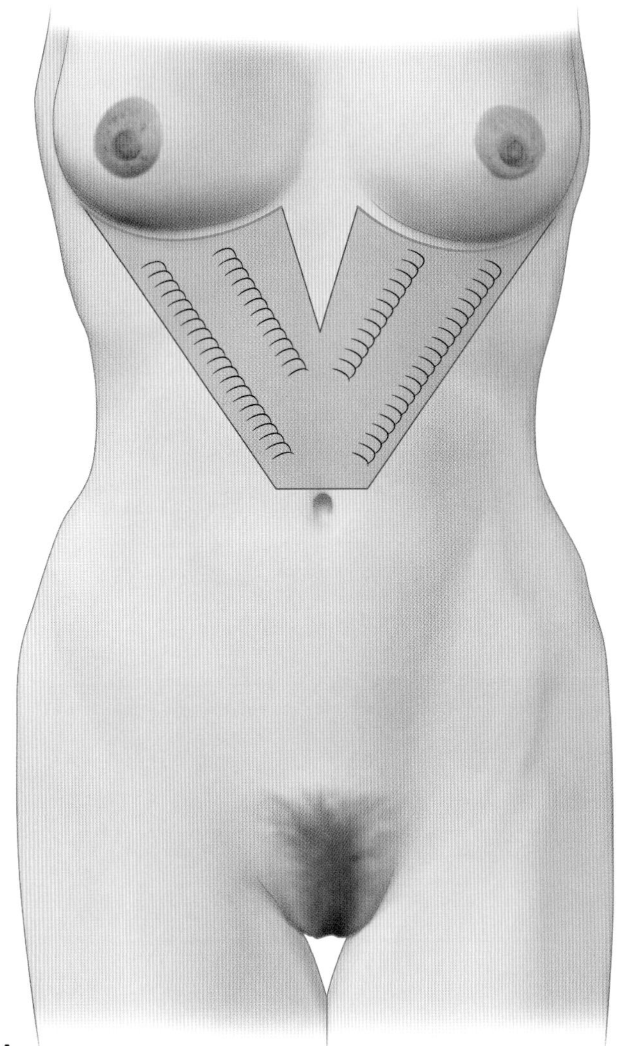

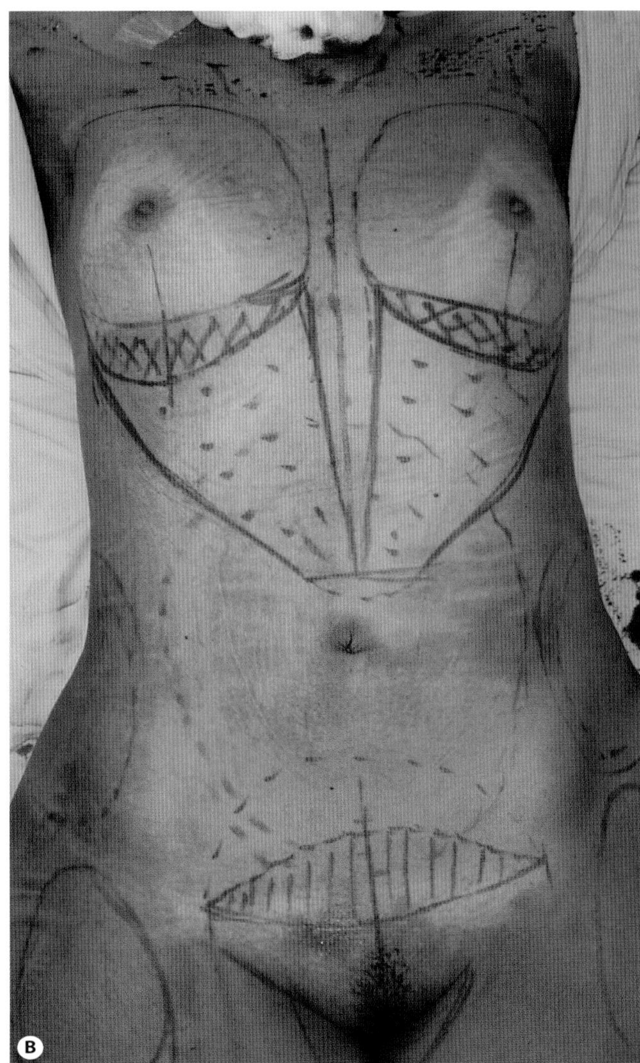

Fig. 10.10 Incomplete inframammary incision limited to the base of the breasts. Two tunnels that lead from the breasts join together inferiorly toward the umbilicus. Two oblique suture lines are noted in each tunnel.

In the midline, the linear scar is broken up into a W or M configuration. Vicryl 4/0 intracuticular sutures are used for final closure. If necessary, the lower abdominal skin can be resected without undermining, as in a mini abdominoplasty, as long as the inferior epigastric vessels are protected. No drains are used. A bulky protective dressing is applied with an abdominal binder. An artist's rendering of the progressive tension sutures is noted in **Fig. 10.11 A**. Note that the rectus plication has already been performed in the midline prior to placement of progressive tension sutures. **Figure 10.11 B** is a clinical photograph taken from the head of the table looking inferiorly beneath the elevated abdominal skin flap. The ellipse drawn in the midline indicates where the rectus plication will be performed. The five vertical lines identify the lines for placement of progressive tension sutures.

Figures 10.12–10.19 are before and after photographs of patients undergoing reverse abdominoplasty with progressive tension sutures. Lean patients (**Figs 10.12, 10.15, 10.17 and 10.19**), and heavier patients (**Figs 10.13, 10.14 and 10.16**) are noted.

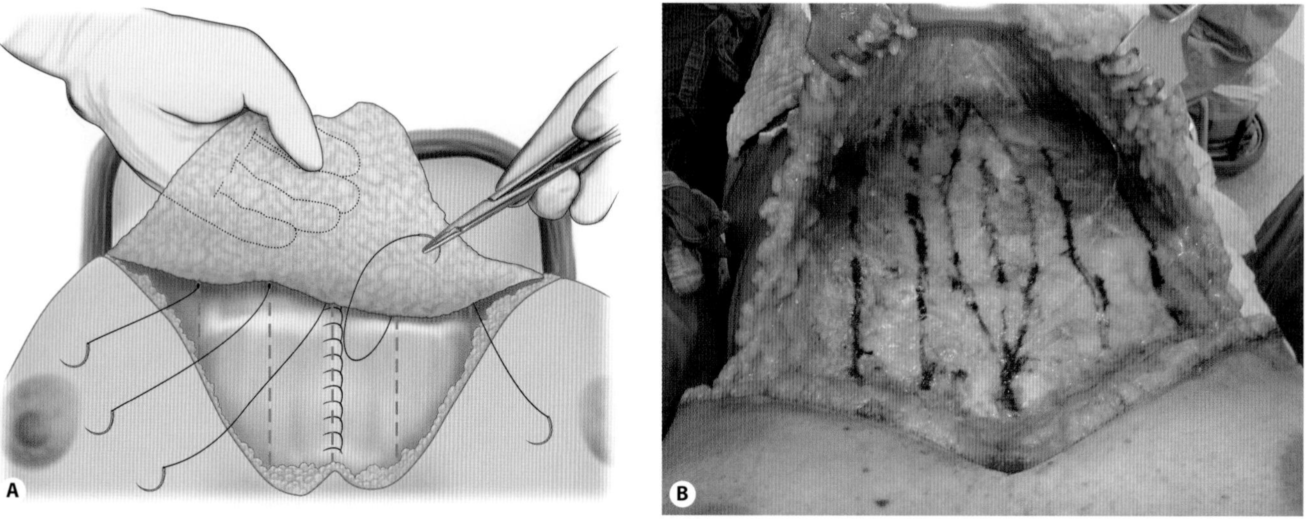

Fig. 10.11 Progressive tension suture in reverse abdominoplasty. Five continuous suture lines are made using 2/0 Vicryl. The assistant elevates the abdominal tissue each time a suture is placed.

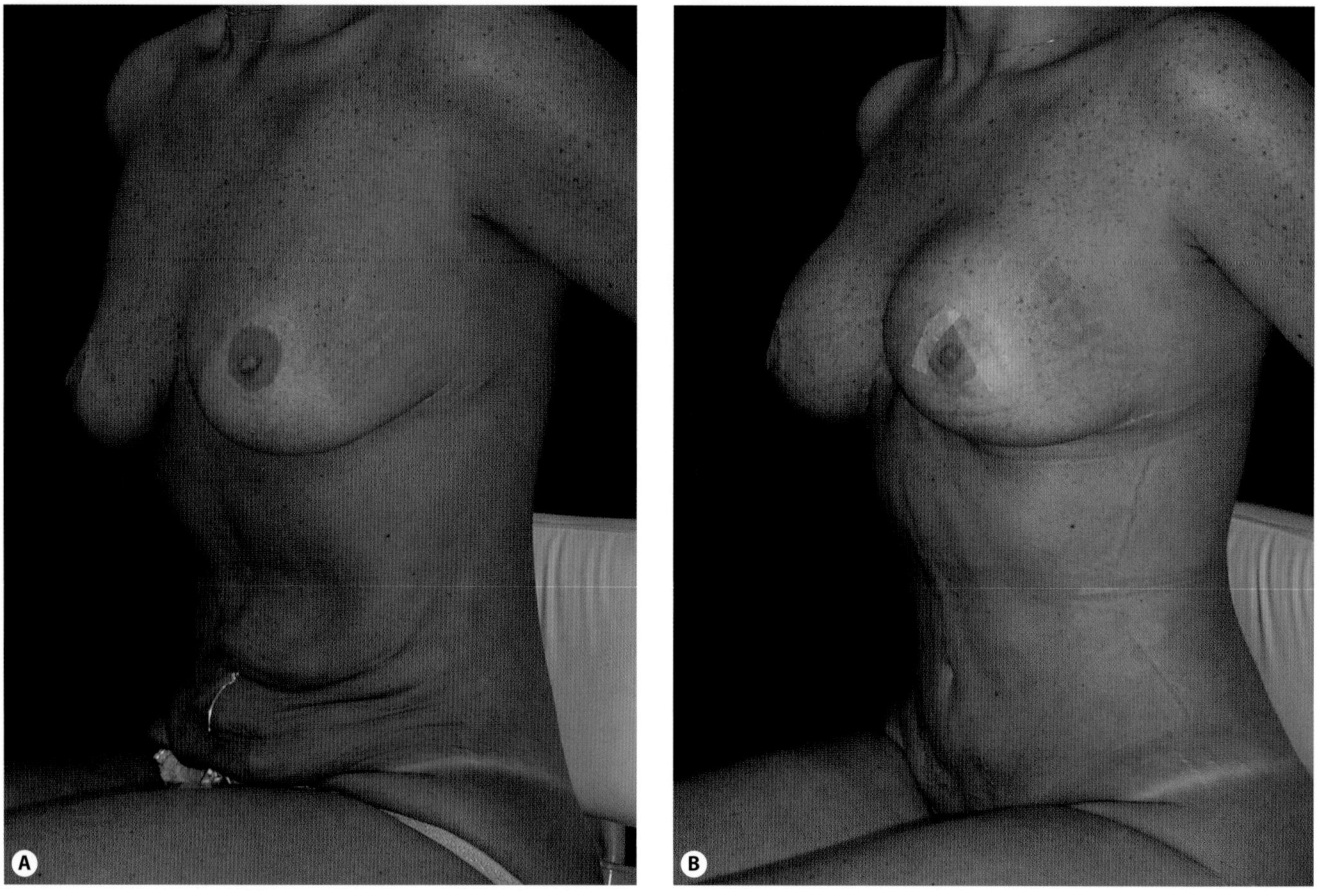

Fig. 10.12 This 35-year-old without prior abdominal surgery but with existing inframammary scars presented with the complaint of flaccidity in the supraumbilical region. Reverse abdominoplasty was performed through a complete incision across both breasts and using five progressive suture lines. Preoperative and 2-week postoperative views.

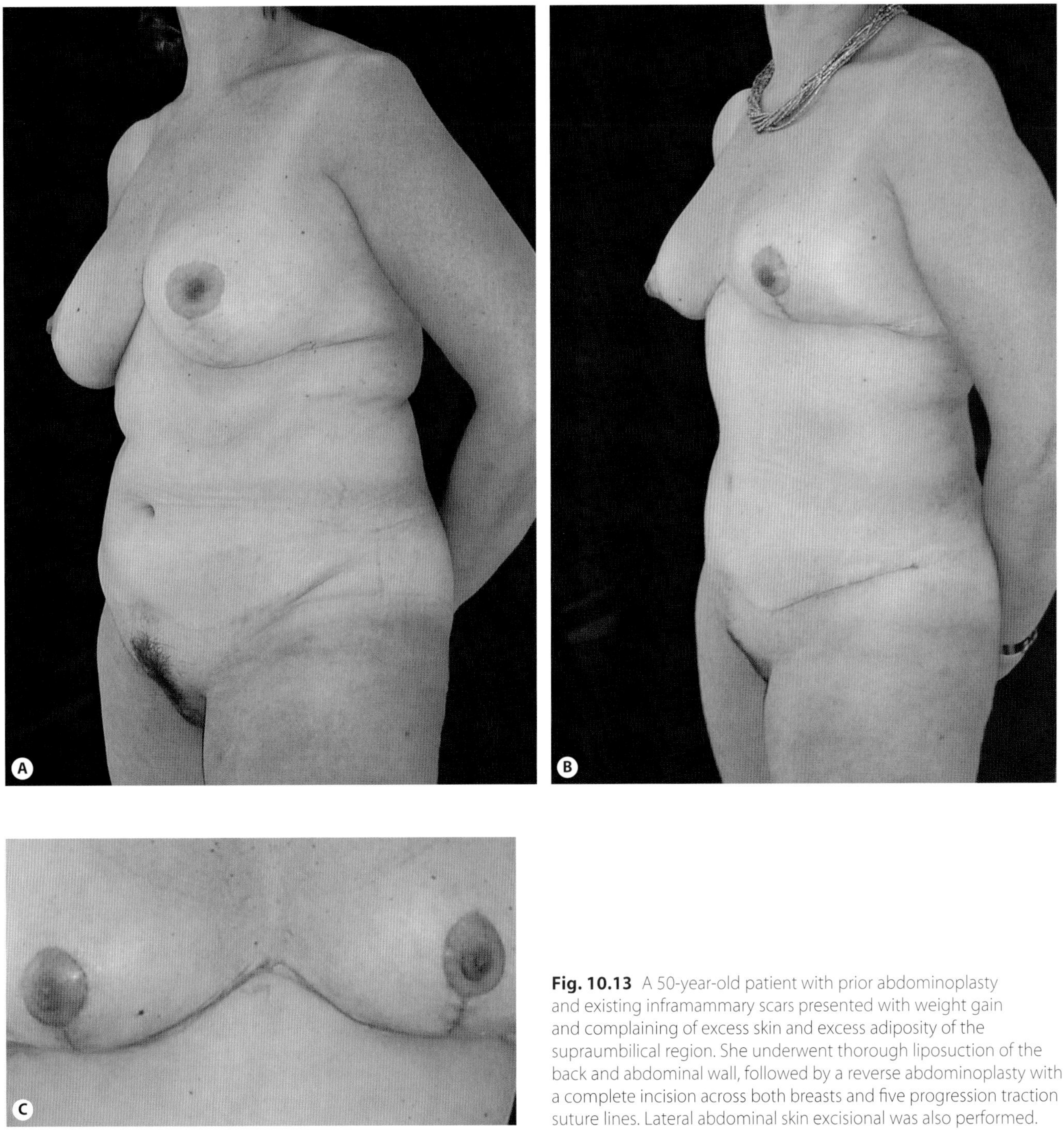

A

B

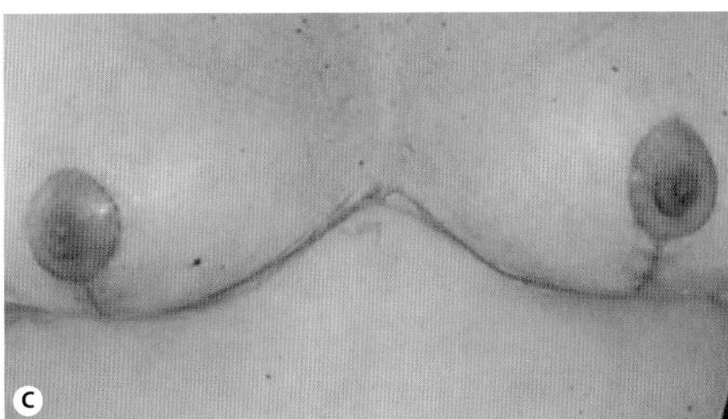

C

Fig. 10.13 A 50-year-old patient with prior abdominoplasty and existing inframammary scars presented with weight gain and complaining of excess skin and excess adiposity of the supraumbilical region. She underwent thorough liposuction of the back and abdominal wall, followed by a reverse abdominoplasty with a complete incision across both breasts and five progression traction suture lines. Lateral abdominal skin excisional was also performed.

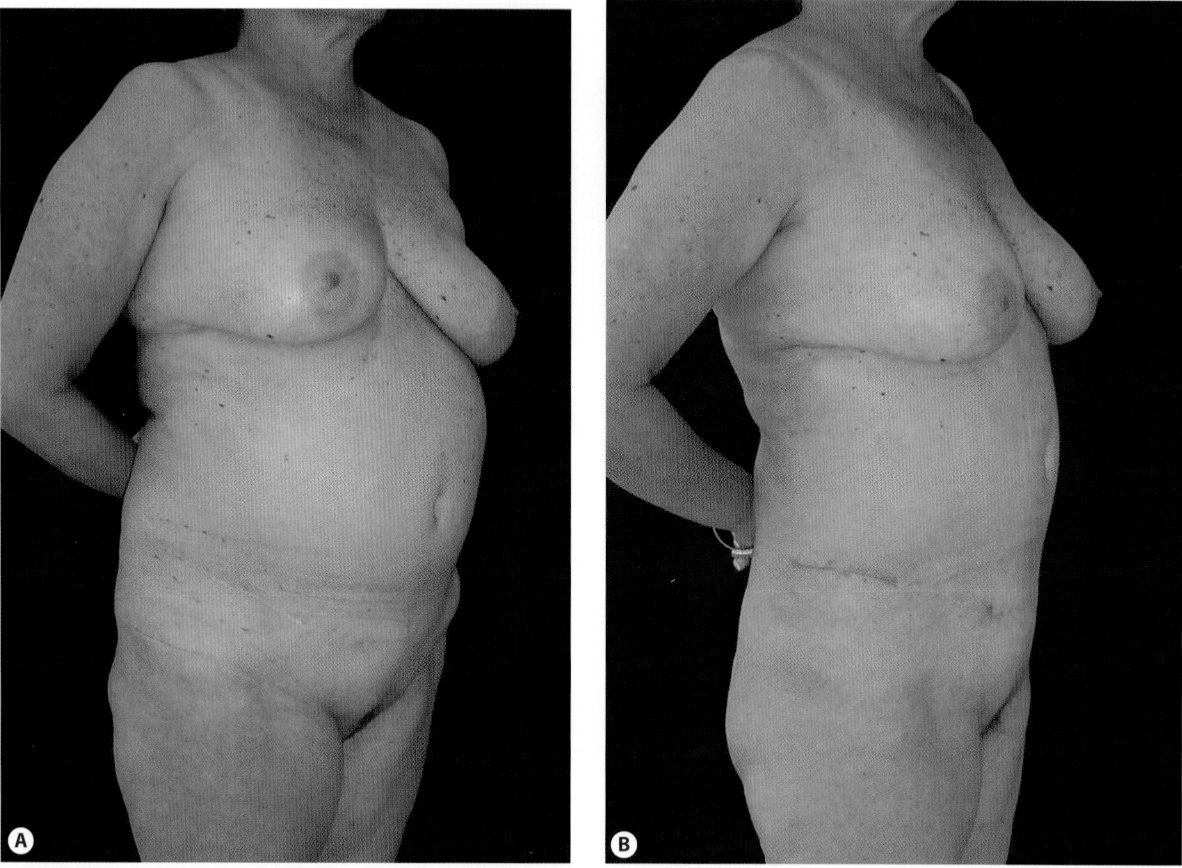

Fig. 10.14 A 58-year-old patient with previous abdominoplasty and mammaplasty scar. She gained weight after surgery and complained about excess adiposity and excess skin in the supraumbilical region. Thorough liposuction of the back and abdomen was performed, followed by a reverse abdominoplasty with a complete incision and using five progressive traction lines. Additional tissue was resected from the lateral abdomen bilaterally.

Fig. 10.15

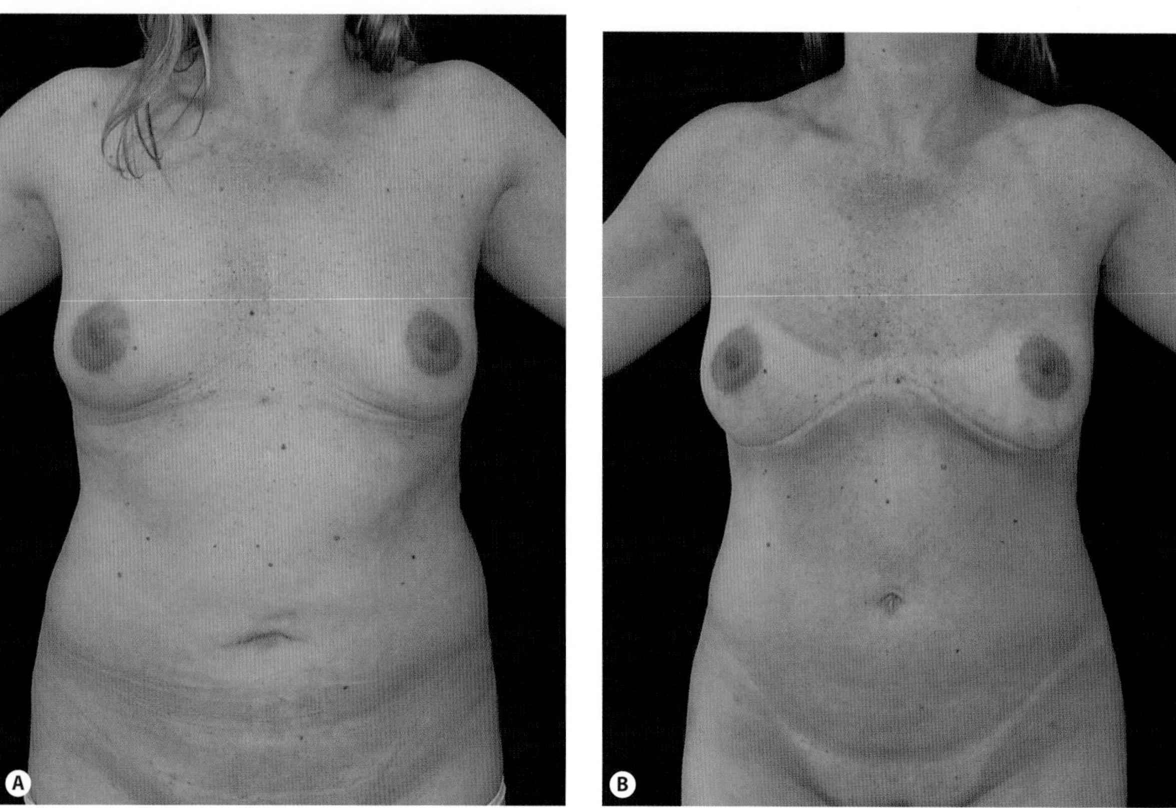

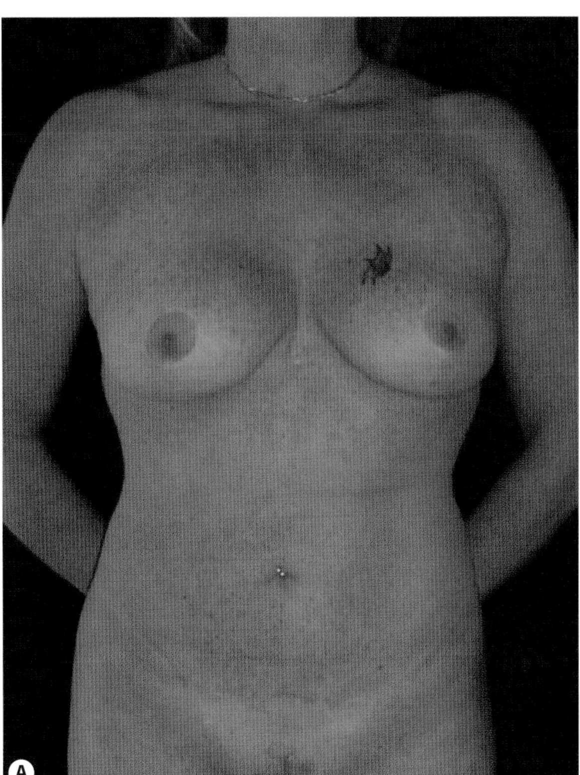

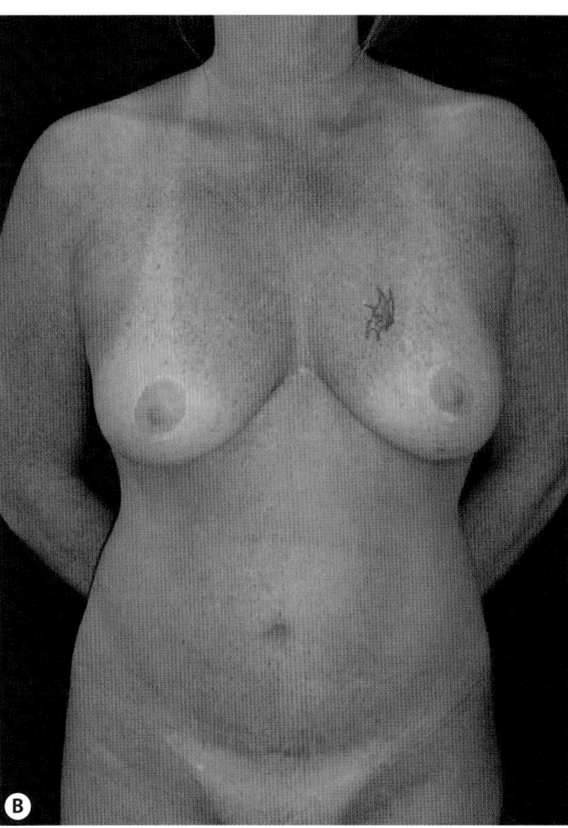

Fig. 10.16 A 43-year-old patient with excess adiposity and excess skin in the upper abdominal region, with small, narrow breast bases. Thorough liposuction of the back and abdominal area was performed, together with reverse abdominoplasty with a complete incision, rectus plication, and three progressive traction suture lines. Breast augmentation was performed with inclusion of the excess dermal fat flap of the abdomen.

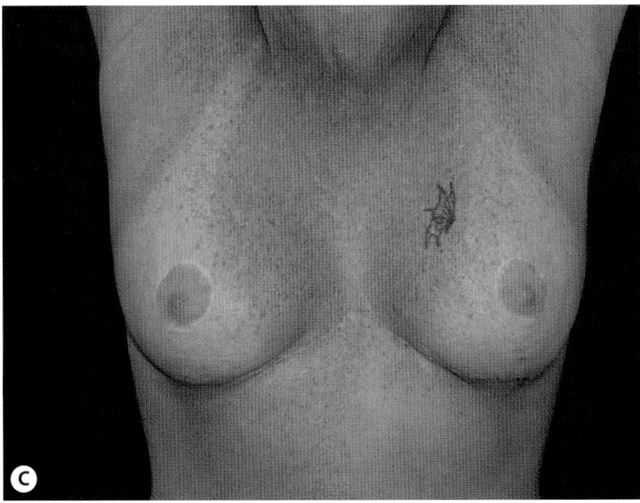

A 37-year-old patient with moderate abdominal lipodystrophy and excess skin in the upper and lower abdominal areas with existing inframammary scars. Thorough liposuction of the back and abdomen was performed followed by a reverse abdominoplasty and a complete skin excision without rectus plication but with three strong progressive traction suture lines. A mini abdominoplasty resection was also performed. Pre-and postoperative views at 2 years.

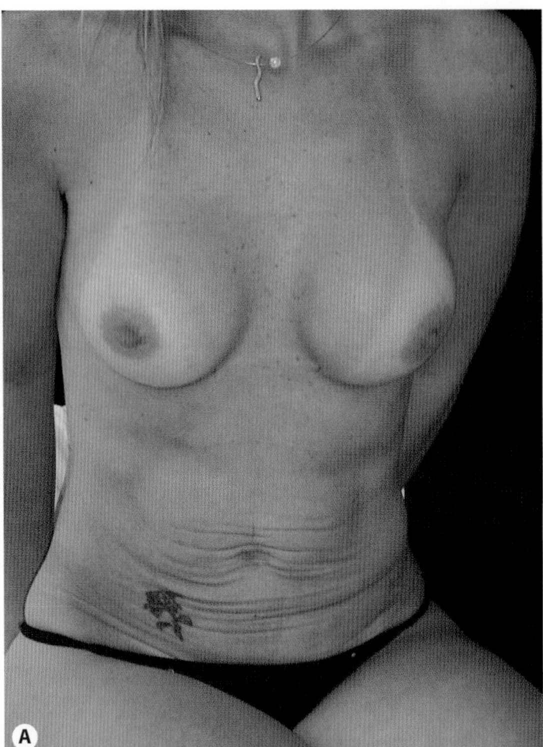

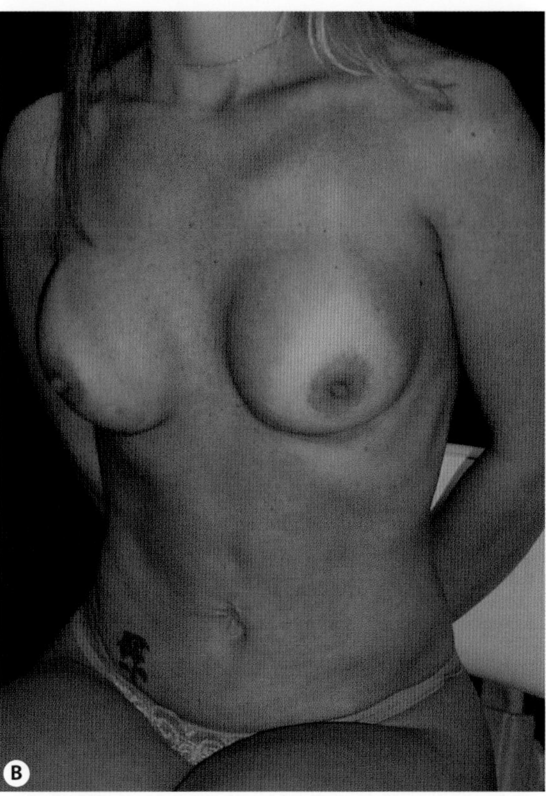

Fig. 10.17 A 37-year-old patient with slight infra- and supraumbilical flaccidity resulting in a severe alteration of the umbilical shape and folds in the skin, especially when sitting. She had an existing inframammary incision. She underwent a reverse abdominoplasty with the creation of two separate tunnels within an incision limited to the base of each breast. Two progressive traction suture lines were placed in each tunnel. No rectus plication was performed. A mini abdominoplasty resection was also performed without liposuction. Pre- and postoperative photographs at 1.5 years are shown.

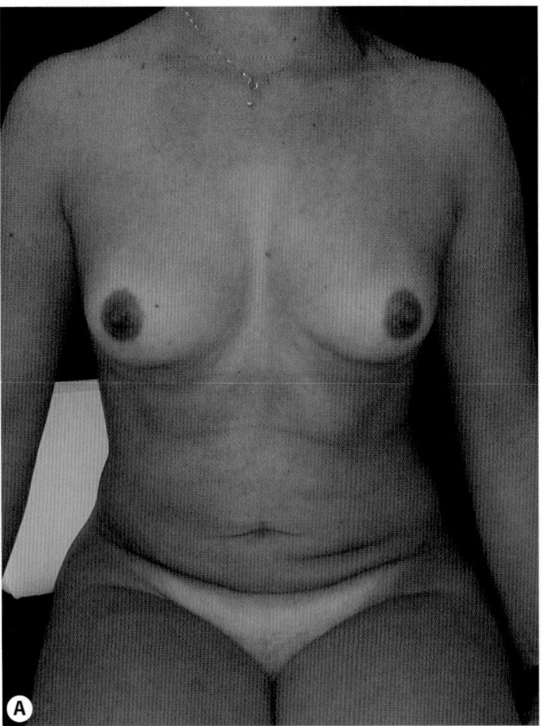

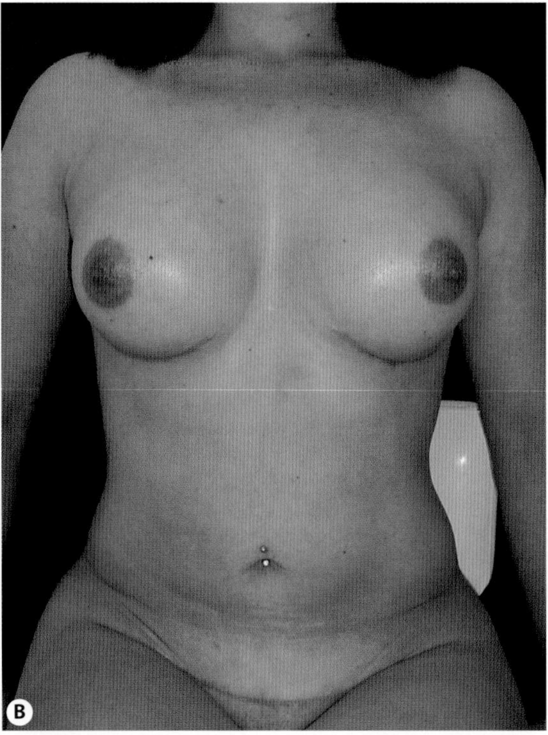

Fig. 10.18 A 30-year-old patient with moderate lipodystrophy and supraumbilical flaccidity. She was very concerned about the skin folds of the abdomen, which were more evident on sitting, and the alteration of her umbilical shape. She underwent liposuction of the back and abdominal area with reverse abdominoplasty and the formation of two discrete tunnels within an incision limited to the base of each breast. No rectus plication was performed. Two progressive traction sutures were placed in each tunnel. A mini-abdominoplasty resection was performed as well as an inframammary silicone breast augmentation. Pre-and postoperative photos at 1 year.

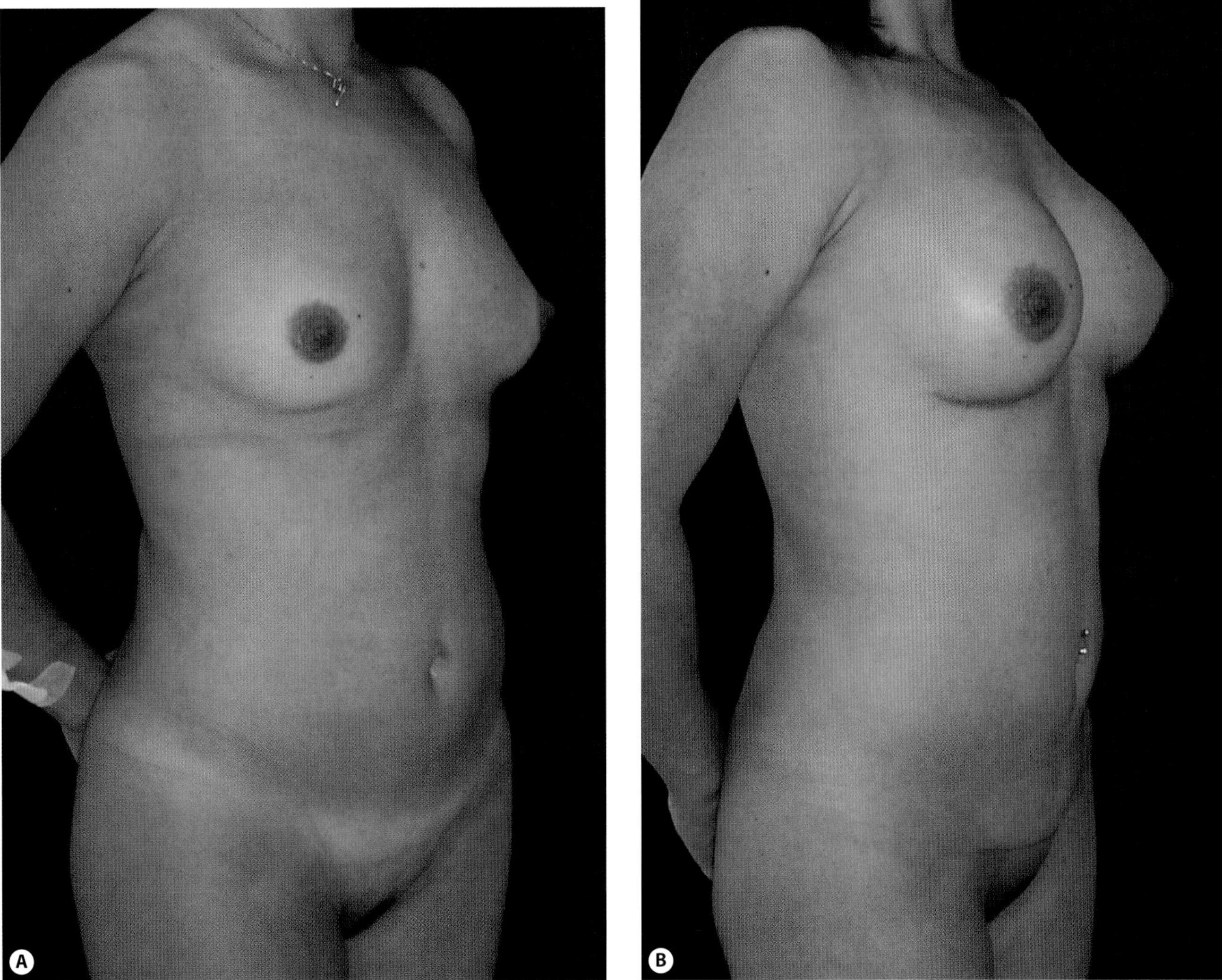

Fig. 10.19 A 30-year-old patient with moderate lipodystrophy and supraumbilical flaccidity. She was very concerned about the skin folds of the abdomen, which were more evident on sitting, and the alteration of her umbilical shape. She underwent liposuction of the back and abdominal area with reverse abdominoplasty and the formation of two discrete tunnels within an complete incision limited to the breast-based bilaterally. No rectus plication was performed. Two progressive traction sutures were placed in each tunnel. A mini-abdominoplasty resection was performed as well as an inframammary silicone breast augmentation. Pre-and postoperative photos at 1 year.

Conclusion

Patients suffering from excess skin and localized adiposity, particularly in the upper abdomen, continue to represent a challenge for most plastic surgeons. Reverse abdominoplasty and reverse abdominoplasty with continuous progressive tension suture can be useful in the treatment of this deformity. Patient selection and education are particularly important: the patient must understand the location and length of the scar. The reverse abdominoplasty is also particularly well suited for patients requesting concurrent breast procedures that require a sizeable inframammary incision, as this will coincide with the final scar for the reverse abdominoplasty. Reverse abdominoplasty with progressive tension sutures results in fixation of the flap widely throughout the entire upper abdomen, with minimal tension on the final inframammary incision line that delivers consistent results.

Clinical Caveats: Reverse Abdominoplasty

- Candidates for reverse abdominoplasty have most of the soft-tissue laxity and deformity located in the upper abdomen.
- Reverse abdominoplasty is more effective than standard abdominoplasty techniques in correcting upper abdominal contour irregularities
- The final scar will be in the inframammary fold, hidden within the confines of the bra
- Patients should be educated about the location and appearance of the final scar
- Breast work can be performed concurrently
- The lateral component of the reverse abdominoplasty can be connected to a bra-line back lift to correct upper and middle back laxity
- The umbilicus is pulled up toward its normal position by the vector of the reverse abdominoplasty pull
- There is a natural tendency for the final scar to migrate inferiorly. A slightly superiorly placed, well-anchored closure is recommended

References

1. Baroudi R, Keppke EM, Carvalho CG. Mammary reduction combined with reverse abdominoplasty. Ann Plast Surg 1979; 2: 368–373.
2. Thorek M. Plastic surgery of the breast and abdominal wall. Springfield Ill: CC Thomas, 1942.
3. Rebello C, Franco T. Abdominoplasty through a submammary incision. Int Surg 1977; 62: 462–463.
4. Akbas H, Guneren E, Eroglu L, et al. The combined use of classic and reverse abdominoplasty on the same patient. Plast Reconstruct Surg 2002; 109: 2595.
5. Craig SB, Faller MS, Puckett CL. In search of the ideal female umbilicus. Plast Reconstruct Surg 2000; 105: 389.
6. Baroudi R, Ferreira C Seroma. How to avoid it and how to treat it. Aesthet Surg J 1998; 18: 439–441.
7. Pollock H, Pollock T. Progressive tension sutures: a technique to reduce local complications in abdominoplasty. Plast Reconstruct Surg 2000; 105: 2583–2586; discussion 2587–2588.

Suggested Reading

Al-Basti HB, El-Khatib HA, Taha A, et al. Intraabdominal pressure after full abdominoplasty in obese multiparous patients. Plast Reconstruct Surg 2004; 113: 2145.

Andrades P, Prado A, Danilla S, et al. Progressive tension sutures in the prevention of postabdominoplasty seroma: a prospective, randomized, double-blind clinical trial. Plast Reconstruct Surg 2007; 120: 935–946; discussion 947–951.

Avelar JM. Upper abdominoplasty: without panniculus undermining and resection. In: Avelar JM, ed. Abdominoplasty: without undermining and resection. São Paulo: Editora Hipócrates, 2002; 183–198.

Deos MF. Lipoabdominoplasty. Bases and classification. In: Saldanha O. Lipoabdominoplasty. São Paulo: Dilivros, 2004; 57–65.

El-Khatib HA, Bener A. Abdominal dermolipectomy in an abdomen with pre-existing scars: a different concept. Plast Reconstruct Surg 2004; 114: 992.

Grazer FM. Abdominoplasty. Plast Reconstruct Surg 1973; 51: 617.

Hakme F, Freitas RR, de Souza BA. Historical evolution in abdominoplasties. In: Saldanha O. Lipoabdominoplasty. São Paulo: Dilivros, 2004; 1–12.

Hester RT Jr., Baird W, Bostwick J III, et al. Abdominoplasty combined with other surgical procedures: Safe or sorry? Plast Reconstruct Surg 1989; 83: 997.

Khan S, Teotia SS, Mullis WF, et al. Do progressive tension sutures really decrease complications in abdominoplasty? Ann Plast Surg 2006; 56: 14–20; discussion 20–21.

Manassa EH, Hertl CH, Olbrisch RR. Wound healing problems in smokers and non-smokers after 132 abdominoplasties. Plast Reconstruct Surg 2003; 111: 2082.

Matarasso A, Swift RW, Rankin M. Abdominoplasty and abdominal contour surgery: a national plastic surgery survey. Plast Reconstruct Surg 2006; 117: 1797.

Nahas FX, Ferreira LM, Ghelfond C. Does quilting suture prevent seroma in abdominoplasty? Plast Reconstruct Surg 2007; 119: 1060–1064; discussion 1065–1066.

Pollock H, Pollock T. Progressive tension sutures: a technique to reduce local complications in abdominoplasty. Plast Reconstruct Surg 2000; 105: 2583.

Pollock T, Pollock H. Progressive tension sutures in abdominoplasty. Clin Plast Surg 2004; 31: 583–589; vi.

Saldanha OR, De Souza Pinto EB, Mattos WN Jr., et al. Lipoabdominoplasty with selective and safe undermining. Aesthet Plast Surg 2003; 27: 322–327.

Shermak AM. Contouring the epigastrium. Aesthet Surg J 2005; 25: 506.

CHAPTER 11

Complete Revision Abdominoplasty

Joseph P. Hunstad & Remus Repta

IN THIS CHAPTER

KEY POINTS

The goal of complete revision abdominoplasty is to improve and optimize the aesthetic appearance of the abdomen following a prior abdominoplasty. It involves full elevation of the abdominal soft-tissue apron, which allows any residual myofascial laxity and soft-tissue excess to be properly addressed. Depending on the needs of the individual patient, complete revision abdominoplasty may include some or all of the normal components of a standard abdominoplasty, including concurrent liposuction of the abdomen, strong myofascial plication, and additional skin and soft-tissue resection. Improvement in the quality and position of the scar, the shape and position of the umbilicus, and correction of any sequelae from the previous procedure are also addressed. The type of procedure performed during complete revision abdominoplasty may differ from that originally performed and should be selected according to the patient's needs and wishes. A detailed examination and discussion is critical for an optimal aesthetic result and high patient satisfaction.

Introduction (Box 11.1)

Complete revision abdominoplasty is the term used to describe a revision abdominoplasty procedure that involves complete dissection and elevation of the abdominal soft-tissue apron. In so doing, residual myofascial laxity can be corrected and residual soft-tissue excess can be resected. This procedure is performed to correct and optimize the aesthetic result of a previous abdominoplasty or abdominal contouring procedure.

Complete revision abdominoplasty may also includes scar revision and scar repositioning, improvement in umbilical shape and location, as well as liposuction of the abdomen and adjacent areas. Candidates for complete revision abdominoplasty may present after having had any of the abdominoplasty procedures previously discussed, including mini, full, extended, and circumferential abdominoplasty. The specific reason for their dissatisfaction may include the presence of contour irregularity, residual abdominal wall laxity, residual excess soft-tissue laxity, and residual excess adiposity.[1] There may also be dissatisfaction with the presence of thick, widened, or poorly positioned scars, an aesthetically unappealing umbilical shape and position, as well as various other sequelae from the initial procedure.

Box 11.1 Factors responsible for suboptimal abdominoplasty result

The abdominoplasty technique was not properly selected or performed, leading to:

- Insufficient correction during the prior abdominoplasty procedure
- Insufficient or no myofascial plication
- Insufficient or no concurrent liposuction
- Insufficient soft-tissue resection
- Poorly designed/executed procedure leading to
  - Poor scars: asymmetry, position, quality
  - Unattractive umbilicus
  - Lateral dog-ears

The goal of complete revision abdominoplasty is similar to that of primary abdominoplasty, namely to improve the shape and appearance of the abdomen by thinning the soft-tissue apron through the use of concurrent liposuction, tightening of the abdominal wall through myofascial plication, and resection of excess soft-tissue laxity. In addition, complete revision abdominoplasty also aims at correcting poor scars, which are often too high, the presence of lateral dog-ears, aesthetically unattractive umbilical shape and position, and other contour irregularities.

The suboptimal result associated with the primary procedure is usually secondary to insufficient correction using an appropriately selected procedure.[2,3] This group of patients present with residual abdominal contour irregularity secondary to insufficient or absent abdominal soft-tissue thinning through liposuction, insufficient or no myofascial plication, and/or insufficient soft-tissue resection. Usually a less aggressive or less extensive procedure was performed, leaving the patient with residual laxity and/or a suboptimal abdominal contour.

There are, however, certain patients who present for secondary abdominoplasty after having had an initial procedure that was not ideal for their specific aesthetic goal. A common example of this is the patient who has significant soft-tissue laxity and undergoes a standard full abdominoplasty. These patients will probably be left with residual lateral and/or posterior soft-tissue laxity, lateral dog-ears, or a combination of the two. Complete revision abdominoplasty using an extended or a circumferential abdominoplasty may be required to achieve the desired result.

Patient Selection

Dissatisfied patients who have previously undergone an abdominoplasty but have not achieved the desired aesthetic result are potential candidates for secondary abdominoplasty. There are two main types of secondary abdominoplasty procedures, based on the need for complete dissection and elevation of the abdominal soft-tissue apron. Patients who require myofascial plication, correction of residual soft-tissue laxity, or significant lowering of the transverse abdominal scar will need to undergo complete dissection and elevation of the abdominal soft tissue. These patients are more accurately categorized as complete revision abdominoplasty candidates, as most or all of the major components of a standard abdominoplasty are performed. Patients who only require scar revision, dog-ear excision, and liposuction touch-up are better defined as revision abdominoplasty candidates, because the process of abdominal soft-tissue elevation is not needed to accomplish this.

Many secondary abdominoplasty patients can clearly benefit from enhanced myofascial plication and a more complete correction of skin and soft-tissue laxity by resection.

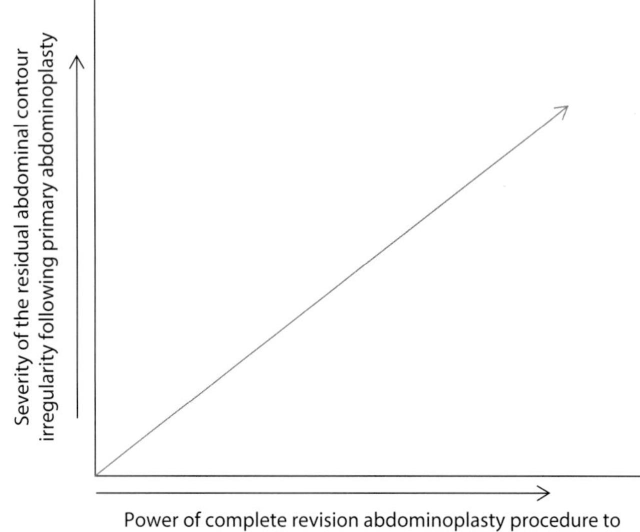

Fig. 11.1 There is a general correlation between the severity of the residual contour deformity following the initial abdominoplasty procedure and the effect of the complete revision abdominoplasty in improving the aesthetic result. Patients who have had an appropriate and complete abdominoplasty but have minor irregularities or complaints are less likely to benefit from a complete revision, and are often more appropriately treated with a problem-focused technique such as liposuction touch-up, excision of lateral dog-ears, or simple scar revision. However, residual myofascial laxity, as well as residual soft-tissue laxity, is best addressed by complete revision abdominoplasty.

Correctly diagnosing the source of the residual deformity will allow better preoperative planning and facilitate appropriate discussion. For patients with smaller deformities, more minor procedures such as scar revision, treatment of dog-ears, and liposuction can be very beneficial and does not require the financial cost and recovery time associated with a complete revision abdominoplasty. Careful discussion of these issues, especially for patients who do not fall specifically into a single category, is critical as the potential improvement from a complete revision abdominoplasty decreases with lesser degree residual contour irregularity. It is important to appreciate the fact that patients who undergo secondary abdominoplasty have chosen to re-invest the time, money, and energy to undergo surgery again in order to improve their aesthetic result (**Fig. 11.1**).

Preoperative History and Considerations (Box 11.2)

A clear understanding of the patient's surgical history, previous weight, pre-abdominoplasty soft-tissue excess, abdominal fascial laxity, and abdominal contour is helpful. Understanding the patient's goal is very important to perform the procedure safely and successfully, and to achieve high patient

Box 11.2 Preoperative recommendation for revision abdominoplasty

The preoperative requirements for revision abdominoplasty procedures are the same as those for primary abdominoplasty. They should be modified based on the needs of the patient and on the specifics of the revision procedure.

- Smoking cessation/avoidance of nicotine exposure for 4–6 weeks prior to surgery
- Multivitamin daily
- Stop aspirin/other blood thinning products with primary care doctor's permission
- Abstain from all dietary/herbal supplements not approved by the surgeon
- Basic laboratory work should be tailored to each patient. It may include a pregnancy test CBC, Chem. 7, factor V Linden and PT/PTT/INR
- Medical clearance if needed
- Wearing abdominal binder for 2 weeks before surgery
- Shower with a gentle antimicrobial soap the night before and day of surgery

Box 11.3 Operative pearls

The operative sequence for complete revision abdominoplasty is largely the same as that listed in each specific primary abdominoplasty chapter.

- Thorough tumescent infiltration will facilitate proper liposuction and tissue dissection.
- Control of the superficial inferior epigastric and superficial circumflex vessels as well as any remaining perforators from the prior abdominoplasty procedure is important to reduce the chance of postoperative hematoma
- Extra care should be taken to ensure that the dissection is performed in the proper tissue plane, as scar tissue can make the dissection less clear
- Excessive scar tissue and foreign bodies (suture) should be removed
- A more aggressive resection and closure is possible if needed, as the initial abdominoplasty procedure functioned in part as a vascular delay procedure for the abdominal soft tissue.

satisfaction. Most patients share similar aesthetic goals, which include a better-looking transverse scar positioned lower on the abdomen, a better-looking umbilicus, correction or reduction of the skin and soft-tissue excess, and a better abdominal contour and silhouette.

A focused physical examination similar to that performed for a primary abdominoplasty is recommended. Specific problem areas related to the previous surgery are also evaluated as indicated. Poor healing, seroma, capsule formation, or a history of infection or hematoma occurring with the prior abdominoplasty require careful examination, as they will potentially affect the ease of dissection secondary to the extent of scar tissue present.

Physical examination, including evaluation of skin quality and the extent of soft-tissue laxity, will aid discussion about the amount of tissue that can or should be removed, which subsequently affects the position of the final scar. As with all abdominoplasty patients, and particularly those undergoing secondary abdominoplasty, preoperative discussion about the possibility that the amount of soft-tissue resection will not safely allow the complete removal of the current umbilical location is important. The patient should be aware that this will result in an additional small vertical midline scar from the former location of the umbilicus. This is particularly common when scar revision is also performed and the transverse scar is positioned lower on the abdomen.

Operative Approach (Box 11.3)

Standard preoperative photographs are obtained with the patient standing (**Fig. 11.2**). Additional preoperative photographs are taken as needed to detail specific areas related to the previous abdominoplasty. These may include localized adiposity, contour irregularities, abdominal wall laxity, or poor scars (**Fig. 11.3**).

Preoperative markings are also made with the patient standing. Often the transverse abdominoplasty scar requires revision, as it may be higher than desired and a more inferior or caudal location of the final scar is planned. This is measured by having the patient lift the lower abdominal soft tissue strongly upwards, as done with a standard primary abdominoplasty (**Fig. 11.4**). The low transverse incision is marked, placing the final scar at the level of the pubic symphysis (**Fig. 11.5**). For complete revision abdominoplasty the position of the final transverse scar will need to be modified as the ideal placement may not be possible without having an inverted 'T' incision. Additional marks, including those identifying areas to be liposuctioned, are made as needed, and photographs showing these marks are taken.

Intraoperatively, a complete revision abdominoplasty mirrors a full primary abdominoplasty. General endotracheal anesthesia is induced, the patient is positioned supine and adequate padding is placed. If a circumferential abdominoplasty or posterior liposuction is planned, the patient is placed in the prone position first following anterior tumescent infiltration. A warming blanket, sequential compression stockings, and a Foley catheter are routinely used as done with primary abdominoplasty procedures. A prophylactic dose of intravenous antibiotics is given prior to the start of the procedure.

The sequence of the complete revision abdominoplasty procedure is the same as that outlined in Chapter 7, Full

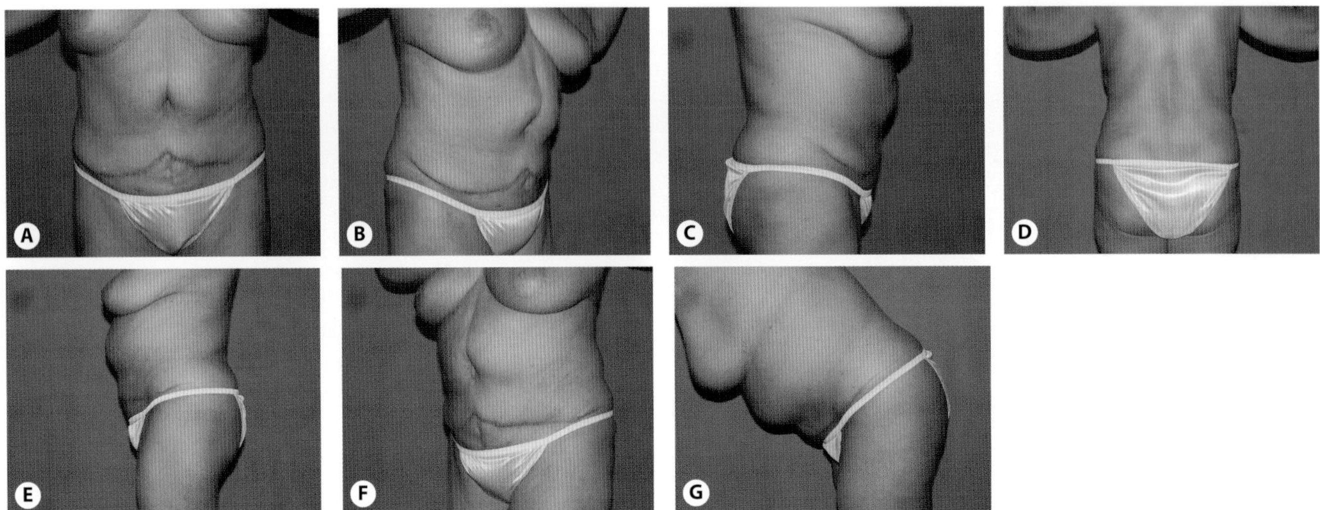

Fig. 11.2 Standard preoperative photographs are obtained with the patient in the standing position as done with primary abdominoplasty procedures. The diver's view (G) is particularly important because residual lower abdominal myofascial laxity and its correction are best shown in this view.

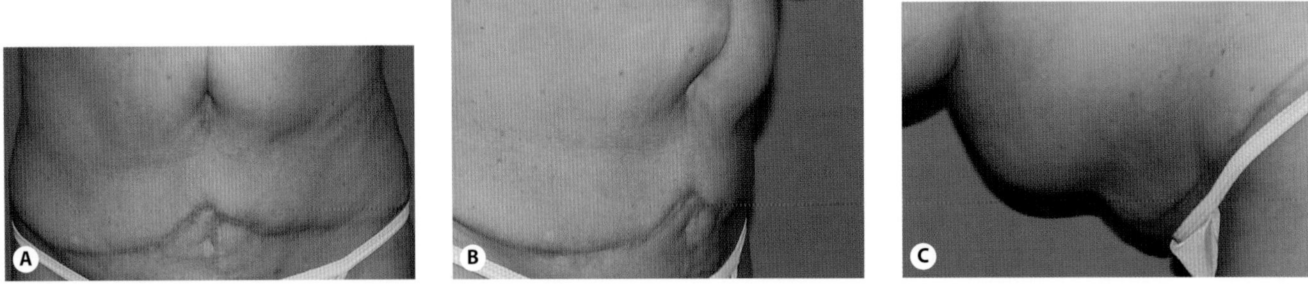

Fig. 11.3 Additional preoperative photographs are obtained as needed that focus on specific problem areas.

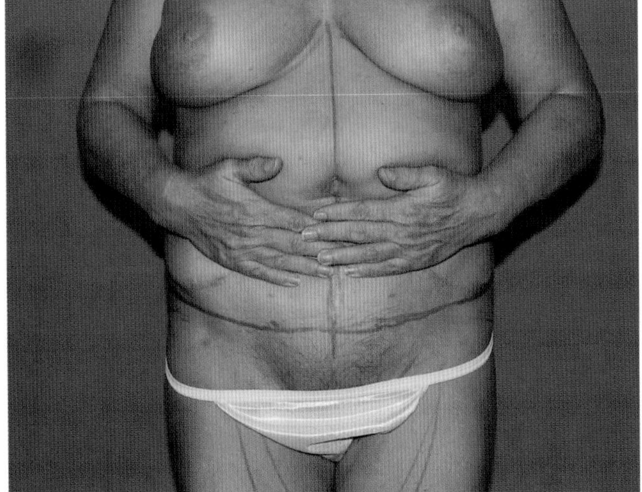

Fig. 11.4 Surgical marking is performed by first having the patient pull strongly upwards on the lower abdominal tissue. This allows the final transverse scar to be located at the level of the pubic symphysis.

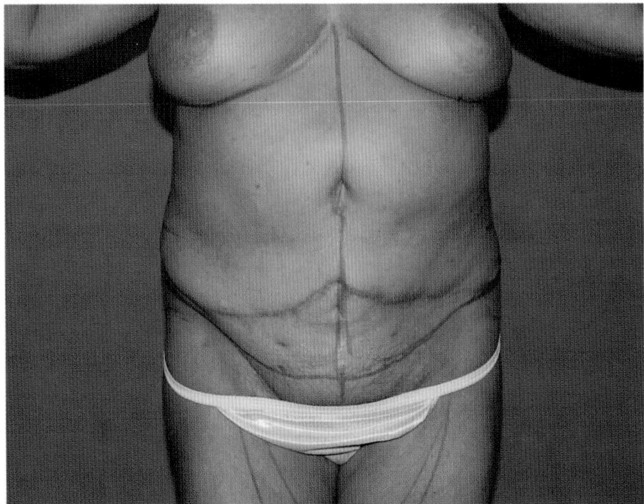

Fig. 11.5 The goal is to have the final transverse scar lie at the level of the pubic symphysis.

Abdominoplasty. Tumescent infiltration is performed in all areas where liposuction is planned (see Chapter 2, Liposuction in Abdominal Contouring) (**Fig. 11.6**). If liposuction is planned it is performed first. The transverse incision is made with a number 10 scalpel partly through the dermis and then completed with electrocautery. The electrocautery is then used to dissect the abdominal soft tissue up to the costal margins and the xiphoid.

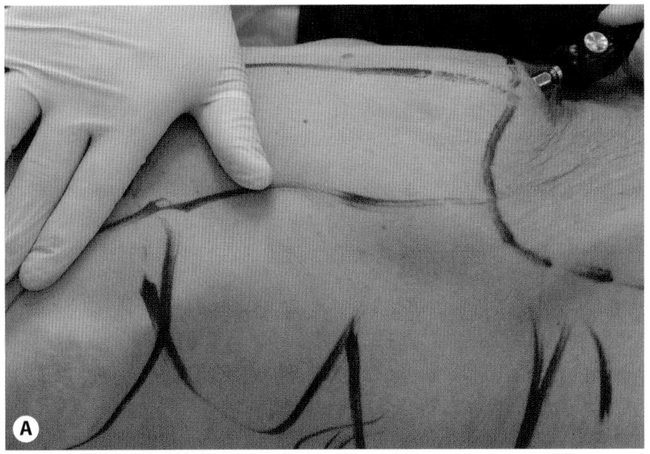

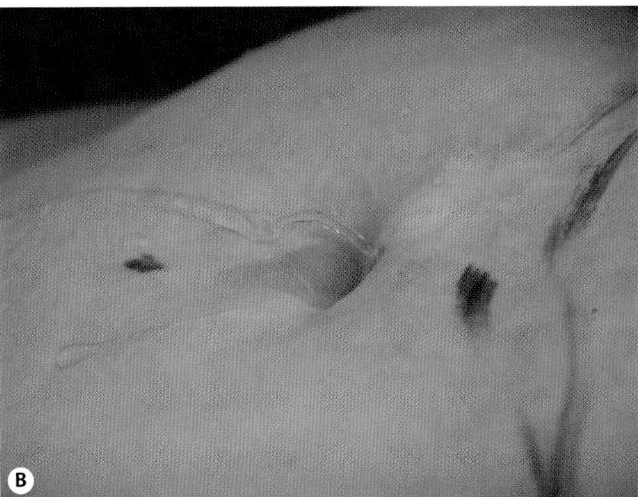

Fig. 11.6 If concurrent liposuction is planned, tumescent infiltration is performed prior to preparation and draping of the patient.

Extra care is needed in secondary abdominoplasties to ensure that dissection is in the correct tissue plane, as previous seromas, hematomas, or infection – among other factors – may have contributed to excess scar tissue formation, making the dissection plane less clear (**Fig. 11.7**). Identification and cautery of perforating vessels is still important. Although the perforators from the deep epigastric arcade have been divided, a new lower transverse incision usually crosses the path of the superficial inferior epigastric and superficial circumflex vessels, which should be identified and controlled (**Fig. 11.8**).

The umbilicus is released from the surrounding soft tissue (see Chapter 12, The Umbilicus in Abdominal Contouring) to allow access to the upper half of the abdominal wall up to the xiphoid (**Fig. 11.9**). If lower abdominal soft-tissue resection is not required, the soft tissue inferior to the umbilicus is not divided as is usually performed during a primary abdominoplasty. If significant scar tissue is encountered it is removed from the abdominal wall fascia and the undersurface of the abdominal soft-tissue apron prior to myofascial plication. This needs to be performed with great

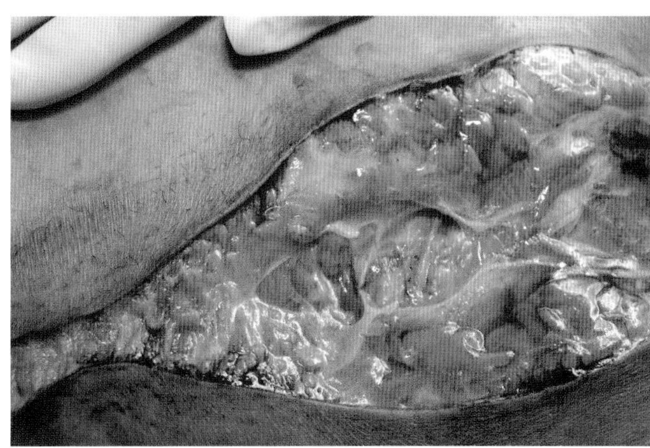

Fig. 11.8 Although the prior abdominoplasty may have eliminated most or all of the perforators from the deep epigastric arcade, the superficial inferior epigastric and superficial circumflex vessels may be encountered, especially when a new incision is placed inferior to the old one. These vessels should be identified and controlled to reduce the chance of postoperative hematoma.

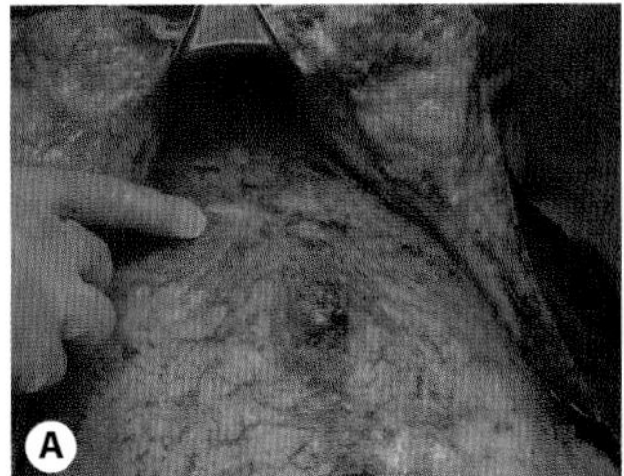

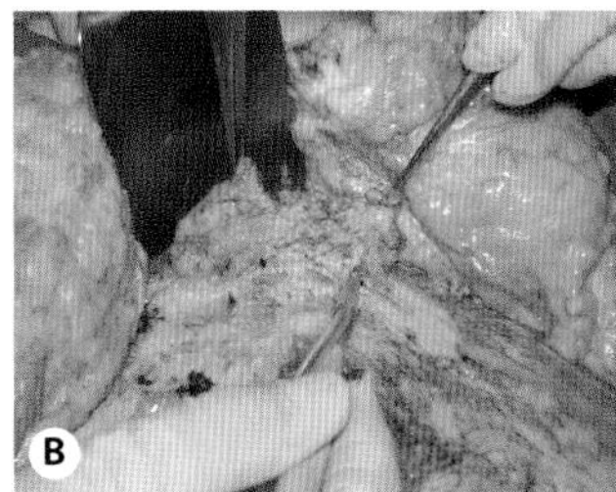

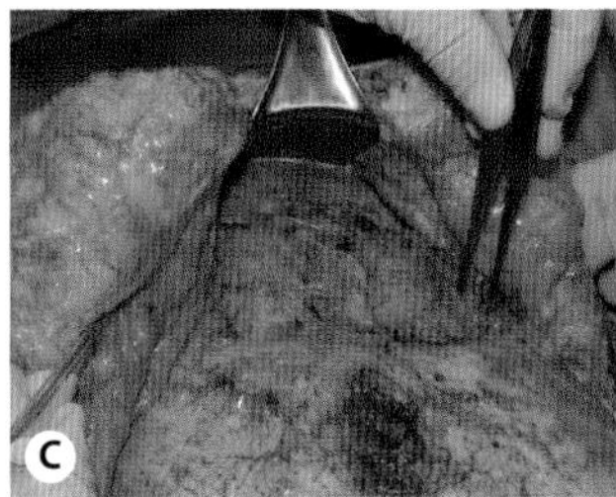

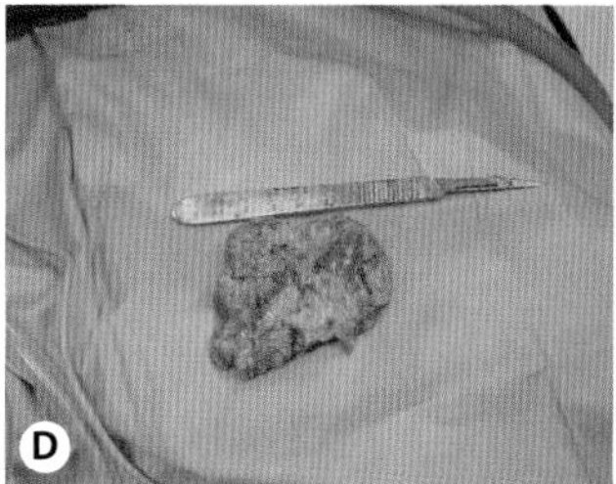

Fig. 11.7 Extra care is required during secondary abdominoplasty procedures, as there may be significant scarring from prior seromas, hematoma, or infection. Excessive scar formation from the previous procedure should be removed (A, B). The removal of a pseudobursae from an untreated localized hematoma (C, D)

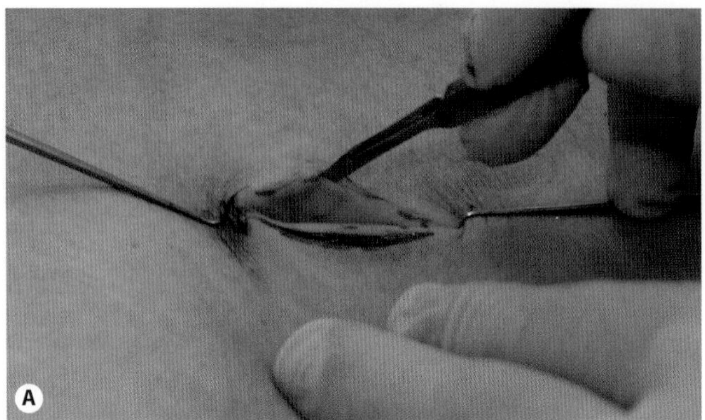

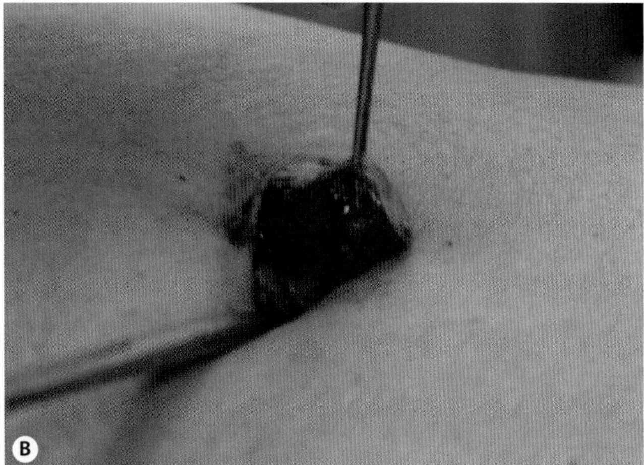

Fig. 11.9 The umbilicus is released in standard fashion as described in Chapter 13. A number 11 blade is commonly used to perform the skin incision, followed by scissors to free the umbilicus from the surrounding soft tissue.

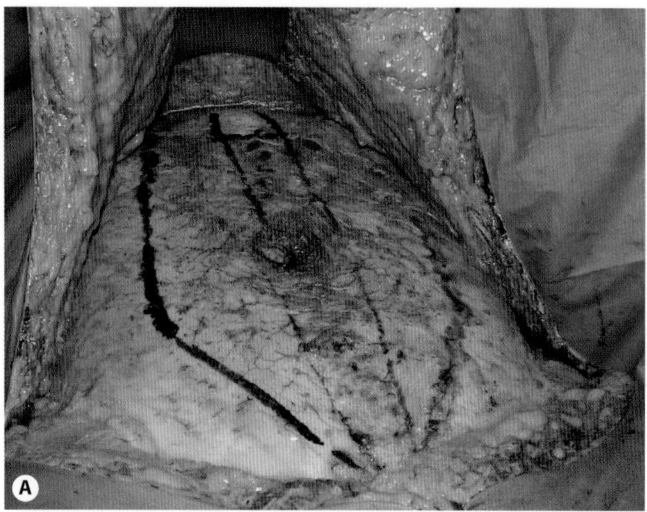

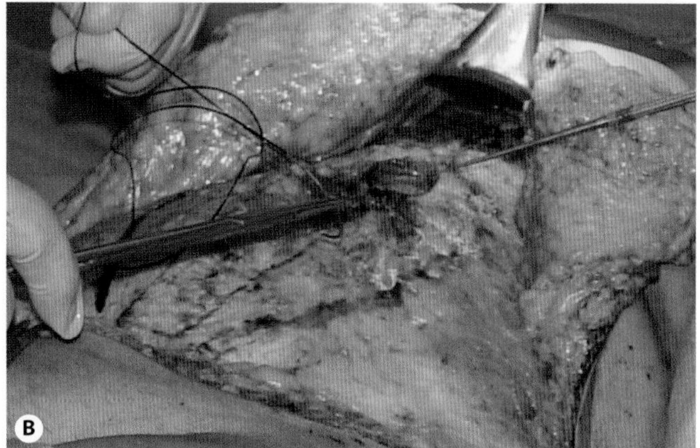

Fig. 11.10 Myofascial plication is performed using size 0 looped nylon suture on a tapered needle. The process starts by estimation of myofascial laxity, followed by marking of the intended plication segment with methylene blue.

care to minimize devascularization of the flap and the creation of unevenness that will be difficult to correct.

Myofascial plication is performed to the extent necessary, guided by the presence of abdominal wall laxity. Often, the complete revision abdominoplasty patient has had inadequate or no myofascial plication. Occasionally, significant weight loss following a primary abdominoplasty has reduced the abdominal fat content, which can also be a source of subsequent abdominal wall laxity. Strong myofascial plication is a key component to the success of both primary and secondary abdominoplasty procedures, and an attempt should be made to properly correct myofascial laxity. Myofascial plication is performed with a number 0 looped nylon suture in a running fashion from xiphoid to pubic symphysis (**Fig. 11.10**).

The soft tissue is resected with the patient in a jack-knife position with the waist flexed. The amount of tissue to be resected is determined with the Pitanguy demarcator (**Fig. 11.11**). Subscarpal fat resection is performed next if needed. A pain pump catheter and a drain are placed after irrigation is performed. Closure is performed by first using skin staples to align the two edges, taking care to advance the lateral portions of the upper edge toward the midline. Prior to wound closure, the new umbilical location is identified with the use of the Pitanguy demarcator (**Fig. 11.12**). A small vertical ellipse of skin and underlying soft tissue is removed and the umbilicus is inset with interrupted deep dermal and continuous intradermal 4/0 Monocryl.[4] The transverse incision is closed in similar fashion to that of a primary abdominoplasty using strong SFS closure with size 0 Vicryl, followed by interrupted deep dermal 2/0 Vicryl and running intradermal 4/0 Monocryl. Tissue adhesive is applied to all incision sites as a water-impermeable dressing.

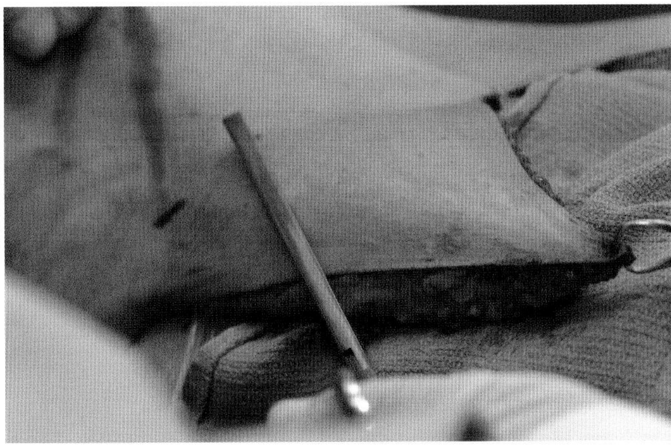

Fig. 11.11 The amount of abdominal soft-tissue to be resected is determined by using the Pitanguy demarcator.

Fig. 11.12 The position of the umbilical inset is also determined by using the Pitanguy demarcator.

Postoperative Care

Postoperative care after complete revision abdominoplasty is similar to that used after primary abdominoplasty. Because the amount of soft-tissue dissection is comparable, proper drain care and use of an abdominal binder are necessary. The same postoperative precautions taken in primary abdominoplasty patients are also taken in complete revision abdominoplasty, including proper hydration, ambulation to decrease the risk of DVT, maintenance of a partially flexed waist, and appropriate follow-up intervals.

Conclusion

Complete revision abdominoplasty is an important procedure for plastic surgeons performing body contouring. It is performed when the aesthetic result of the primary abdominoplasty has left residual myofascial laxity, residual soft-tissue excess, and/or residual excess adiposity. Complete revision abdominoplasty is fundamentally different from basic revision abdominoplasty as it encompasses all or most of the major components of a primary abdominoplasty, including complete dissection and elevation of the abdominal soft-tissue apron. The negative

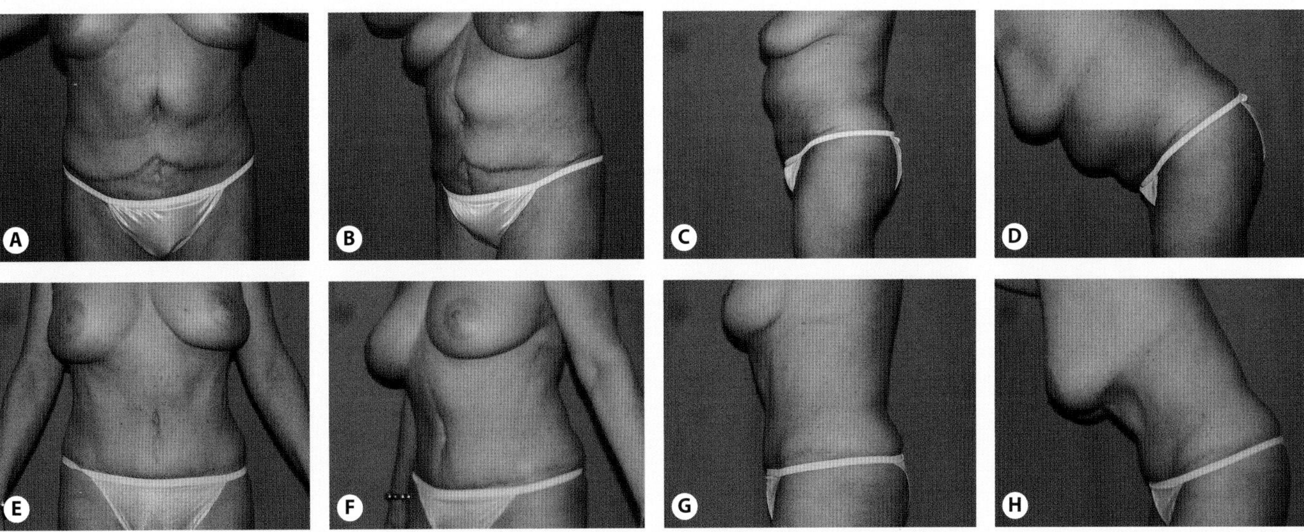

Fig. 11.13 This patient underwent a full abdominoplasty several years earlier by another plastic surgeon and now requested correction of the fullness in her upper abdomen, as well as improvement in the appearance of the transverse scar. In order to lower her scar, a complete revision abdominoplasty was performed, together with concurrent abdominal liposuction and myofascial plication. Postoperative photographs demonstrate reduced adiposity, a lower and improved transverse scar, and a better profile on lateral and divers' views.

sequelae of the initial procedure may also be addressed, including lowering a high transverse scar, correcting the presence of lateral dog-ears, reducing localized adiposity, and improving the appearance of the umbilicus. Thorough preoperative evaluation and discussion with the patient is important to establish a common vision of the final aesthetic result. Preoperative and postoperative photographs are shown in **Figs 11.13–11.15**.

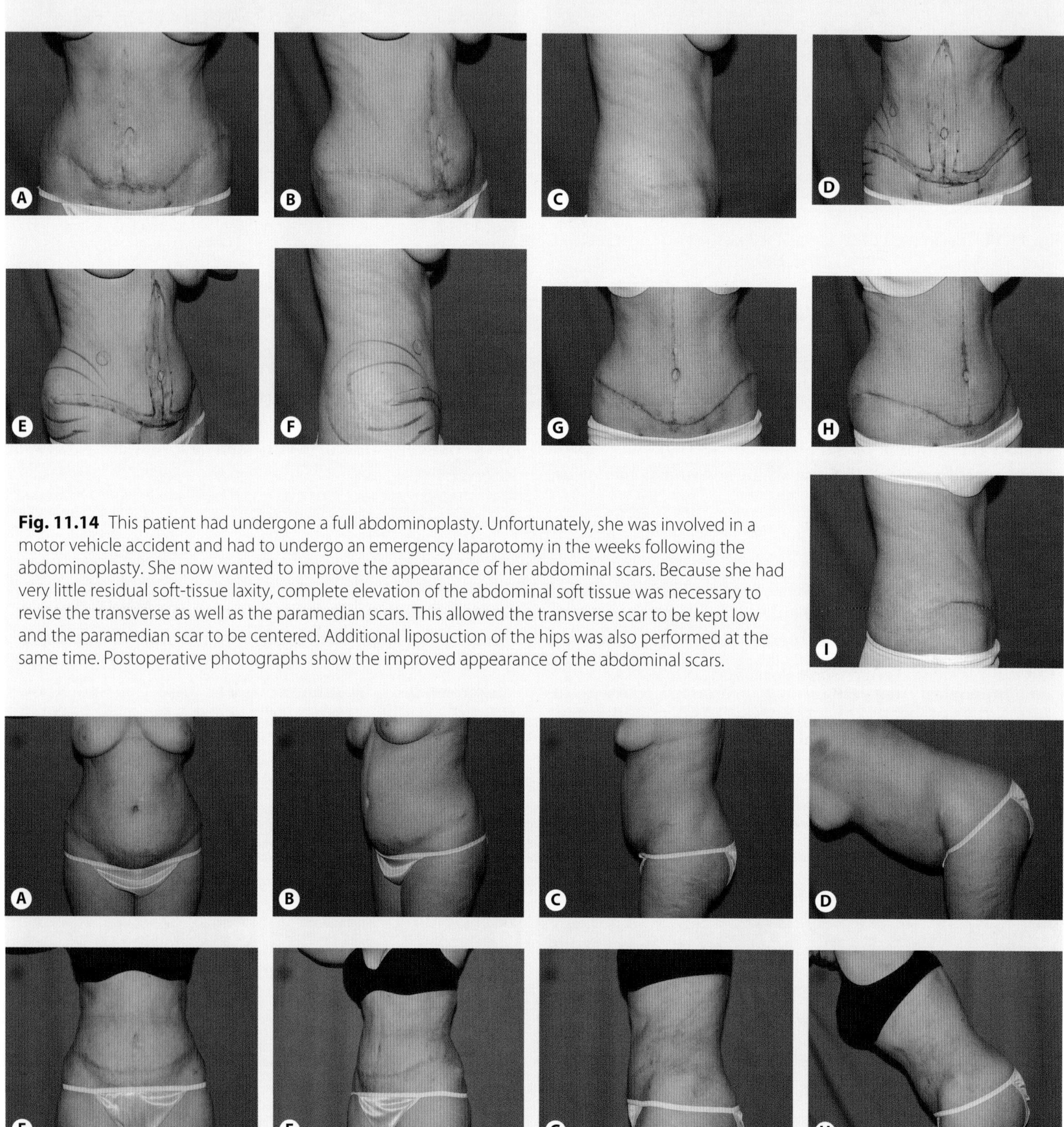

Fig. 11.14 This patient had undergone a full abdominoplasty. Unfortunately, she was involved in a motor vehicle accident and had to undergo an emergency laparotomy in the weeks following the abdominoplasty. She now wanted to improve the appearance of her abdominal scars. Because she had very little residual soft-tissue laxity, complete elevation of the abdominal soft tissue was necessary to revise the transverse as well as the paramedian scars. This allowed the transverse scar to be kept low and the paramedian scar to be centered. Additional liposuction of the hips was also performed at the same time. Postoperative photographs show the improved appearance of the abdominal scars.

Fig. 11.15 This patient had also undergone a full abdominoplasty elsewhere. The scar was kept low, but residual adiposity, soft-tissue laxity, and myofascial laxity are evident, as well as small lateral dog-ears. The patient desired an improved abdominal contour. As there was significant excess soft-tissue laxity and residual myofascial laxity present, a complete revision abdominoplasty was performed. Concurrent abdominal liposuction and myofascial plication were also performed. Postoperative photographs demonstrate an improved abdominal contour in the AP, lateral, and divers' views.

Clinical Caveats: Complete revision abdominoplasty

- The need for complete soft-tissue elevation fundamentally differentiates complete revision abdominoplasty from other abdominoplasty revision procedures
- Complete revision abdominoplasty may involve some or all of the major surgical components of a primary abdominoplasty, including full abdominal soft-tissue elevation, concurrent liposuction, myofascial plication, and soft-tissue resection
- Understanding the patient's desired goal is key to choosing the ideal revision abdominoplasty technique
- Thorough discussion will allow the surgeon and patient to share a common vision of the expected results. This is particularly important for revision abdominoplasty patients
- Inability to incorporate the umbilical site into the resection segment is more likely in complete revision abdominoplasty. Preoperative discussion about this is critical, as many patients do not anticipate additional scarring
- The intraoperative sequence and postoperative care are largely the same as for primary abdominoplasty

References

1. Hensel JM, Lehman JA Jr., Tantri MP, et al. An outcomes analysis and satisfaction survey of 199 consecutive abdominoplasties. Ann Plast Surg 2001; 46: 357.
2. Matarasso A, Wallach SG, Rankin M, Galiano RD. Secondary abdominal contour surgery: a review of early and late reoperative surgery. Plast Reconstruct Surg 2005; 115: 627.
3. Chaouat M, Levan P, Lalanne B, et al. Abdominal dermolipectomies: early postoperative complications and long-term unfavorable results. Plast Reconstruct Surg 2000; 106: 1614.
4. Guerrerosantos J, Dicksheet S, Carrillo C, Sandoval M. Umbilical reconstruction with secondary abdominoplasty. Ann Plast Surg 1980; 5: 139.

Suggested Reading

Dillerud E. Abdominoplasty combined with suction lipoplasty: A study of complications, revisions, and risk factors in 487 cases. Ann Plast Surg 1990; 25: 333.

El-Khatib HA, Bener A. Abdominal dermolipectomy in an abdomen with pre-existing scars: a different concept. Plast Reconstruct Surg 2004; 114: 992.

Grazer FM, Goldwyn RM. Abdominoplasty assessed by survery with emphasis on complications. Plast Reconstruct Surg 1977; 59: 513.

Hester RT Jr., Baird W, Bostwick J III, et al. Abdominoplasty combined with other surgical procedures: Safe or sorry? Plast Reconstruct Surg 1989; 83: 997.

Hunstad JP. Advanced concepts in abdominoplasty. Perspect Plast Surg 1998; 12: 13.

Hunstad JP. Body contouring in the obese patient. Clin Plast Surg 1996; 23: 647.

Kim J, Stevenson TR. Abdominoplasty, liposuction of the flanks, and obesity: analyzing risk factors for seroma formation. Plast Reconstruct Surg 2006; 117: 77.

Lee MJ, Mustoe TA. A simplified version to achieve aesthetic results for the umbilicus in abdominoplasty. Plast Reconstruct Surg 2002; 109: 2136.

Manassa EH, Hertl CH, Olbrisch RR. Wound healing problems in smokers and non-smokers after 132 abdominoplasties. Plast Reconstruct Surg 2003; 111: 2082.

Matarasso A. Abdominoplasty: A system of classification and treatment for combined abdominoplasty and suction-assisted lipectomy. Aesthet Plast Surg 1991; 15: 111–121.

Matarasso A. Awareness and avoidance of abdominoplasty complications. Aesthet Surg J 1997; 17: 256.

Matarasso A. The male abdominoplasty. Clin Plast Surg 2004; 31: 555.

Matarasso A, Swift RW, Rankin M. Abdominoplasty and abdominal contour surgery: a national plastic surgery survey. Plast Reconstruct Surg 2006; 117: 1797.

Nahas FX, Ferreira LM, Augusto SM, Ghelfond C. Long-term follow-up of correction of rectus diastasis. Plast Reconstruct Surg 2005; 115: 1736–1741; discussion 1742–1743.

Netscher DT, Wigoda P, Spira M, Peltier M. Musculoaponeurotic plication in abdominoplasty: How durable are its effects? Aesthet Plast Surg 1995; 19: 531.

CHAPTER **12**

The Umbilicus in Body Contouring

Joseph P. Hunstad and Remus Repta

IN THIS CHAPTER

KEY POINTS

The umbilicus is an aesthetically important component of the abdomen. Extra care should be taken in planning and executing the release and inset of the umbilicus during abdominoplasty procedures to provide the best result possible. The size, shape, contour, position, and appearance of the umbilicus and umbilical scars should be carefully planned to optimize the final aesthetic appearance of the umbilicus.

Introduction

The umbilicus is the central focus of the abdomen and an important aesthetic component of the body. It has been represented throughout history and across cultures as a sign of youth and beauty. The eye is naturally drawn to this point of the abdomen, which makes the appearance and location of the umbilicus critical. As such, an aesthetically pleasing umbilicus is necessary for an attractive abdomen, and vice versa. Far too often, great effort is made to keep the abdominoplasty incisions hidden only to have an umbilicus that is left unrejuvenated, with poor visible scars, or with a displeasing shape.

In order to create an aesthetically pleasing umbilicus one must first identify the characteristics that define it (**Table 12.1**). Despite anatomical variability among patients, as well as particular surgeon and patient preference, there is a general consensus as to the characteristics that add to the aesthetic beauty of an umbilicus as well as those that detract from it.[1,2] The vertical position of the umbilicus, the amount of depression compared to the periumbilical soft tissue, and the shape and size of the umbilicus should all be taken into account in abdominal contouring surgery.

The vertical position of the umbilicus varies according to the length of the patient's torso and the degree of soft-tissue laxity associated with aging and weight loss. An aesthetically pleasing umbilicus should have a shape that is vertically oriented and located in the midline, just cephalad to an imaginary line connecting the superiormost portions of the iliac crests. That said, in traditional abdominoplasty procedures, where the umbilicus is released from the surrounding soft tissue and inset into the abdominal flap, there is only a limited ability to change the vertical position of the umbilicus. This small variation is determined largely by the length of the umbilical stalk. As most abdominoplasty procedures involve some form of myofascial plication, the umbilical stalk is usually shortened and the variability in the vertical position of the umbilical inset is further reduced, essentially making it a relatively fixed position. Attempting to inset the umbilicus at a point much further cephalad or caudal from this will result in an unnatural shape and appearance and potentially lead to poor healing.

The umbilicus can present with a diverse variety of shapes and sizes in the body contouring population. Many factors combine to create each individual umbilical shape, including skin quality, soft-tissue laxity, body type, weight gain and loss, amount of adiposity, age, previous surgery/trauma, and genetics. Despite this variety, there are general characteristics of umbilical size, shape, and periumbilical contour that are more consistent with youth and beauty.

Table 12.1 Desirable umbilical characteristics

Small is preferable to large
A vertical ellipse is preferable to a circle
An 'inny' is more desirable than an 'outie'

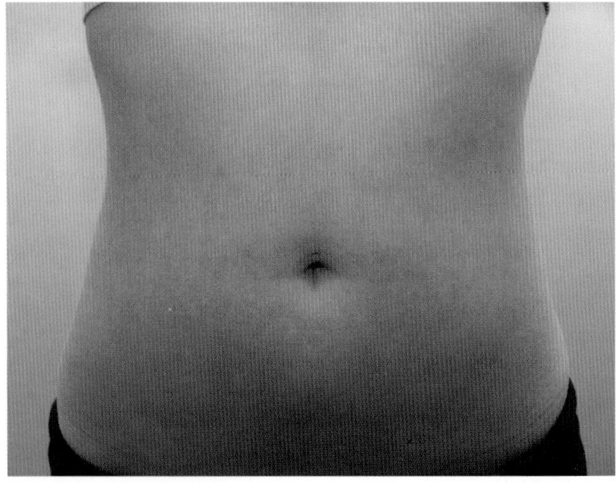

Fig. 12.1 The youthful umbilicus is often vertically oval or elliptical, as opposed to round.

The youthful umbilicus is often vertically oval or jewel-shaped (**Fig. 12.1**). The ideal size should match the patient's body and preference, and therefore an exact measurement cannot be used for all patients. However, when the opportunity allows, it is better to err on the small side since, as aging and weight fluctuation usually result in an umbilicus that appears wider and larger than desired. A smaller umbilicus is usually judged to be more youthful in appearance.

A woman with a thin, toned abdomen usually presents with an umbilicus that also has a mild amount of superior hooding and a faint but appreciable depression or 'washout' area at the inferior pole (**Fig. 12.2**). The superior hooding is largely a result of gravity pulling inferiorly on the upper skin and soft tissue when the patient is standing, leading to gathering of the skin and soft tissue at the superior portion of the umbilicus, which is firmly anchored by its stalk. This can easily be verified when patients are placed supine with a little Trendelenburg position. With reversal of the direction of the pull of gravity on the abdominal skin and soft tissue, the superior hooding is reduced or eliminated and inferior umbilical hooding becomes evident.

Surgical Approach (Box 12.1)

The umbilicus can be released in various ways, depending on surgeon preference and patient needs. The goal of release is to create a symmetric cutaneous component and to release it from the surrounding tissue in a manner that

Box 12.1 Umbilical release

- The skin of the umbilicus should be released at the junction of the umbilicus with the abdominal skin
- The use of skin hooks and a number 11 blade facilitates skin incision
- Dissection down to the anterior rectus sheath is performed sharply with scissors
- The remainder of the umbilical release is performed with electrocautery after the lower abdominal flap is transected

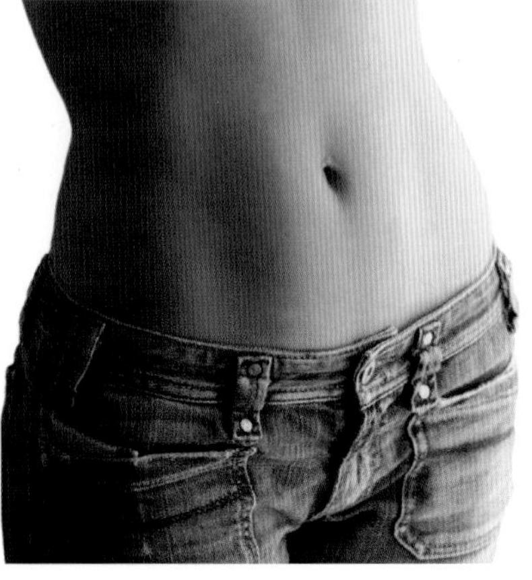

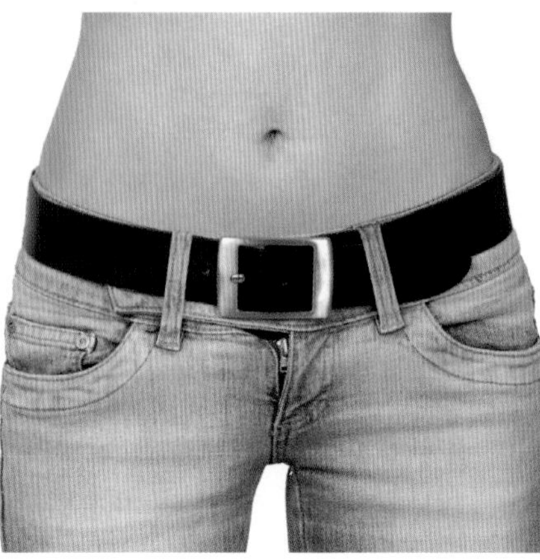

Fig. 12.2 Women who are athletic and toned and present with an aesthetically pleasing umbilicus usually have a mild amount of superior hooding and a lower umbilical 'washout' area. These characteristics are seen when the effect of gravity on the periumbilical skin and soft tissue is greater than on the relatively fixed umbilicus. Above the umbilicus the skin and soft tissue are pulled on top of the umbilicus to create hooding, and below the umbilicus they are pulled down to create the 'washout' area.

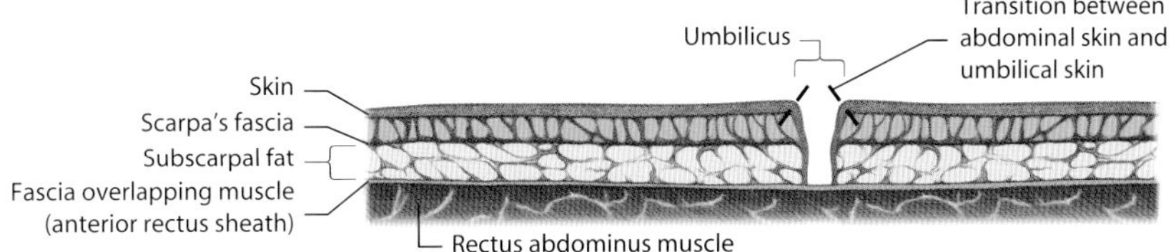

Fig. 12.3 A cross-section of the abdominal soft tissue and skin at the level of the umbilicus shows the transition between the umbilical skin and the abdominal skin. These two surfaces are at 90° to each other. In most abdominoplasty patients the umbilicus is released at this transition. The exact level of the skin incision for the release should be tailored to each patient.

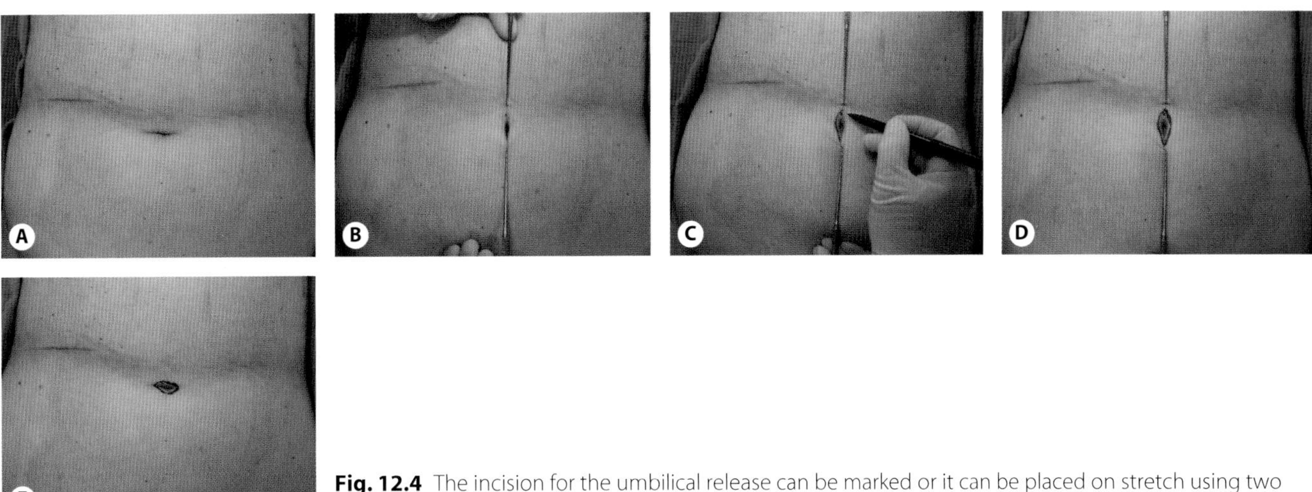

Fig. 12.4 The incision for the umbilical release can be marked or it can be placed on stretch using two opposing skin hooks at the 12 o'clock and 6 o'clock positions.

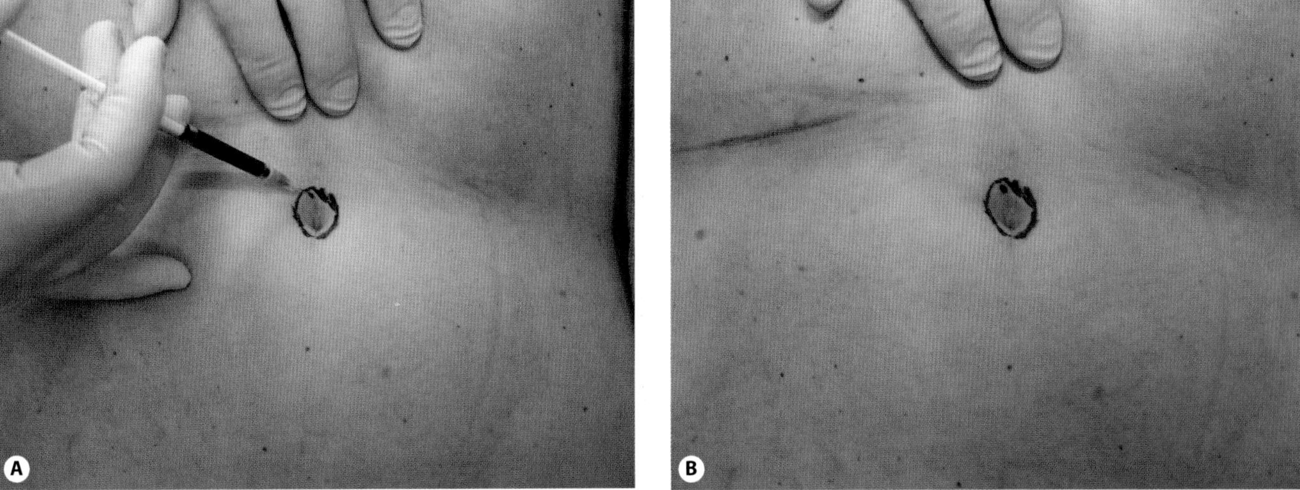

Fig. 12.5 A methylene blue tattoo mark placed at the 12 o'clock position before the umbilical release will help orient the umbilicus during inset to prevent twisting of the stalk.

protects the blood supply but does not leave a large amount of excess adipose tissue. The size of the cutaneous component created when the umbilicus is released can be varied to suit the patient. Often, there is a transition zone where the umbilical skin becomes the abdominal skin, in a dorsoventral direction from the umbilicus to the coronal plane of the abdominal skin (**Fig. 12.3**).

The skin incision can be marked, or the umbilical opening can be placed on stretch using skin hooks to create the folds delineating the area to be incised (**Fig. 12.4**). Using a methylene blue tattoo placed at the 12 o'clock position will identify this location during insetting (**Fig. 12.5**). The incision can be made with either a number 15 or a number 11 scalpel. The number 11 is best used via a pushing motion (**Fig. 12.6**). Once the skin has been incised, curved Metzenbaum scissors are used to sharply release the soft tissue around the umbilicus down to the deep fascia (**Fig. 12.7**). The periumbilical perforators are usually within a centimeter or so from the umbilical stalk, so scissor dissection is performed down to the abdominal wall fascia near the stalk (**Fig. 12.8**). The remainder of the periumbilical soft-tissue release is performed with electrocautery under

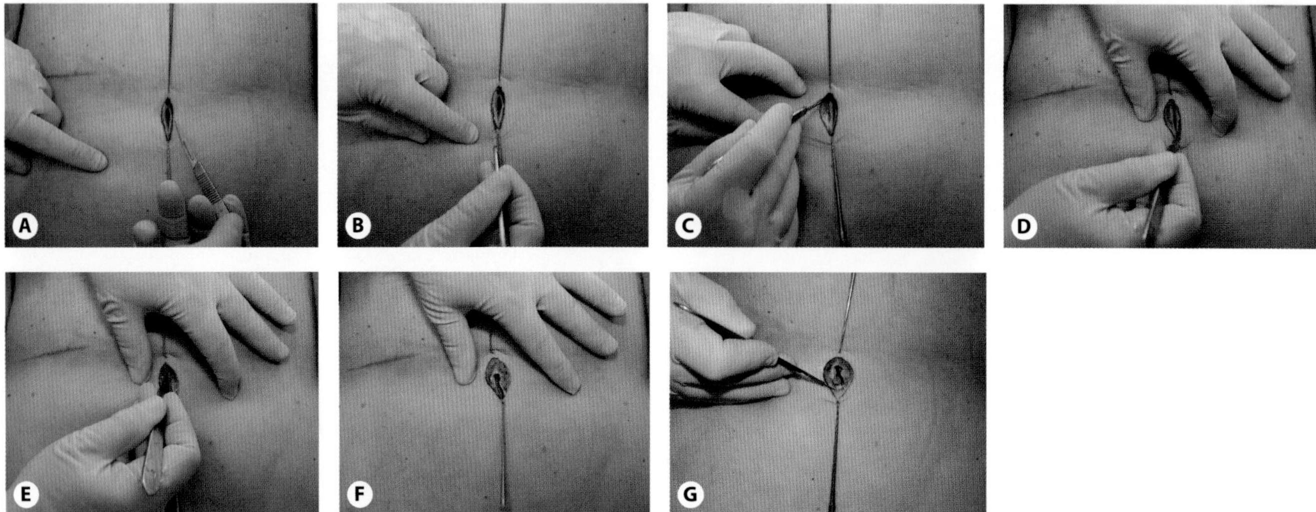

Fig. 12.6 The skin incision can be performed in a variety of ways. We prefer a number 11 scalpel for the skin incision of the umbilical release. This blade performs best when it is used in a pushing motion.

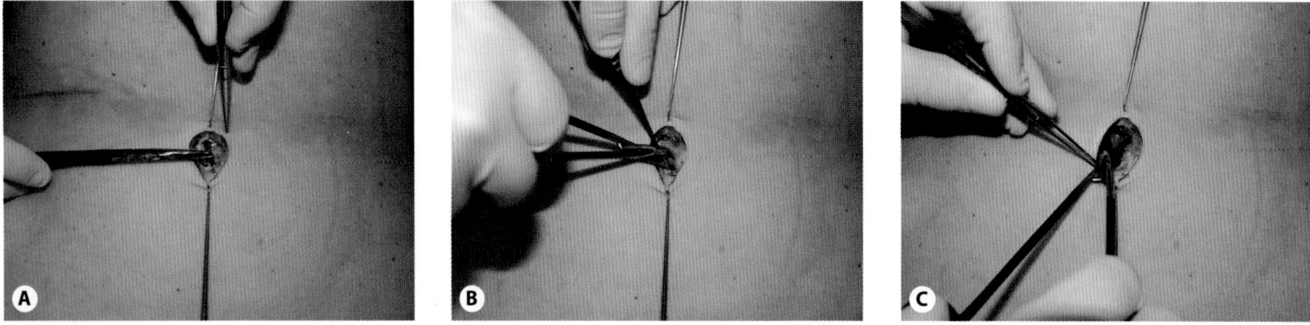

Fig. 12.7 The soft tissue surrounding the umbilical stalk is released sharply with curved Metzenbaum scissors. The goal is to release the stalk without leaving a large amount of fat attached. There is a loose areolar plane surrounding the stalk that provides a good plane of dissection.

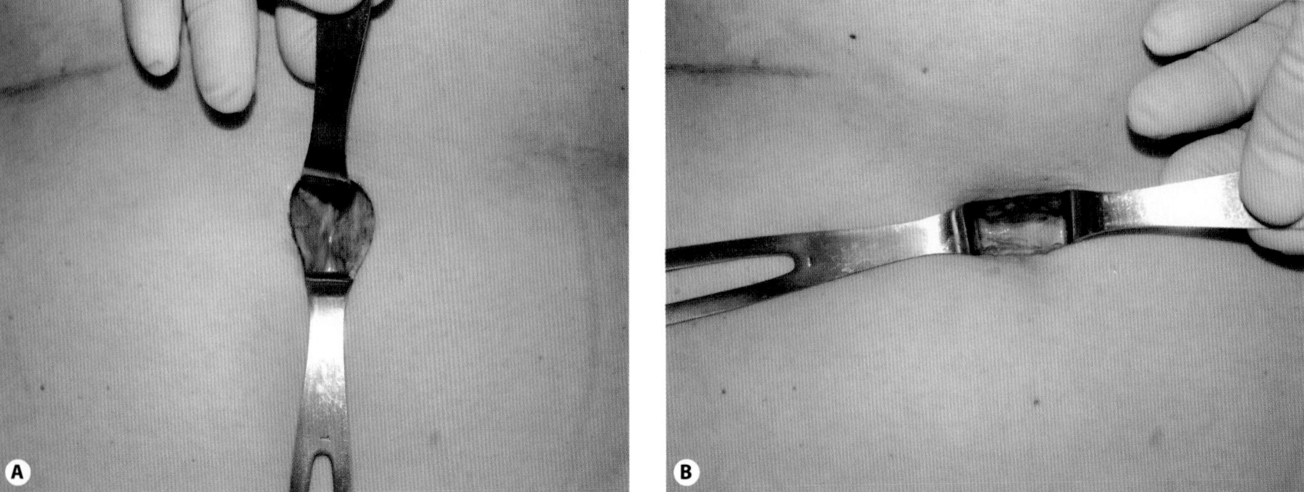

Fig. 12.8 Dissection is performed down to the anterior rectus sheath, taking care to stay relatively close to the base of the umbilical stalk, as there is usually one or more umbilical perforators in the vicinity.

direct vision once the abdominal soft-tissue apron inferior to the umbilicus has been transected (**Fig. 12.9**).

The length of the umbilical stalk should be given some consideration. Patients who have experienced massive weight loss usually have an elongated, stretched-out umbilical stalk. Fortunately, the process of myofascial plication usually shortens the stalk by invagination of the midline tissues (**Fig. 12.10**). If the stalk remains excessively long, for example in patients with massive weight loss, it can be shortened by resecting the excess length or it can be secured down to the anterior rectus sheath. Great care should be taken when resection is performed, because the cutaneous lining of the stalk quickly narrows and excessive resection will produce a very small-diameter umbilicus. An alternate method is to anchor the mid-portion of the stalk down to the rectus sheath, resulting in a 'telescoped' stalk that is effectively shortened (**Box 12.2**).

Box 12.2 Myofascial plication and the umbilicus

- The attractive umbilicus is slightly concave or recessed from the surrounding abdominal skin and soft tissue
- Myofascial plication shortens the umbilicus through imbrication of the midline tissue, and helps create a recessed umbilicus at the time of inset
- Periumbilical myofascial plication should correct fascial laxity and leave enough space around the stalk to safely avoid perfusion problems
- Verification that this periumbilical space is sufficient should be performed during plication by using the back end of the dermal forceps or tip of the gloved index finger
- Asymmetric myofascial plication can be used to correct an umbilicus that is noted to be off-midline preoperatively

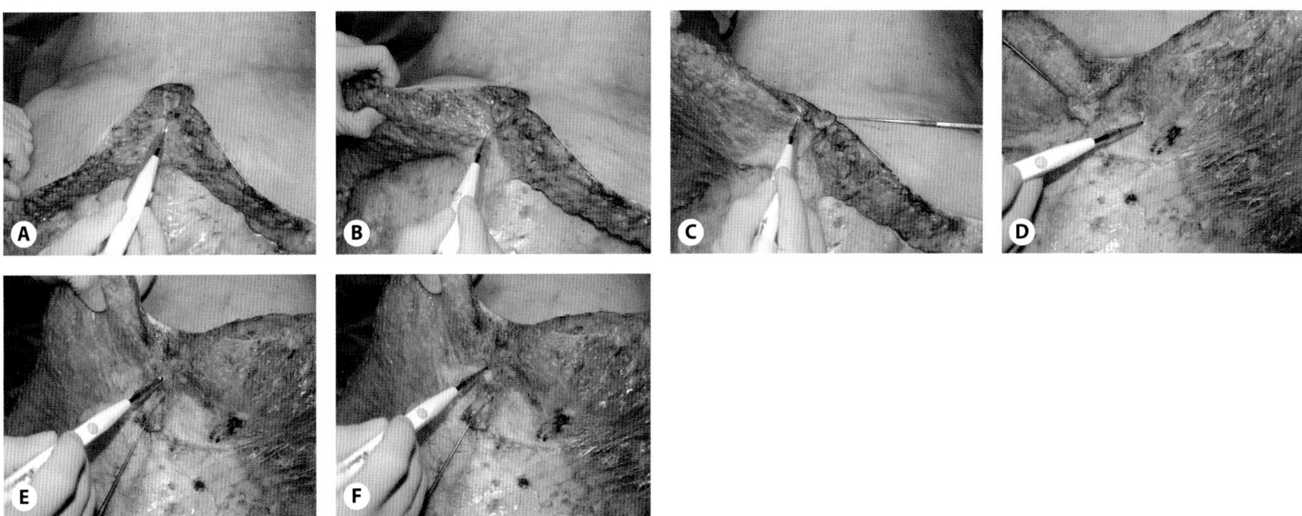

Fig. 12.9 The umbilical release is completed with electrocautery after the inferior abdominal soft-tissue apron is divided. The umbilicus is retracted away from the dissection area with a single hook placing the soft tissue in the dissection area under tension. This allows efficient use of the electrocautery without creating excessive heat near the stalk. There are a number of periumbilical perforators in this area, so careful dissection and control of these vessels is recommended.

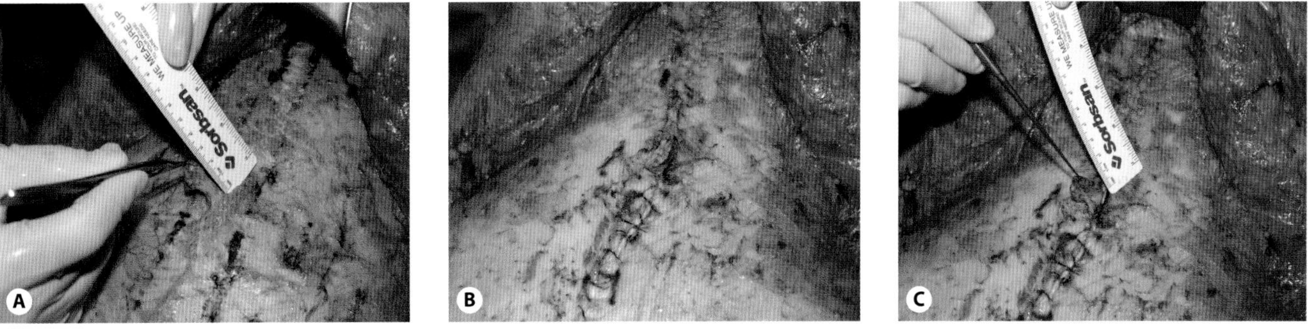

Fig. 12.10 The process of myofascial plication produces invagination of the midline tissue. This pulls the umbilical stalk deeper within the imbricated tissue and the umbilicus is in essence shortened. How much the stalk is shortened depends on the degree of myofascial laxity and the extent of myofascial plication.

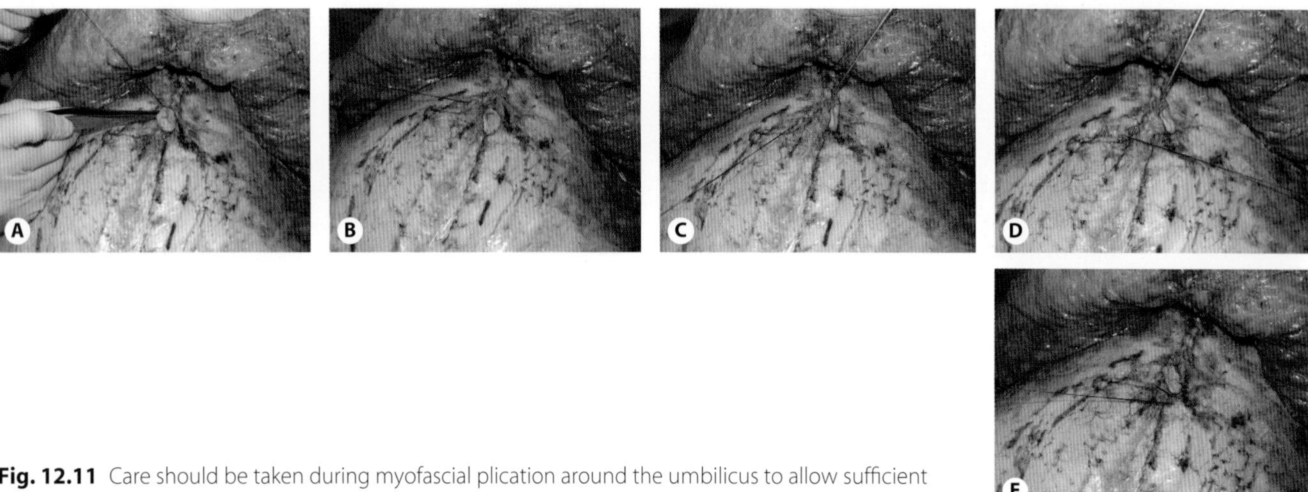

Fig. 12.11 Care should be taken during myofascial plication around the umbilicus to allow sufficient space for postoperative soft-tissue swelling without endangering the perfusion to the umbilicus.

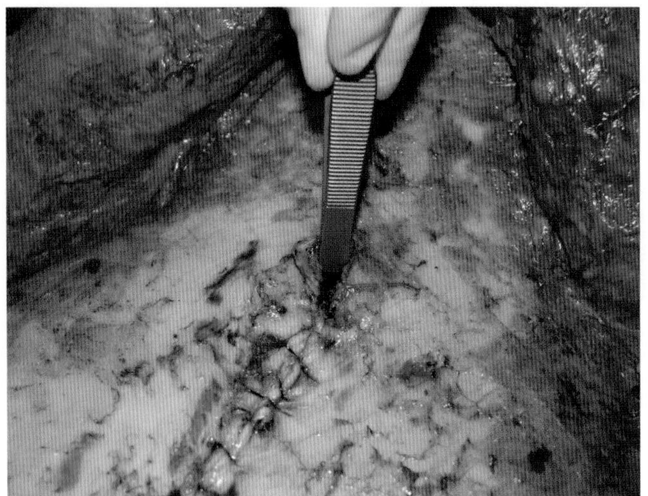

Fig. 12.12 There is a fine line between adequate umbilical perfusion and adequate correction of fascial laxity during myofascial plication. Determining the appropriate amount periumbilical fascial tightening may be hard at times. If the tip of the gloved index finger or the back end of the dermal forceps can be easily introduced between the plicated fascial edge and the umbilical stalk, there is good evidence that the space provided around the umbilicus is sufficient.

Box 12.3 Umbilical inset

- The midline of the abdomen can be verified by spanning a taut suture from the xiphoid to the pubic symphysis
- The vertical position of the umbilical inset is largely set after myofascial plication is performed
- A skin ellipse is incised slightly smaller than the umbilicus
- The underlying soft tissue is excised down to the anterior rectus sheath, making sure there is sufficient room for the umbilicus to pass without constriction
- Removing soft tissue under the abdominal flap in the periumbilical area can help produce a slight depression around the umbilicus, which is attractive
- The umbilical inset is completed with buried interrupted dermal and intradermal 4/0 Monocryl suture

Enough space should be left around the base of the umbilical stalk during myofascial plication to allow for some soft-tissue swelling without resulting in excessive compression of the stalk (**Fig. 12.11**). Myofascial plication of the periumbilical area that is too loose may result in some fullness in the central or periumbilical abdomen secondary to uncorrected fascial laxity. Conversely, plication that is too tight may lead to strangulation, ischemia, and possible loss of the umbilicus. The goal is therefore to tighten the abdominal fascia sufficiently to correct the fascial laxity but to allow enough space for umbilical stalk perfusion. In general, if the stalk can be manipulated easily, or if the tip of the gloved index finger or the back end of a dermal forceps can be partially introduced, then there is sufficient space (**Fig. 12.12**, **Box 12.3**).

Insetting the umbilicus is fairly straightforward. The location of inset should be in the midline, which is easily demonstrated by pulling a suture taut between the xiphoid and the center of the pubic symphysis (**Fig. 12.13**). An appreciable number of patients have an off-center umbilicus preoperatively, so this must be taken into account[3] (**Fig. 12.14**). Noting this asymmetry preoperatively and discussing it with the patient will help determine the best course of action. Patients are usually unaware that their umbilicus is not perfectly in the midline. Often there is some degree of scoliosis or musculoskeletal asymmetry present if there is no history of prior soft-tissue trauma. Prior pregnancy and the resulting abdominal wall laxity or previous surgery may also be the source of the malpositioned umbilicus. Eccentric or intentionally asymmetric myofascial plication can be performed to help correct the malpositioned umbilicus (**Fig. 12.15**).

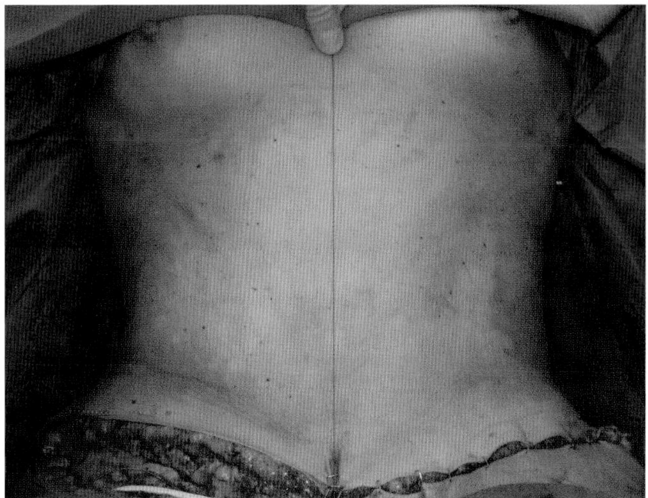

Fig. 12.13 The midline is usually determined by identifying the xiphoid and the middle of the mons pubis or pubic symphysis. Pulling a suture taut between these two points will help delineate the midline of the abdomen.

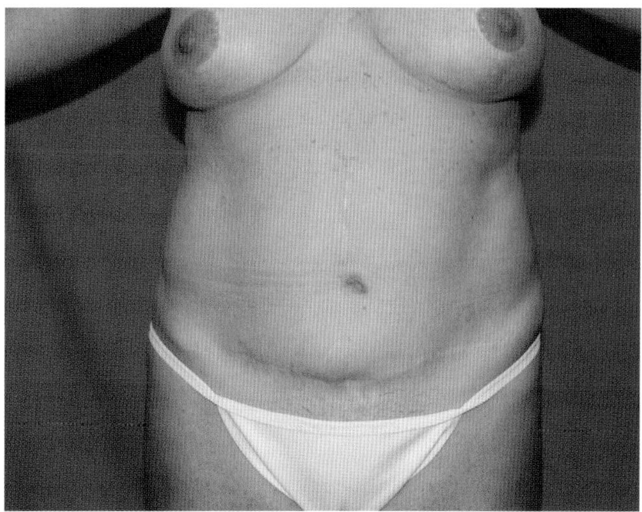

Fig. 12.14 An appreciable number of patients have an umbilicus that is off-midline to some degree. This discrepancy should be discussed with the patient preoperatively.

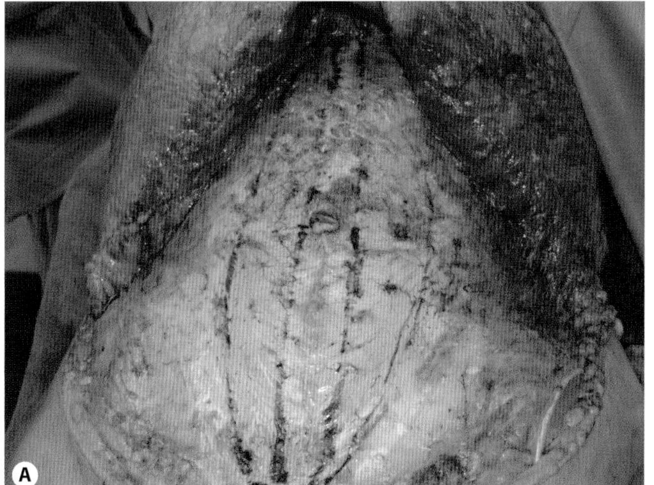

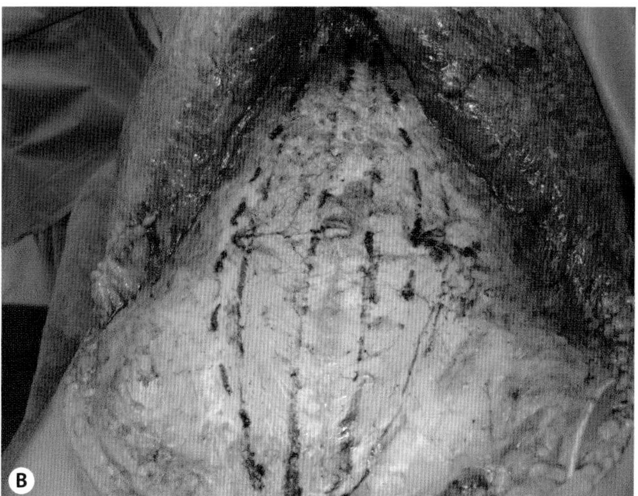

Fig. 12.15 The malpositioned umbilicus can be brought closer to the midline by performing an eccentric or intentionally asymmetric myofascial plication. The medial solid lines indicate the medial borders of the rectus abdominis muscles. The lateral solid lines are equally spaced from the midline and represent the standard myofascial plication path with a midline umbilicus. The dashed lines and arrows indicate the asymmetric shift in the myofascial plication performed when the umbilicus is off-midline.

As mentioned above, the vertical position of the umbilical inset is often largely predetermined by the length of the umbilical stalk. Use of a Pitanguy demarcator and verification of this mark prior to closing the abdominoplasty flap will help fine-tune the vertical position of the umbilical inset (**Fig. 12.16**). The skin of the abdominal flap is marked in a vertical ellipse that is slightly smaller in the vertical and transverse dimensions than the umbilicus (**Fig. 12.17**). This will permit the creation of a vertically oblong umbilicus that is closed without skin tension. Following skin removal, the new umbilical site immediately enlarges (**Fig. 12.18**). The subcutaneous tissue of the abdominal flap at the umbilical inset is resected to correspond to the skin ellipse removed, except at the superior portion of the ellipse, where it is maintained to add to superior umbilical hooding (**Fig. 12.19**). The surgeon must verify that the soft-tissue resection for the inset is sufficient to deliver the umbilicus without constriction, particularly by the superficial fascia.

Defatting the undersurface of the abdominal flap in the periumbilical area is appropriate for virtually all patients to create a mild amount of periumbilical depression. Maintenance

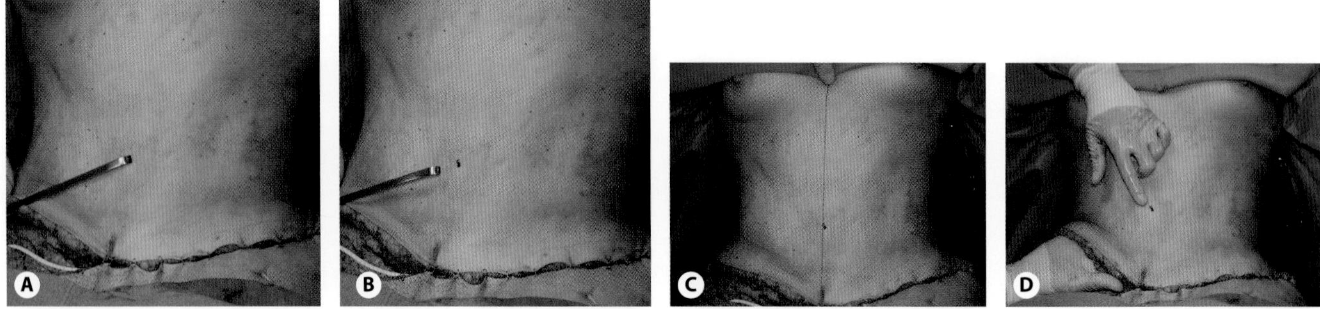

Fig. 12.16 The Pitanguy demarcator is used to translocate the position of the umbilicus to the overlying abdominal skin in preparation for insetting. The position of the umbilical inset is further verified by spanning a suture from the xiphoid to the midline symphysis pubis.

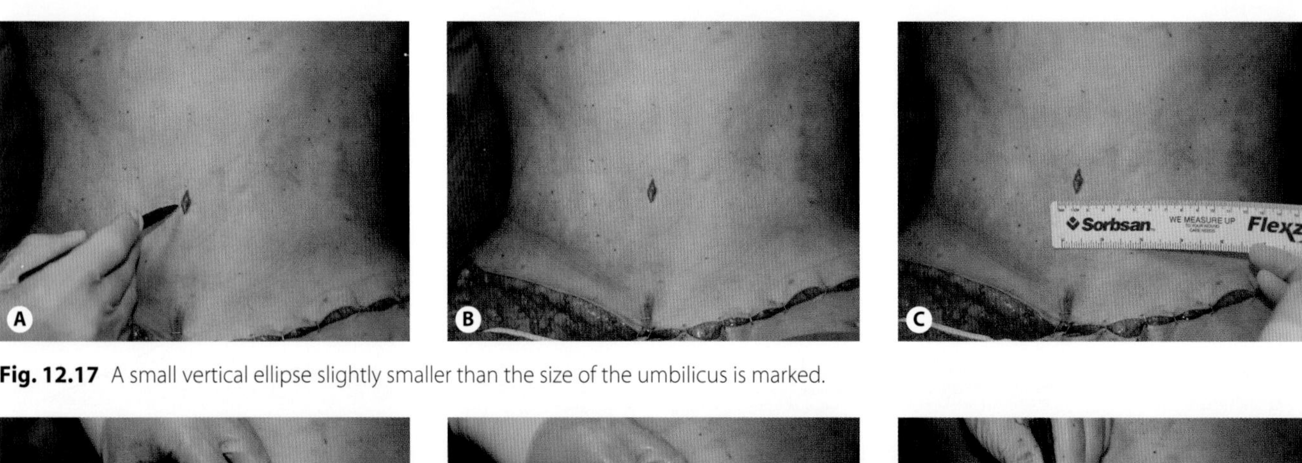

Fig. 12.17 A small vertical ellipse slightly smaller than the size of the umbilicus is marked.

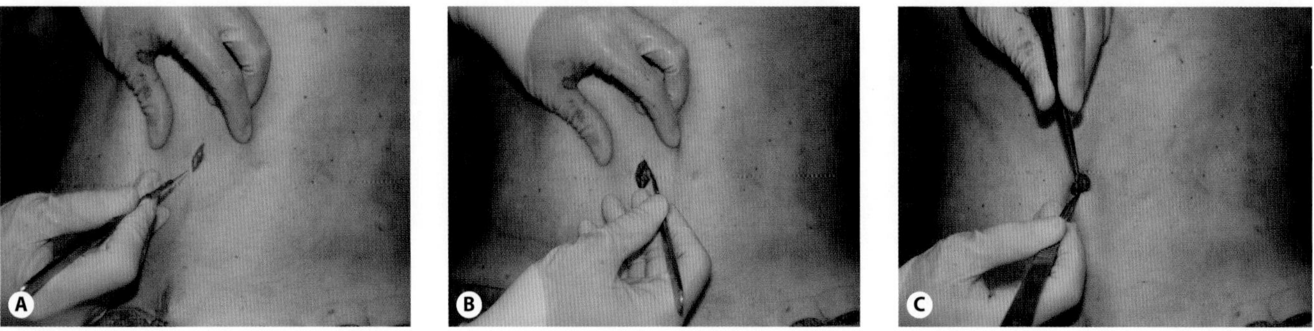

Fig. 12.18 A number 11 scalpel is used to incise the ellipse. Once the skin is completely incised, the opening often enlarges slightly depending on the amount of soft-tissue tension present.

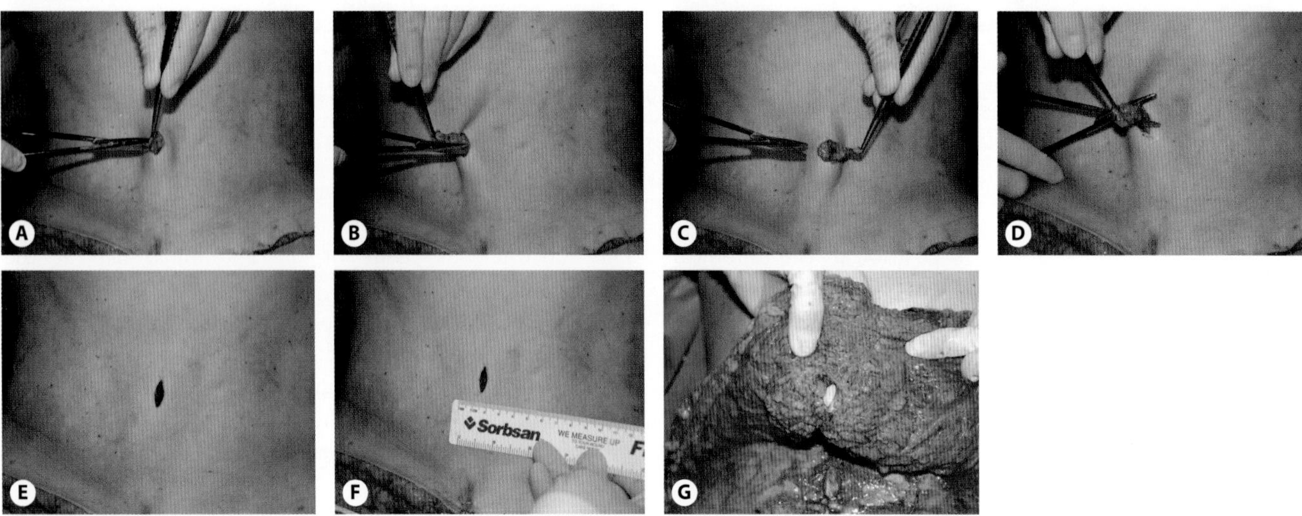

Fig. 12.19 The subcutaneous and underlying soft tissue of the abdominal flap is resected to allow the umbilicus to be pulled out through the opening without tension. Ample tissue should be resected, especially at the level of the superficial fascia, to prevent constriction of the umbilical stalk. Some soft tissue is left superiorly to add to superior umbilical hooding.

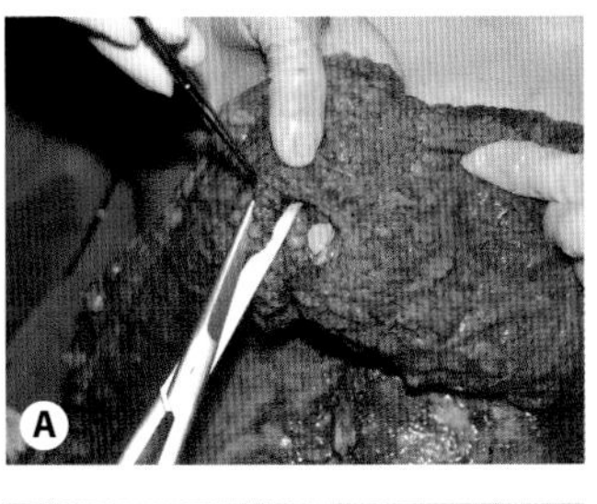
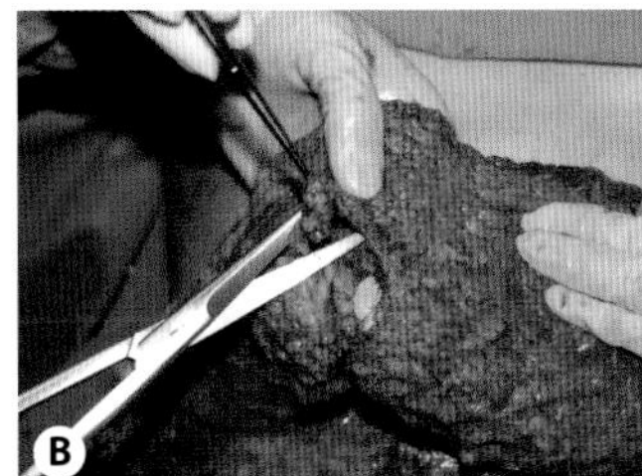
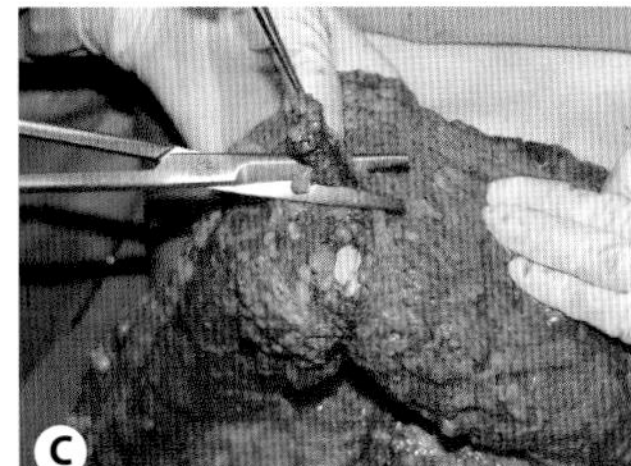
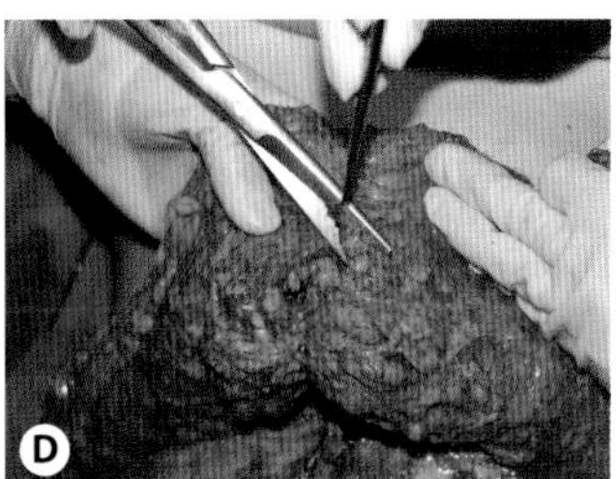
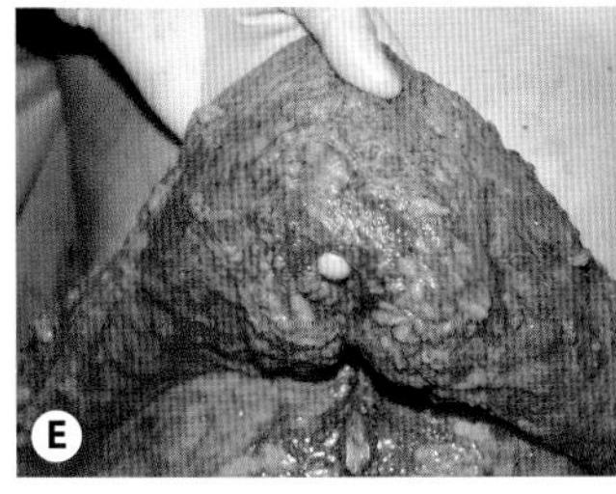

Fig. 12.20 The undersurface of the abdominal flap in the periumbilical area can also be defatted. This creates a relative periumbilical depression or hollow, which can be attractive. Defatting is performed on the undersurface in the inferior half of the umbilical opening, preserving soft tissue at the 12 o'clock position to add to superior umbilical hooding.

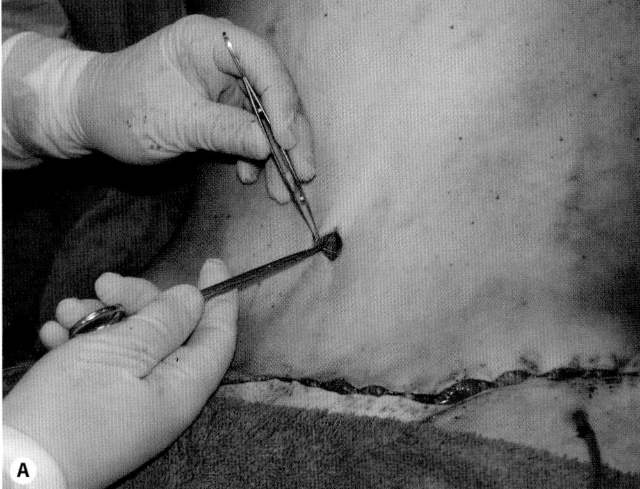
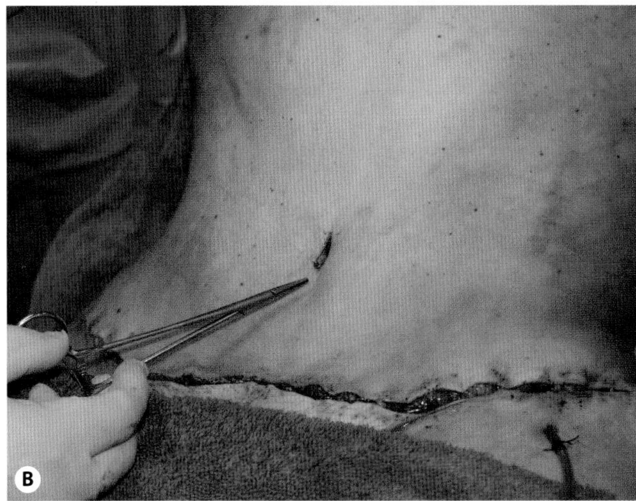

Fig. 12.21 Insetting of the umbilicus is completed with interrupted deep dermal and running intradermal 4/0 Monocryl sutures.

of the soft tissue at the 12 o'clock position will help augment superior hooding. Careful trimming of fat from the 3 o'clock to the 9 o'clock position will benefit the final umbilical insetting and appearance (**Fig. 12.20**). The umbilical inset is completed using interrupted and running intradermal 4/0 Monocryl sutures (**Fig. 12.21**). During the actual inset, care should be taken to assure that the umbilicus is not twisted. Verification of the methylene blue tattoo mark that was placed at the superior margin of the umbilicus at the beginning of the case will help ensure correct orientation (**Fig. 12.22**).

The final appearance of the umbilicus should be a vertically orientated opening with the base of the stalk somewhat superior to the skin opening to help conceal the final scars and contribute to superior hooding (**Fig. 12.23**). Because myofascial plication will effectively shorten the umbilical stalk, the umbilicus should be pulled inward and the final incision internalized within the umbilical opening (**Fig. 12.24**). We often use tissue adhesive to treat the final

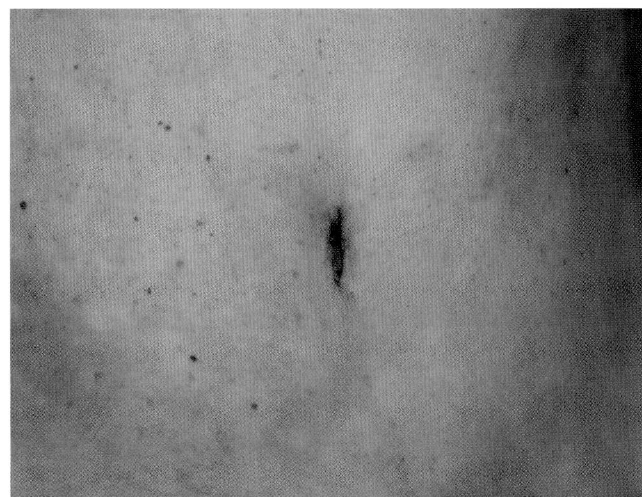

Fig. 12.22 Care should be taken during insetting to ensure that the umbilicus is not twisted or rotated. This can be verified by identifying the methylene blue tattoo mark that was place at the 12 o'clock position prior to umbilical release.

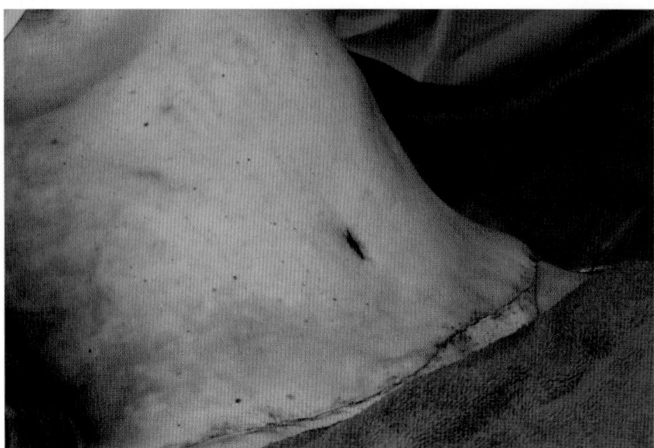

Fig. 12.23 The final intraoperative appearance shows an appropriately sized umbilicus with a vertical ellipse shape and superior hooding.

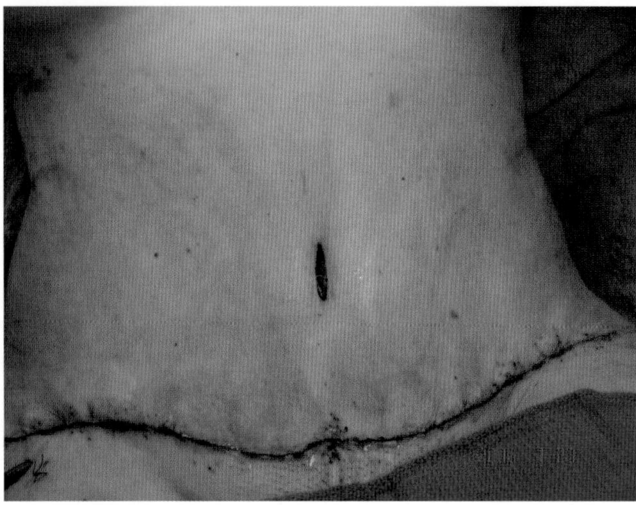

Fig. 12.24 The process of myofascial plication pulls the stalk of the umbilicus deep into the invaginated midline, effectively shortening it. This will allow the scar to be concealed within the opening.

incision at this point (**Fig. 12.25**). Vaseline- or antibiotic-impregnated gauze is placed in the opening to prevent it from filling with fluid and to keep the incision areas apart. It is usually removed within a day or two postoperatively. The umbilicus should be carefully inspected at each post-operative visit.

Reconstruction

Loss of the umbilicus can be very disturbing to the patient. Loss can occur secondary to ischemia or necrosis, or to intentional removal during various surgical procedures. Regardless of the reason for the loss, the patient should be consulted preoperatively regarding the desired shape, size,

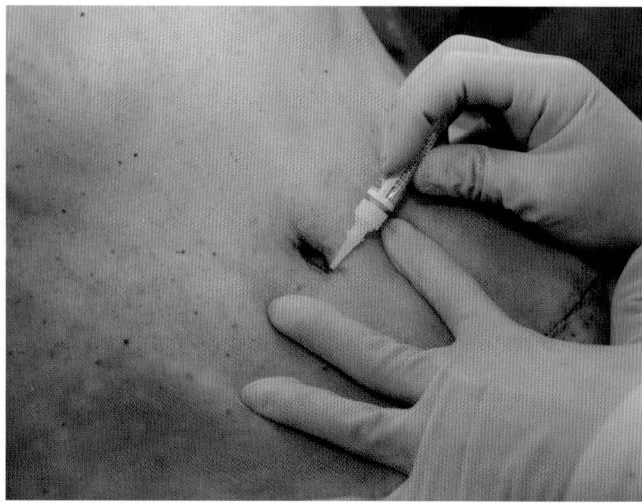

Fig. 12.25 Tissue adhesive is routinely used on the incision of the umbilical inset as a water-impermeable dressing.

and location of the umbilicus. With this in mind, umbilical reconstruction, or neoumbilicoplasty, can be performed to establish a new umbilicus for these patients.

Neoumbilicoplasty

Many techniques have been introduced for reconstruction of the umbilicus. Most are based on recruiting skin from the surrounding abdomen and rotating or advancing these small flaps to provide skin for the walls of the neoumbilicus. One of earliest references on the subject is from Baroudi.[4] Many plastic surgeons use some variant of this technique; some have advocated the use of free cartilage grafts to add shape to the neoumbilicus. To date, we have not felt the need to do so. The best method should be determined by the surgeon based on the patient's tissue characteristics and their desired goal. Regardless of the technique chosen, the goal should always be to have a well-proportioned umbilicus, that is centered, vertically oblong, with well-concealed scars, and some degree of periumbilical contour depression leading to an 'inny.' Naturally, the exact appearance should take into account the final appearance desired by the patient.

We have found that a simple four-flap reconstruction technique is useful and effective (**Fig. 12.26**). During this procedure, the midline is established by drawing a vertical line between the xiphoid and the middle of the symphysis pubis. With the patient as an active participant, the vertical location for the new umbilicus is selected and its desired size determined. Anesthetic options include local anesthesia with or without sedation. Local anesthesia is usually effective because this area is often hyposensitive or insensate. The new umbilical shape is outlined, within which are the four proposed flaps (**Fig. 12.27**). Lidocaine with epinephrine

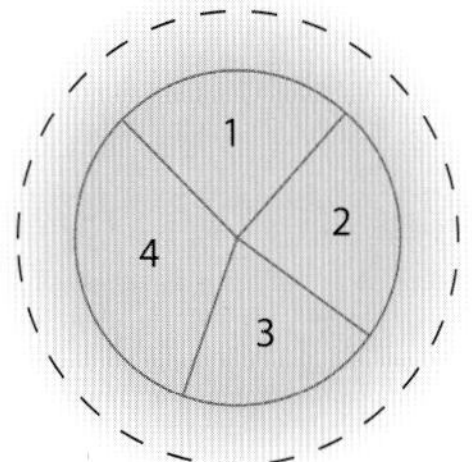

Fig. 12.26 Many neoumbilicoplasty procedures exist. We prefer the use of a four flap technique.

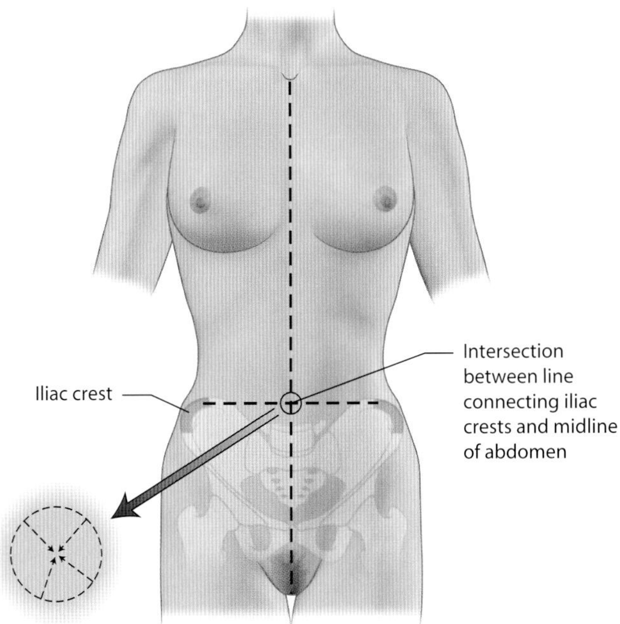

Fig. 12.27 The site of the neoumbilicus is identified and marked. Within this designated area the four flaps that will become the walls of the neoumbilicus are drawn.

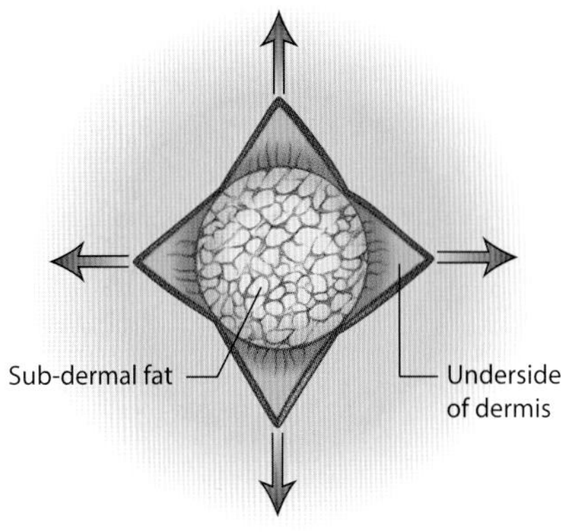

Fig. 12.28 The preoperatively marked flaps are incised and elevated.

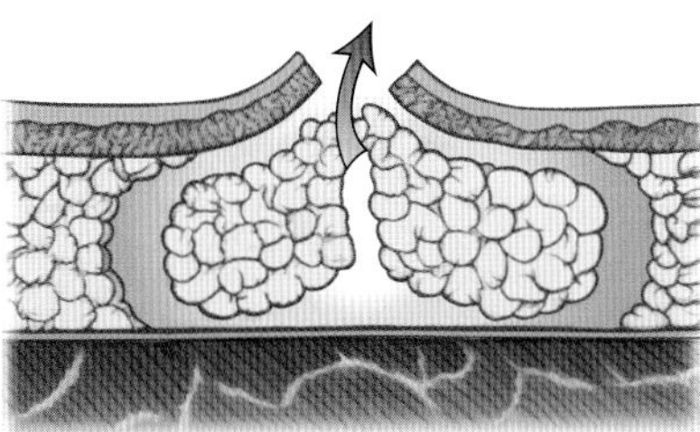

Fig. 12.29 The flaps are defatted down to the rectus sheath.

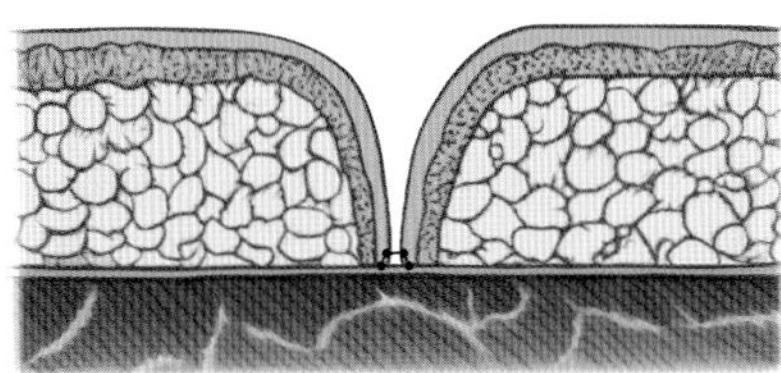

Fig. 12.30 The flaps are secured with permanent sutures down to the underlying rectus sheath in a slightly super-positioned location. This will augment the superior umbilical hooding.

is infiltrated into the surrounding region for anesthesia and vasoconstriction. The four flaps are incised and elevated (**Fig. 12.28**), and all are defatted. The soft tissue is resected down to the linea alba (**Fig. 12.29**). Flap insetting is then performed with permanent or longer lasting absorbable sutures. The location of the flap inset is usually slightly superior to the center of the new umbilicus to help create superior hooding (**Fig. 12.30**). A Dacron or cotton ball is coated with antibiotic ointment and used as a stent. It should be removed frequently during the postoperative period to assess flap viability and healing. Any external sutures are removed when healing is assured. A normal and aesthetically pleasing umbilicus can be created in this fashion (**Fig. 12.31**).

Umbilical Stenosis

Umbilical stenosis is usually a result of ischemia secondary to excessive umbilical stalk skeletonization or excessive tension during closure. An umbilical inset opening that is very small and circular can also result in stenosis. This can become a hygiene problem if the stenosis is so severe that normal epithelial desquamation results in buildup within the umbilicus. Multiple Z-plasties can be performed along the stenotic rim of the umbilicus (**Fig. 12.32**). If the stenosis is severe enough that Z-plasties would not sufficiently correct the deformity, slits can be made into the umbilicus and abdominal skin recruited and inset to enlarge the

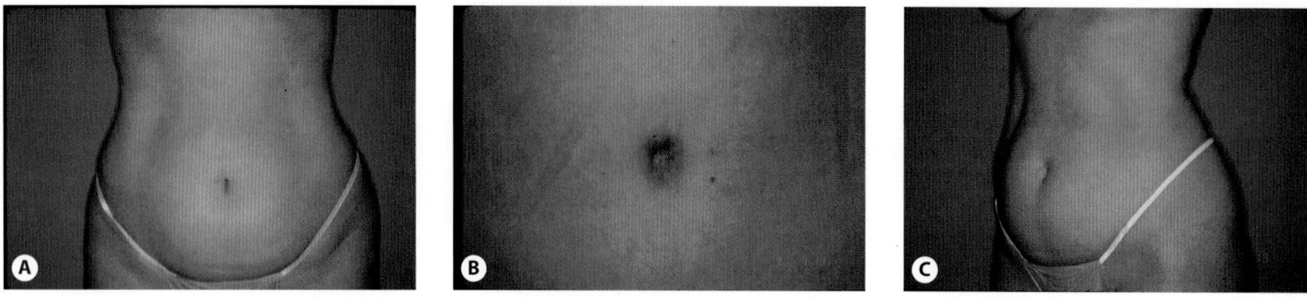

Fig. 12.31 Result following miniabdominoplasty with umbilical float with infection (A). The four-flap technique for neoumbilical reconstruction can yield a normal and aesthetically pleasing umbilicus (B, C).

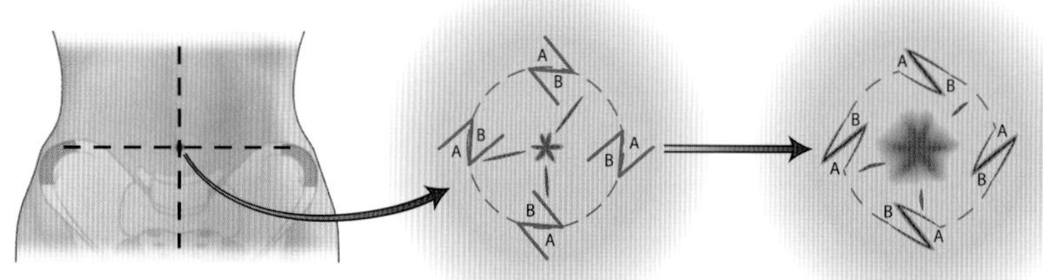

Fig. 12.32 Correction of mild umbilical stenosis can be achieved by performing multiple Z-plasties along the stenotic rim.

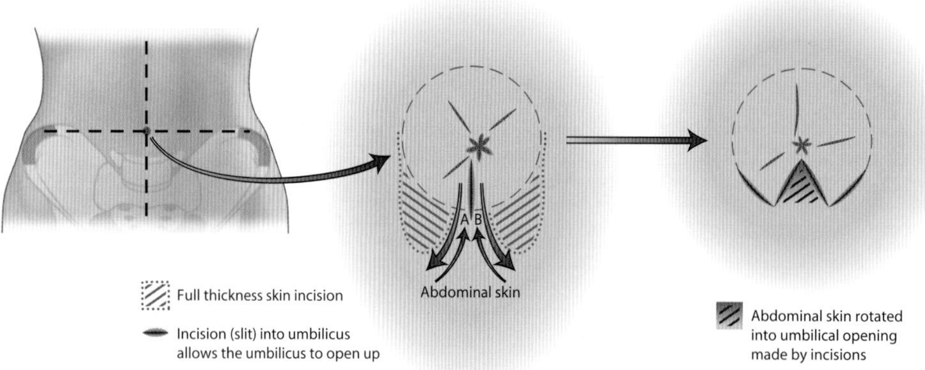

Fig. 12.33 For moderate umbilical stenosis where multiple Z-plasties will not be sufficient to correct the deformity, slits can be made into the umbilicus and abdominal skin recruited and inset into the openings to expand the umbilicus.

opening (**Fig. 12.33**). If these efforts are unsuccessful, the stenotic umbilical remnant can be excised and a neoumbilicoplasty performed.

Umbilical Flattening

Occasionally the umbilicus remains flat, without adequate inward concavity, following abdominoplasty (**Fig. 12.34**). This can be seen in thin athletic patients who have a minimal amount of subcutaneous fat. If this is the case, a purse-string type procedure on the periumbilical abdominal fascia can be useful (**Fig. 12.35**). Dissection is performed down to the anterior rectus sheath all the way around the umbilicus. A permanent purse-string suture is then placed into the rectus sheath around the umbilical stalk, and tightened to promote invagination of the umbilicus (**Fig. 12.36**). The skin around the umbilicus is closed with an intracuticular absorbable suture (**Fig. 12.37**).

Umbilical Delay

Umbilical delay is an unusual procedure that is performed when the umbilical stalk has been divided during a previous surgery, such as a mini abdominoplasty, and formal abdominoplasty is now planned. The full abdominoplasty procedure will require release and inset of the umbilicus. Because the umbilicus has been previously detached, extra care is needed to ensure its viability and in such cases an umbilical delay should be considered.

Fig. 12.34 Exceptionally thin patients with minimal fascial laxity which require little myofascial plication may be prone to developing a flat, non-concave-appearing umbilicus.

The proposed umbilical incision is marked and infiltrated with lidocaine containing epinephrine (**Fig. 12.38**). The patient is prepped and draped, and then the incision is made through the full thickness of the skin, dividing the cutaneous blood supply to the umbilicus (**Fig. 12.39**). Limited soft-tissue spreading should be performed around the umbilical stalk to reduce the vascular supply to the umbilicus (**Fig. 12.40**). A simple closure is then undertaken to allow the periumbilical incision to heal in anticipation of the subsequent full abdominoplasty, which should take place approximately 2 weeks later. Theoretically, the umbilicus will achieve its maximum vascularity at this point.

During the full abdominoplasty, the sutures are removed and the umbilical incision opened by spreading. Abdominal flaps are elevated in the usual fashion up to the costal margins. During the dissection, care should be taken to maintain the subcutaneous tissue at the base of the umbilical stalk. After muscle plication, the umbilicus can be inset in the normal fashion, with great care being taken to avoid excessive tension on the closure. A very normal-appearing umbilicus can be obtained using this technique (**Fig. 12.41**).

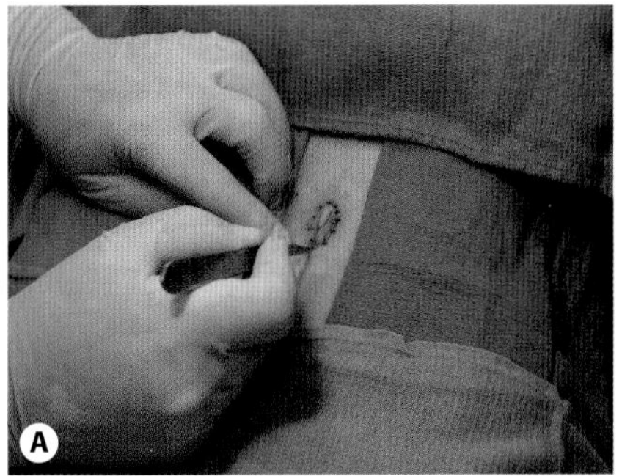

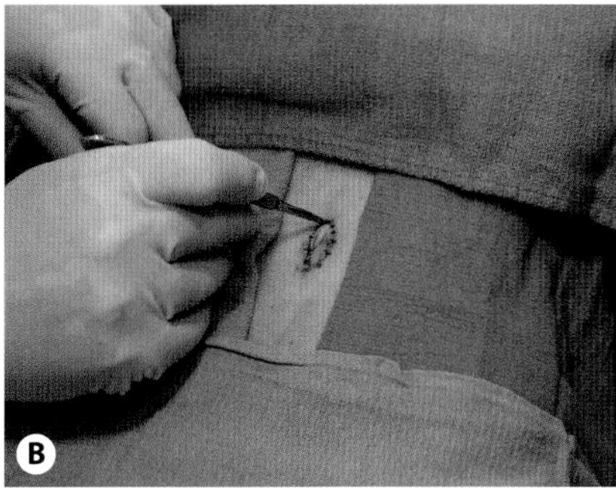

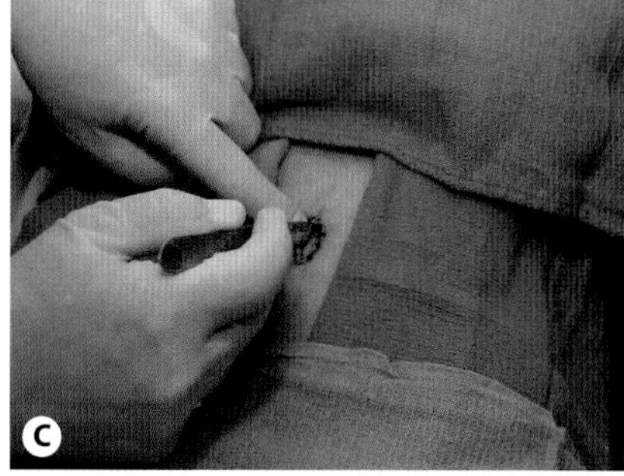

Fig. 12.35 The process of correcting the flat or non-concave umbilicus begins by incising the existing periumbilical scar.

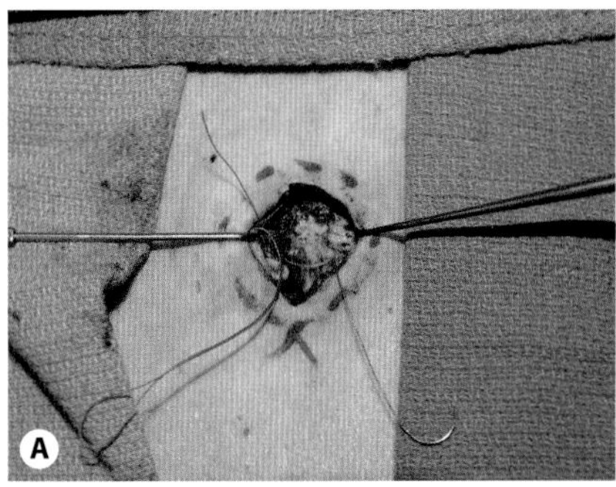

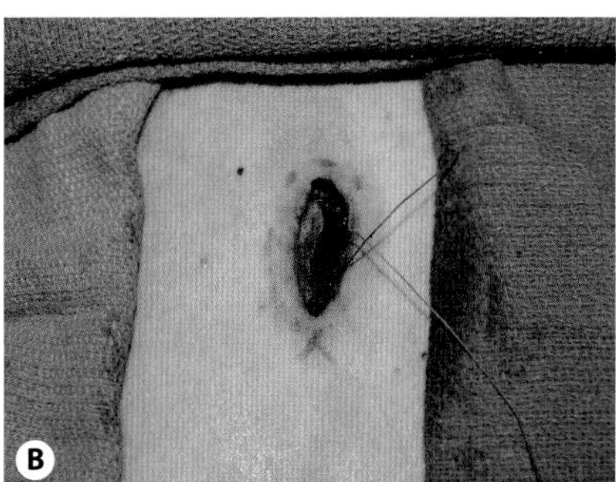

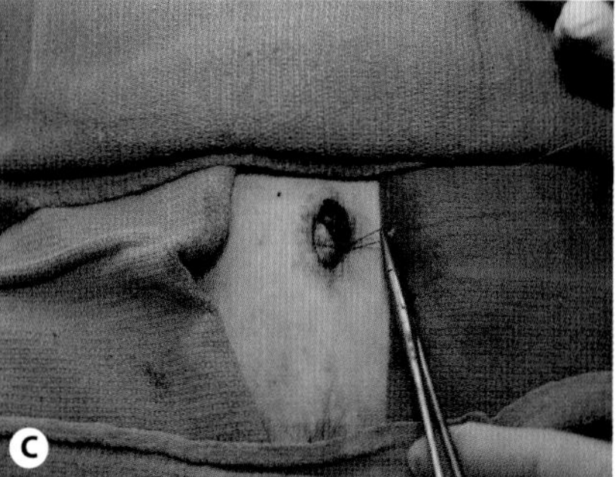

Fig. 12.36 A permanent purse-string suture in the rectus sheath around the umbilical stalk is performed to increase the midline invagination of the periumbilical area.

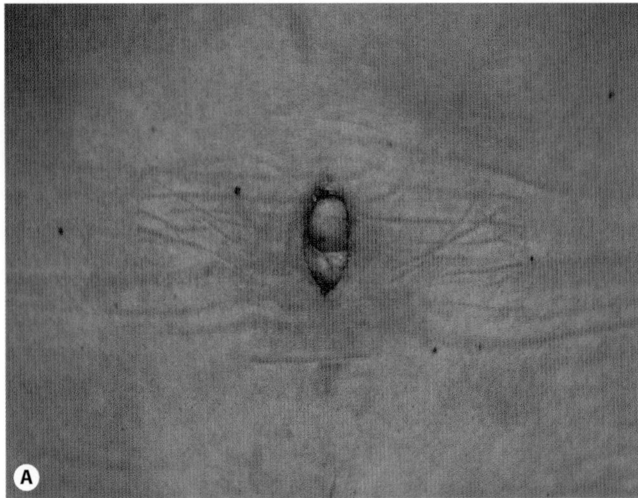

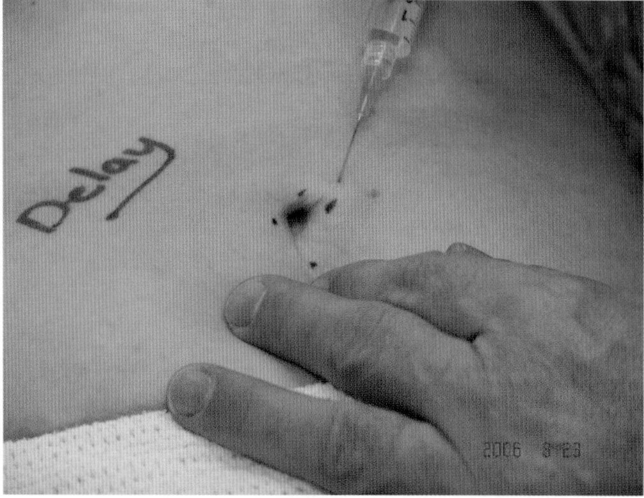

Fig. 12.38 Umbilical delay is performed approximately 2 weeks before the abdominoplasty procedure. The proposed umbilical incision is infiltrated with lidocaine containing epinephrine.

Fig. 12.37 The use of a permanent suture in a purse-string technique to help recess the umbilicus can help correct the flat, non-concave appearing umbilicus in the thin abdominoplasty patient.

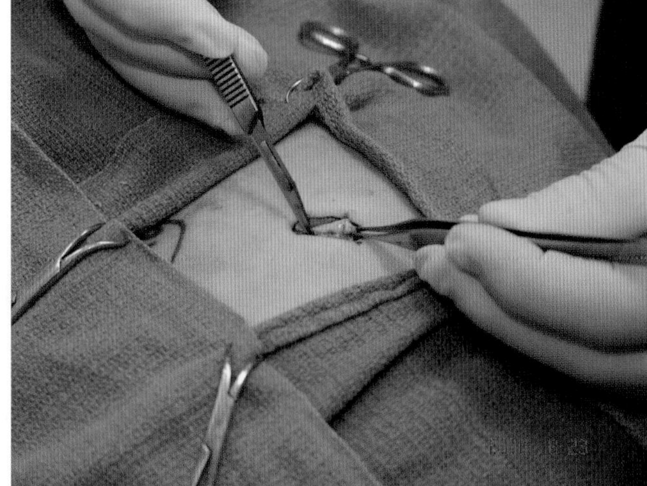

Fig. 12.39 The proposed umbilical incision is then incised completely into the subcutaneous tissue, dividing the dermal blood supply to the umbilicus.

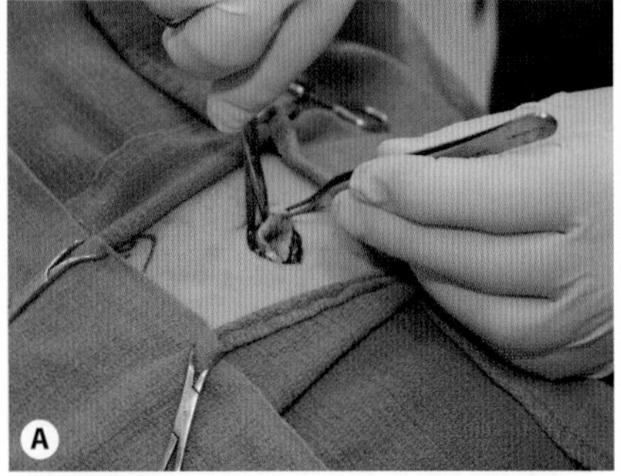

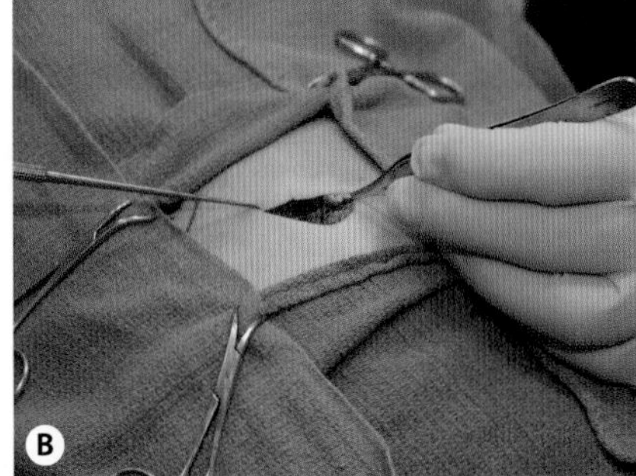

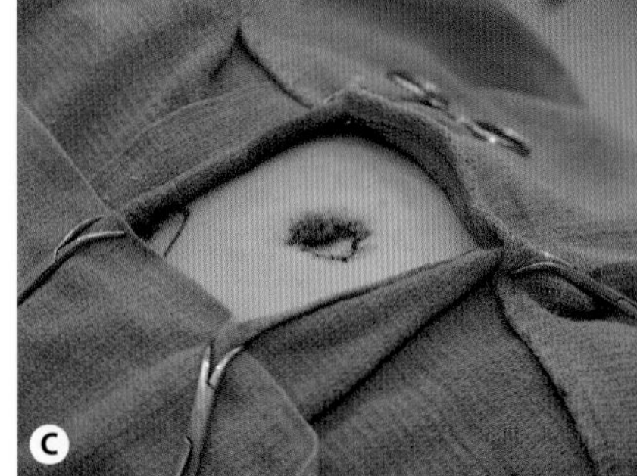

Fig. 12.40 Limited soft-tissue dissection around the umbilical stalk is performed next. This process eliminates all of the vascular supply to the umbilicus except for the deep soft-tissue perforators. Discussion with the patient about the possibility of ischemic injury and loss of the umbilicus is recommended. This cutaneous skin division will result in enhanced vascularity coming from the stalk and deep tissues.

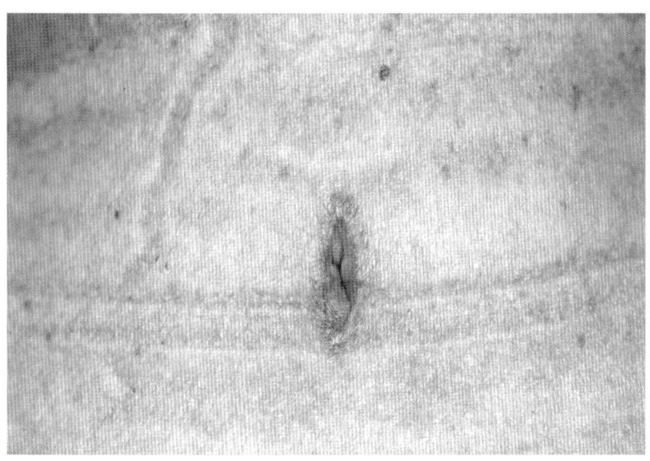

Fig. 12.41 A well-perfused, normal-appearing umbilicus can be achieved during a standard abdominoplasty following umbilical delay. The umbilicus is shown several weeks after the full abdominoplasty procedure was performed following the umbilical delay.

Summary

The aesthetic significance of the umbilicus is commonly underappreciated during many of the abdominal contouring procedures. Because the eye naturally focuses on the umbilicus as the center of the abdomen, the plastic surgeon should be particularly mindful of its appearance. Rejuvenating the umbilicus to a normal location, shape and appearance, with well-concealed scars, should be part of the overall goal when performing abdominoplasty.

Clinical Caveats: The umbilicus in body contouring

- The umbilicus is the center of focus of the abdomen and an important sign of health and beauty
- The rejuvenated umbilicus should be in harmony with the rejuvenated abdomen
- Shape and size should be tailored to each patient, bearing in mind that a small, vertically oval umbilicus is often preferred
- Myofascial plication shortens the umbilical length, creating a desirable concave appearance during final inset
- The vertical position of the umbilicus is fairly restricted after myofascial plication. If there is some umbilical stalk laxity, placing the umbilicus higher rather than lower is almost always preferable
- The midline of the abdomen can be accurately determined by spanning a suture from the xiphoid to the center of the pubic symphysis
- An umbilicus that is off-midline preoperatively can be corrected intraoperatively by asymmetric myofascial plication
- The incisions of the umbilical inset should be well hidden
- Umbilical delay should be performed prior to a full abdominoplasty if an umbilical float has been performed with a previous mini abdominoplasty
- Mild umbilical stenosis can be corrected by multiple Z-plasties. Moderate to severe stenosis requires longitudinal opening of the umbilicus and advancement of abdominal skin or neoumbilical reconstruction
- A flat, non-concave umbilicus can be corrected secondarily by further imbricating the fascia around the umbilical stalk in standard or purse-string type fashion

References

1. Craig SB, Faller MS, Puckett CL. In search of the ideal female umbilicus. Plast Reconstruct Surg 2000; 105: 389.
2. Weir E. Navel gazing: a clinical glimpse at body piercing. CMAJ 2001; 164: 864.
3. Rohrich RJ, Sorokin ES, Brown SA, Gibby DL. Is the umbilicus truly midline? Clinical and medicolegal implications. Plast Reconstruct Surg 2003; 112: 259.
4. Baroudi R. Umbilicoplasty. Clin Plast Surg 1975; 2: 431.

Suggested Reading

Dini GM, Ferreira LM. A simple technique to correct umbilicus vertical malposition. Plast Reconstruct Surg 2007; 119: 1973–1974.

Juri J, Juri C, Raiden G. Reconstruction of the umbilicus in abdominoplasty. Plast Reconstruct Surg 1979; 63: 580.

Kirianoff TG. Making a new umbilicus when none exists. Plast Reconstruct Surg 1975; 61: 603.

Kurul S, Uzunismail A. A simple technique to determine the future location of the umbilicus in abdominoplasty. Plast Reconstruct Surg 1997; 100: 753–754.

Lee MJ, Mustoe TA. A simplified version to achieve aesthetic results for the umbilicus in abdominoplasty. Plast Reconstruct Surg 2002; 109: 2136.

Lim TC, Tan WT. Managing the umbilicus during abdominoplasty. Plast Reconstruct Surg 1996; 98: 1113.
Massiha H, Montegut W, Phillips R. A method of reconstructing a natural-looking umbilicus in abdominoplasty. Ann Plast Surg 1997; 38: 228–231.
Marconi F. Reconstruction of the umbilicus: a simple technique. Plast Reconstruct Surg 1995; 95: 1115–1117.
Nahas FX. How to deal with the umbilical stalk during abdominoplasty. Plast Reconstruct Surg 2000; 106: 1220–1221.
Onishi K, Yang YL, Maruyama Y. A new lunch box-type method in umbilical reconstruction. Ann Plast Surg 1995; 35: 654–656.
Otto A, Wechselberger G, Schoeller T, Lille S. A method of reconstructing a natural-looking umbilicus in abdominoplasty. Ann Plast Surg 1997; 39: 435.

CHAPTER **13**

Ancillary Procedures in Body Contouring

Joseph P. Hunstad & Remus Repta

IN THIS CHAPTER

KEY POINTS

The process responsible for developing abdominal contour irregularity, including soft-tissue laxity, excess adiposity, and skin redundancy, also affects the appearance of other parts of the body. Ancillary procedures, including brachioplasty, vertical thighplasty, bra-line back lift, purse-string gluteoplasty method of autologous buttocks augmentation, and mons remodeling, can all play a very important role in optimizing overall body contour as well as improving harmony following abdominoplasty. These procedures can be performed in conjunction with or following the abdominal contouring procedure.

Introduction

Patients seeking abdominal contouring may be good candidates for ancillary procedures that can help rejuvenate and reshape other areas of the body. The forces that contribute to abdominal contour irregularity are also responsible for the undesirable appearance of the arms, the upper back, buttocks, mons area, and the thighs. These areas may have similar undesirable characteristics to the abdomen, including soft-tissue laxity, skin redundancy, excess adiposity, and striae. When ancillary procedures are combined with abdominoplasty, a more comprehensive and harmonious body contouring result can be achieved.

Ancillary procedures can be performed concurrently with abdominoplasty or as standalone operations. A side-benefit of performing ancillary procedures after the abdominoplasty is that it provides the opportunity to modify or refine components of the previously performed operation.

Patient Selection (Box 13.1)

Most patients presenting for abdominal contouring are good candidates for the additional ancillary procedures discussed above. Our role as plastic surgeons is to provide the appropriate information and to help the patient feel better about their body and themselves by correcting the areas of concern. Therefore, a fine balance is required between addressing only the topics presented by the patient, and offering opinion and recommendation about other areas and procedures. Frequently, after the initial consultation it is the patient who asks what can be done to improve the appearance of other areas of the body, and so the process is largely decided by the patient. The surgeon must then decide which procedure is

Box 13.1 Brachioplasty

- Patients desiring improved contour of the arm can undergo liposuction, resection, or a combination of the two
- The resection design can be limited to a scar in the axilla only, along the length of the arm, or extended to include the lateral chest area
- The procedure best suited to the patient depends on the amount of excess adiposity, the amount of soft-tissue laxity, and the extent of the scar the patient is willing to accept in return for the degree of contour improvement possible
- The final scar position and location should be marked and reviewed with the patient in order to avoid any misunderstanding and postoperative disappointment

suited best for the particular concern and whether it should be performed concurrently or following the abdominal contouring procedure.

Upper Extremity

Patients who present with concerns about soft-tissue laxity of the upper arms are frequently candidates for some form of brachioplasty. Occasionally the amount of adiposity is significant and the amount of soft-tissue laxity is only moderate. In these cases, liposuction of the arms alone is a reasonable choice. More often, however, the presence of soft-tissue laxity requires an excisional component to achieve the desired result. If the patient cannot tolerate a long longitudinal arm scar, a mini brachioplasty, with the final scar concealed within the axilla, may be appropriate if they have only moderate soft-tissue laxity and are willing to accept the more modest improvement offered by this procedure. For those with significant laxity of the arm, axilla, and flanks, an extended brachioplasty encompassing the upper arm, axilla, and lateral breast or flank area may be appropriate.

Upper and Middle Back

Because of the posterior midline zone of adherence, the excision of soft tissue in the lower back as an isolated procedure to correct buttock ptosis, or as a part of a body life or circumferential abdominoplasty, will not improve the soft-tissue laxity of the middle and upper back. This is often disappointing to patients who have had a circumferential abdominoplasty but still have back laxity with rolls and folds near the bra area. For these patients, the bra-line back lift can be tremendously rewarding. It can be performed as a standalone procedure or in combination with a reverse abdominoplasty, mastopexy, or breast reduction. The procedure is described and shown in greater detail in the specific operative approach section of this chapter.

Buttocks

For patients with mild or modest buttock laxity and excess adiposity of the hip rolls, lower back, and abdomen, autologous fat grafting is an ideal solution. Instead of discarding the fat obtained from liposuction of the adjacent areas, it can be used as autologous soft-tissue filler. The combination of suctioning adjacent areas such as the hip rolls and lumbar area and concurrently fat-grafting the buttocks can achieve a very desirable contour and shape.

Deflational buttock ptosis is commonly seen in patients with massive weight loss. In these patients, excision of the excess soft tissue laxity to correct buttock ptosis will often result in tighter, lifted, but overall volume-deficient buttocks. Using the tissue that would otherwise be discarded in this procedure can be highly effective in augmenting gluteal volume. Although many rotational flaps have been described for autologous gluteal augmentation, we have found that using the central gluteal tissue is more efficient, effective, and reliable. To accomplish this we have developed the purse-string gluteoplasty. The procedure is described and shown in greater detail in the specific operative approach section of this chapter.

Lower Extremity

Patients can present with various amounts of soft-tissue laxity, excess adiposity, and concerns about surgical scars. Because of this, the exact thighplasty procedure should be tailored to each patient based on their desired goal and how tolerant they are of surgical scars. The upper inner or crescent medial thigh lift is usually ineffective for patients with significant soft-tissue laxity. Most patients who have experienced moderate or significant weight loss have an appreciable amount of soft-tissue laxity in the medial thighs that may exist all the way to the knee. The vertical thigh lift is the ideal procedure to treat significant circumferential thigh laxity. However, patients must accept a long vertical scar on the medial thigh in return for the often dramatic results this procedure can provide. As many of these patients have undergone circumferential or extended abdominoplasty procedures they are usually accepting of long scars in return for a significantly improved contour.

Preoperative Considerations

A clear understanding of the patient's surgical history, previous weight, and final target weight is useful. Understanding the patient's overall aesthetic goal is very important to perform these procedures safely and successfully, and to achieve high patient satisfaction. Most patients share similar aesthetic goals, including correction or reduction of the skin and soft-tissue excess and an improved contour and silhouette. For buttocks augmentation using autologous fat, it should be emphasized that a significant volume of harvested fat is necessary to achieve an appreciable degree of augmentation, and that the procedure may have to be repeated to achieve the desired buttock volume.

In addition to the standard focused history and physical examination, each specific area should be carefully evaluated and discussed. Specific problem areas related to the previous surgery are also discussed. Poor healing, seroma formation, or a history of infection or hematoma occurring with the any of the previous procedures requires careful consideration. A review of the proposed length and position of the final incision is also important and must be agreed upon by the patient. Physical examination, including evaluation of skin quality and the extent of soft-tissue laxity, will aid discussion about the amount of tissue that can or should be removed. Preoperative laboratory analysis is performed as discussed in the earlier chapters. This is particularly relevant for patients with massive weight loss, as certain metabolic and physiologic abnormalities can impair normal healing.

Operative Approach

Mini Brachioplasty

The mini or axillary brachioplasty is a useful procedure for patients with mild or moderate arm laxity who do not want a longitudinal scar.[1] However; it is limited in the amount of soft-tissue tightening and contour correction possible, which is often proportional to the length of the scar. The ideal candidate is usually young, with moderate soft-tissue laxity, and interested in improving the tone of their arm.

The markings are made within the axilla and reviewed with the patient (**Fig. 13.1**). They should not be visible anteriorly with the arm at the patient's side. The amount of tissue to be removed is estimated by bimanual palpation. Under either intravenous (IV) sedation or general anesthesia, dilute lidocaine containing epinephrine is used to infiltrate this region. The skin is resected full thickness and hemostasis achieved. A layered closure is performed. The deep layer is secured with 2/0 PDS or Maxon. These initial sutures should grasp the deep dermal layer of both incision lines and the axillary fascia at the apex of the axilla, and should pull the skin up into the axilla. The skin is closed with interrupted 3/0 PDS and 4/0 intradermal Monocryl or equivalent. The incision line can be taped, treated with skin adhesive, or covered with a simple dressing.

Postoperative Care

No overhead lifting is suggested for 4–6 weeks to prevent disruption of the deep sutures. Occasionally, all or most of the hair-bearing axillary skin can be removed with this procedure, which eliminates the need for shaving.

Before and After Figures for Mini Brachioplasty (Figs 13.2–13.13)

Full Brachioplasty

The full brachioplasty procedure is indicated for patients with moderate to significant laxity of the arm: it is not necessarily ideal for patients with significant excess adiposity of the arms. In most patients the extent of soft-tissue laxity and contour deformity exists from the axilla to the

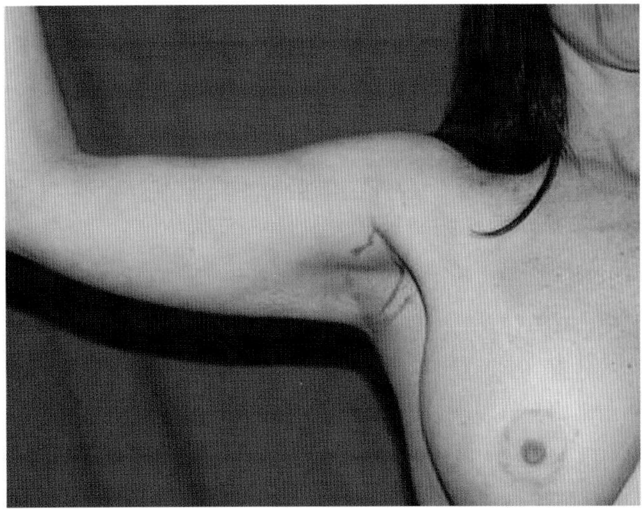

Fig. 13.1 Mini arm lift The markings for the mini arm lift should stay within the axilla. The pinch test is used to determine how much skin can be removed, and often it is the entire hair-bearing region. This is very desirable for the patient. After the marks are made the patient should have their arm relaxed by their side to ensure that the incision anteriorly is not visible. Because this is an exaggerated elliptical excision, the incision length will actually increase as it is closed. This needs to be taken into account when performing the markings and the most anterior point should be well within the nonvisible axilla with the arm adducted.

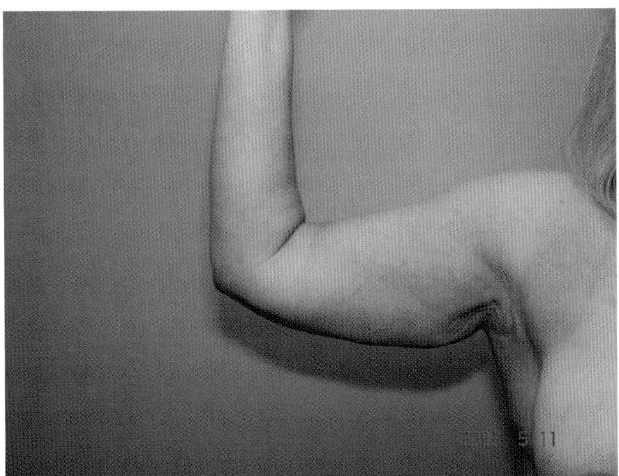

Fig. 13.2

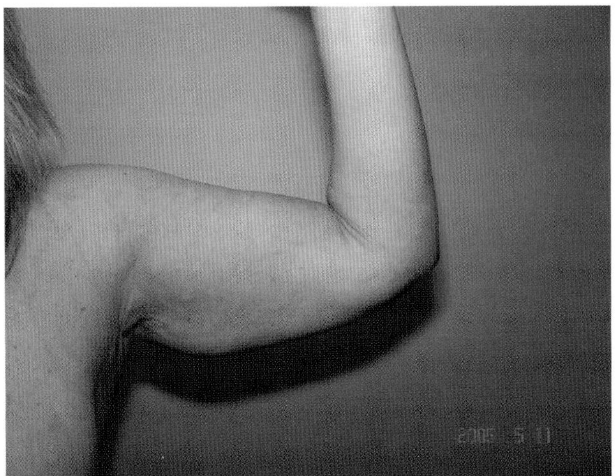

Fig. 13.3

Figs 13.2 and 13.3 Mini Arm Lift Preoperative Images The preoperative anterior view demonstrates moderate laxity, particularly within the axilla. Axillary laxity is usually improved with a mini arm lift.

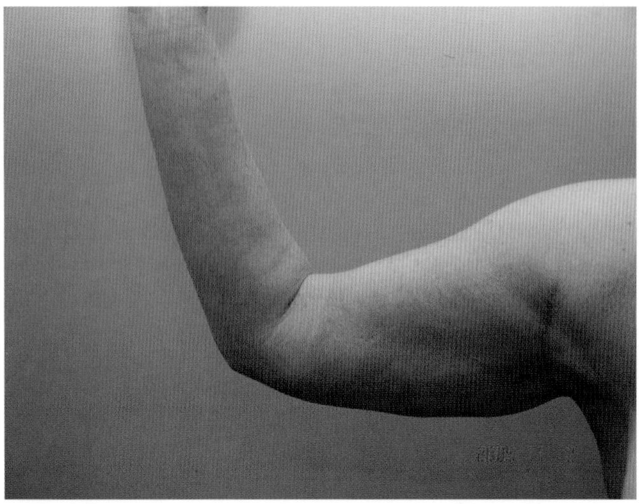

Fig. 13.4

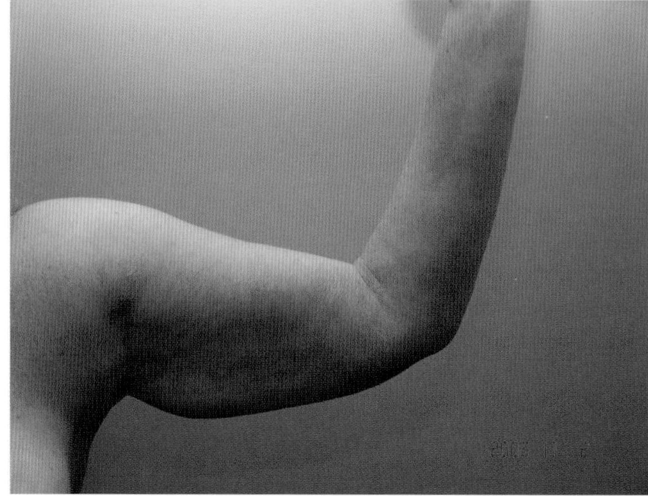

Fig. 13.5

Figs 13.4 and 13.5 Mini Arm Lift Postoperative Images Postoperative anterior view of the mini arm lift. The axillary laxity has been corrected and the incision is relatively narrow.

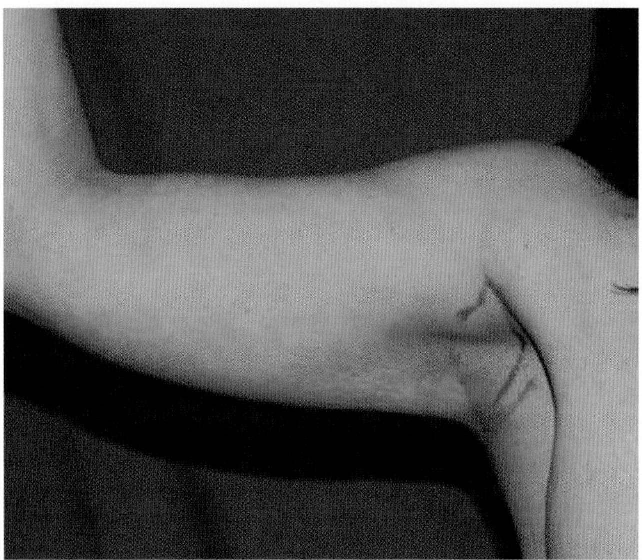

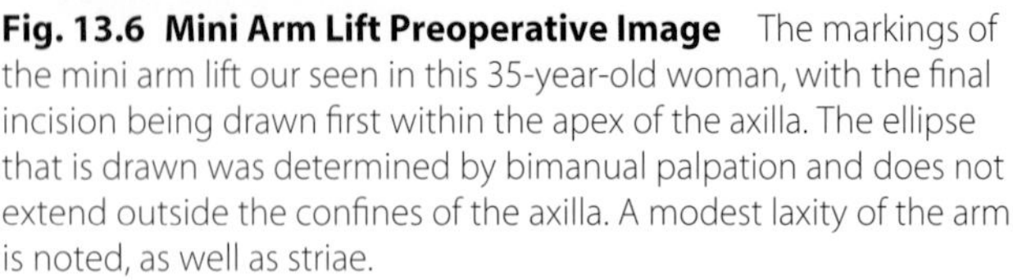

Fig. 13.6 Mini Arm Lift Preoperative Image The markings of the mini arm lift our seen in this 35-year-old woman, with the final incision being drawn first within the apex of the axilla. The ellipse that is drawn was determined by bimanual palpation and does not extend outside the confines of the axilla. A modest laxity of the arm is noted, as well as striae.

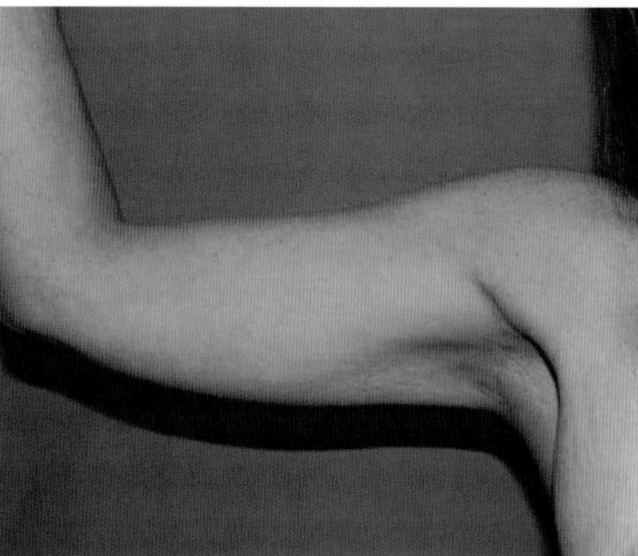

Fig. 13.7 Mini Arm Lift Postoperative Image Postoperative view, with the incision thin, nicely healed, and situated in the apex of the axilla. It is not visible anteriorly. The overall contour of the arm is improved.

elbow. The fishtail brachioplasty, advocated by Regnault,[2] has been a useful procedure for these patients. For patients with massive weight loss or with residual excess adiposity, the extended brachioplasty, as described by Aly, Soliman, and Cram,[10] can be very useful and is described in greater detail in the next section. For patients with incomplete weight loss but with significant excess adiposity, a staged procedure of thorough liposuction followed by brachioplasty 3–6 months later should be considered.

Patients are marked while standing. The final scar placement is marked between the posterior and medial brachial surfaces with the patient's arms at their side. The amount of soft-tissue resection needed is estimated and marked. The final length and position of the incision is viewed and agreed by the patient. The excess tissue in the axilla is also gathered up and this redundancy marked. Because of the tension in the axilla, the amount of tissue to be

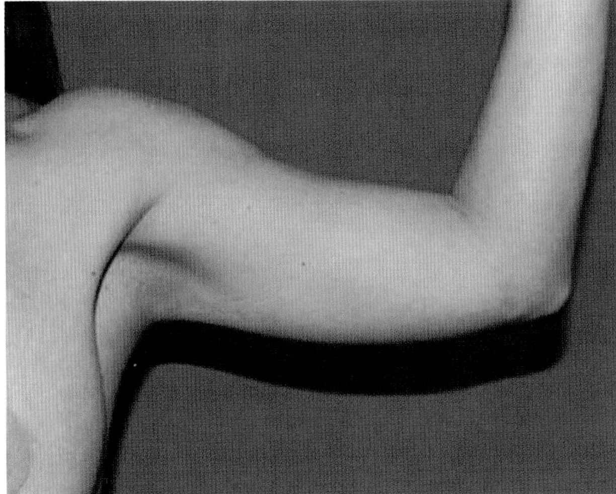

Fig. 13.8 Mini Arm Lift Preoperative Image The preoperative view of the left arm is noted again, with striae of the skin and moderate laxity.

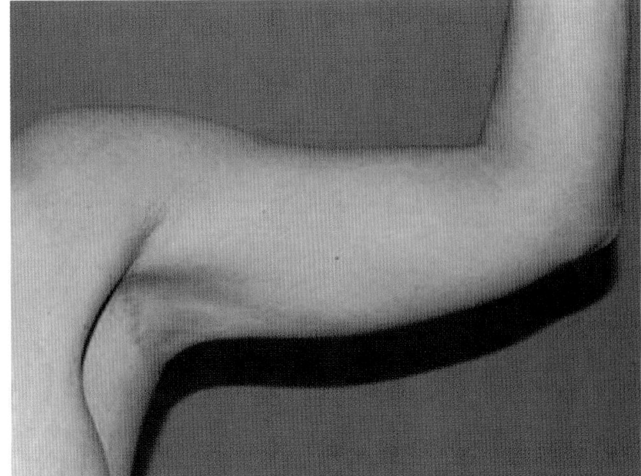

Fig. 13.9 Mini Arm Lift Postoperative Image The postoperative view reveals a well-healed incision within the confines of the axilla, with an improved shape and contour of the arm.

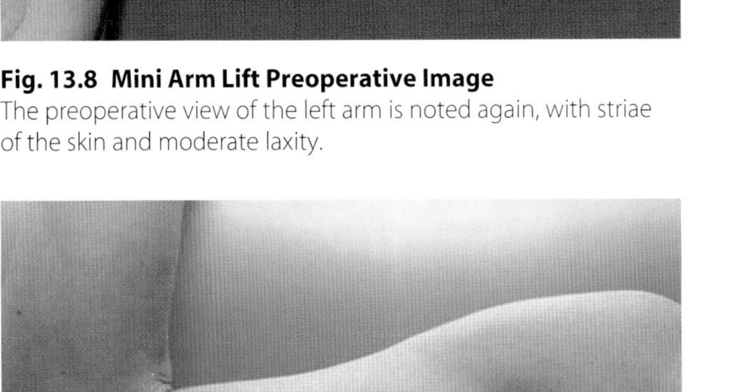

Fig. 13.10

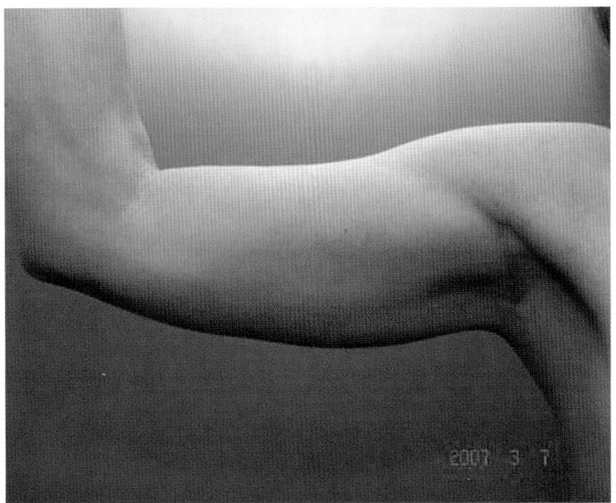

Fig. 13.11

Figs 13.10 and 13.11 Mini Arm Lift Pre- and Postoperative Images Preoperative view of this 42-year-old woman with moderate arm laxity.

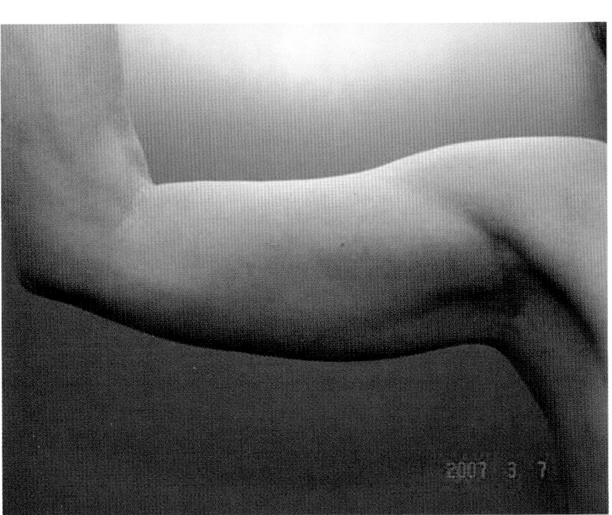

Fig. 13.12

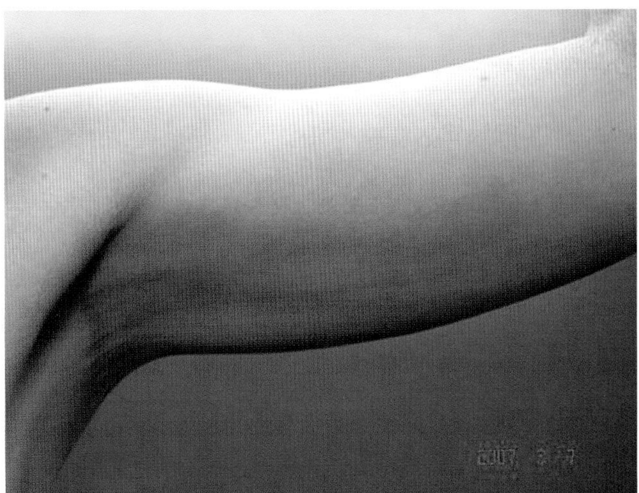

Fig. 13.13

Figs 13.12 and 13.13 Mini Arm Lift Postoperative Images Postoperative view with the incision within the axilla and the shape and appearance of the armed improved.

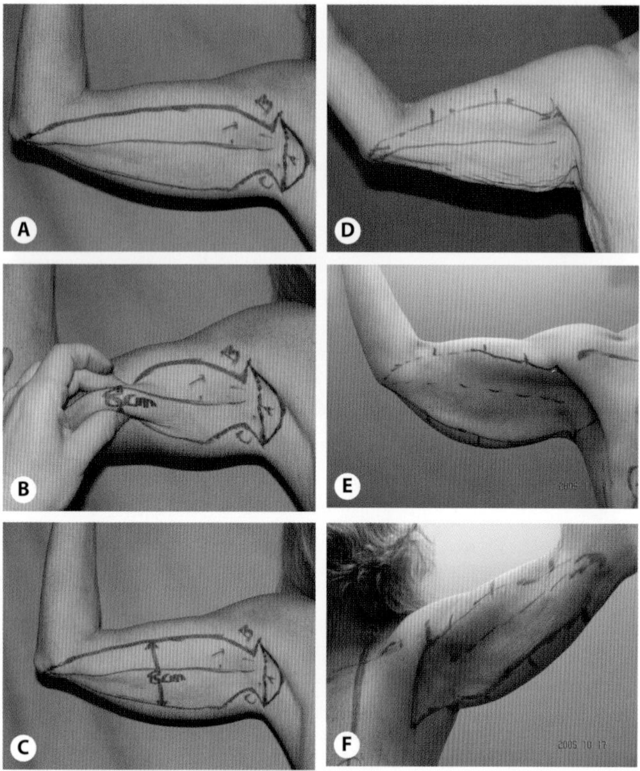

Fig. 13.14 Full Brachioplasty Images **A** Fishtail brachioplasty drawings. The mid-brachial final incision line is marked first, and then bimanual palpation is used to identify the amount of skin to be removed. The marking in the apex of the axilla is used for orientation. Because a greater tension in the axilla the markings at B and C remove less skin to reduce the risk of dehiscence. **B** The pinch test demonstrates that this tissue can be readily removed. It measures 8 cm. **C** The final markings are noted, with a resection width of 8 cm. The removal of tissue in the axilla will pull the skin up, tightening the lateral breast area. The excision extends to the elbow to improve contour all the way down the arm. **D** Fishtail brachioplasty marked in a patient with a greater skin laxity. The final incision is posterior to the bicipital groove. Realignment marks are noted in purple. A significant amount of tissue will be taken up in the axilla because of the patient's laxity. **E** Another example of a similar lift, again with the final midline marking posterior to the bicipital groove with multiple realignment marks. A significant axillary resection will be performed, improving the laxity of the lateral breast and flank area. **F** A patient's final markings are noted, with additional tissue to be removed in the axilla because of skin laxity.

removed here should be more conservative (**Fig. 13.14 A–F**). Realignment marks are placed to facilitate proper closure.

In the operating room under general anesthesia, penetrating towel clamps can be used to double-check that the amount of skin marked for removal is not excessive. It is not unusual to find that the preoperative markings may be too aggressive, and new markings should be placed within the previous pattern to ensure that closure is possible without undue tension. Dilute lidocaine containing epinephrine is used to infiltrate the incision lines. Tumescent infiltration can also be performed superficially to help hydrodissect the tissue plane. The incisions are made with a number 10 scalpel and the electrocautery is used to continue the incision and dissection down through the superficial fascia. A liposuction cannula without suction can be used to thoroughly undermine the skin through multiple tunnel passes. This releases many of the soft-tissue attachments, allowing the skin and soft-tissue resection segment to literally be avulsed off proximal to distal in a clean manner in the proper plane of dissection. It also preserves the medial brachial and antebrachial cutaneous nerves, as well as many small veins and lymphatic vessels. Electrocautery can also be used to remove the skin and soft tissue, but extra care should be taken to avoid injury to these structures.

Closure is performed with interrupted 2/0 or 3/0 PDS or equivalent suture, and intradermal 4/0 Monocryl. Drains are not routinely used. Final incision line treatment can include Steristrips, taping, or tissue adhesive. We frequently wrap the upper extremity with Kerlix and Ace wraps from the fingertips to the axilla for 24–48 hours. Care should be taken to ensure that these are not too tight and that there will be sufficient room for swelling.

Postoperative Care

Arm elevation is very helpful and is recommended especially in the first 24 hours. No vigorous activity or strenuous activity is recommended for the first 2 weeks, to permit the healing process to continue with as little swelling as possible. Scar Guard is useful on the incisions during the healing and maturation process.

Before and After Figures for Full Brachioplasty (Figs 13.15–13.38)

Extended Brachioplasty

The extended brachioplasty is useful for patients with significant weight loss and soft-tissue laxity that extends into the axilla and lateral chest. The design of this procedure as described by Aly[3] places the anterior incision just posterior to the bicipital groove, thereby shifting the resection posterior or dorsal to the location of the medial antebrachial cutaneous nerve. The posterior incision is marked by using bimanual palpation to estimate the amount of tissue to be

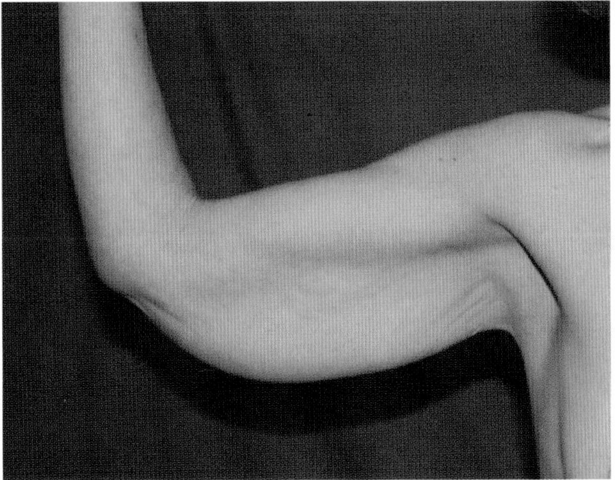

Fig. 13.15

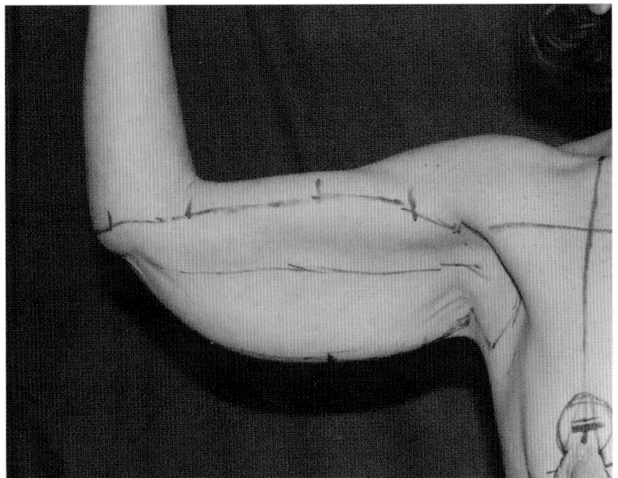

Fig. 13.16

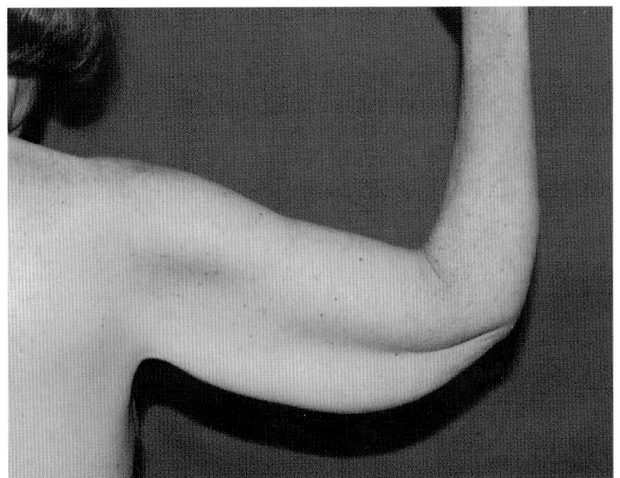

Fig. 13.17

Figs 13.15 , 13.16 and 13.17 Full Brachioplasty Postoperative Images Preoperative view of the right arm showing significant soft-tissue laxity. Preoperative markings show the extent of the arm laxity extending into the axilla as well as the planned resection. Realignment marks are placed to help facilitate closure.

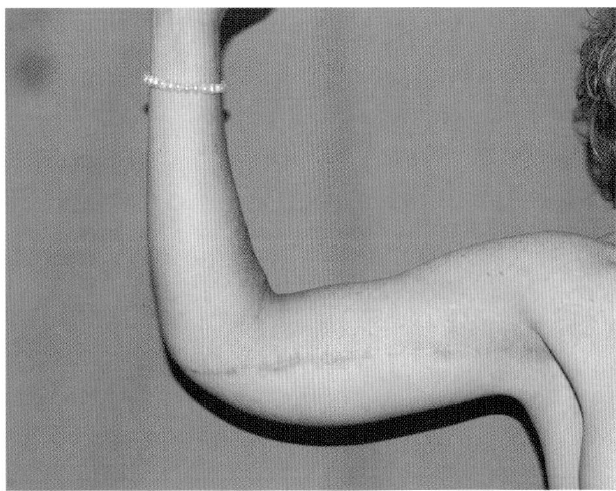

Fig. 13.18 Full Brachioplasty Pre- and Postoperative Images Postoperative view with excellent shape and contour and a well-healing incision.

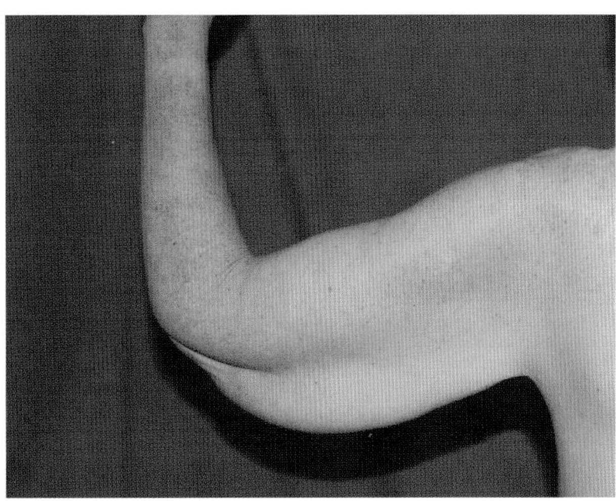

Fig. 13.19

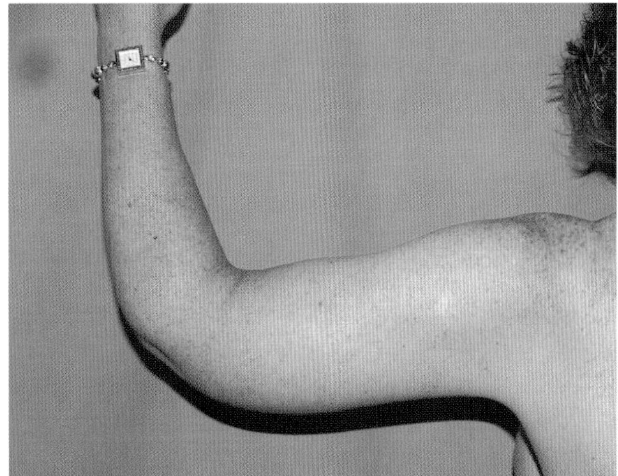

Fig. 13.20

Figs 13.18, 13.19 and 13.20 Full Brachioplasty Pre- and Postoperative Images Pre- and postoperative posterior views of the same patient, with a dramatic improvement in the shape and contour of the arm.

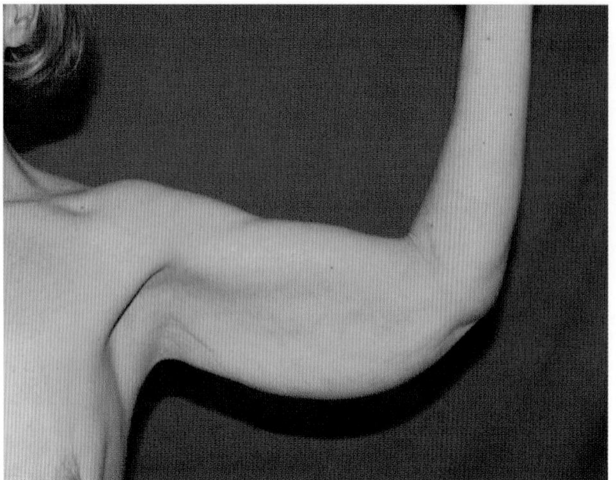

Fig. 13.21

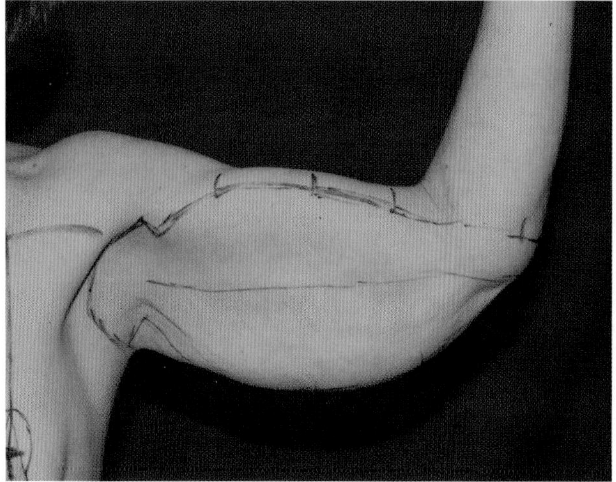

Fig. 13.22

Figs 13.21 and 13.22 Full Brachioplasty Preoperative Images Preoperative view of a patient following massive weight loss with significant arm laxity, where preoperative markings indicated a significant amount of planned skin resection.

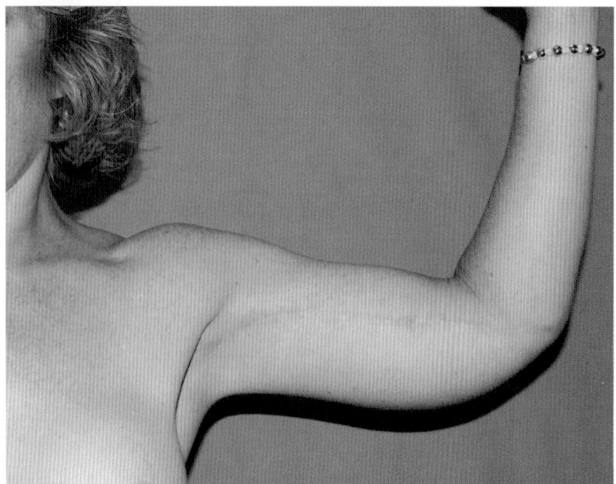

Fig. 13.23

Fig. 13.23 and 13.24 Full Brachioplasty Postoperative Images The postoperative result reveals a very nice shape and contour and a well-healed incision.

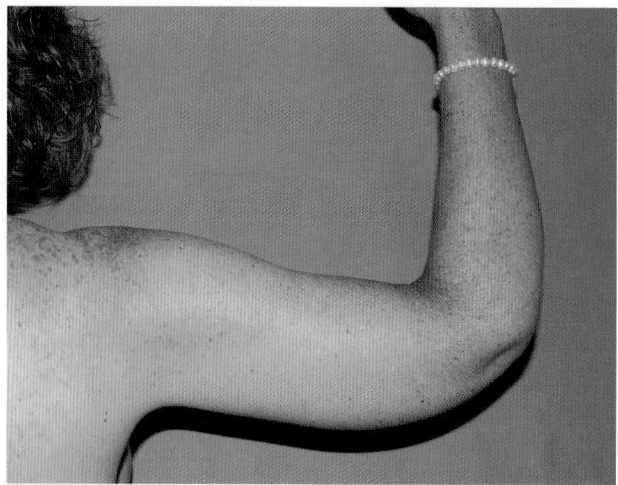

Fig. 13.24

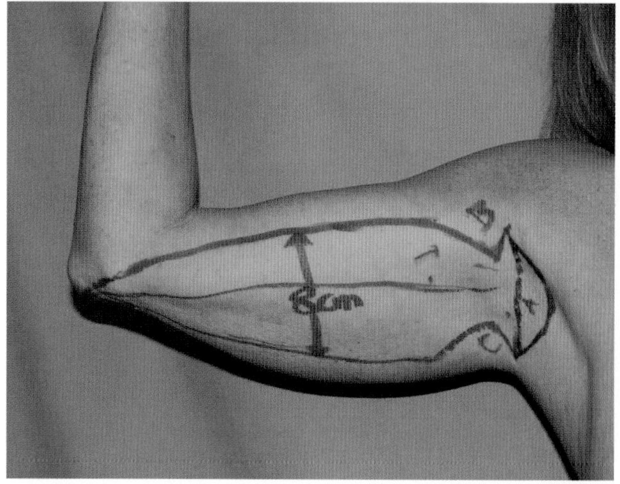

Fig. 13.25

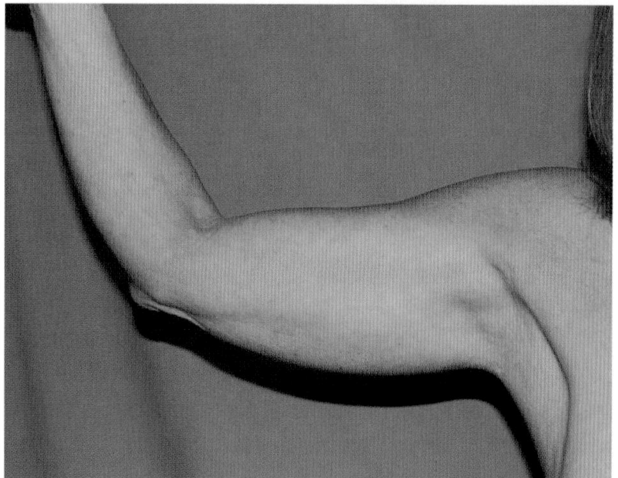

Fig. 13.26

Figs 13.24–13.26 Full Brachioplasty Pre- and Postoperative Images This patient reveals moderate laxity. The markings identify a significant tissue resection, and the postoperative view demonstrates a youthful shape and contour following the brachioplasty with high-quality incisions.

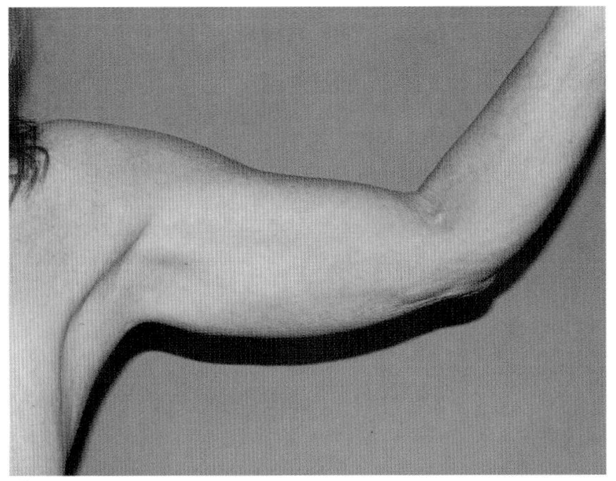

Fig. 13.27

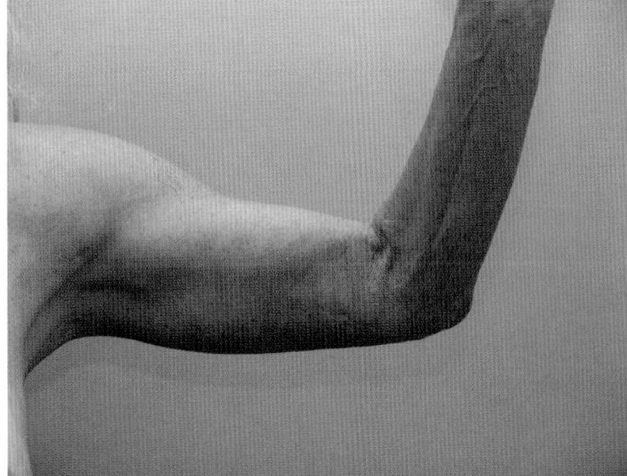

Fig. 13.28

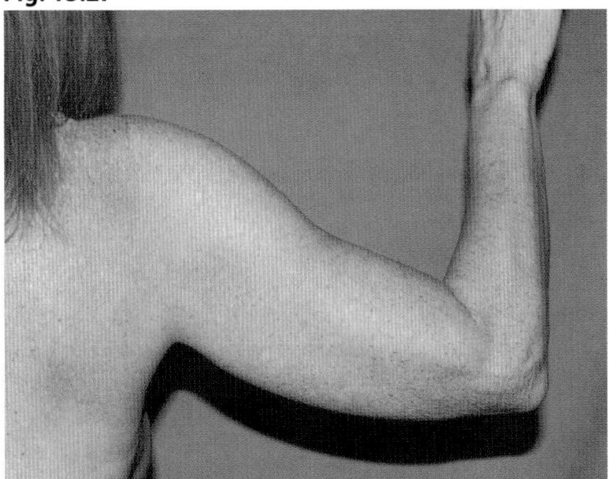

Fig. 13.29

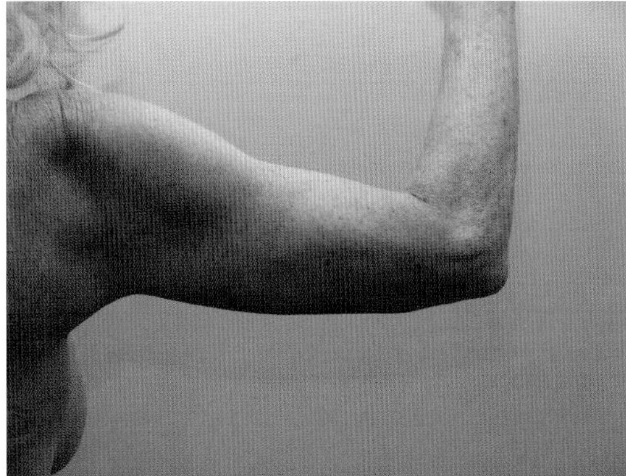

Fig. 13.30

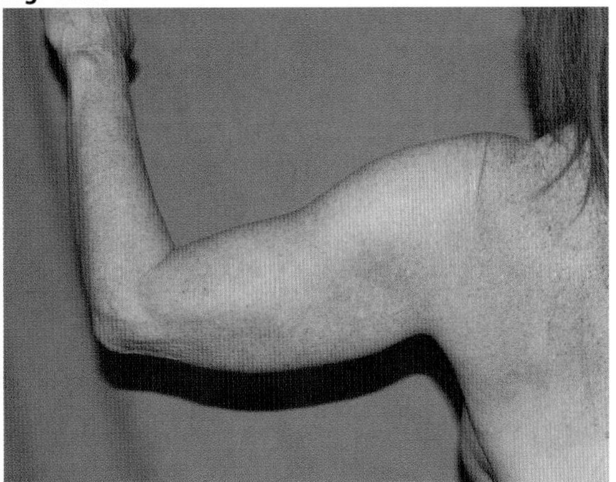

Fig. 13.31

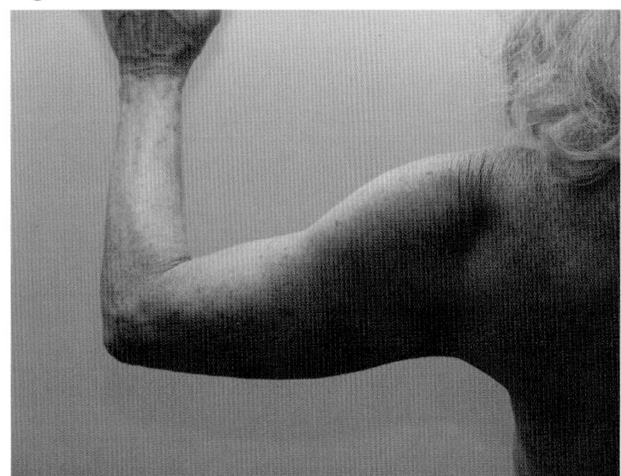

Fig. 13.32

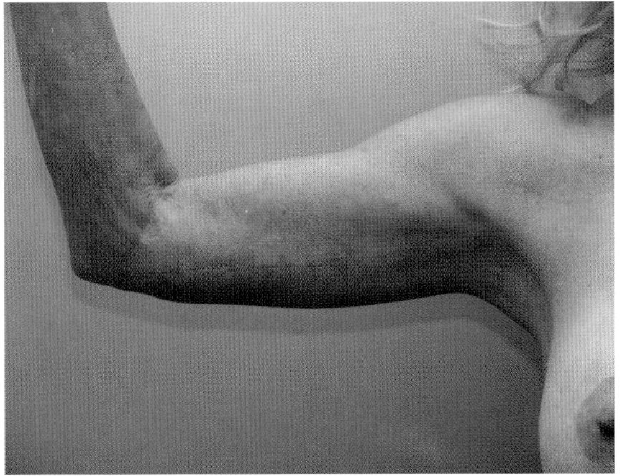

Fig. 13.33

Figs 13.27–13.33 Full Brachioplasty Pre- and Postoperative Images This patient reveals moderate laxity secondary to age and sun exposure. The postoperative view demonstrates a very youthful shape and contour following the brachioplasty with high-quality incision line.

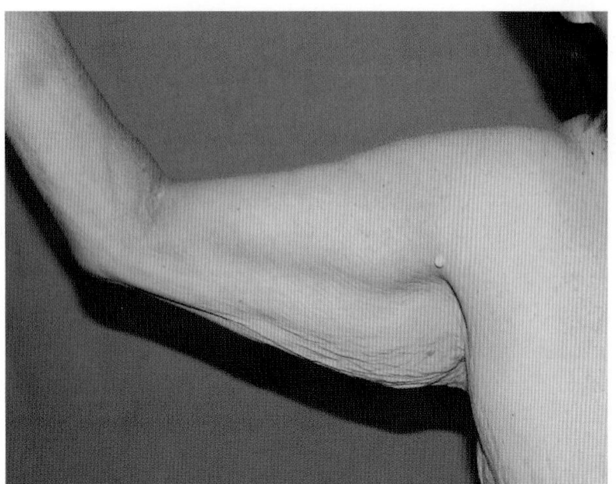

Fig. 13.34

Figs 13.34–13.38 Full Brachioplasty Pre- and Postoperative Images This 57-year-old experienced significant weight loss and was concerned with the soft-tissue laxity and redundancy and shape of the arms. Following a fishtail brachioplasty, the contour and shape of the arm is dramatically improved and the final incision line is of high quality.

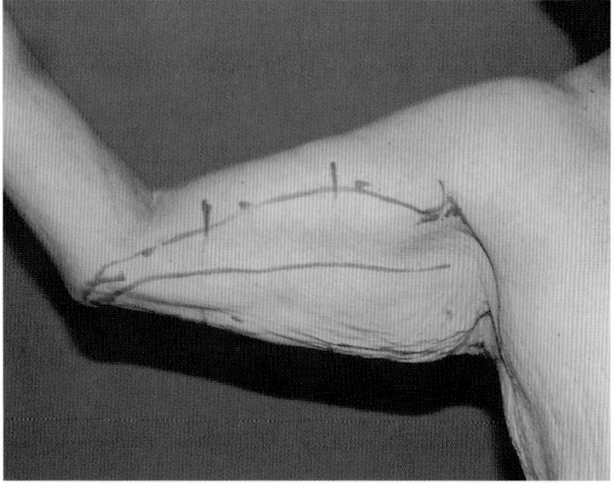

Fig. 13.35

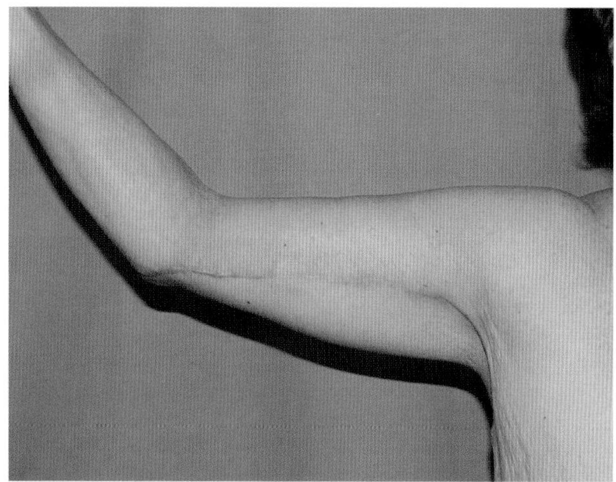

Fig. 13.36

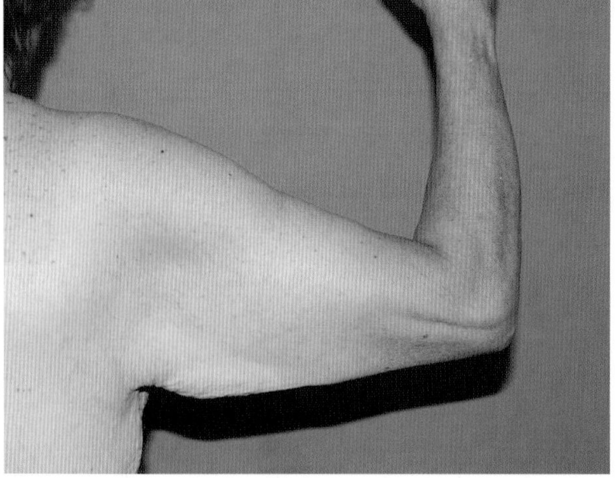

Fig. 13.37

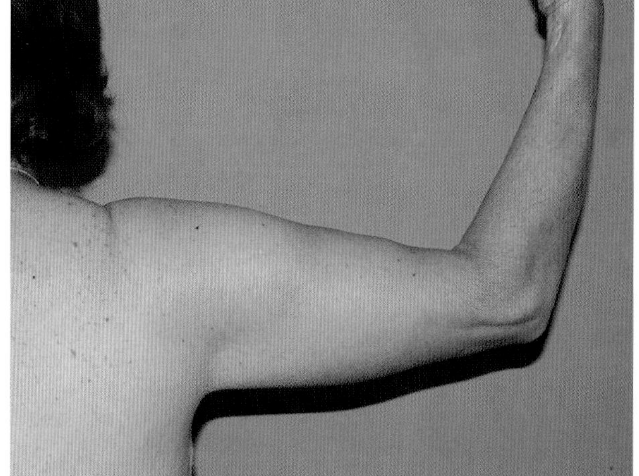

Fig. 13.38

resected. The amount of skin resection now determined is actually drawn more conservatively, placing the incision about a centimeter inside the point determined by bimanual palpation to avoid an excessively tight closure. Doing so takes into account the amount of adipose tissue between the intervening segments during bimanual estimation. A notch placed in the axilla breaks up the linear incision and prevents postoperative bandings (**Fig. 13.39 A–C**).

The distal extent of the resection is dependent on the amount of soft-tissue resection planned. If the excision extends across the elbow, a notch is placed at this level to

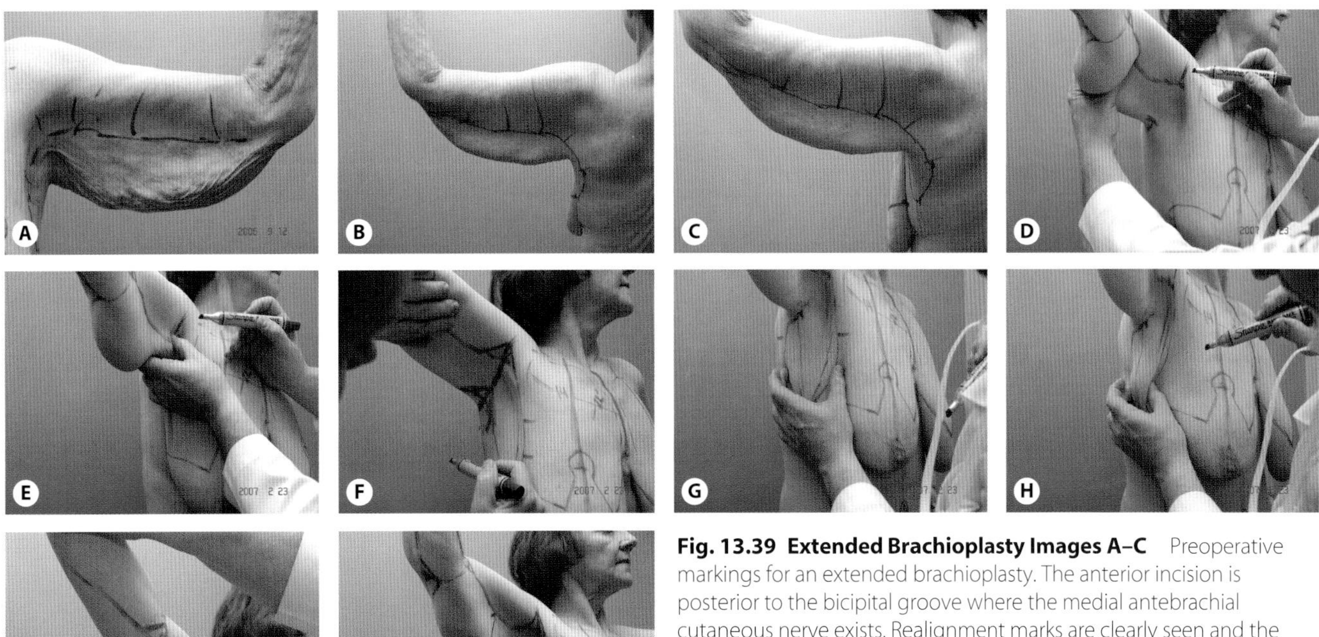

Fig. 13.39 Extended Brachioplasty Images A–C Preoperative markings for an extended brachioplasty. The anterior incision is posterior to the bicipital groove where the medial antebrachial cutaneous nerve exists. Realignment marks are clearly seen and the resection extends down to the lateral breast and flank area. These markings are made using bimanual palpation, and the final incision is placed just inside the markings to take into account the thickness of the soft-tissue. **D–J** In the axilla an anterior notch is drawn, avoiding a linear scar that could form postoperative webbing or banding in the axilla. Bimanual palpation identifies the tissue accessed, which is marked in the axilla and in the lateral breast and flank. If the incision extends distal to the elbow, as here, an anterior notch is placed at the elbow as well, breaking up the linear scar.

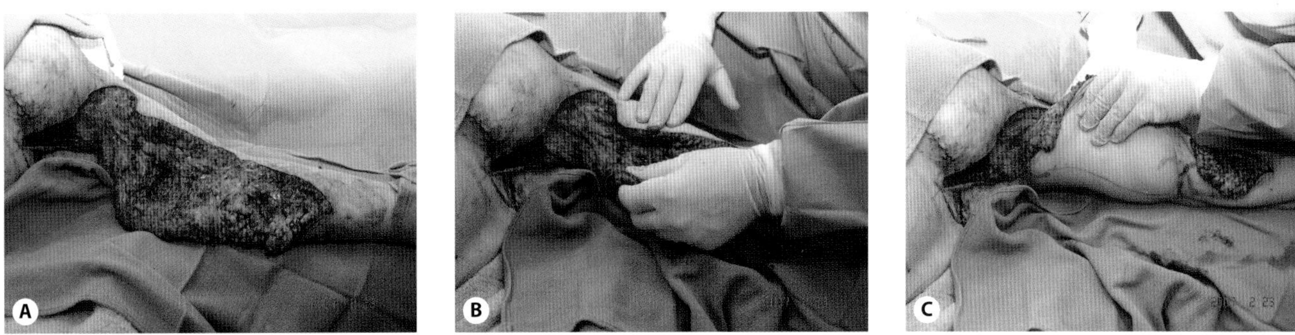

Fig. 13.40 Extended Brachioplasty Images A–C The anterior incision of the extended brachioplasty has been created. Posterior undermining has been incrementally performed and then, using bimanual palpation, the final extent of resection is identified. This demarcation identifies the excess skin and soft-tissue to be resected. Note the axillary notch placed to avoid postoperative banding.

avoid a linear scar across the surface of the joint. The resection extends down the axilla and can be connected to either the inframammary fold/breast procedure anteriorly or the transverse section of the bra-line back lift procedure posteriorly (**Fig. 13.39 D–J**).

In the operating room, dilute lidocaine containing epinephrine is used to infiltrate the incision lines. Cannula undermining as performed with the full brachioplasty and vertical thigh lift (discussed below) is not necessary in this procedure because the tissue resection is full thickness skin and subcutaneous fat down to the investing brachial fascia. A safe approach to this resection is to make the anterior incision first, followed by posterior dissection. The appropriate amount of tissue to be resected is then evaluated incrementally, and only then is the posterior incision made

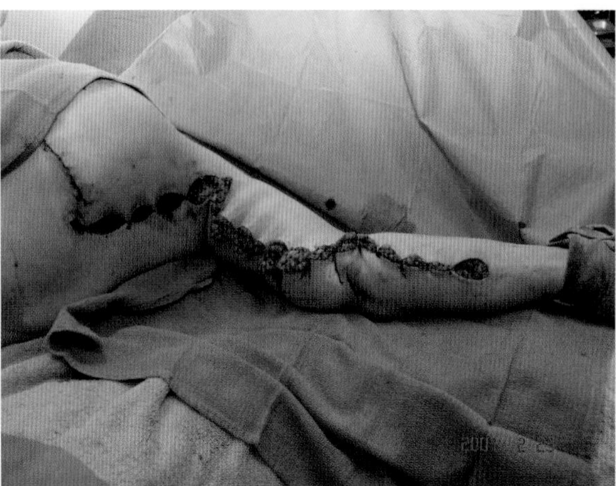

Fig. 13.41 Extended Brachioplasty Images Closure with interrupted PDS sutures. This is prior to final Monocryl intracuticular suturing and skin adhesive closure.

(**Fig. 13.40 A–C**). After hemostasis is obtained, deep dermal closure is performed with interrupted 2/0 or 3/0 PDS or equivalent sutures (**Fig. 13.41**). A final 4/0 Monocryl or equivalent intradermal suture is used. Final incision line treatment can include Steristrips, taping, or tissue adhesive.

Postoperative Care

Compressive ace wraps from the base of the fingers to the axilla are suggested and can usually be removed within 24–48 hours. The patient may find these comfortable, and they can be used in the following postoperative days as well. Arm elevation is very helpful and is recommended, especially in the first 24 hours, but it is frequently beneficial for the first full postoperative week. No vigorous activity or strenuous activity is recommended for the first 2 weeks to allow the healing process to continue with as little swelling as possible. Scar Guard is useful on the incisions during the healing and maturation process.

Before and After Figures (Figs 13.42–13.63)

Bra-Line Back Lift (Box 13.2)

Patients who are good candidates for a bra-line back lift are usually fairly fit, but may have soft-tissue laxity of the middle and upper back associated with aging and weight loss. They are frustrated with the persistence of this laxity despite proper diet and exercise, and hate the way they look in tight-fitting clothing. The bra-line back lift procedure is ideal for correcting soft-tissue laxity of the middle and upper back, and can be performed either as an isolated procedure or in combination with mastopexy, breast reduction, or a reverse abdominoplasty.[4]

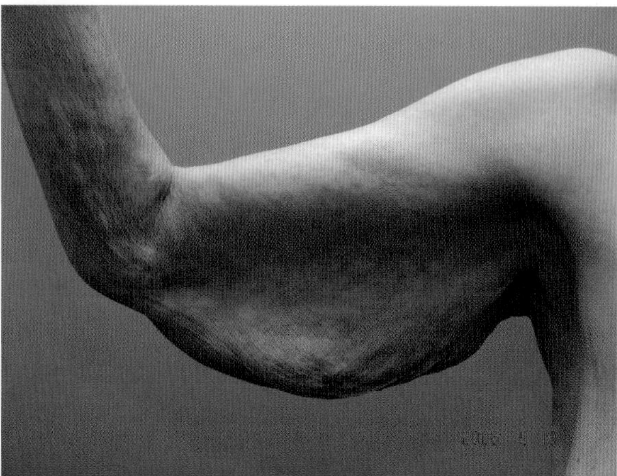

Fig. 13.42

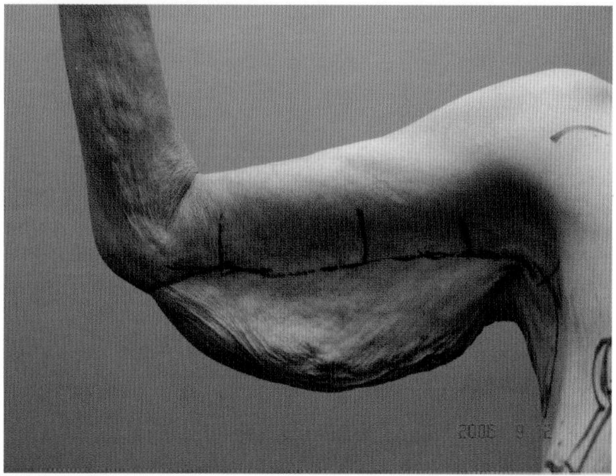

Fig. 13.43

Figs 13.42 and 13.43 Extended Brachioplasty Preoperative Images This patient shows significant soft-tissue laxity following massive weight loss. Preoperative surgical marking of the planned extended brachioplasty is shown.

Box 13.2 Bra-line back lift

- Candidates for the bra-line back lift procedure have graspable soft-tissue laxity in the middle and upper back secondary to aging or to weight loss/fluctuation
- These patients are fairly fit and are often frustrated that proper diet and exercise have not improved this area
- Outlining the border of the bra will help facilitate placement of the final scar in a well concealed location
- The resection usually extends to the anterior axillary line at the level of the inframammary fold
- Preservation of the loose areolar tissue over the underlying muscle fascia will help minimize pain and swelling
- Unless concurrent liposuction is performed or the patient has an excessively thick layer of adipose tissue, a drain is not usually placed
- Restriction from heavy lifting and vigorous activity are the only postoperative limitations that we recommend

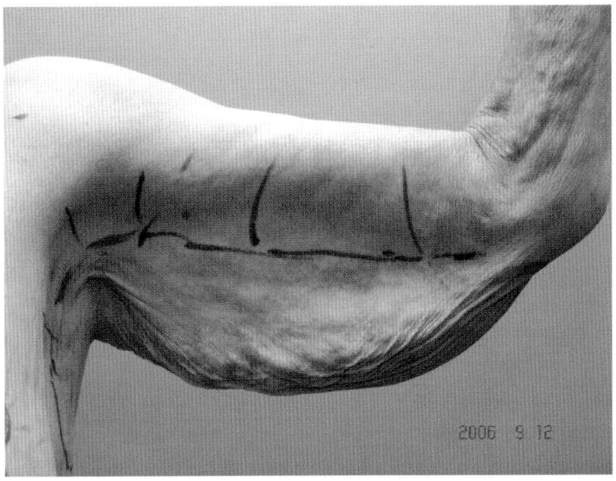

Fig. 13.44

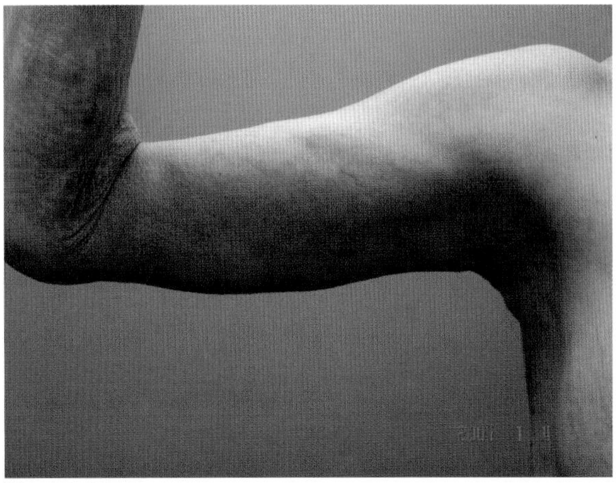

Fig. 13.45

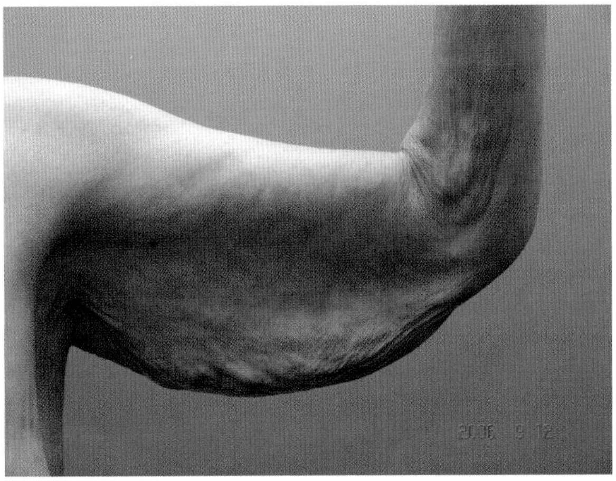

Fig. 13.46

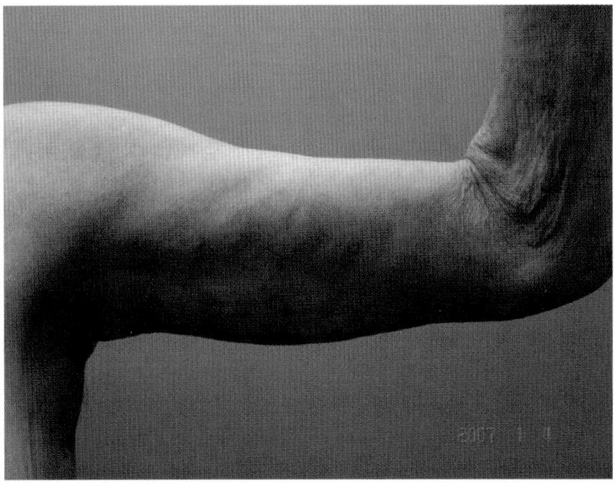

Fig. 13.47

Figs 13.44–13.47 Extended Brachioplasty Pre- and Postoperative Images These images demonstrate a patient following significant weight loss who suffered from marked the laxity of the skin of the arm and lateral breast. The markings for extended brachioplasty can be seen, with realignment marks. The postoperative result is dramatic, eliminating all redundancy and giving the arm a smooth, youthful contour.

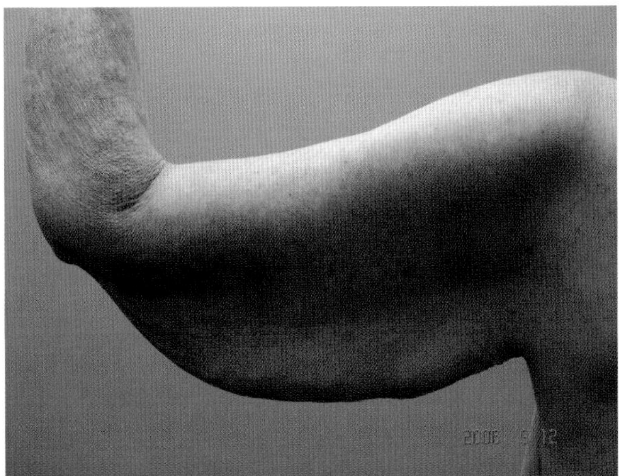

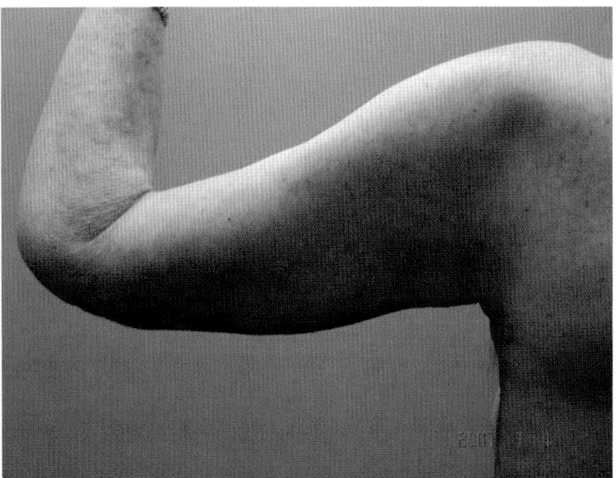

Figs 13.48–13.49 Extended Brachioplasty Pre- and Postoperative Images The posterior aspect of the left arm of this same patient is noted before and after an extended brachioplasty. The dramatic improvement in shape and contour is obvious posteriorly, with the final incision line being placed properly so it is not visible from behind.

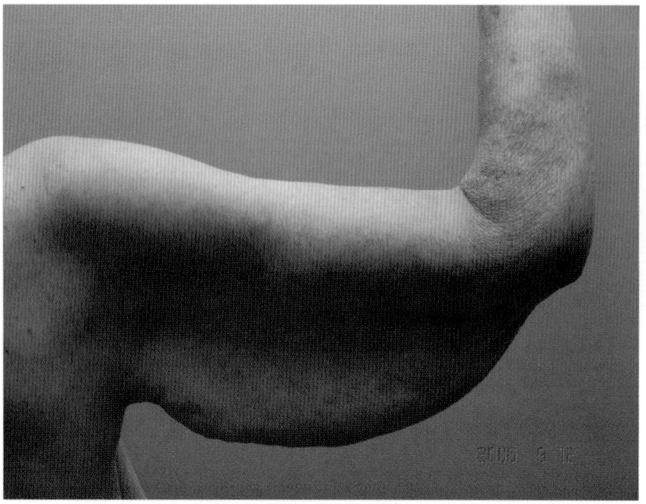

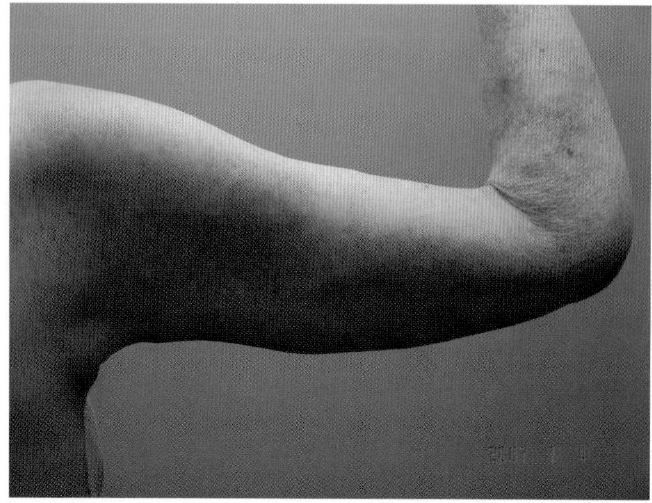

Figs 13.50–13.51 Extended Brachioplasty Pre- and Postoperative Images The posterior aspect of the right arm of this same patient is noted before and after an extended brachioplasty. The dramatic improvement in shape and contour is obvious posteriorly, with the final incision line being placed properly so it is not visible from behind.

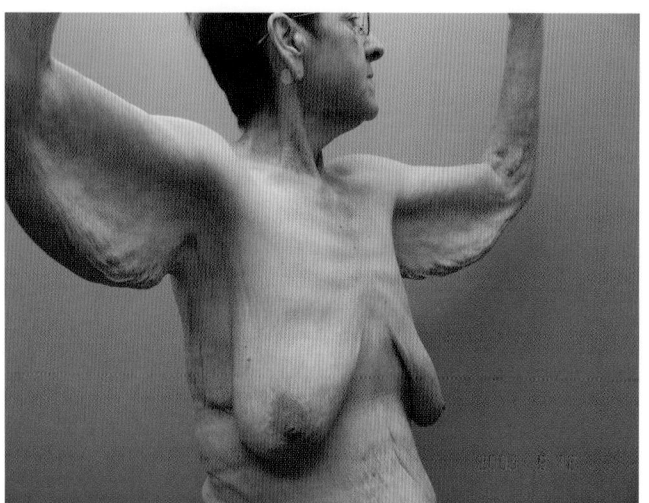

Fig. 13.52

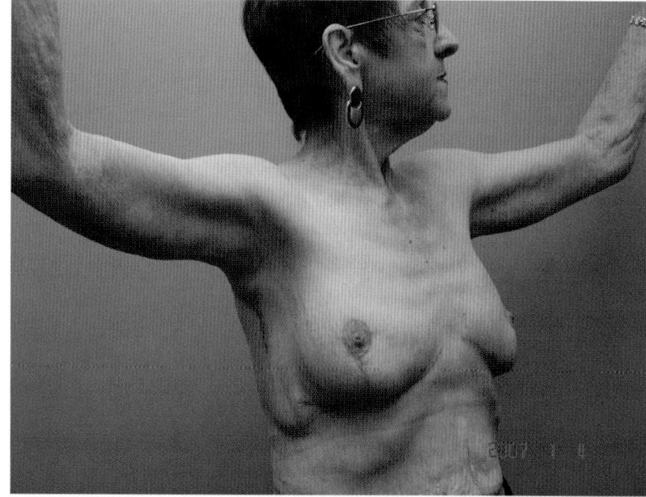

Fig. 13.53

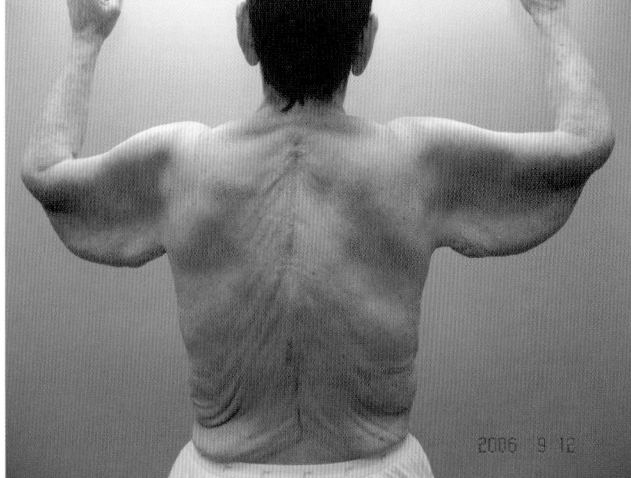

Fig. 13.54

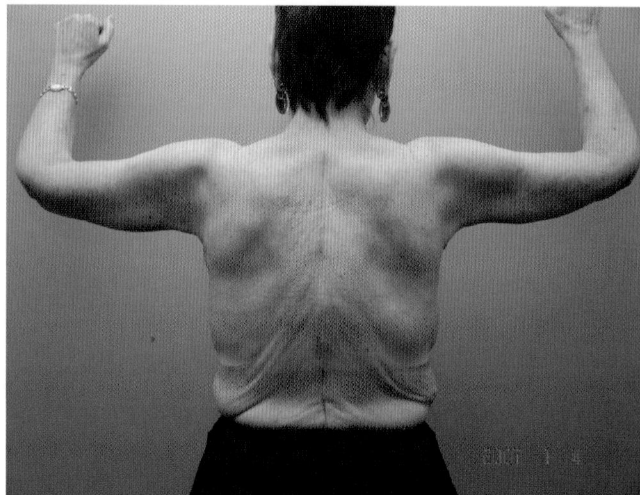

Fig. 13.55

Figs 13.52–13.55 Extended Brachioplasty Pre- and Postoperative Images With the arms up, the true extent of the arm laxity is appreciated. The 'batwing' deformity is easily visualized. The final results reveal a complete correction of this deformity, returning this patient to a more youthful appearance.

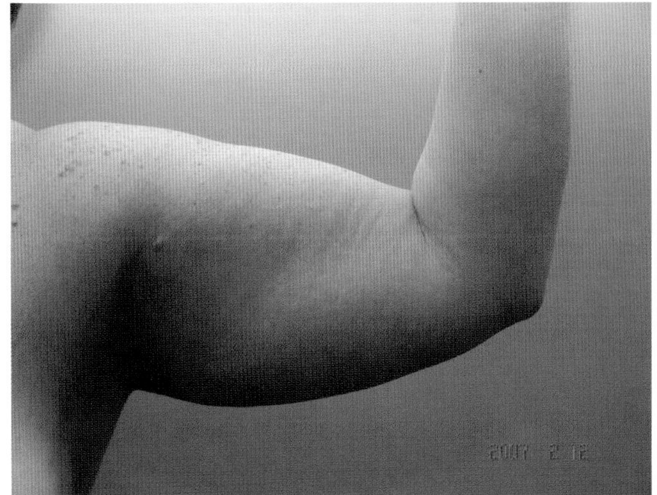

Fig. 13.56

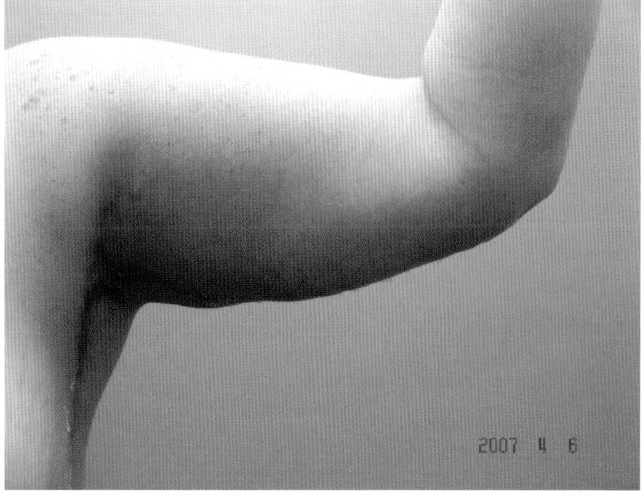

Fig. 13.57

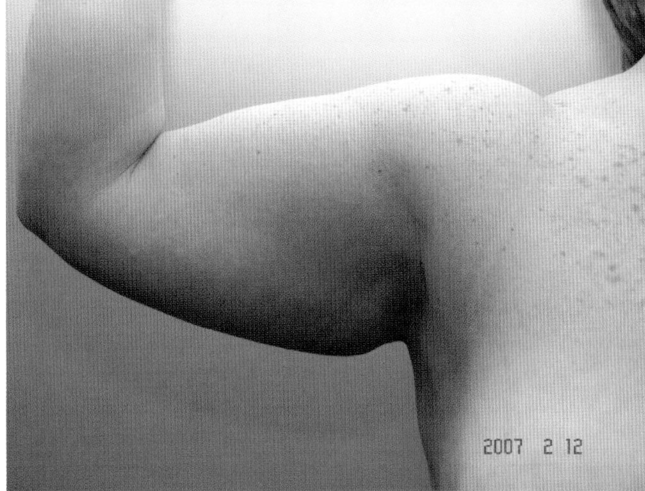

Fig. 13.58

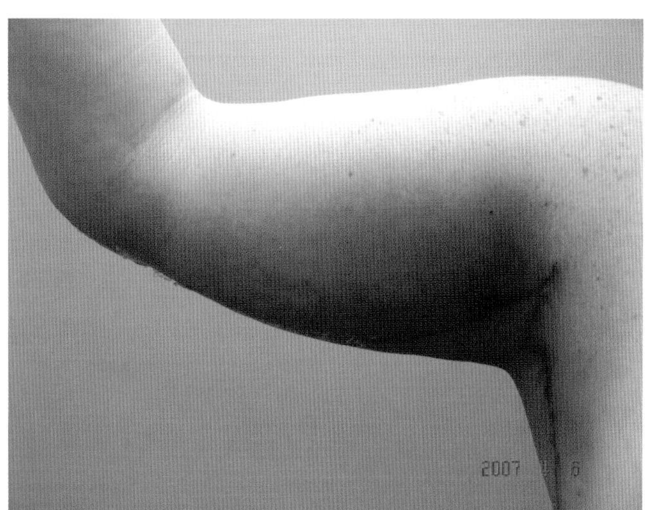

Fig. 13.59

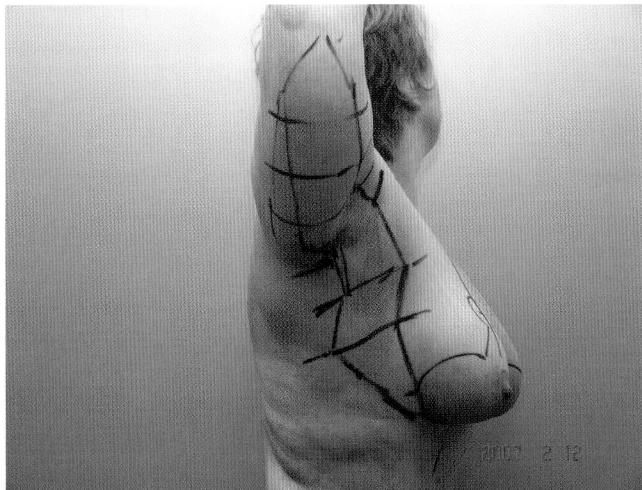

Fig. 13.60

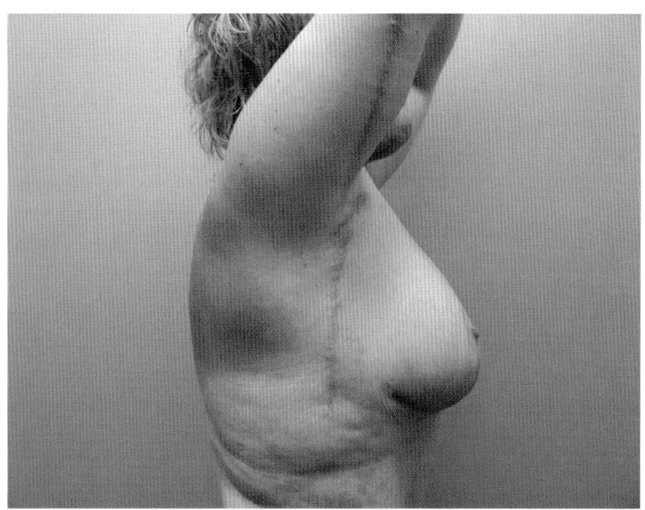

Fig. 13.61

Figs 13.56–13.61 Extended Brachioplasty Pre- and Postoperative Images This patient has experienced incomplete weight loss and still has persistent excess adiposity in the arms and lateral breast. By performing an extended brachioplasty including the lateral breast, the redundancy is corrected, resulting in improvement in the shape and contour of the arm and lateral breast area. The notch at the axilla eliminates scar banding and tethering across this area.

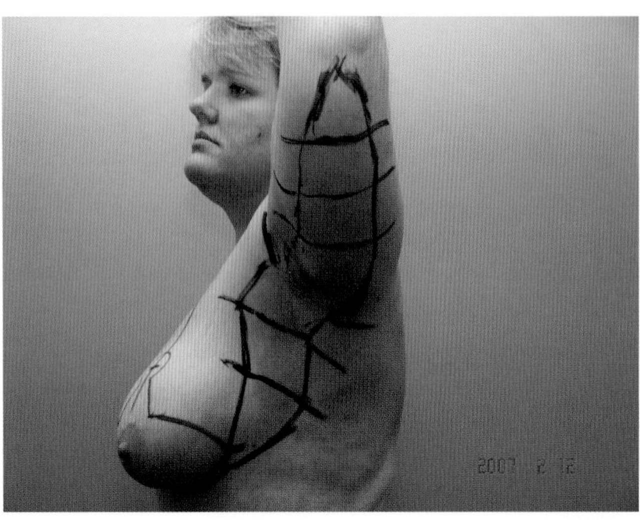

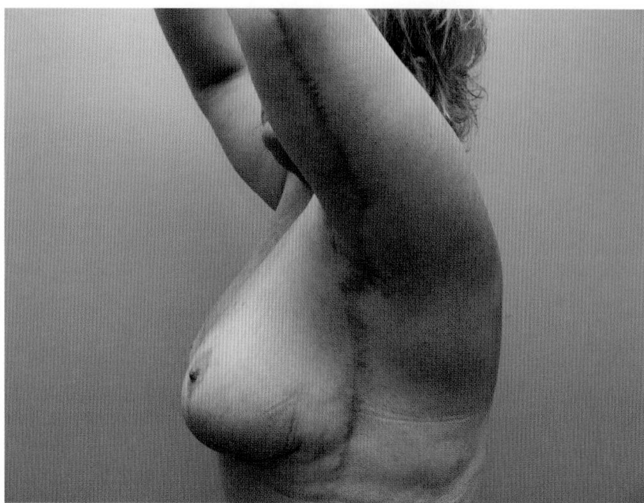

Figs 13.62–13.63 Extended Brachioplasty Pre- and Postoperative Images An additional view of the same patient shows the left arm and left lateral chest before and after extended brachioplasty.

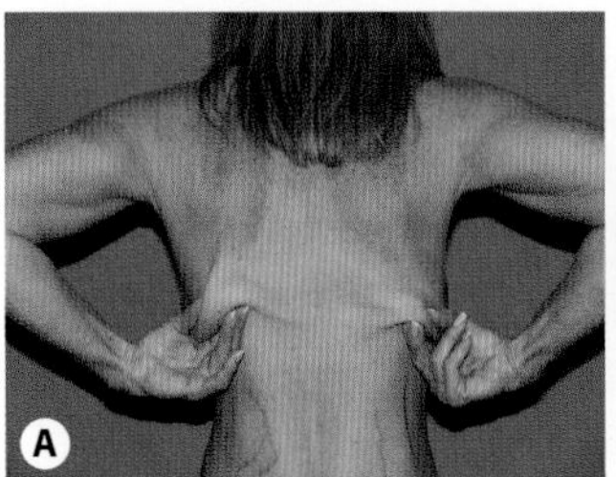

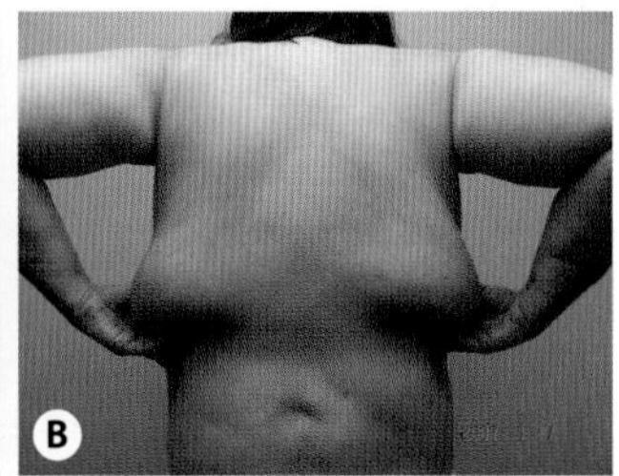

Fig. 13.64 A and B Bra-line Back Lift Images Patients will often grasp the redundant tissue of the upper back when communicating what they want removed. For the normal-weight individual, age and environmental factors can create laxity that cannot be improved with diet or exercise. For the incomplete weight-loss patient the redundant tissue is skin and fat.

Operative Approach

Patients usually demonstrate their displeasure with the laxity of their back by actually pinching the tissue that they would like to have removed (**Fig. 13.64 A and B**). The outline of the patient's bra is marked, and the position of the final scar is placed within these borders (**Fig. 13.65 A–C**). The incision line usually extends to the inframammary fold at the anterior axillary line. The amount of soft-tissue resection is determined using bimanual palpation across the entire incision line (**Fig. 13.66 A–F**). Having the patient review the final incision line is helpful to avoid disappointment with the size and location of the final scar. After general anesthesia is initiated, the patient is placed prone. A penetrating towel

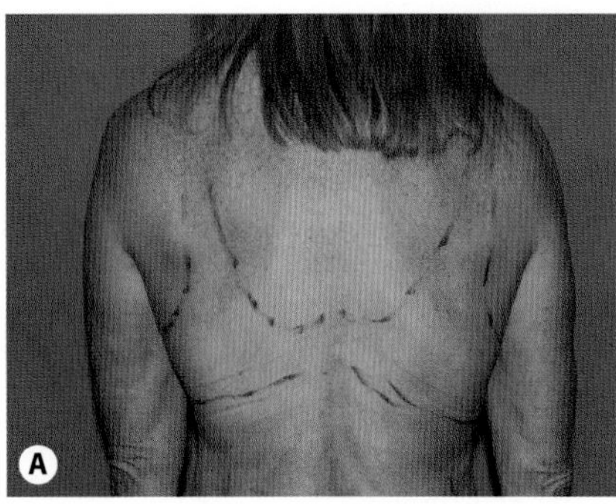

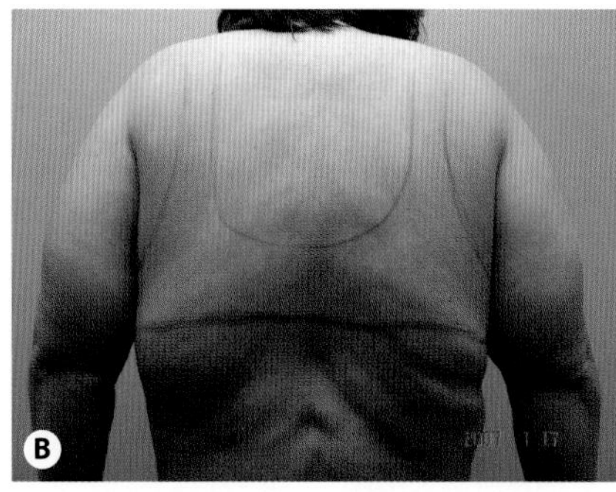

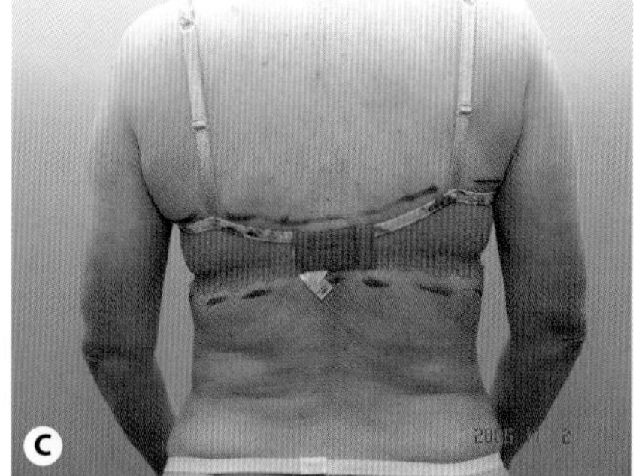

Fig. 13.65 Bra-line Back Lift Images For the patient with incomplete weight loss, significant excess tissue still exists following a body lift because the zone of adherence does not allow for the transmission of tension and tightening. These patients also benefit from the removal of the back skin and the underlying excess adiposity. When patients grasp the upper back area it usually suggests that a bra-line back lift would be a reasonable procedure to correct this problem. The outline of the bra is marked and the final incision line is placed within the borders of this marking. The marking should be agreed upon by the patient.

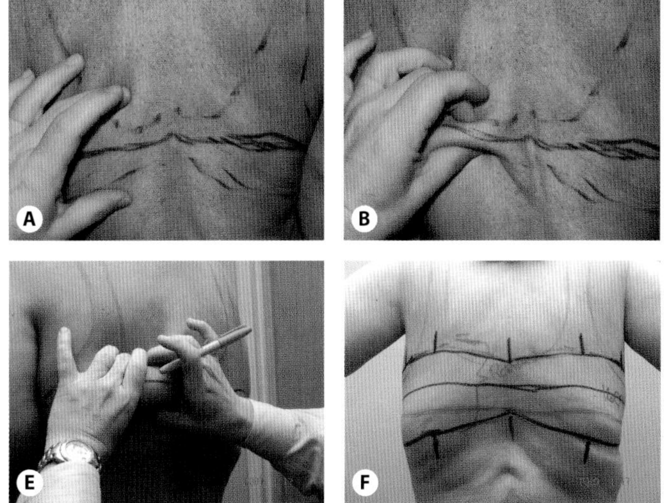

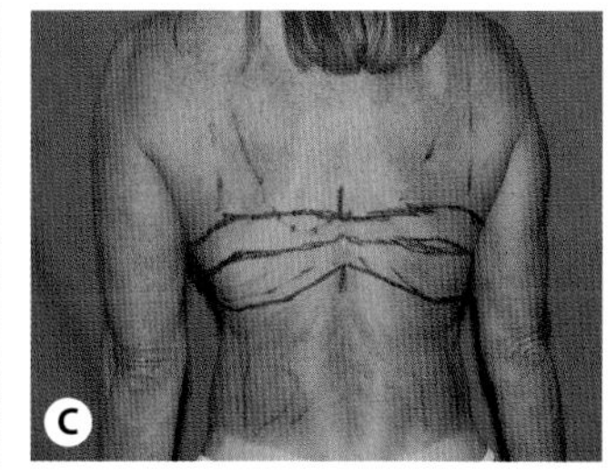

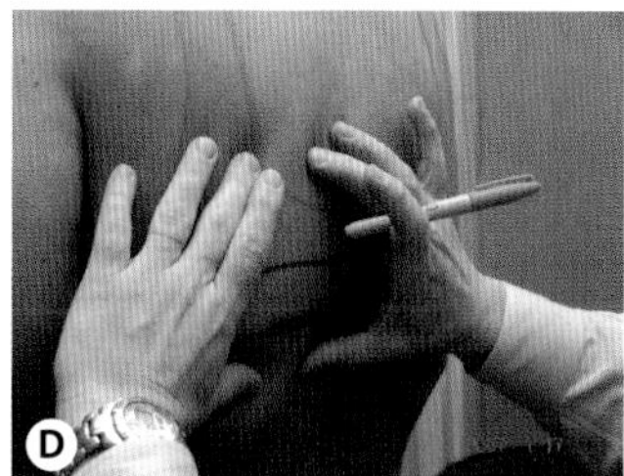

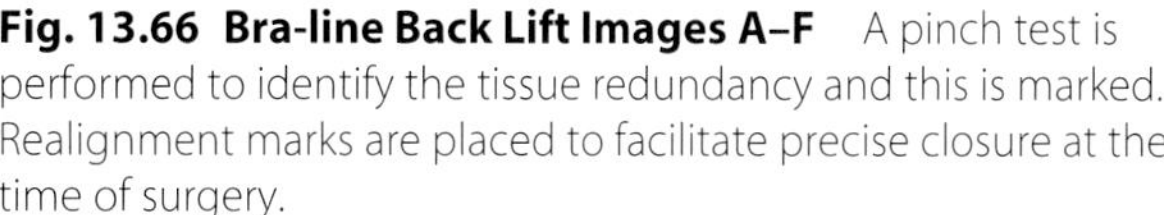

Fig. 13.66 Bra-line Back Lift Images A–F A pinch test is performed to identify the tissue redundancy and this is marked. Realignment marks are placed to facilitate precise closure at the time of surgery.

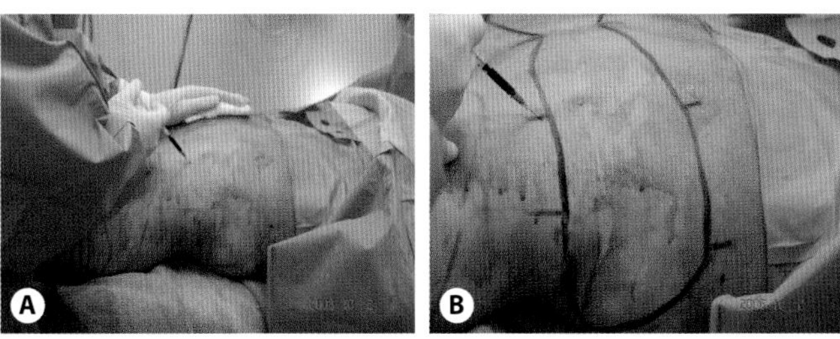

Fig. 13.67 Bra-line Back Lift Images A, B Methylene blue tattoos are placed in the realignment marks. These will stay in place throughout the procedure to facilitate precise closure.

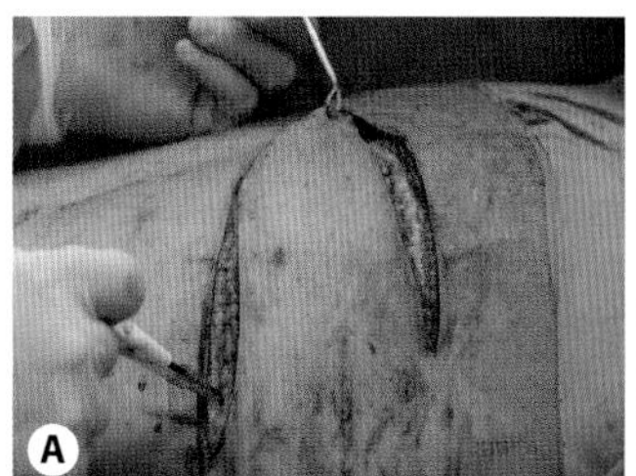

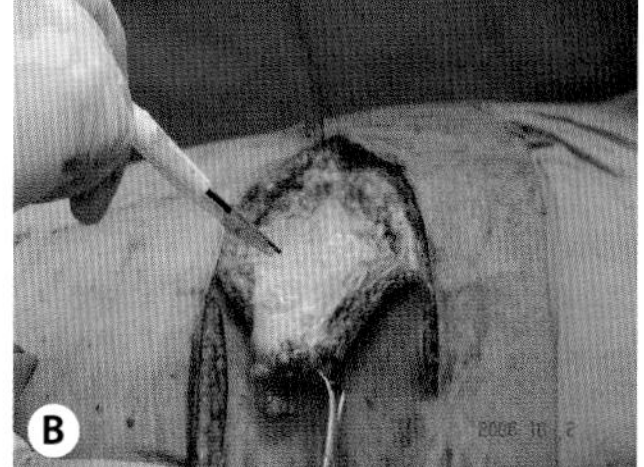

Fig. 13.69 Bra-line Back Lift Images A, B The incision is made partially through the dermis and electrocautery is used to complete the incision through the dermis and subcutaneous tissue to the loose areolar plane superficial to the muscle fascia. This is the proper plane of dissection proper plane.

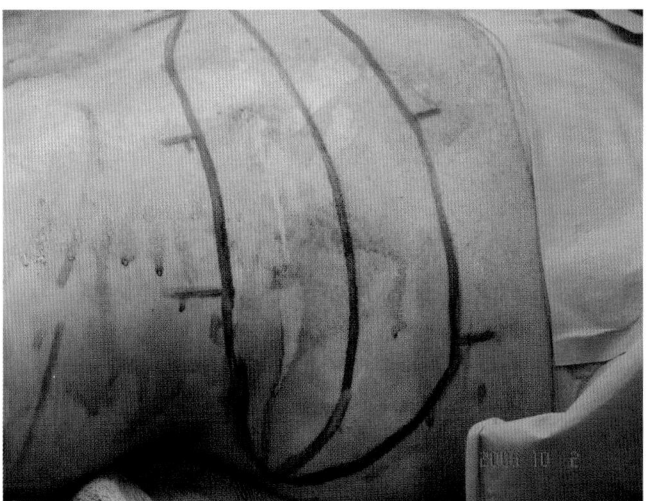

Fig. 13.68 Bra-line Back Lift Image The tissues for resection are infiltrated with dilute epinephrine-containing solutions to promote vasoconstriction and facilitate dissection.

clamp can be used to approximate the upper and lower incision lines, ensuring that closure will not be under excessive tension. Methylene blue ink is used to tattoo realignment marks to help facilitate precise closure (**Fig. 13.67 A, B**). The incision lines should be infiltrated with dilute lidocaine containing epinephrine to minimize bleeding and bruising (**Fig. 13.68**). The incision lines are made with a number 10 scalpel partly through the dermis, and electrocautery is used to complete the skin incision, sealing the subdermal plexus (**Fig. 13.69 A**). Electrocautery is then used to carefully dissect the intervening tissue away from the underlying chest wall musculature, preserving the muscle fascia and the loose areolar tissue superficial to it (**Fig. 13.69 B**). Dissection is continued to the middle or anterior axillary line, usually ending at the inframammary crease. If this cannot be completed in the prone position, a temporary V–Y closure can be performed and the procedure completed after the patient is repositioned supine (**Fig. 13.70 A–E**).

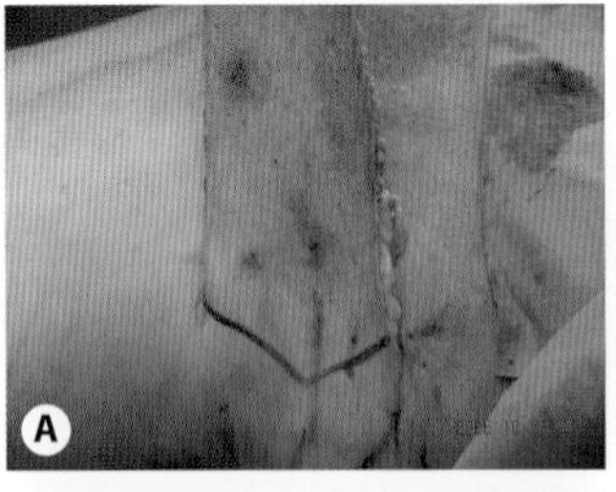

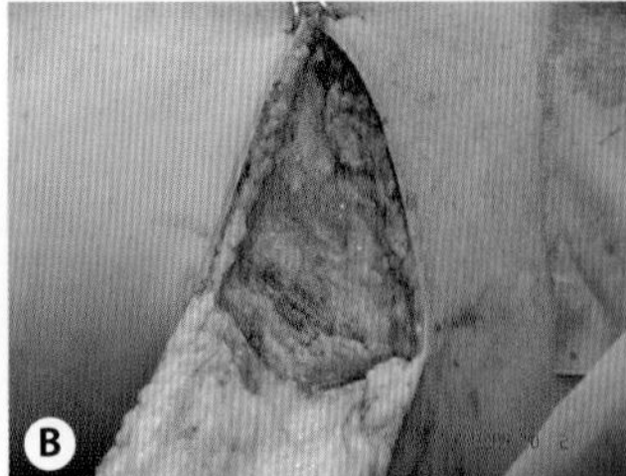

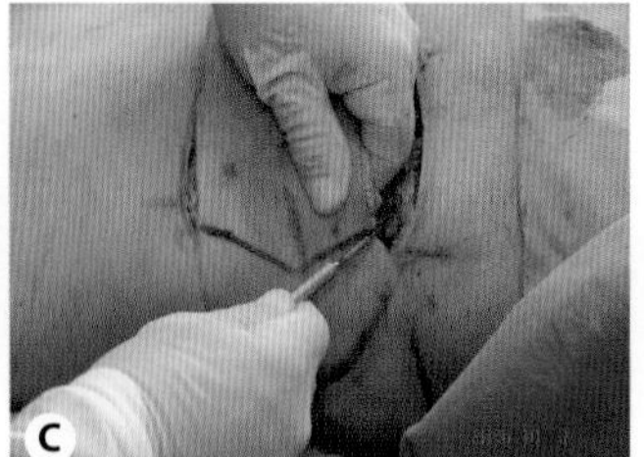

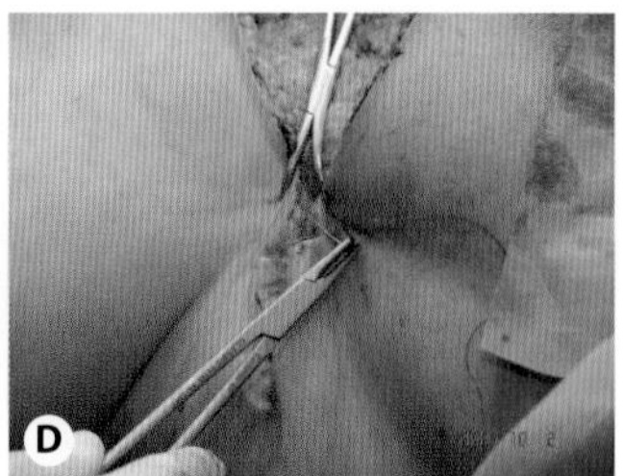

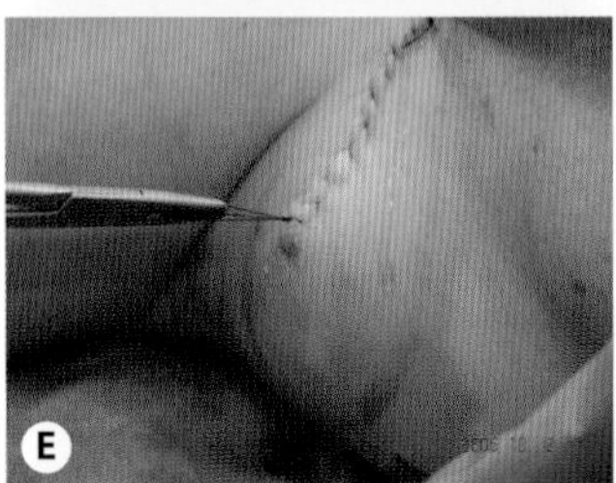

Fig. 13.70 Bra-line Back Lift Images A, E The dissection continues laterally to the inframammary fold. **C–E** If this procedure is to be combined with a reverse abdominoplasty, mastopexy, or breast reduction, a temporary V–Y closure is performed before the patient is turned supine.

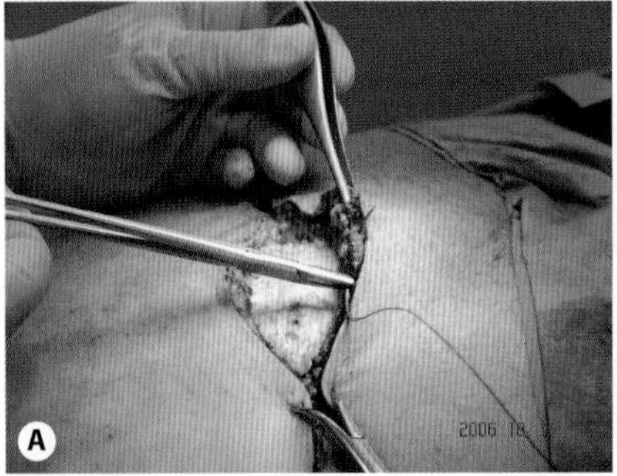

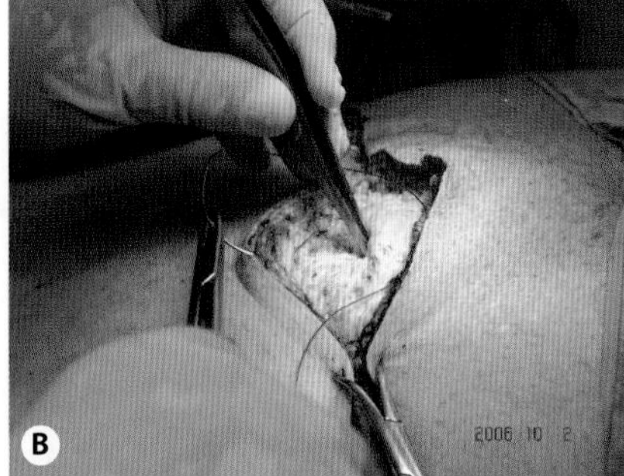

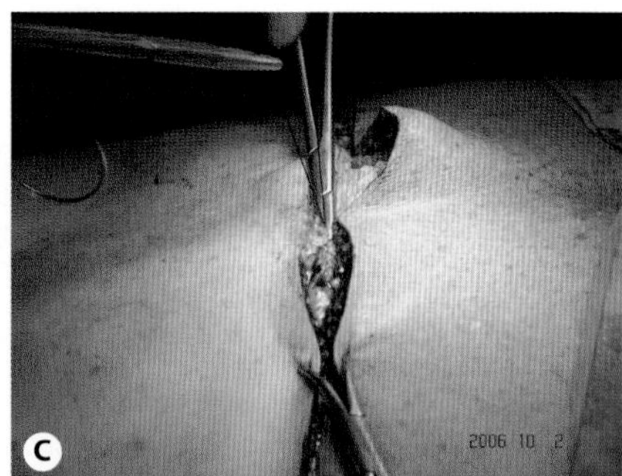

Fig. 13.71 A–C

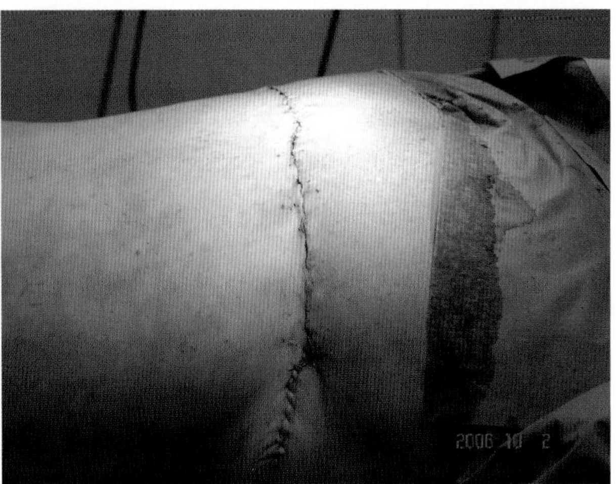

Fig. 13.72

Figs 13.71 A–C and 13.72 Bra-line Back Lift Images Closures performed with 0 or 1 Vicryl, through the SFS. A space-obliterating technique is used which eliminates the need for a drain, except in obese patients which may still benefit from having drain. 2/0 Vicryl closes the deep dermis and 4/0 Monocryl intracuticular sutures are used for final closure. Skin adhesive or tape is then applied.

The incision is closed, placing the tension of the closure at the level of the superficial fascia (**Fig. 13.71 A–C**). Number 1 or 0 Vicryl is used to close the superficial fascia in interrupted fashion, although PDS would be a reasonable alternative. Size 2/0 Vicryl or PDS is used to close the deep dermis, and a 4/0 Monocryl is used for final intradermal closure (**Fig. 13.72**). Tissue adhesive is usually applied to the incision, and if necessary the patient is placed in the supine position for completion of the residual anterior resection and closure.

Postoperative Care

Drains are not routinely used. The exception is the patient who has a thick layer of subcutaneous tissue, or if concurrent upper back liposuction is performed. Heavy lifting and strenuous activity should be avoided. Otherwise there are no additional positional or activity restrictions. The patient is allowed to shower after the first postoperative day. Normal walking, driving, and activities of daily living can be performed within 24–48 hours, but any activity that causes pain or pulling on the back, should be avoided. Sun avoidance is cautioned until the incision line has matured and is no longer red. We recommend Scar Guard on the incision for approximately 6 weeks to help achieve the best scar possible.

Before and After Figures for Bra-line Backlift (Figs 13.73–13.107)

Autologous Buttocks Augmentation

Purse-string Gluteoplasty (Box 13.3)

During a circumferential abdominoplasty, if the volume and projection of the buttocks are adequate the redundant tissue is resected, effectively treating the laxity and achieving correction of ptosis. Following massive weight loss, or in patients with a significant component of gluteal soft-tissue atrophy, the tissue that is usually resected can be used to create a fuller, more youthful buttocks shape. There have been many descriptions of the use of this redundant tissue in the form of a pedicled flap for autologous gluteal augmentation. We prefer the purse-string gluteoplasty because

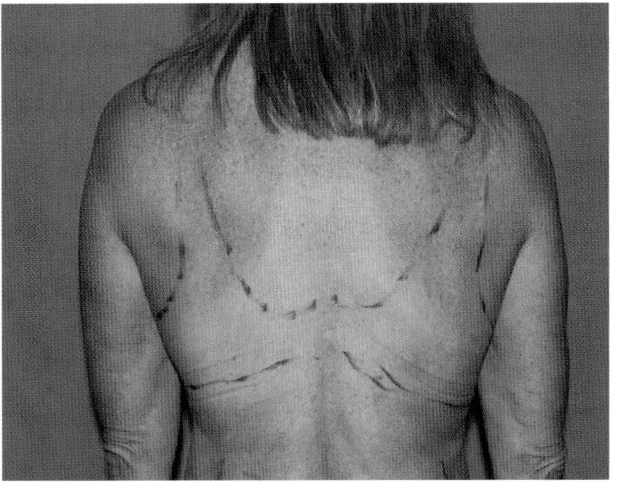

Fig. 13.73

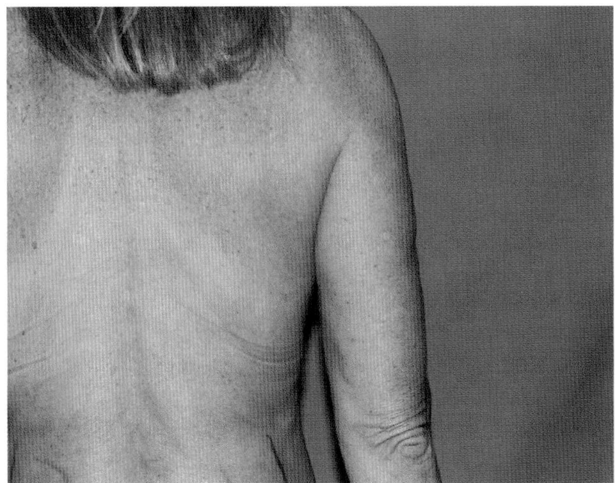

Fig. 13.74

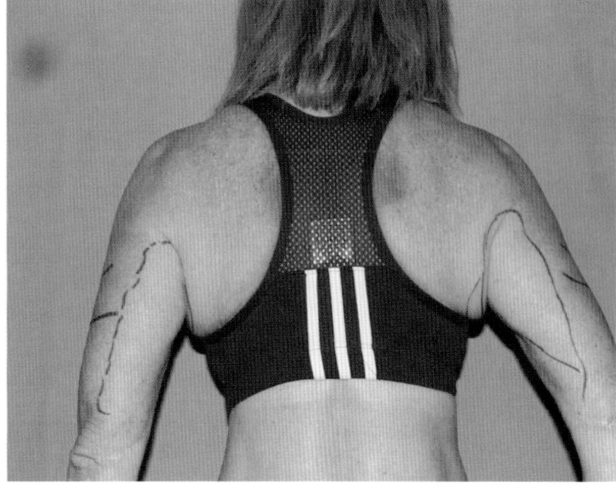

Fig. 13.75

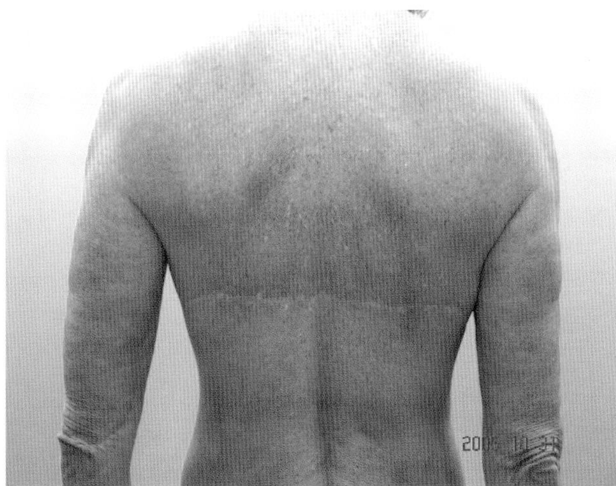

Fig. 13.76

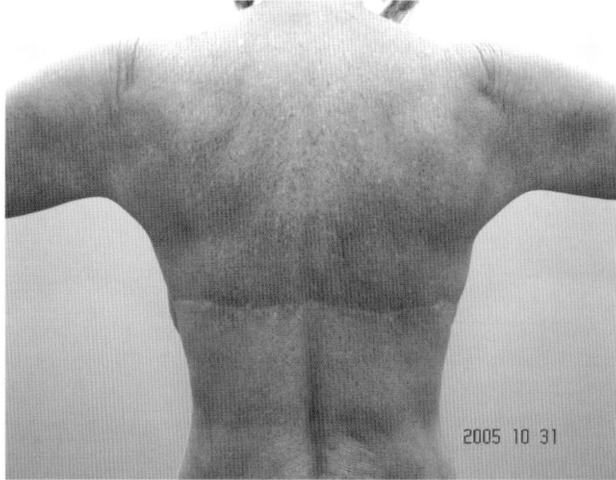

Fig. 13.77

Figs 13.73–13.77 Bra-line Back Lift Pre- and Postoperative Images This patient is an aerobics instructor who was in excellent physical condition. She was very frustrated with her inability to 'exercise her skin' and presented with laxity of the upper back that she wished to have treated. The bra-line back lift procedure was performed, which is easily concealed within her workout attire. The final contour reveals a smooth and even silhouette with a high-quality fine line scar.

Box 13.3 Autologous gluteal augmentation

- Autologous gluteal augmentation can be a powerful body contouring procedure for patients who have a significant amount gluteal atrophy
- Patients with significant amount of truncal soft-tissue laxity are candidates for a circumferential abdominoplasty. The central gluteal mound of the posterior component of the procedure can be used to provide additional volume to the buttocks
- The purse-string gluteoplasty is a straight-forward and reliable technique for providing increased buttock volume and projection
- Patients with excess adiposity of the lumbar area, back, hips, and thighs are particularly good candidates for autologous gluteal augmentation using fat grafting
- Few postoperative restrictions are needed following autologous buttock augmentation. Postoperative antibiotics and ample cushioning when sitting are recommended. Periodic ambulation lessens the chance of DVT as well as limiting the length of time continuous pressure is applied to the buttocks

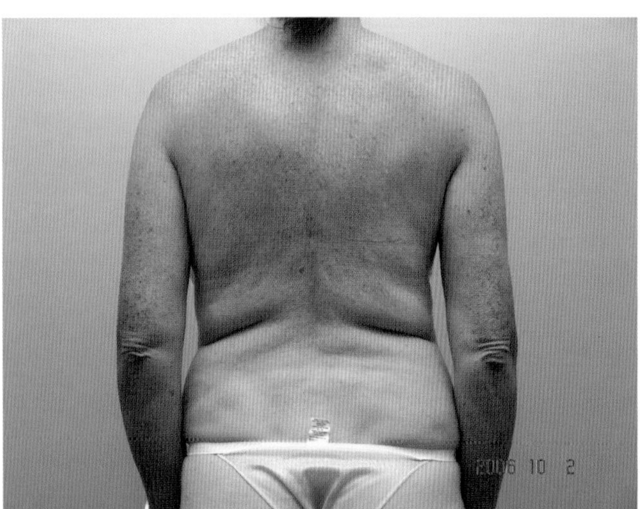

Fig. 13.78

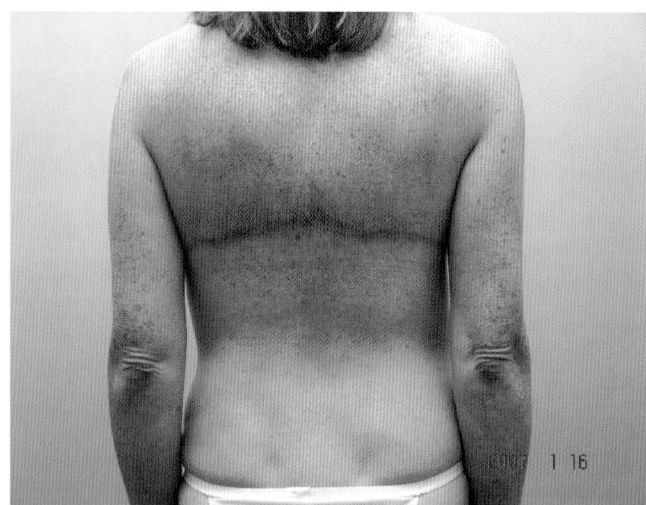

Fig. 13.79

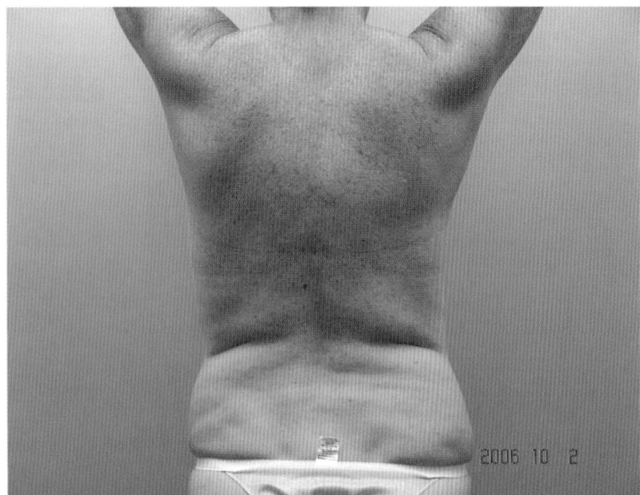

Fig. 13.80

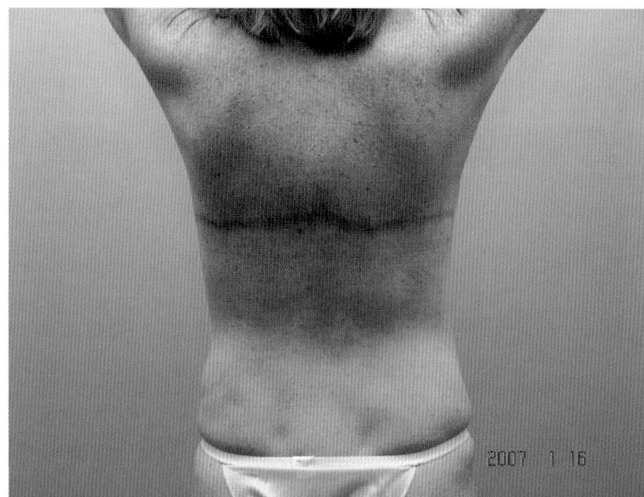

Fig. 13.81

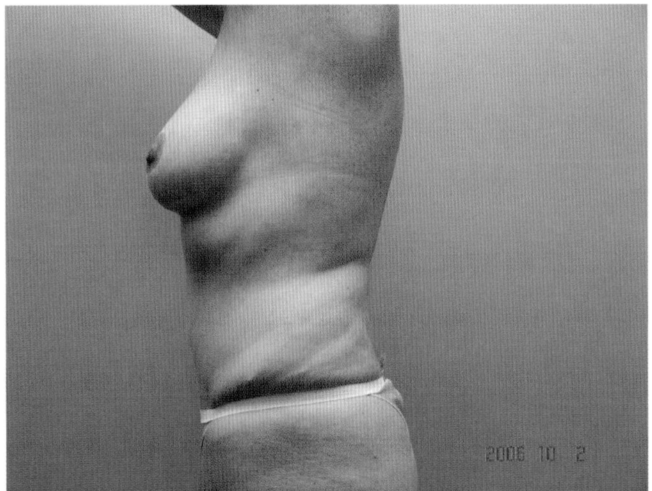

Fig. 13.82

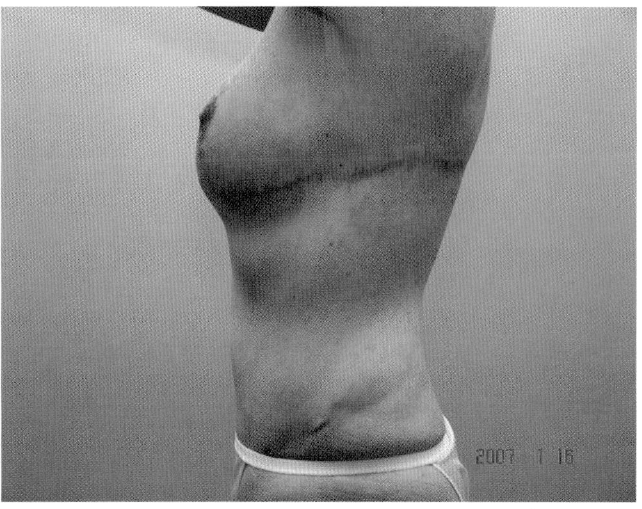

Fig. 13.83

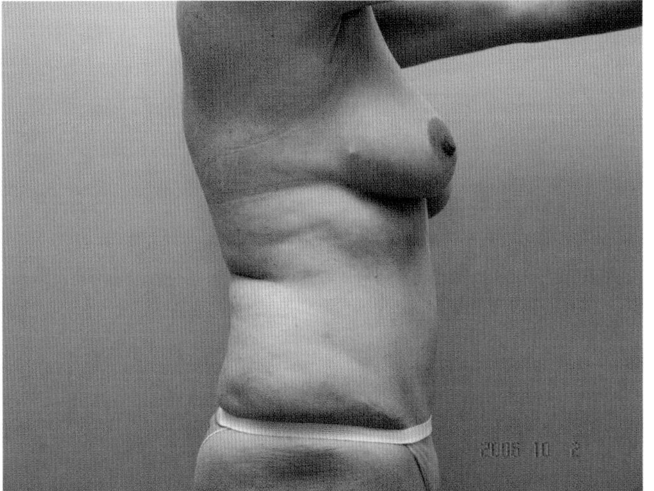
Fig. 13.84

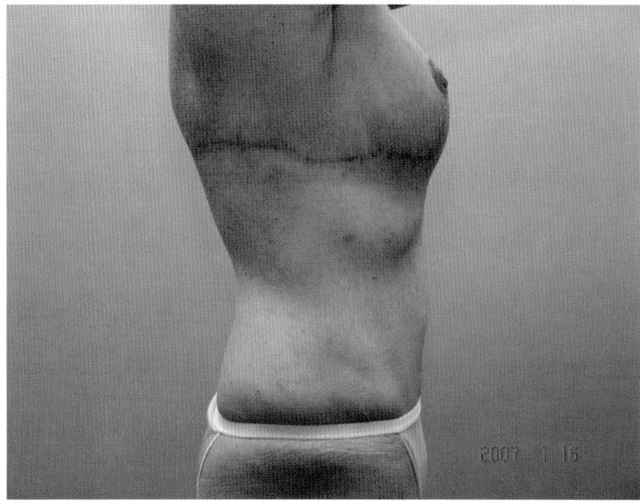
Fig. 13.85

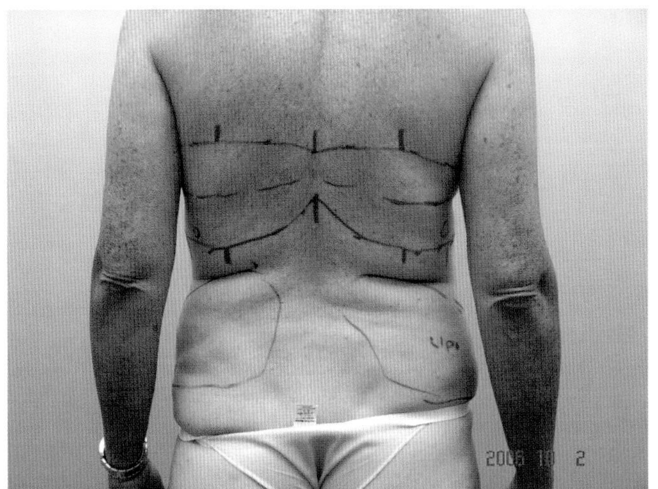
Fig. 13.86

Figs 13.78–13.86 Bra-line Back Lift Pre- and Postoperative Images This 35-year-old woman had previous liposuction of the back but was still left with redundancy and laxity. Hip roll liposuction and a bra-line back lift were suggested to treat her concerns. The result created a beautiful youthful silhouette that corrected all of her preoperative complaints.

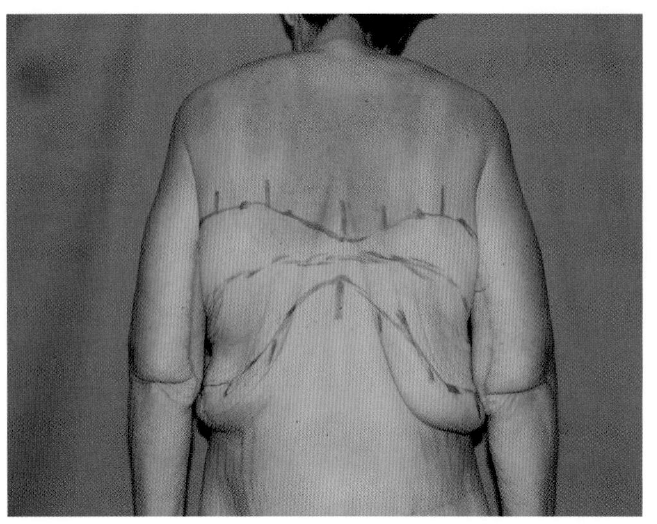

Fig. 13.87

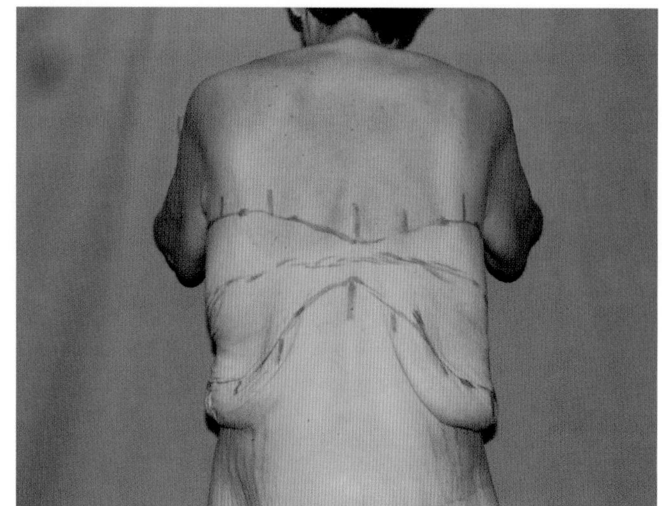

Fig. 13.88

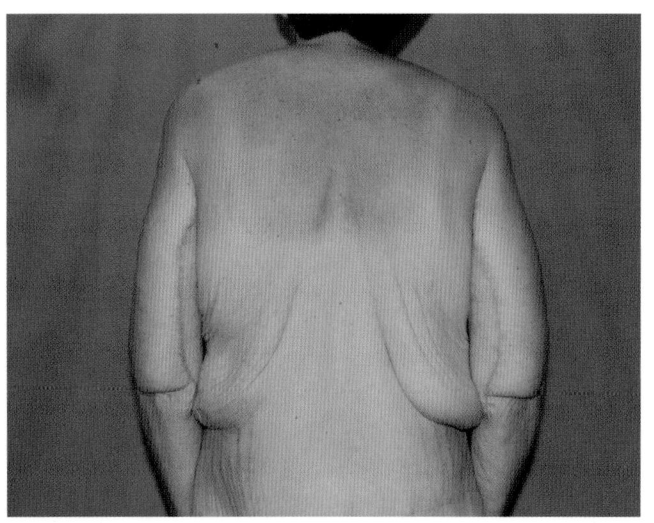

Fig. 13.89

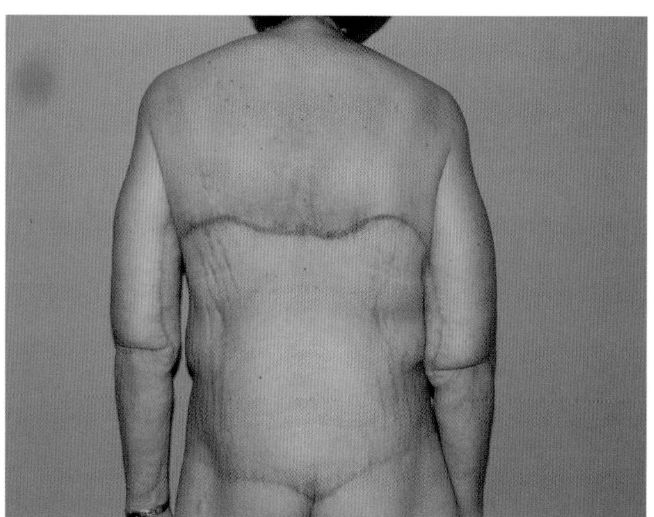

Fig. 13.90

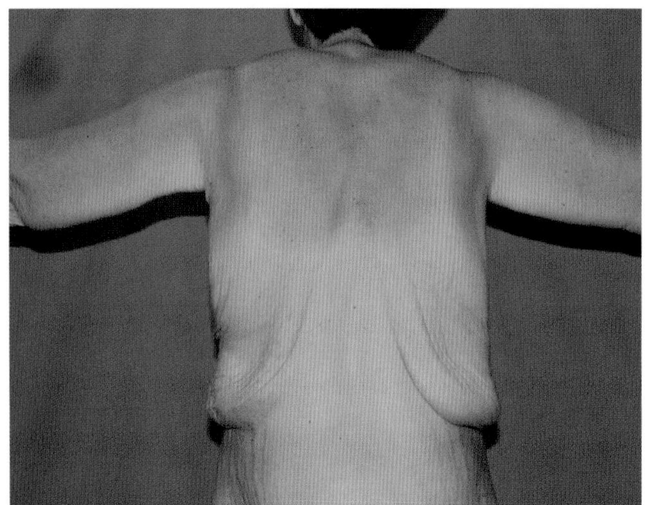

Fig. 13.91

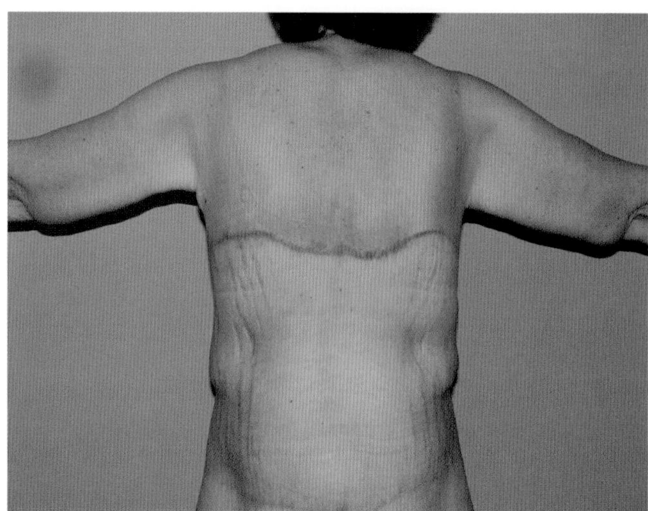

Fig. 13.92

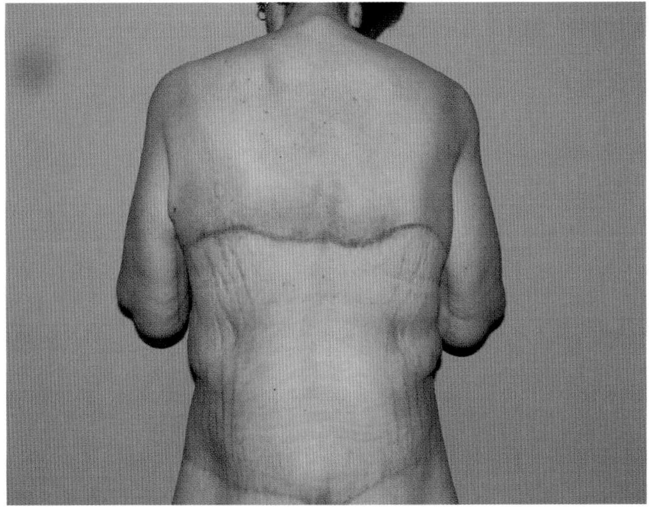

Fig. 13.93

Figs 13.87–13.93 Bra-line Back Lift Pre- and Postoperative Images This massive weight loss patient had previously undergone a circumferential abdominoplasty. This corrected the abdomen and buttocks but had minimal effect on the upper and mid-back. She had massive "festoons" of tissue hanging from the side that were incorporated into an extended bra-line back lift. This procedure dramatically improved her profile, giving her an improved upper body shape and contour.

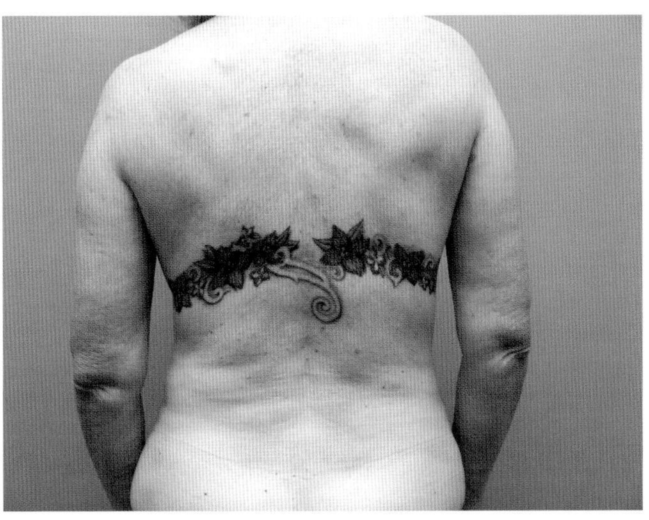

Fig. 13.94

Figs 13.94–13.96 Bra-line Back Lift Pre- and Postoperative Images This patient was concerned about the laxity of the mid and upper back and was treated successfully with a bra-line back lift. She subsequently had a tattoo placed over the posterior incision, which completely obscured it. The improvement in the silhouette and shape can easily be seen.

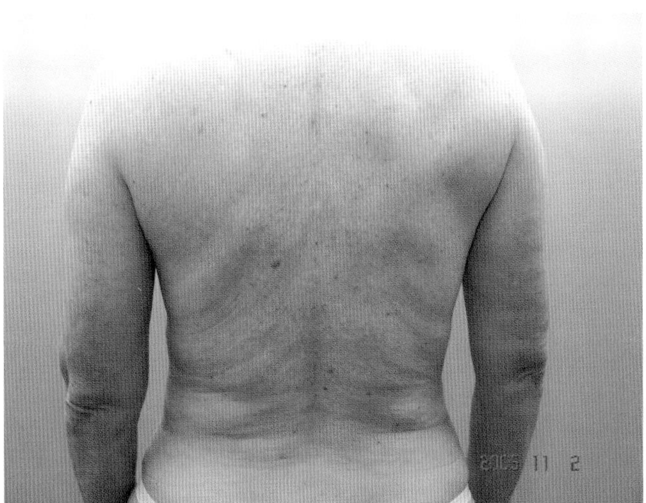

Fig. 13.95

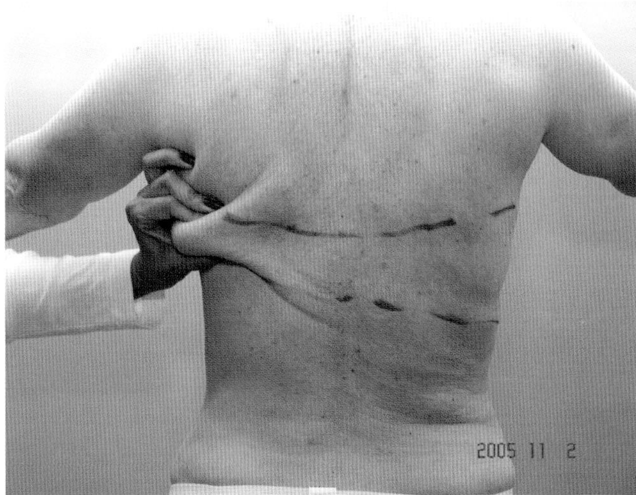

Fig. 13.96

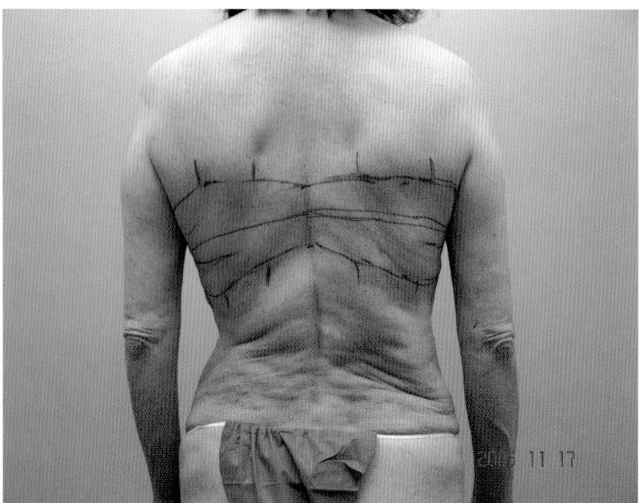

Fig. 13.97

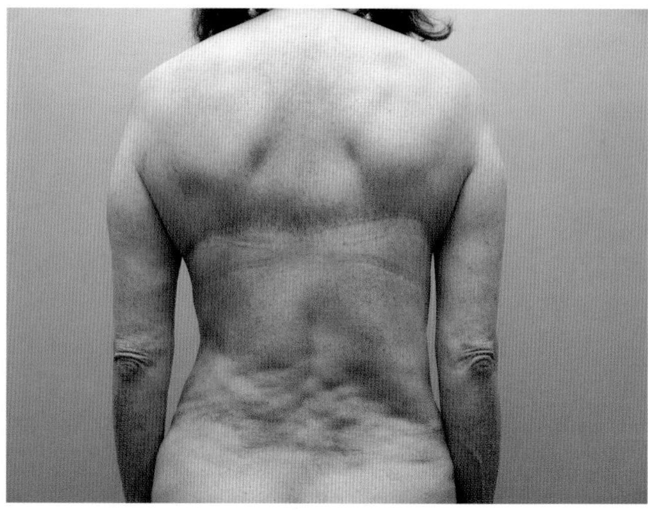

Fig. 13.98

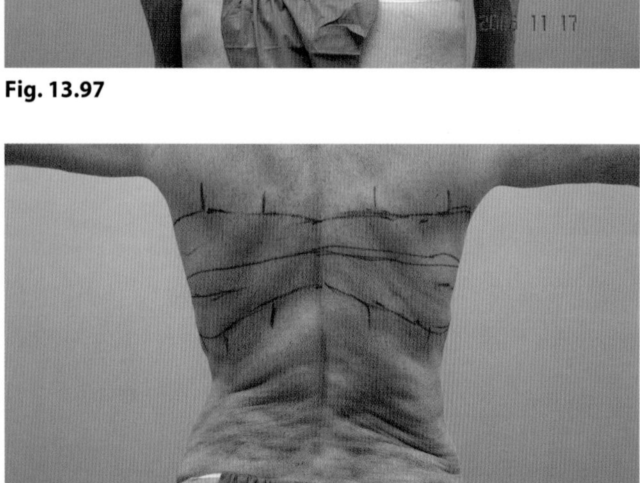

Fig. 13.99

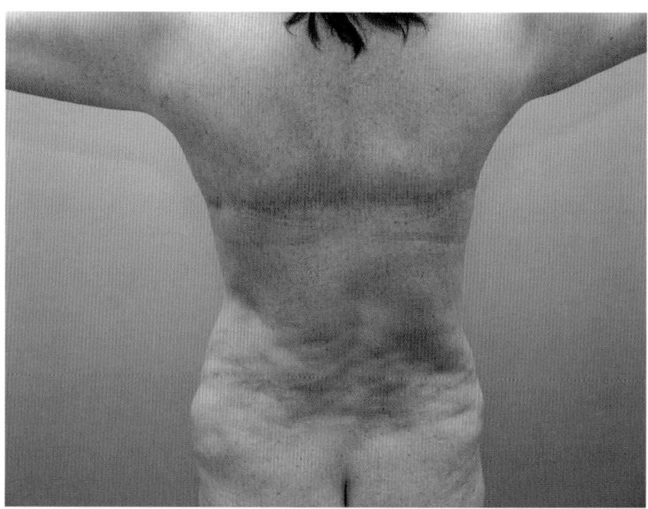

Fig. 13.100

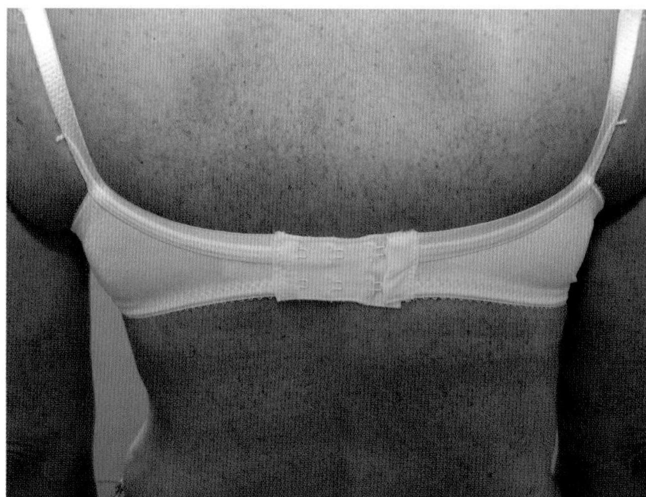

Fig. 13.101

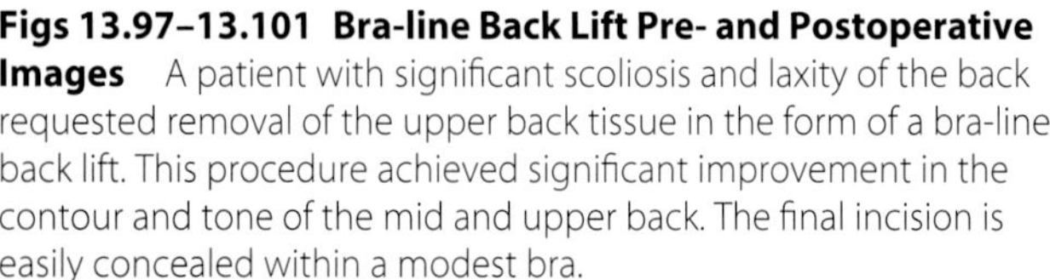

Figs 13.97–13.101 Bra-line Back Lift Pre- and Postoperative Images A patient with significant scoliosis and laxity of the back requested removal of the upper back tissue in the form of a bra-line back lift. This procedure achieved significant improvement in the contour and tone of the mid and upper back. The final incision is easily concealed within a modest bra.

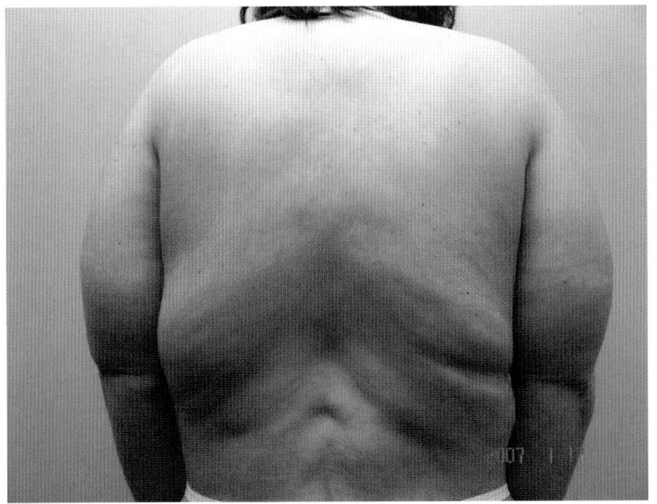

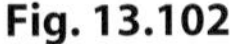

Fig. 13.102

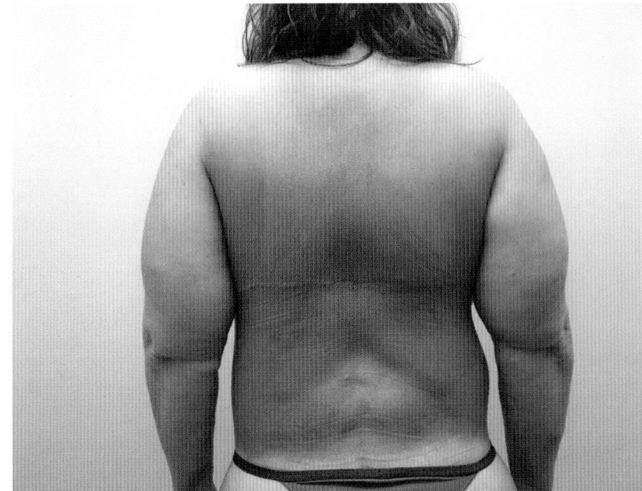

Fig. 13.103

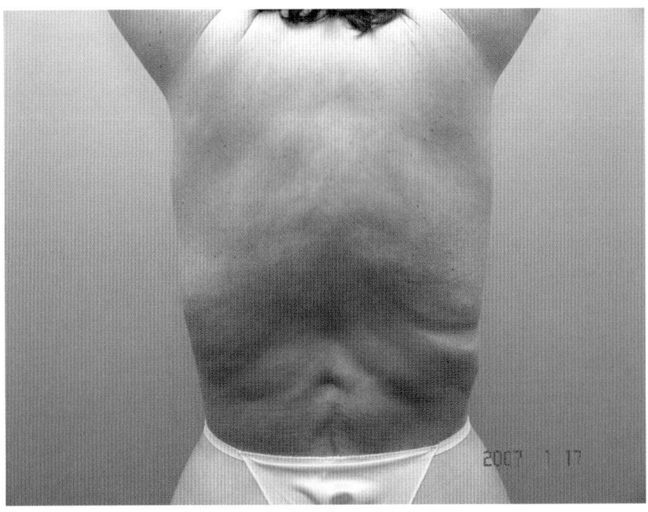

Fig. 13.104

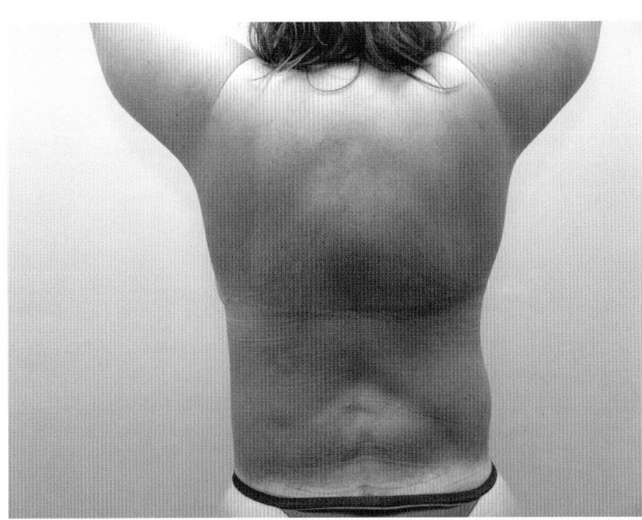

Fig. 13.105

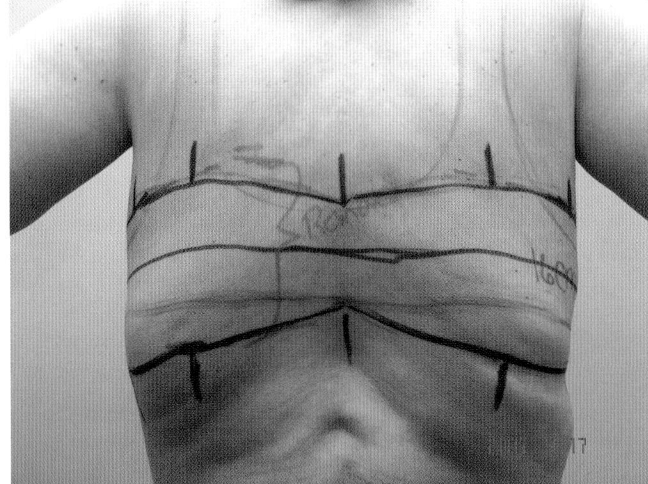

Fig. 13.106

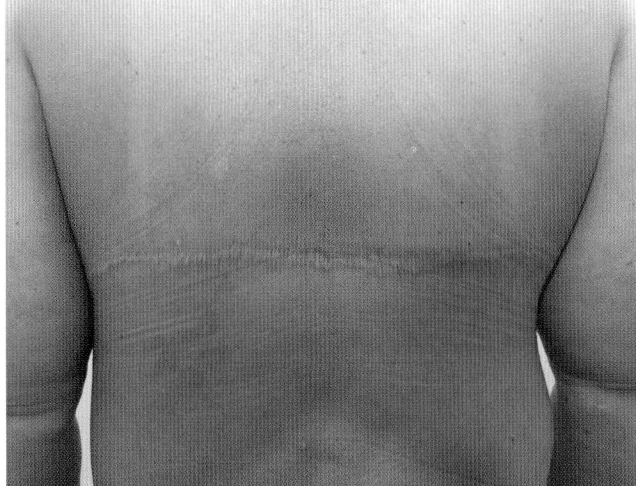

Fig. 13.107

Figs 13.102–13.107 Bra-line Back Lift Pre- and Postoperative Images For the patient with incomplete weight loss with residual laxity and excess adiposity, a bra-line back lift can also be highly effective. The removal of redundant skin and underlying subcutaneous tissue has a pleasing thinning effect that improves the overall shape and contour. The final scar is easily concealed within the bra.

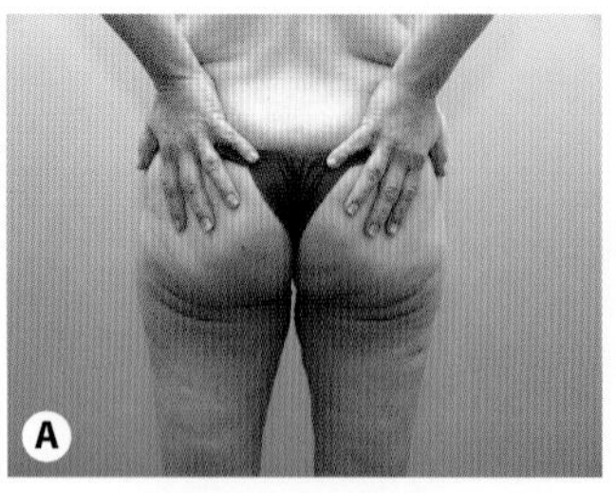
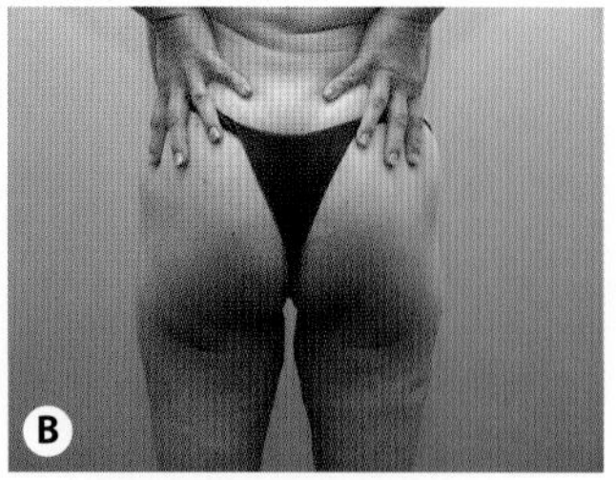
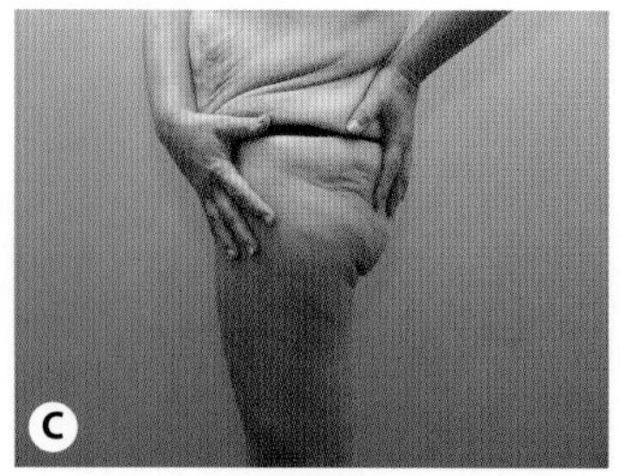
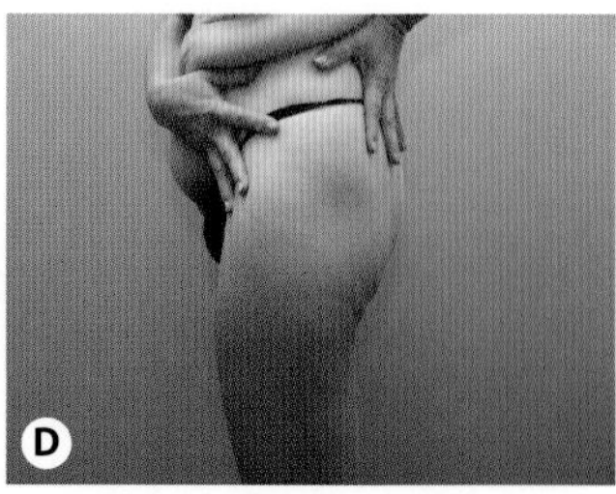

Fig. 13.108 Autologous Buttocks Augmentation Images A–D Patients interested in autologous buttocks augmentation and body lift will demonstrate their desire by strongly lifting their buttocks and thigh soft tissue to demonstrate their desired final appearance.

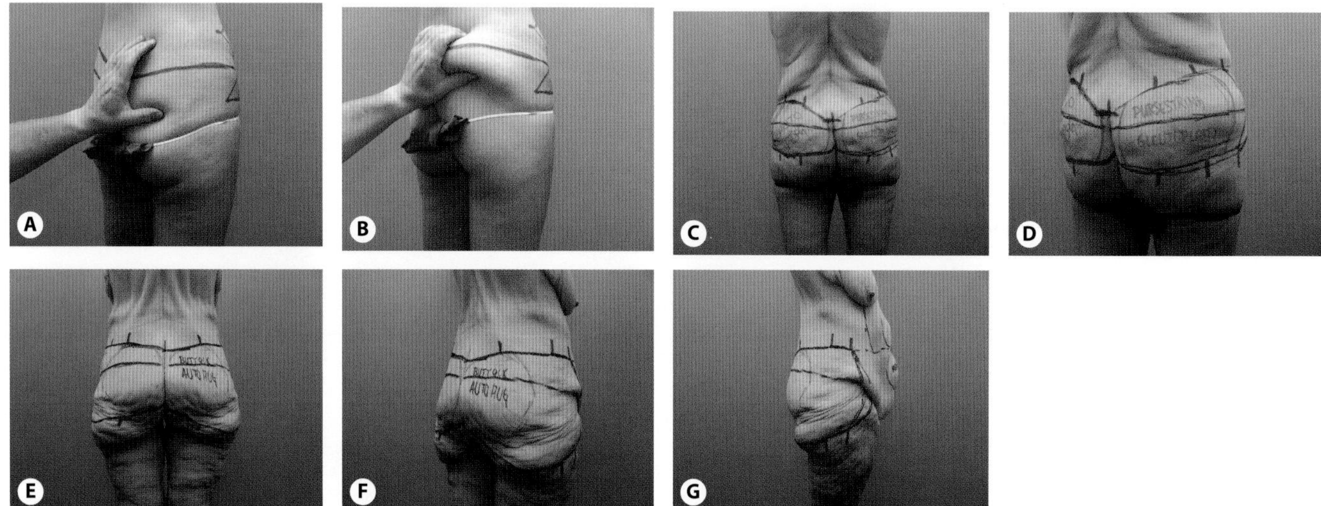

Fig. 13.109 Autologous Buttocks Augmentation Images A–G The final incision line for the buttocks lift as an isolated procedure, or the posterior part of the circumferential abdominoplasty, is marked, ending at the gluteal apex. If the buttocks laxity is significant, the incision can be placed relatively high. If the laxity is less, the final incision should be placed lower. Strong bimanual palpation is used to determine the excess tissue that will be utilized for autologous buttocks augmentation. Realignment marks are placed to facilitate closure. The autologous buttocks tissue is marked within the resection margins, with the inner and outer edges of the central mound marked to correspond to the desired buttock shape. The tissue medial and lateral to the central mound will be resected.

it uses the central mound of soft tissue with completely reliable vascularity. We have found that the central mound technique is simple and reliable, and the purse-string component provides the increased projection needed to achieve excellent results.[5]

Operative Approach

Patients will often demonstrate their desire for buttocks augmentation and lifting by pulling up on their buttocks and thigh tissue, demonstrating their desired result (**Fig. 13.108 A–D**). The markings are made in a fashion similar to the posterior component of a circumferential abdominoplasty. The position of the final scar is marked, usually somewhat more caudally than usual, so that the central tissue mound will be in a better location for buttock augmentation. For this procedure the final incision line is usually oriented horizontally, as opposed to a 'gull wing' configuration, which is often described for the posterior component of a circumferential abdominoplasty (**Fig. 13.109 A–G**). An estimate of the amount of tissue to be incorporated into the autologous buttocks augmentation is made using bimanual palpation. Vertical realignment marks are placed to facilitate proper closure. The lateral extent of the tissue to be maintained corresponds to the outer contour of the buttocks.

The patient is brought to the operating room and placed in the prone position. Appropriate padding and sequential compression pumps on the lower extremities are used. Penetrating towel clamps can be used to check that the markings are correct and that closure can be performed without undue tension (**Fig. 13.110 A–E**). The realignment marks are then tattooed with methylene blue, which further assures proper realignment on closure (**Fig. 13.111 A, B**).

Dilute lidocaine containing epinephrine is infiltrated into the incision lines and under the skin overlying the gluteal mound to facilitate hemostasis (**Fig. 13.112 A, B**). This is done prior to full prepping and draping to allow the epinephrine to take maximum effect before the procedure begins (**Fig. 13.113**). The incisions are made with a number 10 scalpel partway through the dermis, then electrocautery is used to complete the incisions and continue the dissection through the subcutaneous tissue down to the muscle

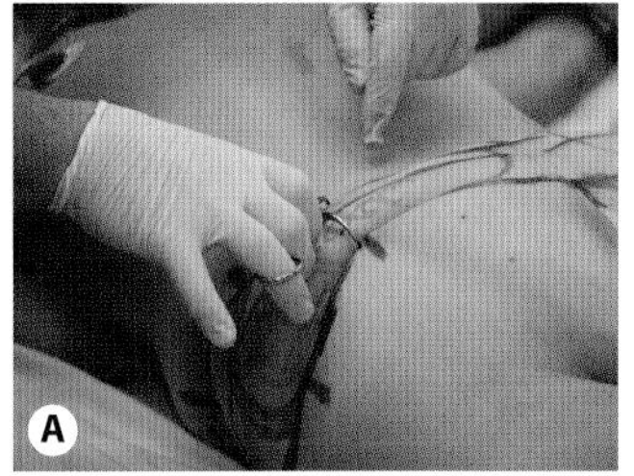
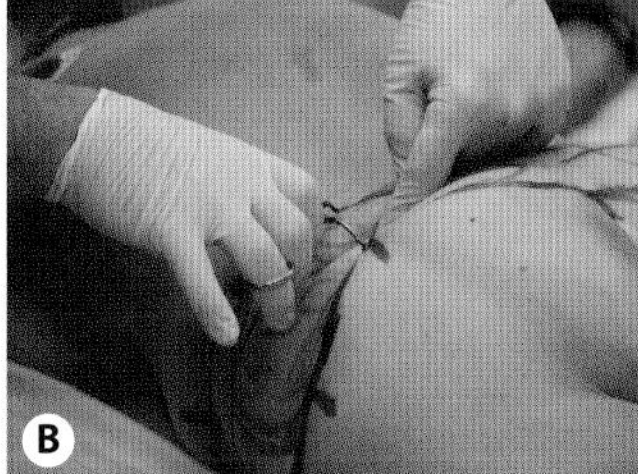
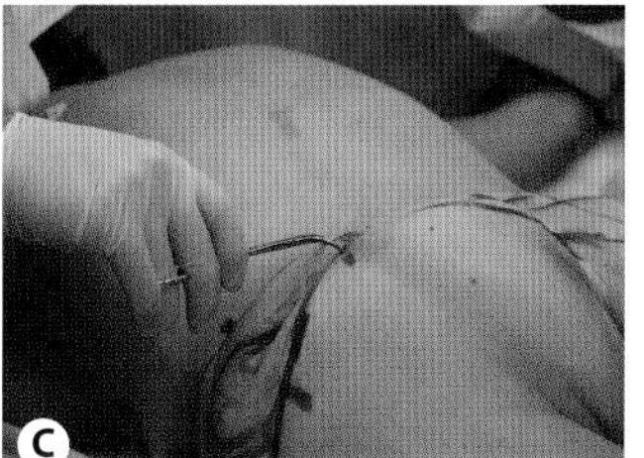
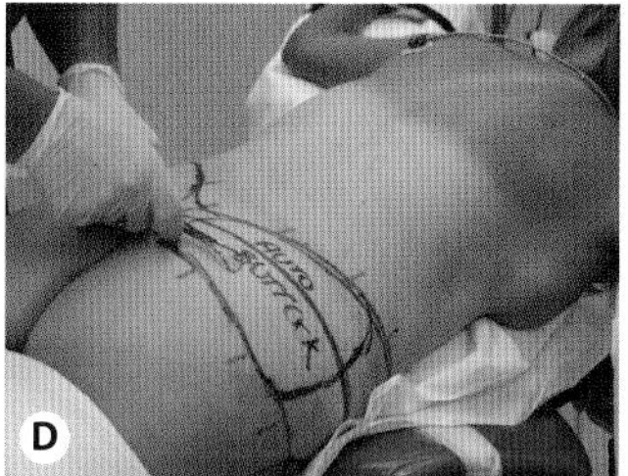
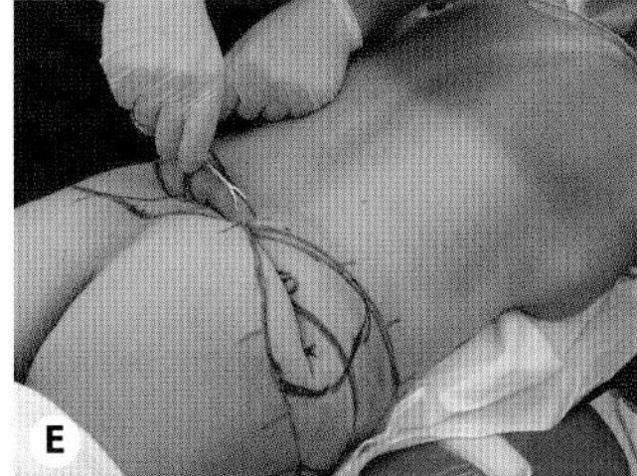

Fig. 13.110 Autologous Buttocks Augmentation Images A–E For a patient undergoing a circumferential abdominoplasty all areas for anterior suctioning are thoroughly infiltrated with tumescent fluid, and the incision line is infiltrated as well before the patient is turned into the prone position. For an isolated buttocks lift and augmentation, the patient is placed in the prone position and infiltration is then performed. With the patient in the prone position, a penetrating towel clamp is used to confirm that the width of the planned resection is appropriate. The estimated tension on closure should not be significant since the intervening tissue will be used for buttocks augmentation.

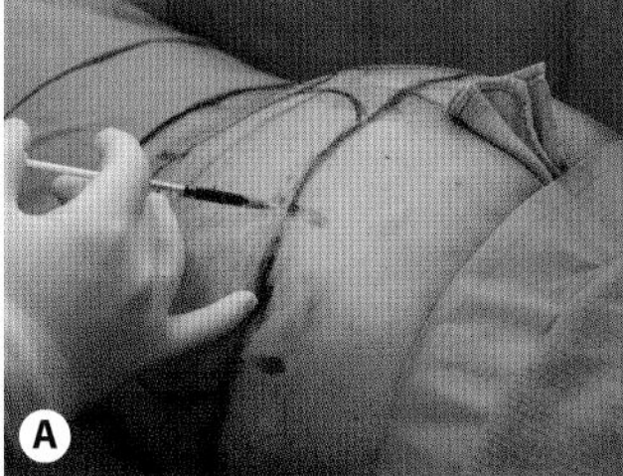
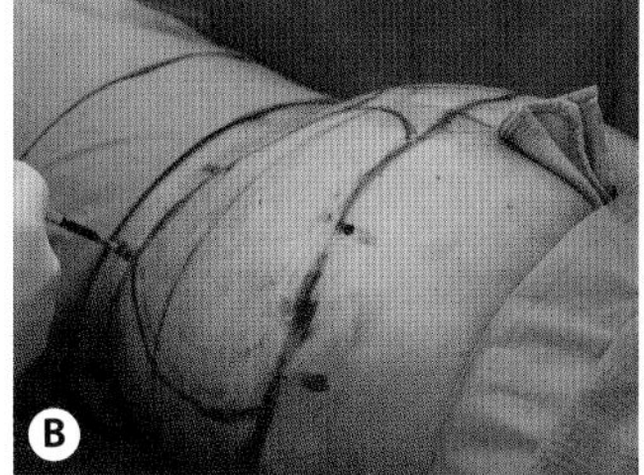

Fig. 13.111 Autologous Buttocks Augmentation Images A, B Methylene blue is used to tattoo the realignment marks to assure precise reapproximation during closure.

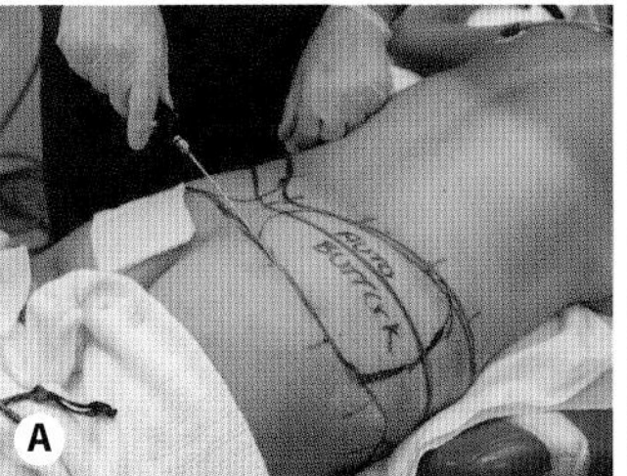
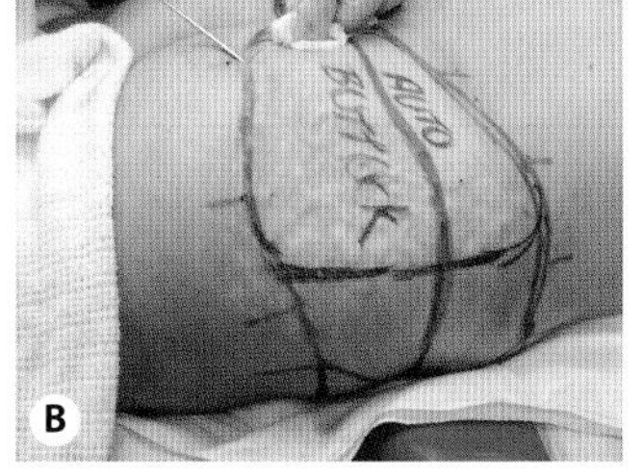

Fig. 13.112 Autologous Buttocks Augmentation Images A, B Infiltration of dilute epinephrine-containing fluid is performed immediately beneath the skin of the buttocks augmentation tissue and in the incision lines. This central mound will be de-epithelialized, and the infiltration facilitates dissection and minimizes bleeding.

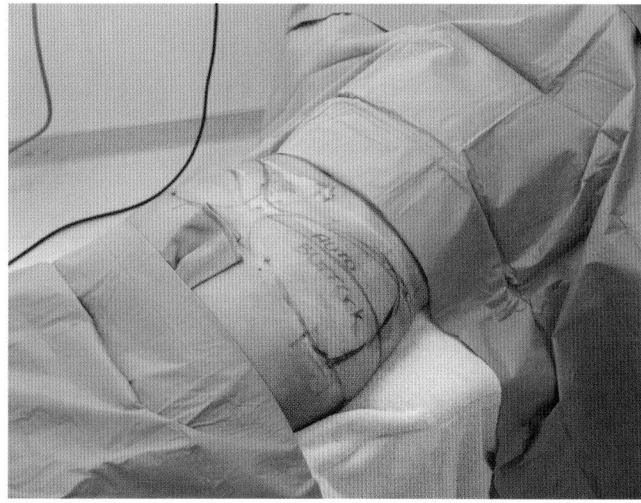

Fig. 13.113 Autologous Buttocks Augmentation Images Following infiltration, profound vasoconstriction of the incision line and the proposed flaps is seen.

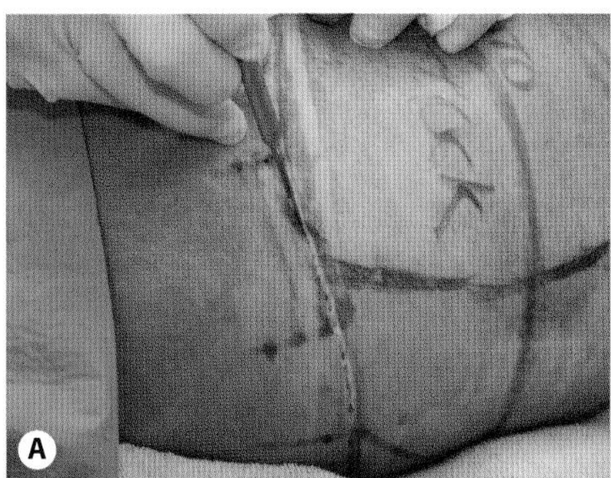
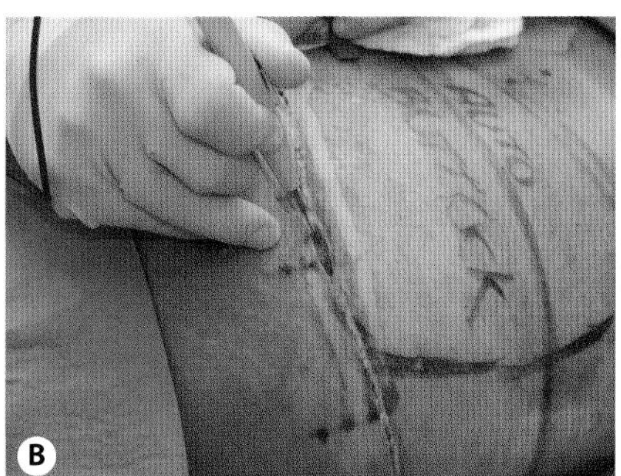
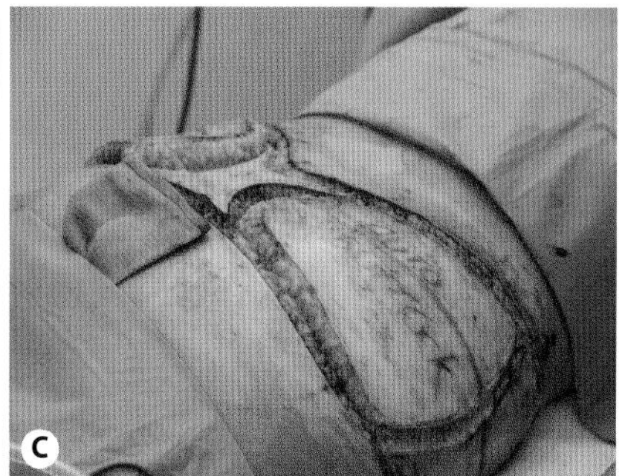

Fig. 13.114 Autologous Buttocks Augmentation Images A–C The incision is made into the dermis with a number 10 blade and then electrocautery is used to deepen the dissection through the dermis and subcutaneous tissue down to the muscle fascia.

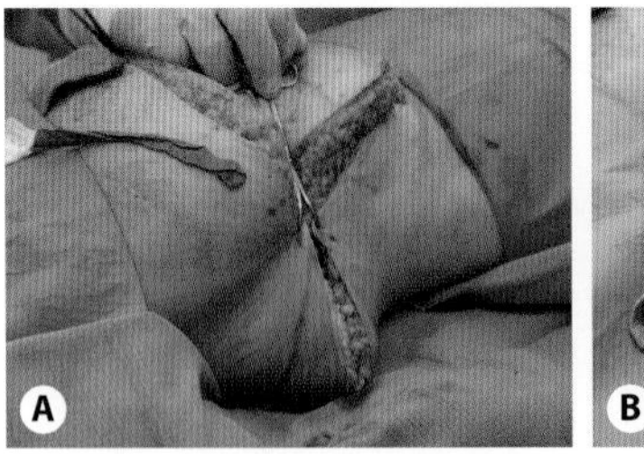

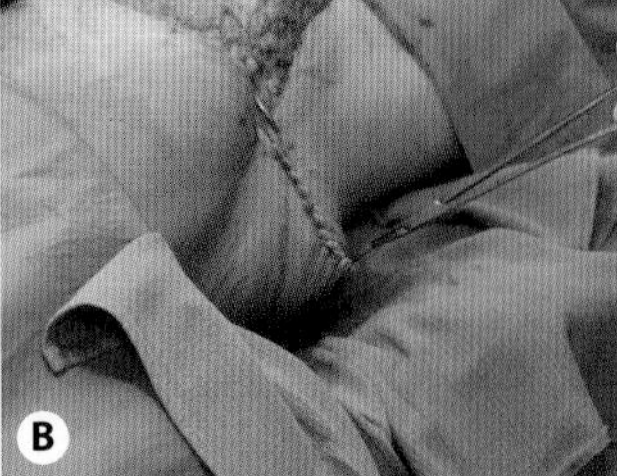

Fig. 13.115 Autologous Buttocks Augmentation Images
A, B When a circumferential abdominoplasty is being performed, a temporary V–Y closure is performed laterally. This signifies the division between the posterior and anterior resections.

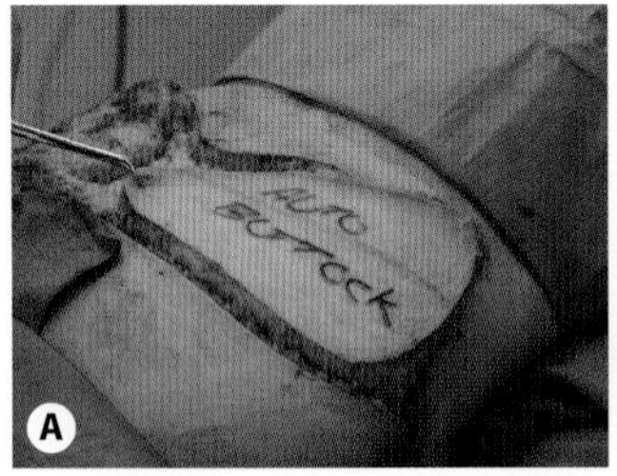

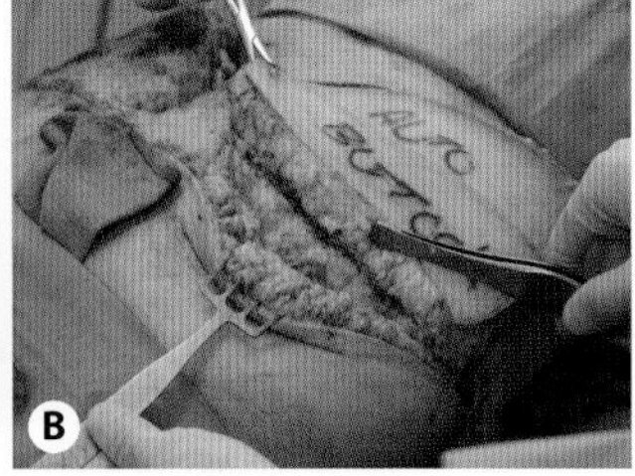

Fig. 13.116 Autologous Buttocks Augmentation Images
A, B The buttocks flaps are dissected down to the muscle fascia. The superficial fascia (SFS) is marked with methylene blue for easy identification.

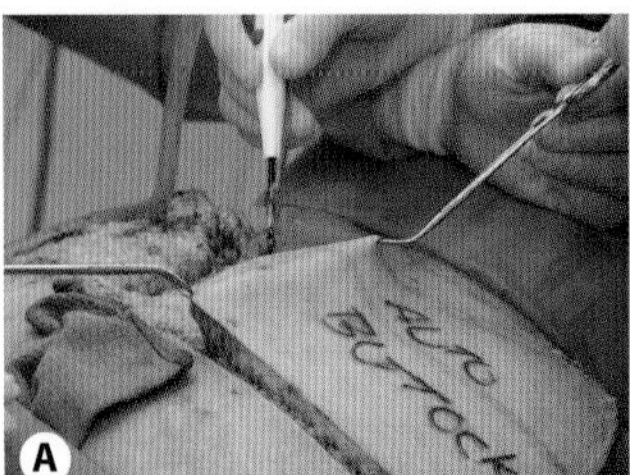

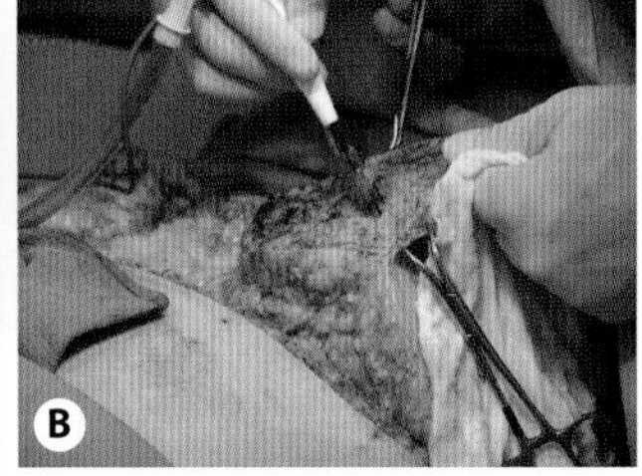

Fig. 13.117 Autologous Buttocks Augmentation Images
A, B The central mound is de-epithelialized or de-skinned using electrocautery.

fascia (**Fig. 13.114 A–C**). The tissue medial and lateral to the autologous flaps is resected and a temporary V–Y closure is performed laterally with number 1 Prolene (**Fig. 13.115 A, B**). The superficial fascia layer is identified and marked (**Fig. 13.116 A, B**). The central mounds are de-epithelialized or de-skinned with electrocautery (**Fig. 13.117 A, B**).

The purse-string suture is then placed at the level of the superficial fascia. Placement at this level is important, as placement at the edge of the de-epithelialized skin will create undesirable invagination of the soft tissue, as opposed to increased projection (**Fig. 13.118**). We use a number 1 braided polyester suture to perform the purse-string component of the procedure, taking equal but substantial bites along the way. Once the entire suture has been placed it is tightened, which narrows the base and increases the projection of the central mound (**Fig. 13.119 A–D**). The importance of the purse-string is immediately obvious on tightening: it creates a beautiful round shape that has impressive projection compared to the opposite side (**Fig. 13.120 A–C**).The dermis of the central mounds is then sutured to the midline at the level of the superficial fascia to prevent lateral or asymmetric displacement (**Fig. 13.121 A–C**).

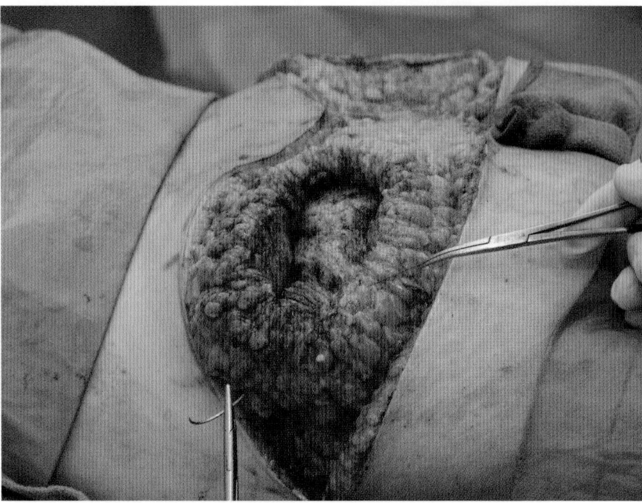

Fig. 13.118 Autologous Buttocks Augmentation Images
If the purse-string suture is placed in the dermis, the tissue everts and creates a 'doughnut' shape.

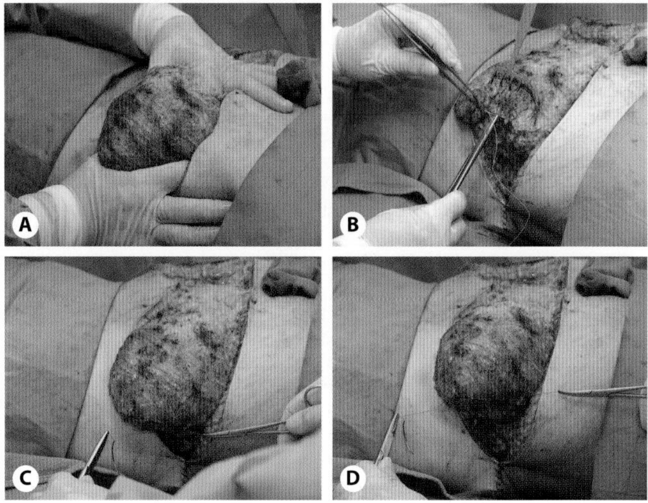

Fig. 13.119 Autologous Buttocks Augmentation Images
A–D The desired shape can be seen by cupping the tissue in the surgeon's hands. Placing the purse-string suture at the level of the superficial fascia and tightening it creates this exact shape. In reality the shape of the purse-stringed tissue is similar to the shape of a buttocks implant.

Undermining is performed as needed inferiorly to allow the autologous tissue to fit properly and to maximize buttock augmentation and shape (**Fig. 13.122 A–E**). Suction drains

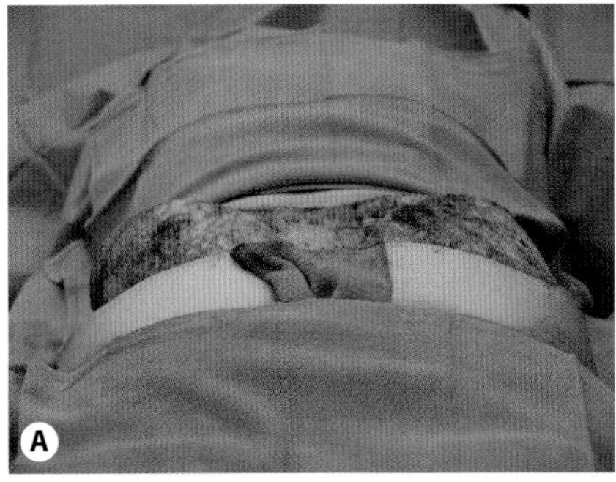
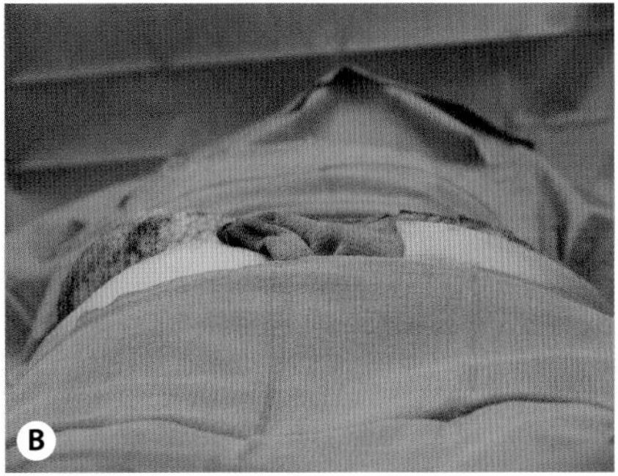
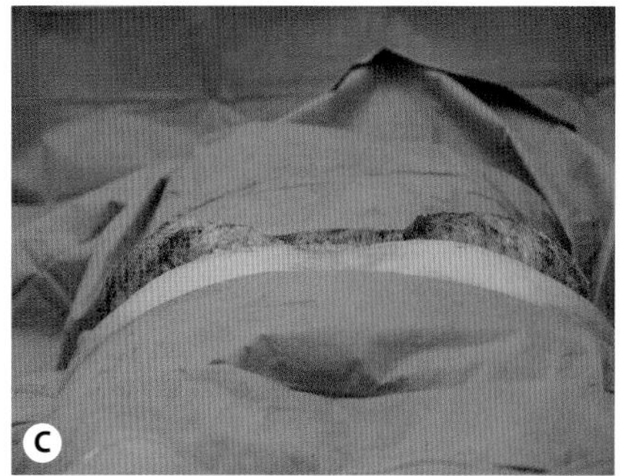

Fig. 13.120 Autologous Buttocks Augmentation Images The left buttocks flap is shaped and the right is not. A distinct difference is noted, with excellent projection and contour on the left side. When the purse-string suture is tightened on both flaps, a wonderful augmented appearance is seen.

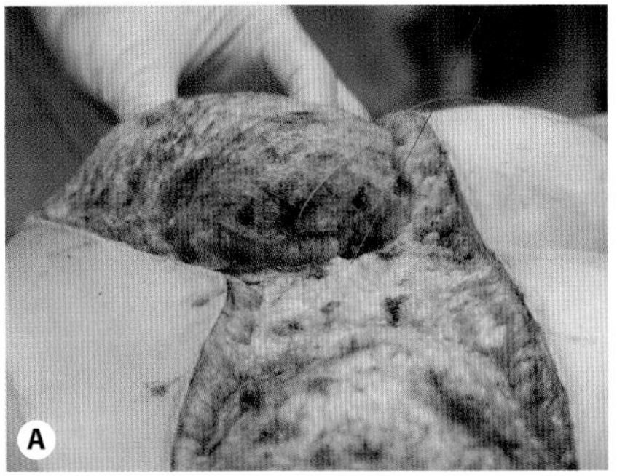
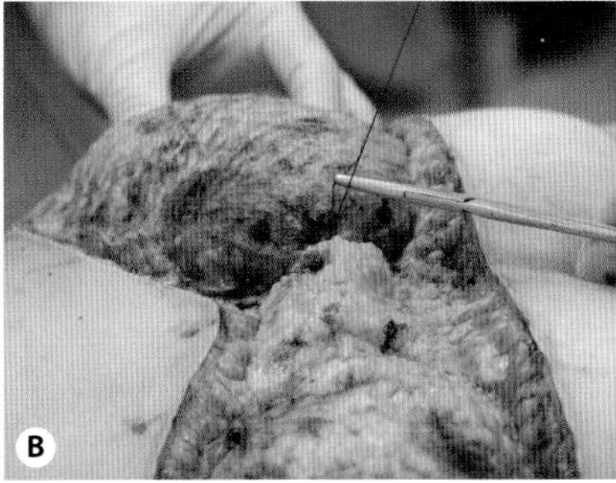
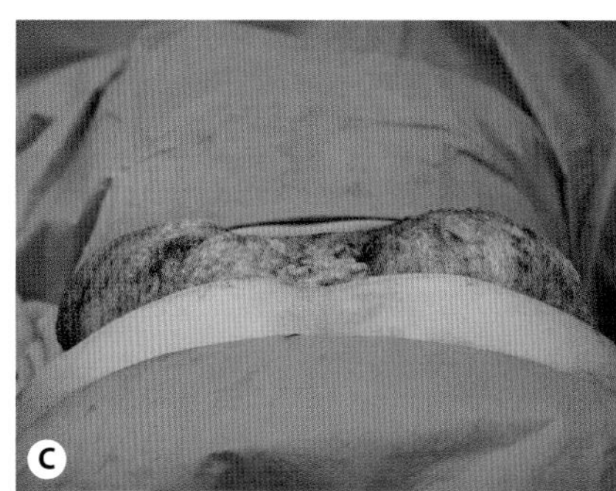

Fig. 13.121 Autologous Buttocks Augmentation Images A–C These flaps must be secured to the midline to prevent lateral displacement. The pressure of the lower buttock skin flap that is brought over the purse-string mound may cause them to move laterally, which is undesirable.

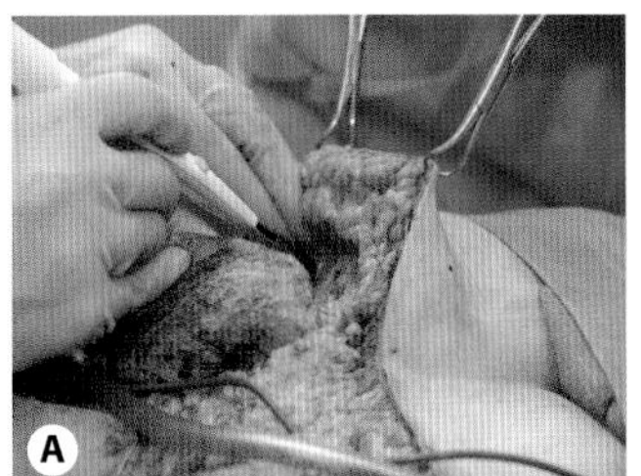
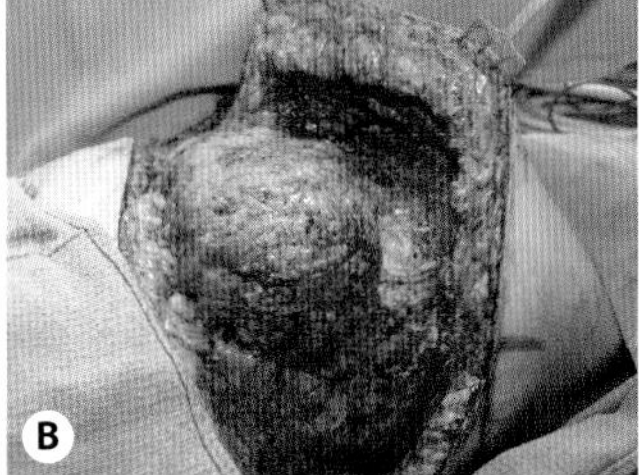
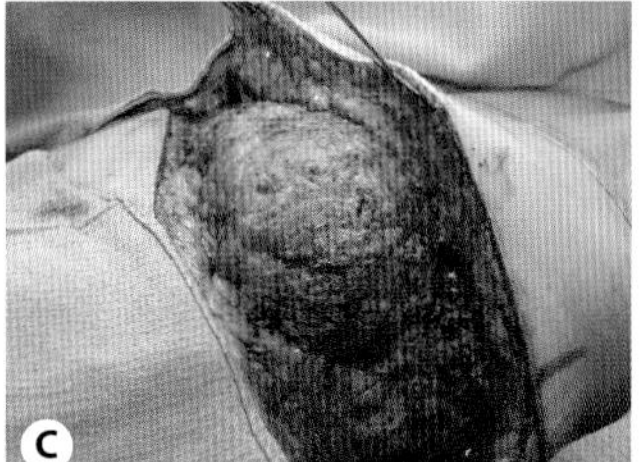
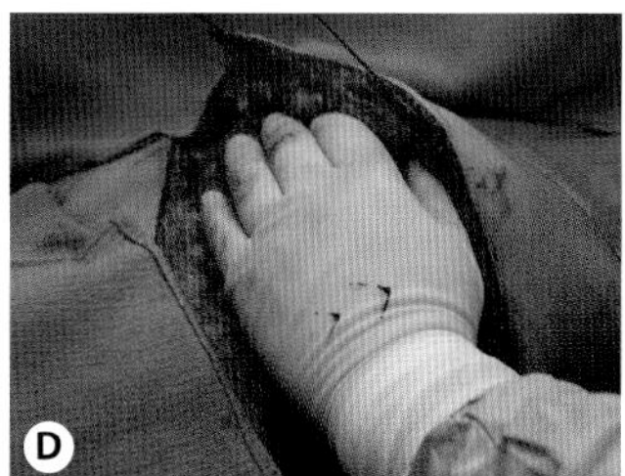
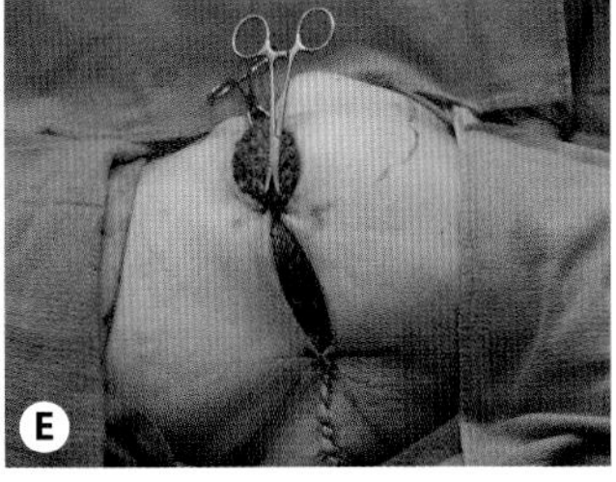

Fig. 13.122 Autologous Buttocks Augmentation Images A–E Undermining is performed as needed to allow for the lower buttocks tissue to be lifted over the newly formed autologous flaps. If the buttocks are extremely lax, undermining may not be necessary. In most cases, however, a moderate degree of undermining enhances the lifting of the lower buttocks tissue over the flaps and places them in an ideal position.

are placed and coiled beneath the temporary V–Y closure (**Fig. 13.123 A, B**). Incision line closure is performed in three layers. Temporary towel clips or staples are used to approximate the tissues, and then the superficial fascia is closed with either 0 or 1 Vicryl. The deep dermis is closed with buried interrupted 2/0 Vicryl, and the final intradermal closure is performed with 4/0 Monocryl. Tissue adhesive is then applied to providing a watertight seal (**Fig. 13.124 A–F**). The immediate result is dramatic and aesthetically pleasing.

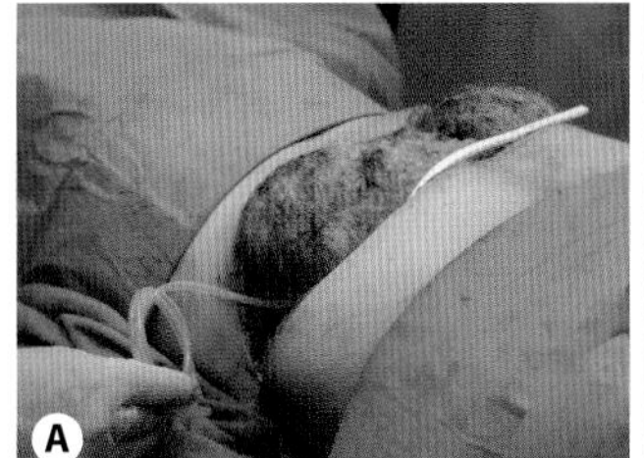
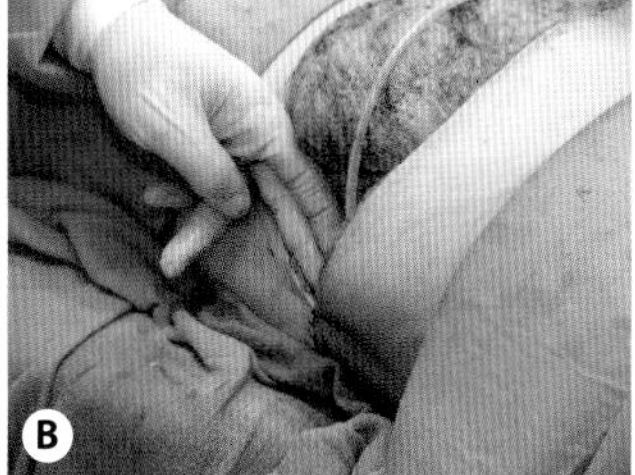

Fig. 13.123 Autologous Buttocks Augmentation Images A, B A Jackson Pratt drain is placed bilaterally, coiled, and placed beneath the temporary V–Y closure.

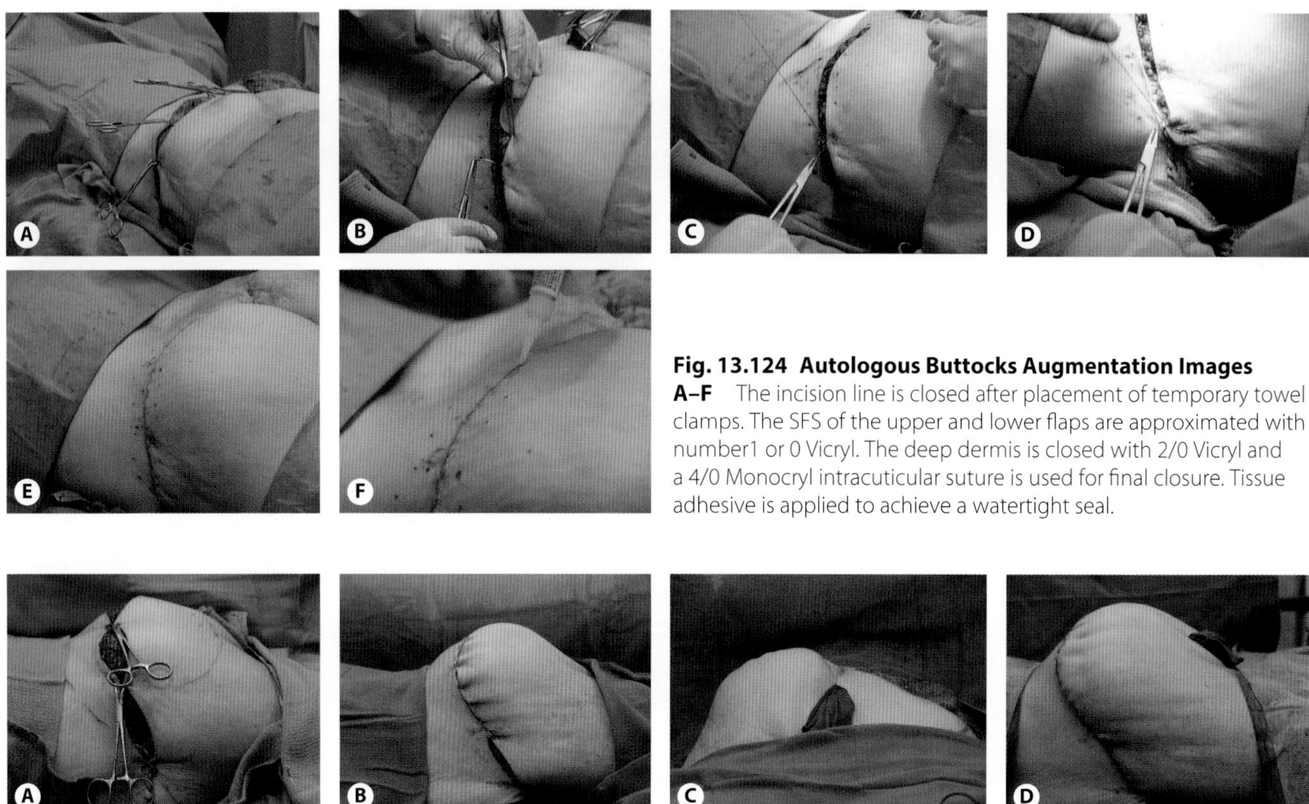

Fig. 13.124 Autologous Buttocks Augmentation Images A–F The incision line is closed after placement of temporary towel clamps. The SFS of the upper and lower flaps are approximated with number1 or 0 Vicryl. The deep dermis is closed with 2/0 Vicryl and a 4/0 Monocryl intracuticular suture is used for final closure. Tissue adhesive is applied to achieve a watertight seal.

Fig. 13.125 Autologous Buttocks Augmentation Images A, B An impressive augmentation is achieved with this technique achieving not only excellent lifting but also dramatic projection. **C, D** The completed left purse-string gluteoplasty. The difference between the left and the right sides is dramatic. The left side is narrow, lifted and projecting, whereas the right side is wide and flat. The final appearance can be very impressive.

A certain amount of relaxation will undoubtedly occur, but this technique has been reliable in achieving and maintaining buttocks volume and projection (**Fig. 13.125 A–D**).

Postoperative Care

No compression garments are used following this procedure. Patients are asked to sit very gently on a pillow or cushion as opposed to a hard surface, and are given prescriptions for antibiotics and pain medication. Periodic ambulation ensures pressure relief on the buttocks as well as reducing the likelihood of deep-vein thrombosis (DVT). Careful follow-up is performed within a few days to make sure healing is progressing as expected, as well as to answer any questions that may arise. Drains are removed when the drainage amount decreases to less than 30–50 mL per 24-hour period.

Before and After Figures for Purse-String Gluteoplasty (Figs 13.126–13.166)

Buttocks Augmentation with Fat Grafting

Buttocks augmentation using autologous fat is appealing to many patients, particularly those who have excess adiposity and those who do not wish to have an alloplastic buttocks implant. Autologous augmentation using a patient's own fat has many advantages. The combination of liposuction of areas of excess adiposity, including the lumbar area, the hips, and the posterior thighs, together with grafting of the harvested fat into the buttocks, is a powerful way to increase the projection of the gluteal area relative to the surrounding areas.[6,7] The grafted fat is soft and pliable, and homogeneous with the surrounding tissues. As opposed to alloplastic gluteal implants, once the initial healing process has occurred and the balance of fat absorption and fat take has been achieved, no further procedures will be needed. The issue of capsule contracture, seroma, infection, and implant malposition are significantly reduced or non-existent with fat grafting.

Operative Approach

The procedure begins as with other liposuction procedures, including careful preoperative photography and marking of all areas for suctioning. The area for buttocks augmentation is also marked, as well as entry sites for both liposuction

Fig. 13.126–13.131

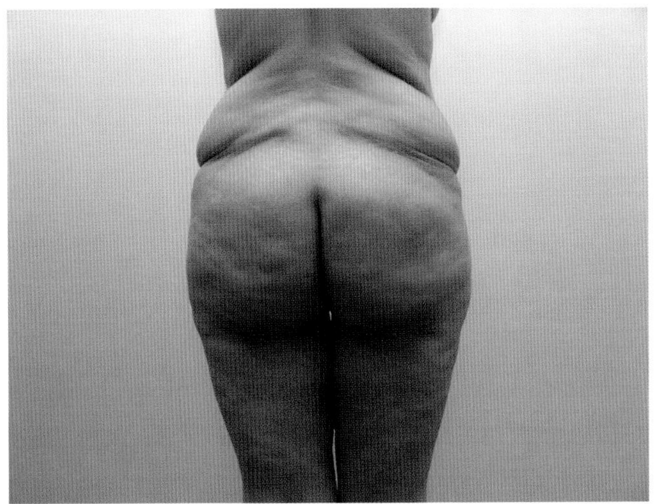

Fig. 13.126

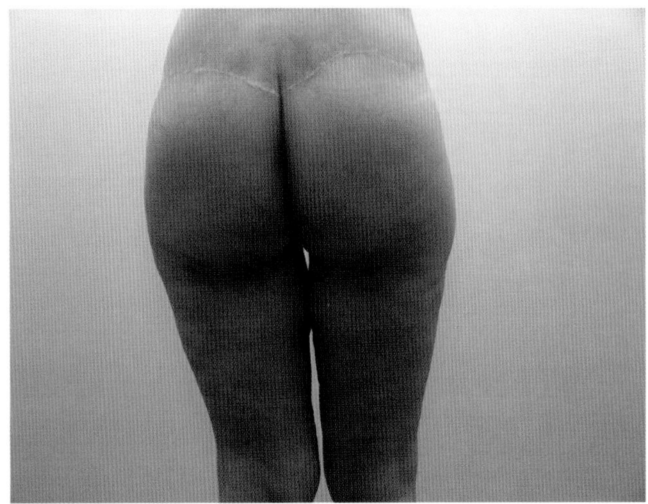

Fig. 13.127

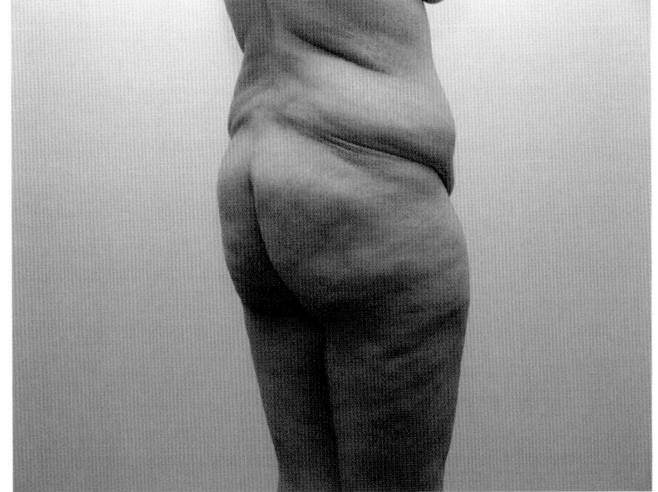

Fig. 13.128

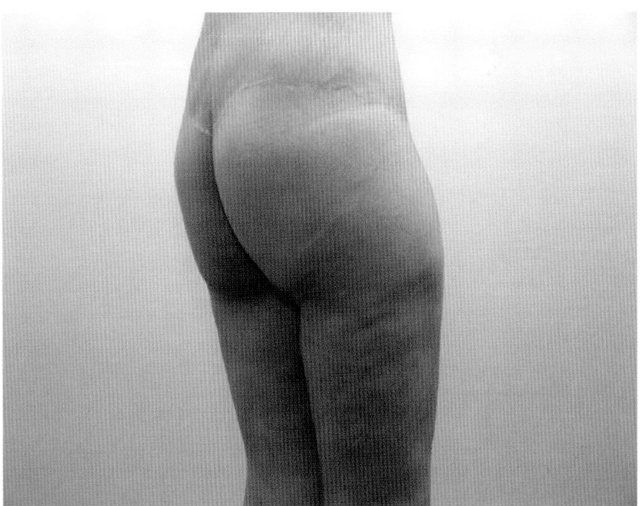

Fig. 13.129

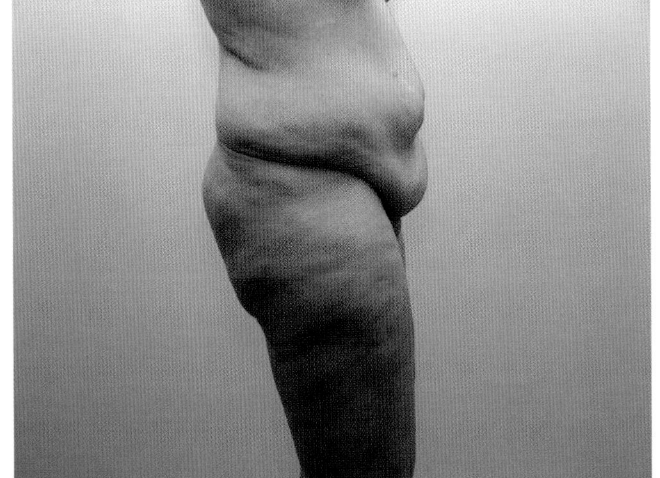

Fig. 13.130

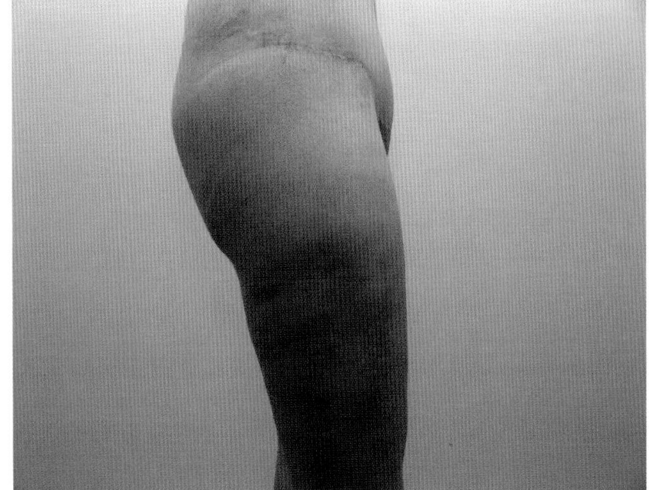

Fig. 13.131

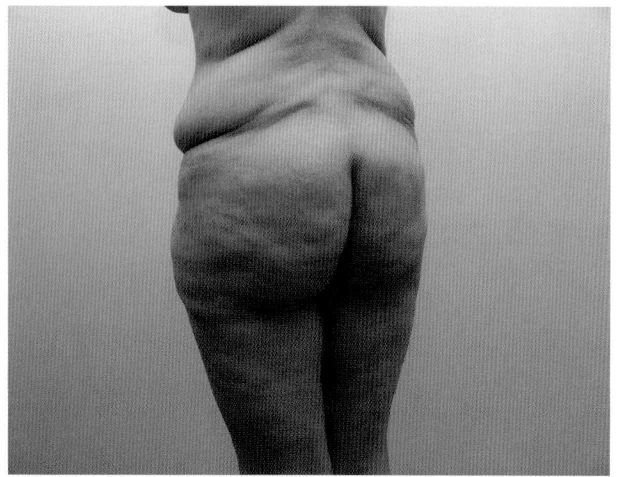

Fig. 13.132

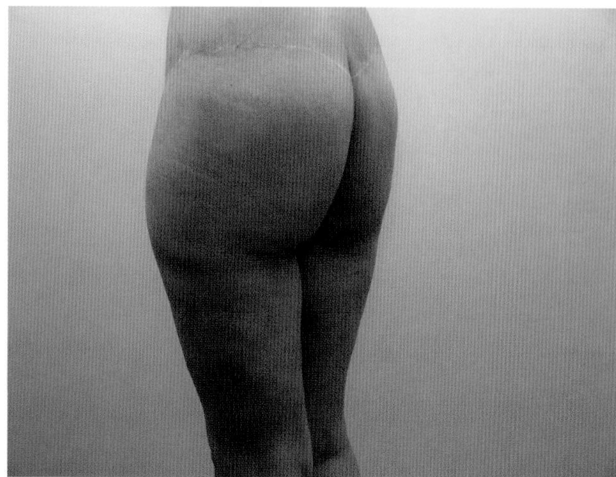

Fig. 13.133

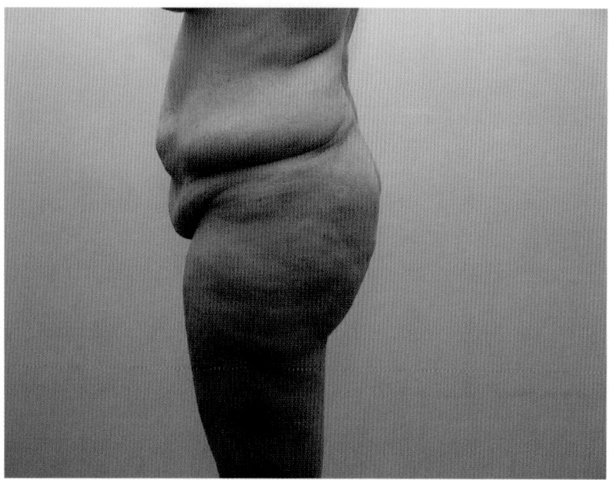

Fig. 13.134

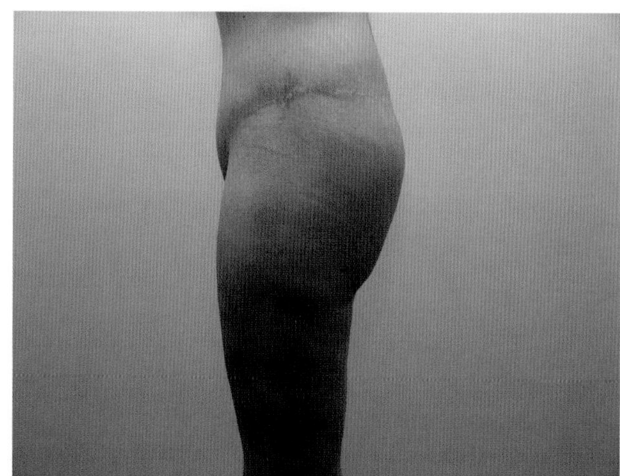

Fig. 13.135

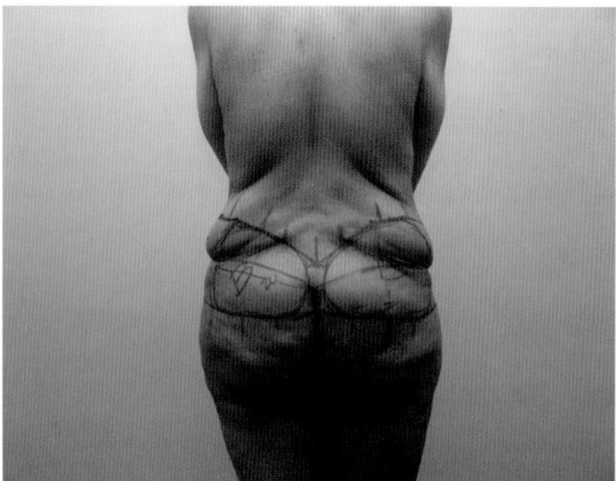

Fig. 13.136

Fig. 13.126–13.136 Autologous Buttocks Pre- and Postoperative Images Pre- and postoperative images of a patient who underwent a circumferential abdominoplasty with autologous purse-string gluteoplasty. The lifting, fullness, projection and shape following this procedure are dramatic. The markings reveal the areas for buttock tissue augmentation as well as the area for resection. The final incision line is well healed and the lifting and projection of the buttocks are excellent.

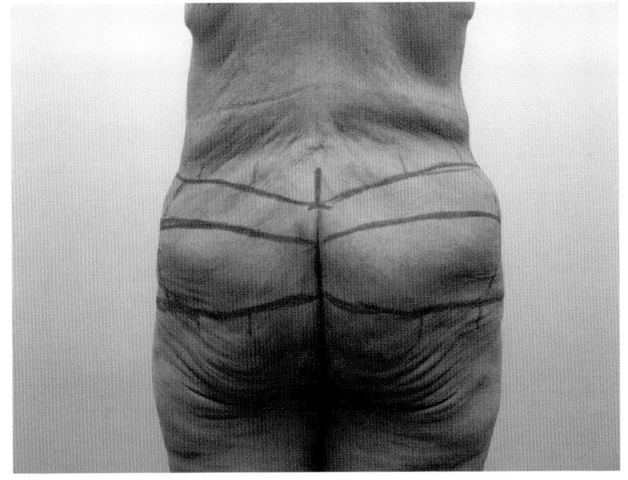

Fig. 13.137

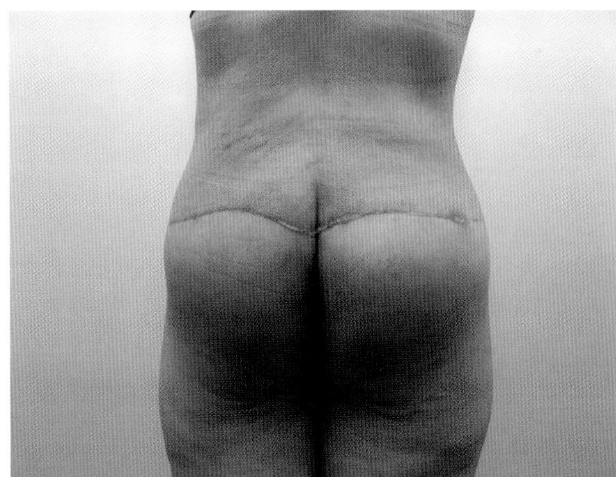

Fig. 13.138

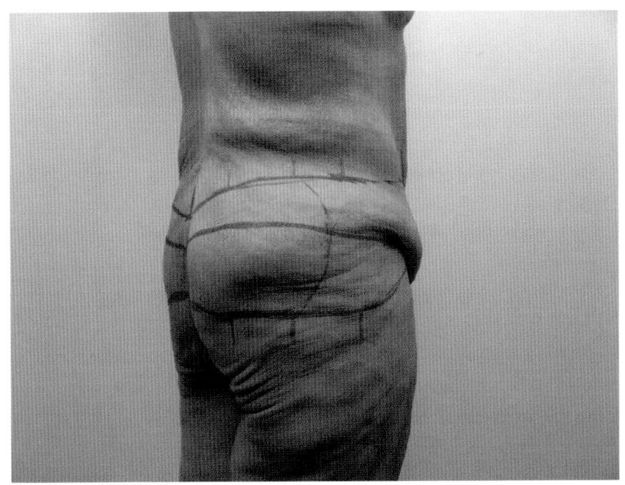

Fig. 13.139

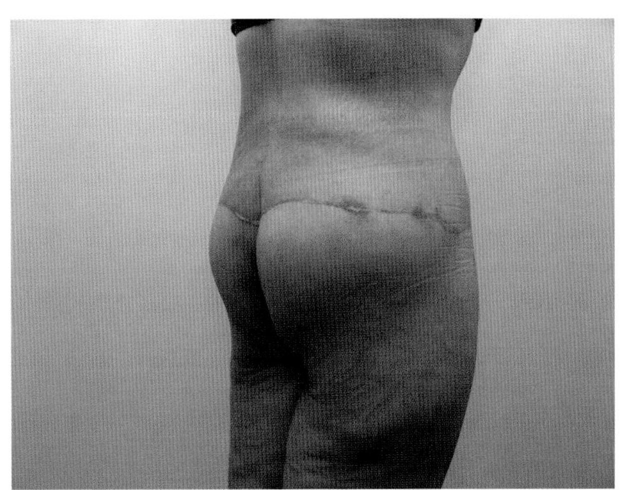

Fig. 13.140

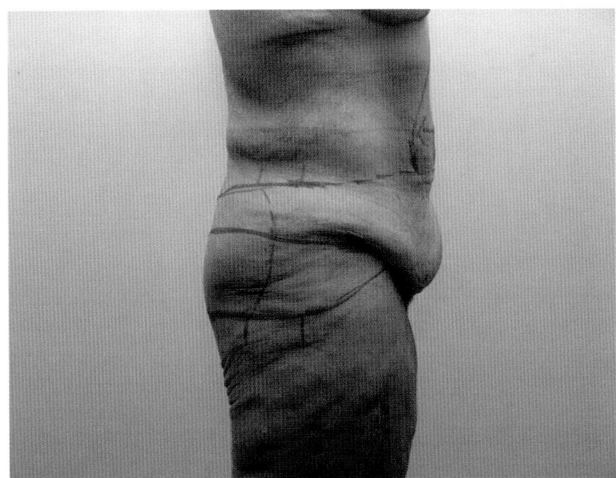

Fig. 13.141

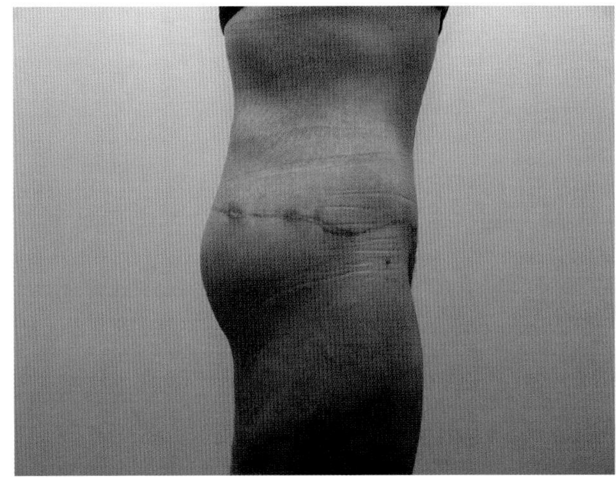

Fig. 13.142

Figs 13.136–13.143

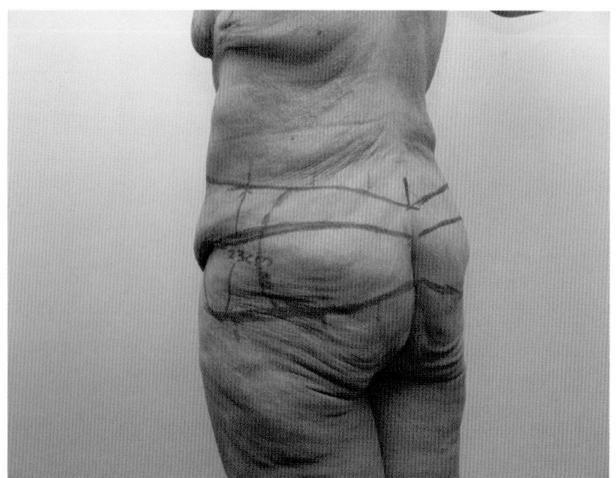

Fig. 13.143

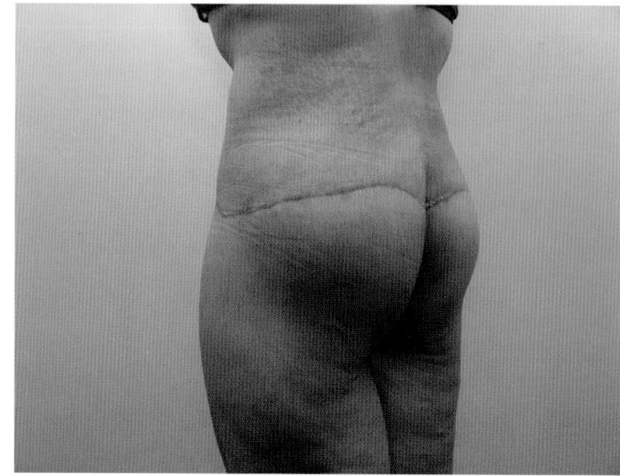

Fig. 13.144

Figs 13.137–13.144 Autologous Buttocks Pre- and Postoperative Images This patient experienced massive weight loss following the successful treatment of Cushing's disease. She was very frustrated with her circumferential body laxity and buttocks flattening and desired buttock augmentation. A circumferential abdominoplasty with autologous purse-string gluteoplasty was performed, allowing lifting, shaping, and projection of the buttocks as well as tightening and smoothing of the buttock skin without the use of silicone implants. A dramatic transformation in overall body shape and contour was achieved.

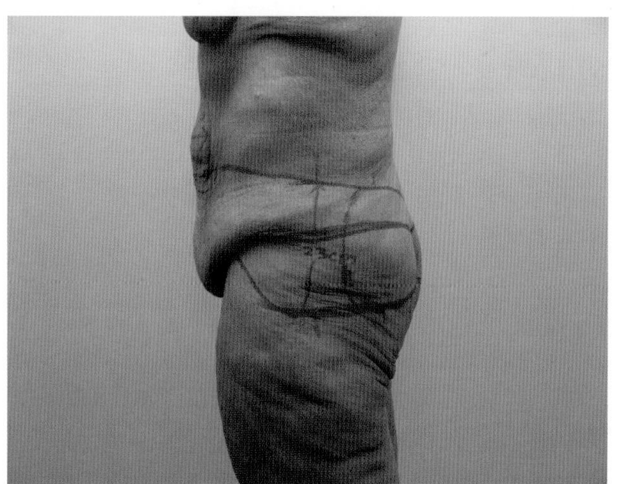

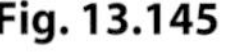

Fig. 13.145

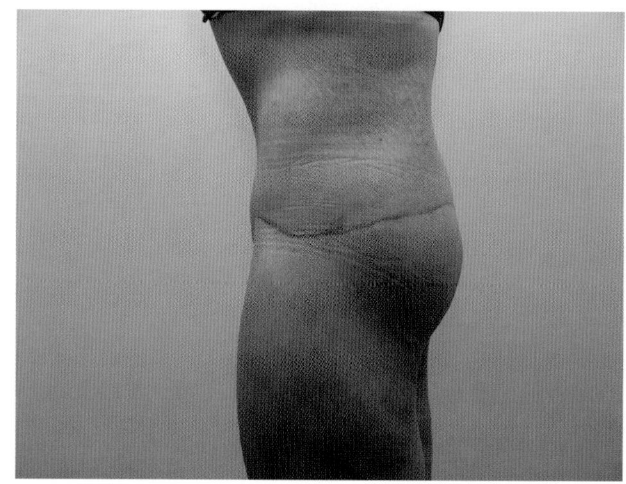

Fig. 13.146

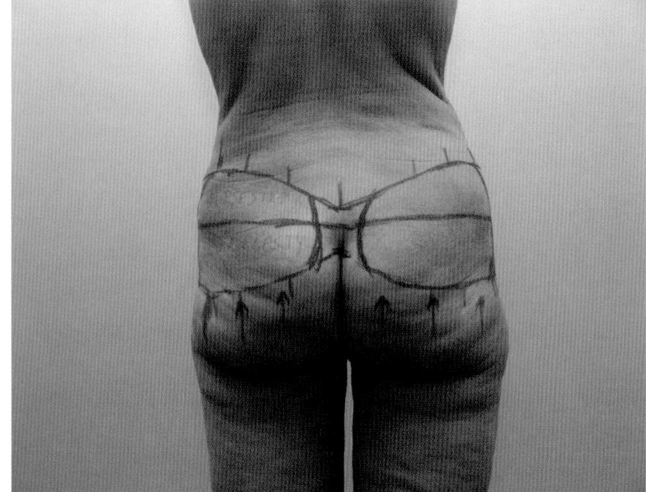

Fig. 13.147

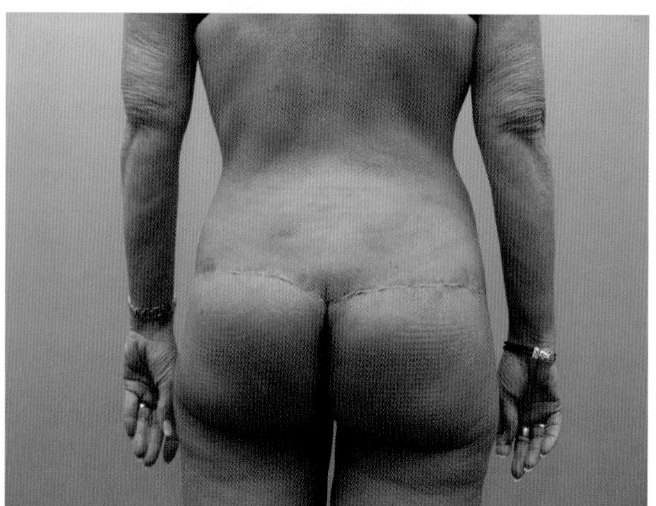

Fig. 13.148

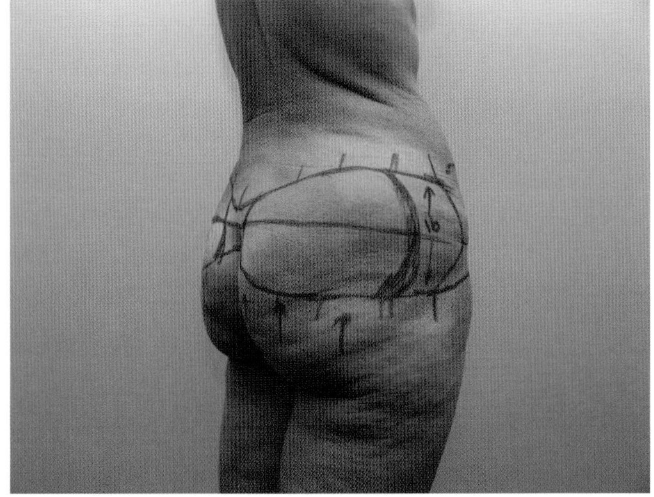

Fig. 13.149

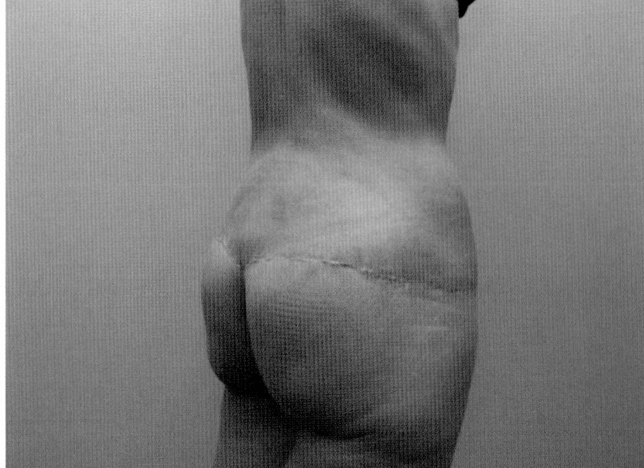

Fig. 13.150

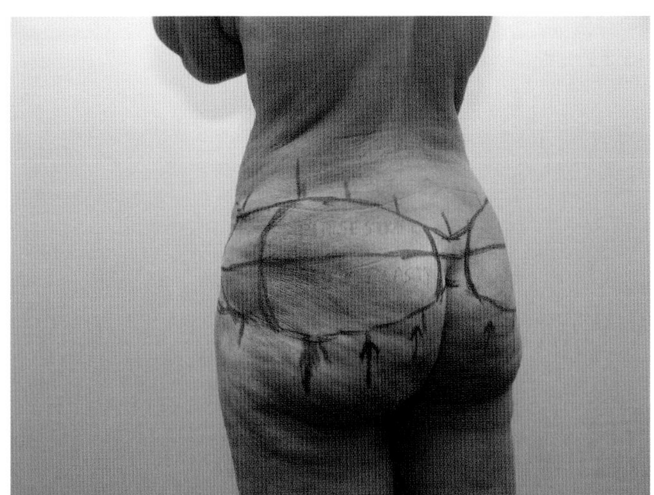

Fig. 13.151

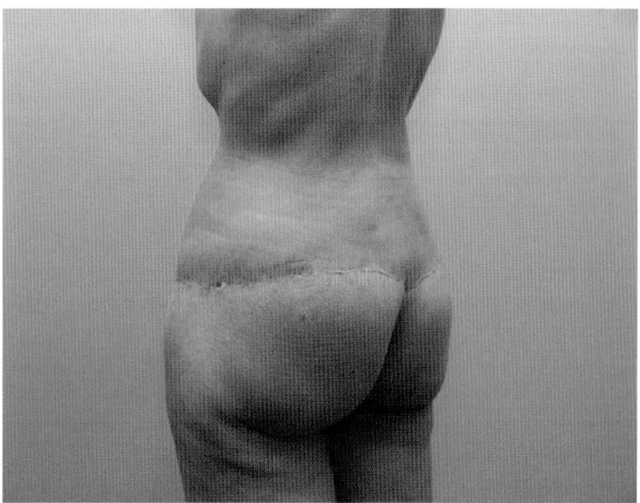

Fig. 13.152

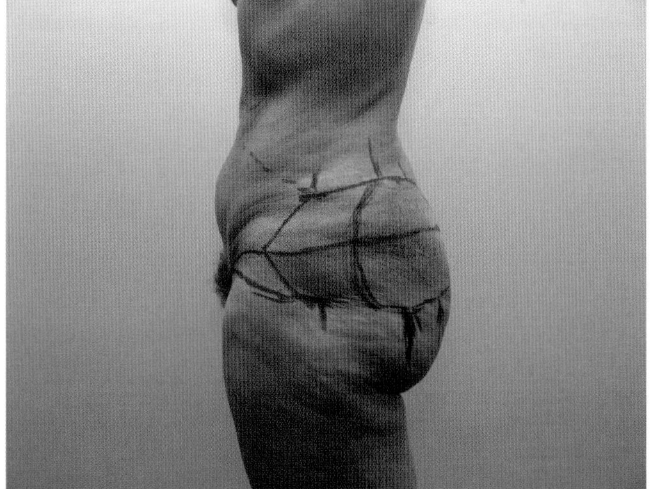

Fig. 13.153

Fig. 13.154

Figs 13.145–13.154 Autologous Buttocks Pre- and Postoperative Images This patient had significant weight loss without surgery. She was concerned about her circumferential laxity and buttock ptosis, and desired enhanced buttock fullness. She underwent a circumferential abdominoplasty with autologous purse-string gluteoplasty, and achieved a significant enhancement in skin tone, silhouette, shape, and contour as well as buttock lifting and projection.

Figs 13.155–13.160

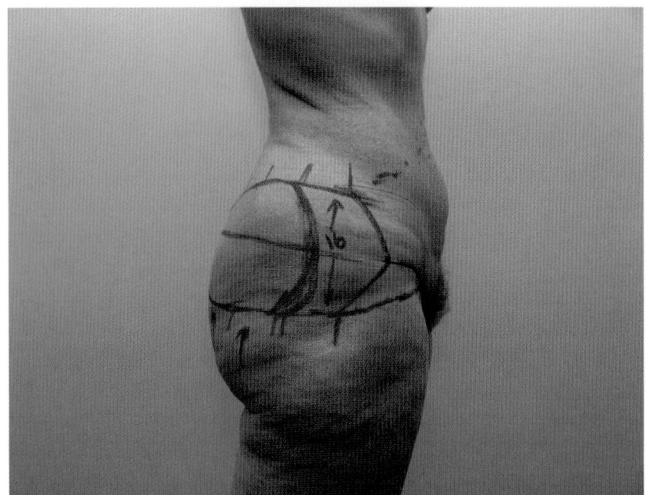

Fig. 13.155

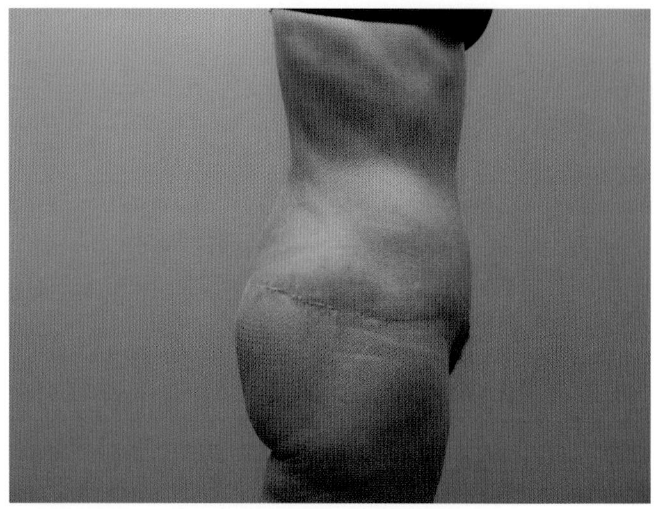

Fig. 13.156

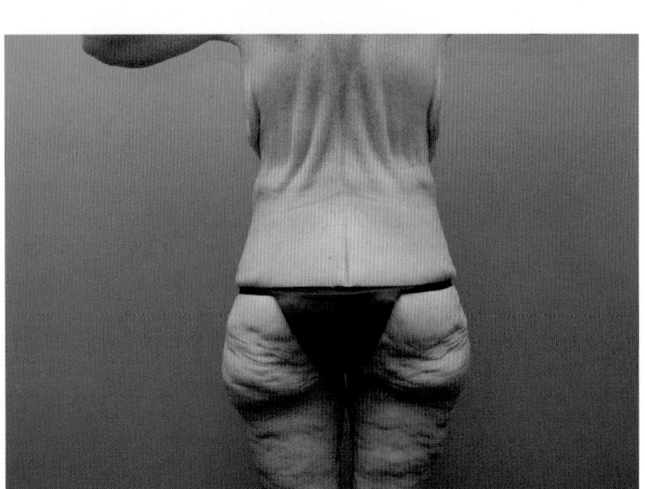

Fig. 13.157

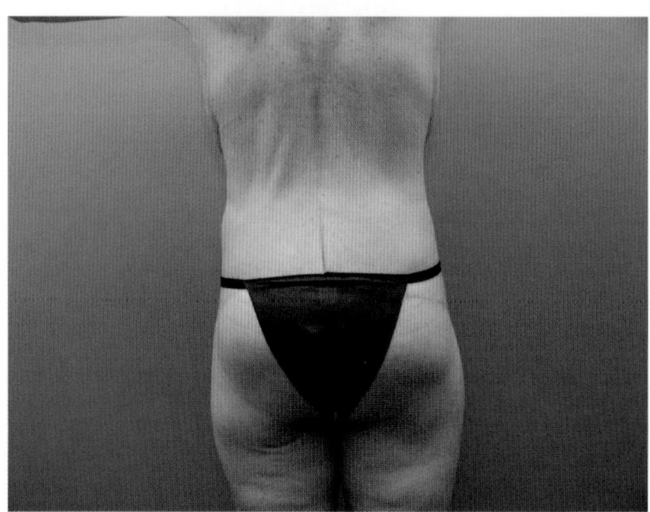

Fig. 13.158

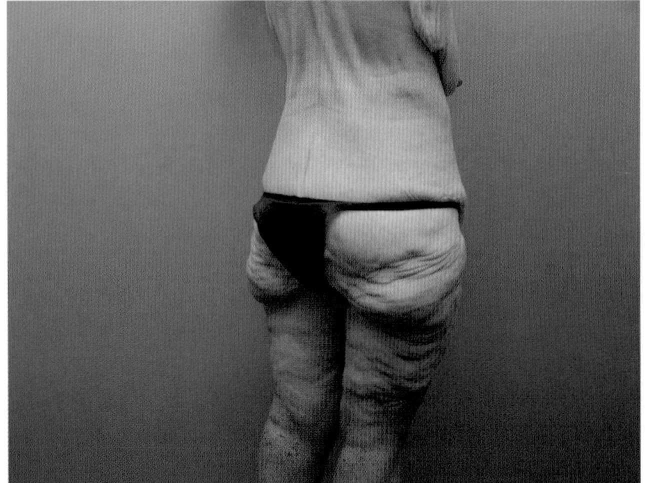

Fig. 13.159

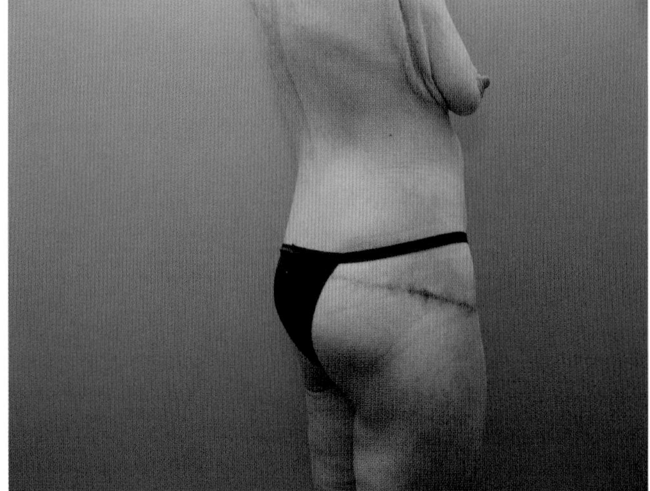

Fig. 13.160

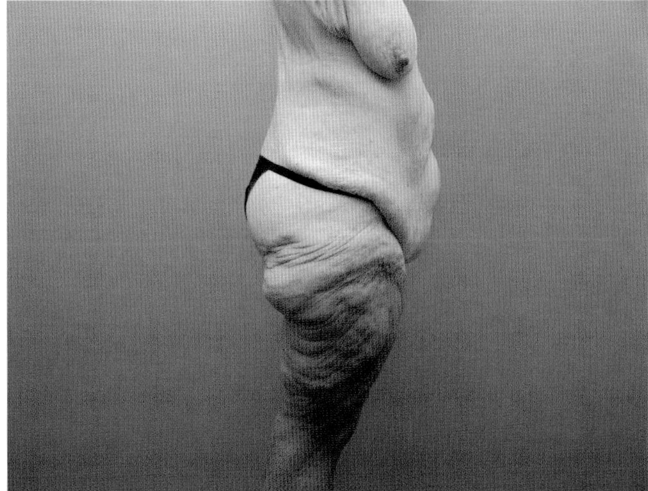

Fig. 13.161

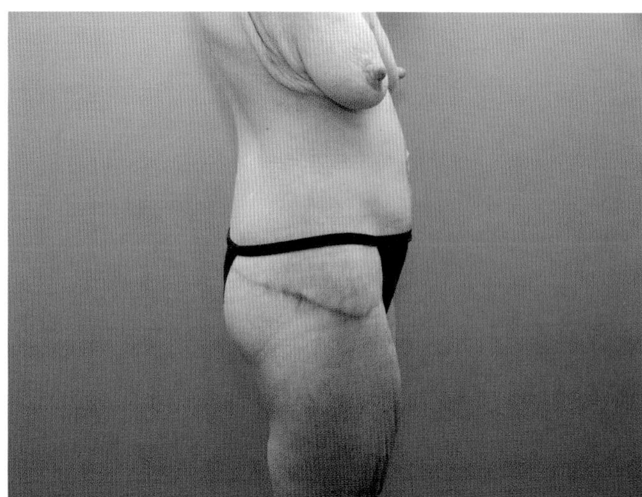

Fig. 13.162

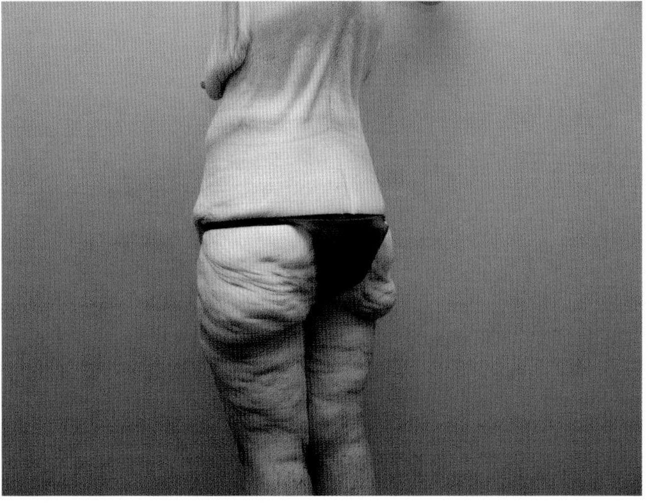

Fig. 13.163

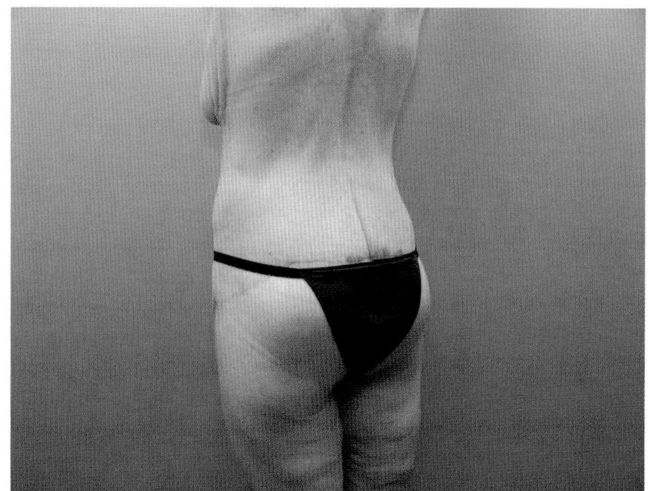

Fig. 13.164

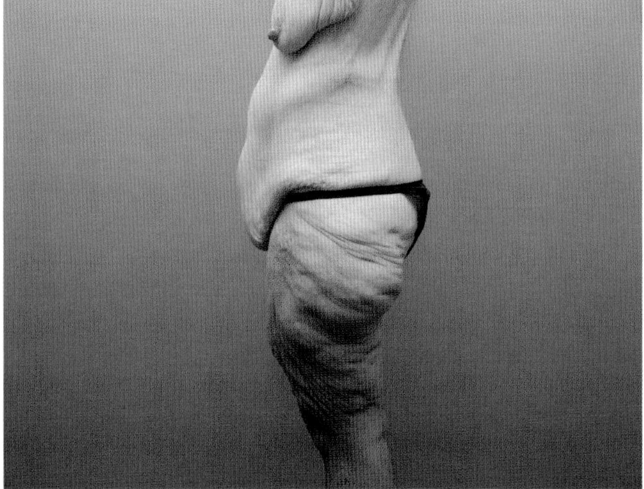

Fig. 13.165

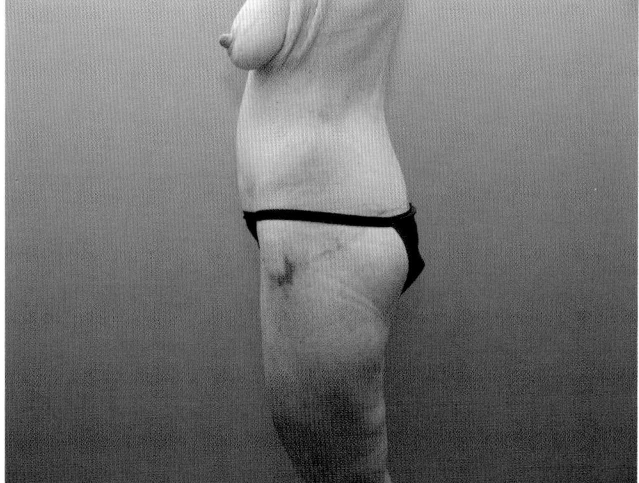

Fig. 13.166

Figs 13.155–13.166 Autologous Buttocks Pre- and Postoperative Images This patient experienced massive weight loss following bariatric surgery. She had significant circumferential laxity, buttocks involution, and ptosis. She underwent a circumferential abdominoplasty with autologous purse-string gluteoplasty, and achieved a dramatic improvement in truncal and buttock contour with correction of laxity, contour deformities, and enhanced buttocks shape, position, and fullness.

and fat grafting (**Fig. 13.167 A–C**). The amount of grafting needed and the approximate amount of fat available should be assessed preoperatively. This can be facilitated by using a 60mL syringe as a representative volume and visualizing that volume added to each buttock.

After general anesthesia is initiated, the anterior liposuction area is thoroughly infiltrated with tumescent fluid. The details of tumescent infiltration are discussed in Chapter 3, Liposuction in Abdominal Contouring. If the fat from the anterior liposuction is needed, then anterior liposuction is performed first. When this is accomplished the patient is repositioned prone and the harvested fat is grafted into each buttock first. More commonly, the fat from the lumbar area, back, and thighs provides sufficient volume for the buttocks augmentation.

To harvest significant volumes of fat, often 300–600mL per buttock or more, we use a Microaire power-assisted liposuction device connected to a sterile in-line trap. This technique was described by Mendieta in 2005 (personal communication). A 4mm Mercedes tip cannula is used to harvest fat efficiently. The in-line trap collects the entire liposuction aspirate (**Fig. 13.168 A–D**), which is allowed to settle out into its supernatant fat and infranatant tumescent fluid components (**Fig. 13.169**). The supernatant fat is then poured into a sterile stainless steel strainer and the liquid component, consisting of residual fluid, oils, and disrupted fat cells, drains from it (**Fig. 13.170 A, B**). If it appears that the fat contains blood and is not pure yellow, it can be

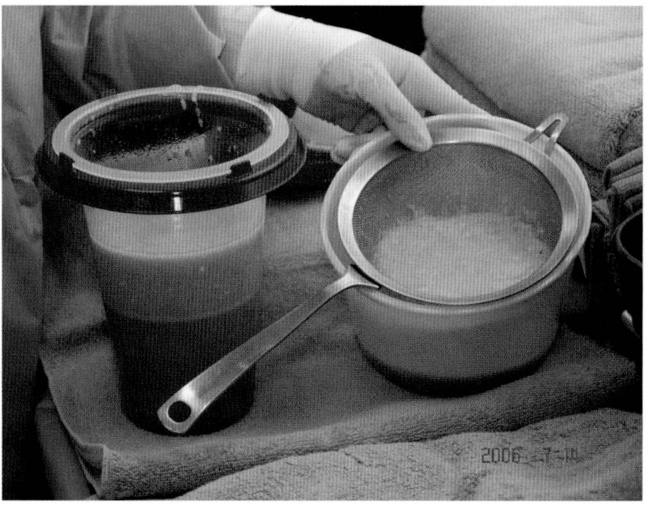

Fig. 13.169 Buttocks Fat Grafting Images The supernatant fat is strained.

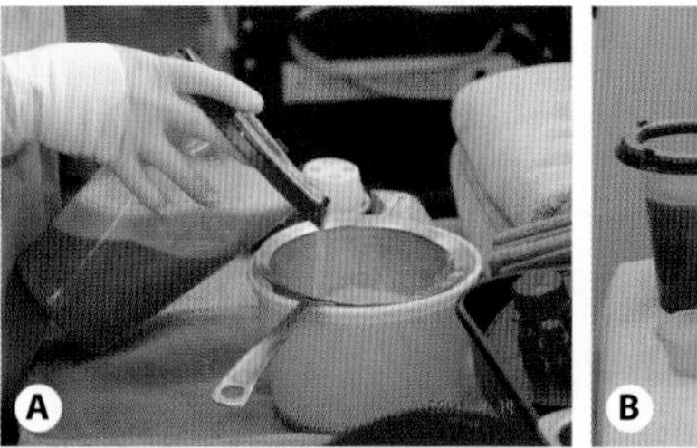

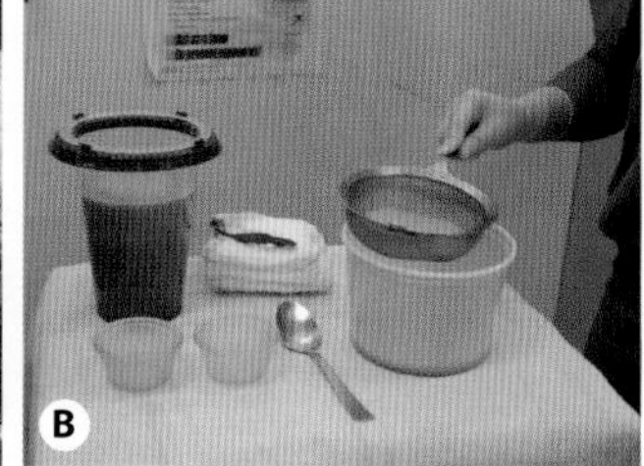

Fig. 13.170 Buttocks Fat Grafting Images A, B The fat is poured into a stainless steel strainer and the fluid is allowed to drain completely.

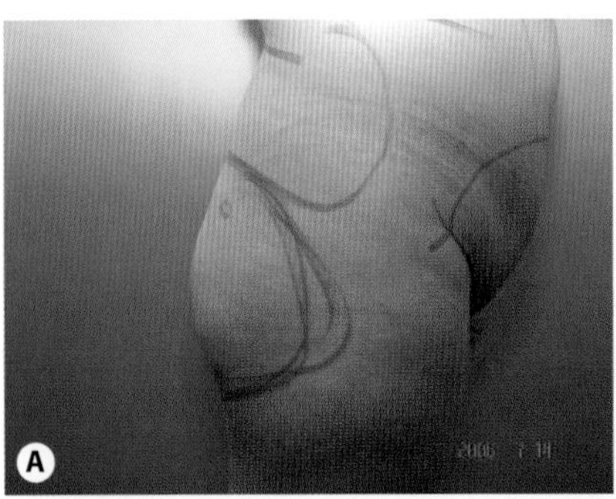

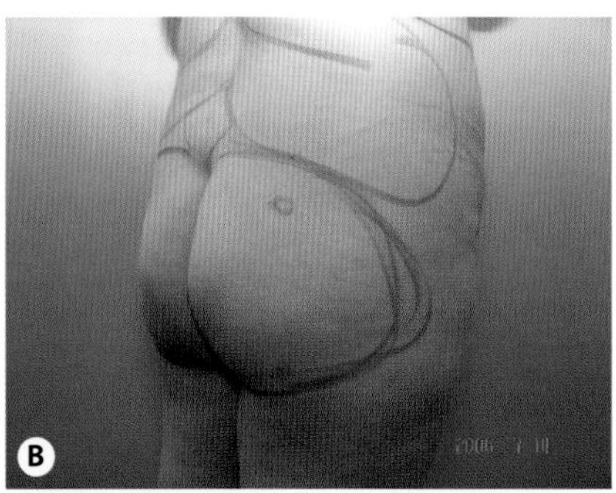

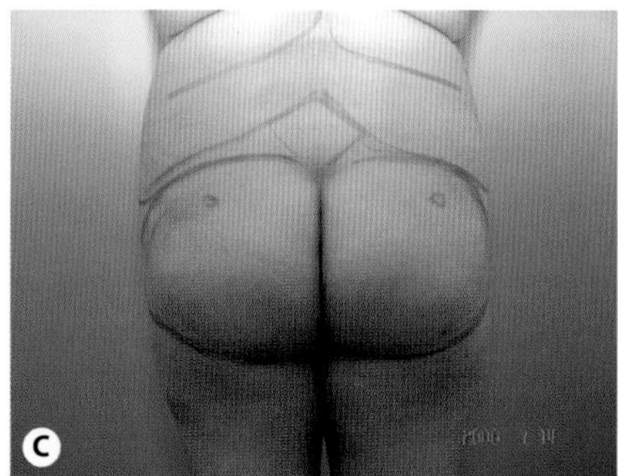

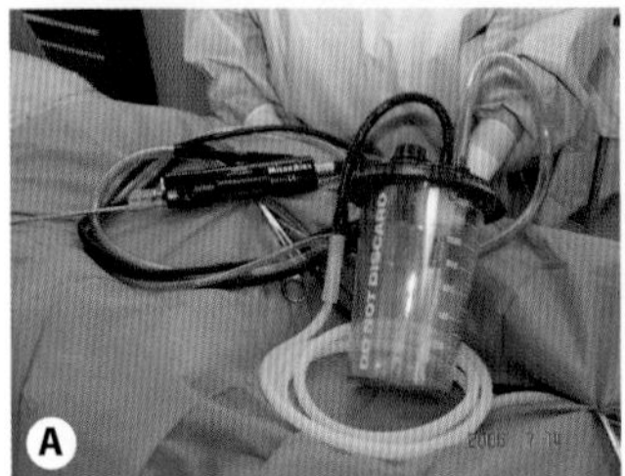

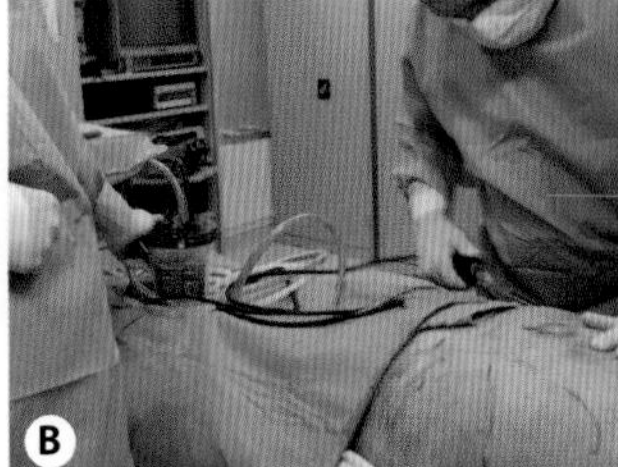

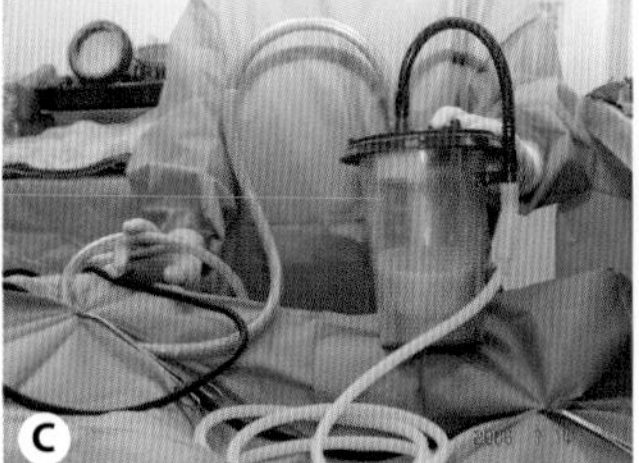

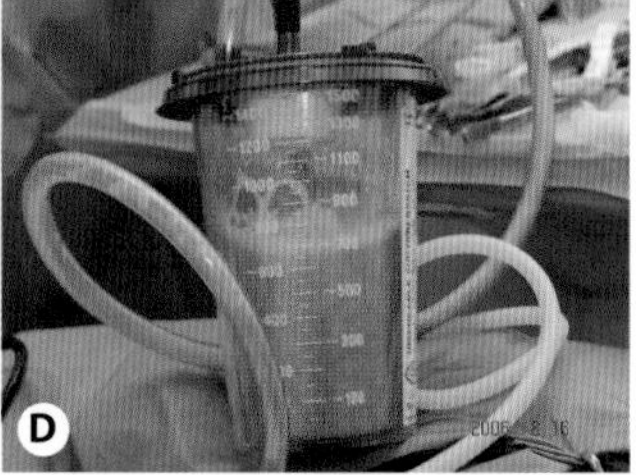

Figs 13.167–13.168 Buttocks Fat Grafting Images For patients who have excess adiposity of the back or abdomen a logical combination is liposuction with concurrent fat grafting. In this patient excess fullness of the hip rolls, back, and abdomen and a paucity of fullness of the buttocks led to a desire for buttock augmentation. A sterile in-line trap is used to collect the aspirated fat. We use MicroAire power-assisted liposuction equipment, but any liposuction equipment is appropriate. The inline trap is helpful because large volumes of fat are needed for effective buttocks augmentation.

rinsed with lactated Ringer's solution to help remove this. The fat is allowed to drain all of this residual fluid to the point where its consistency is semi-solid (**Fig. 13.171**). This process takes only a minute or two, so the harvested fat is exposed to the environment only briefly.

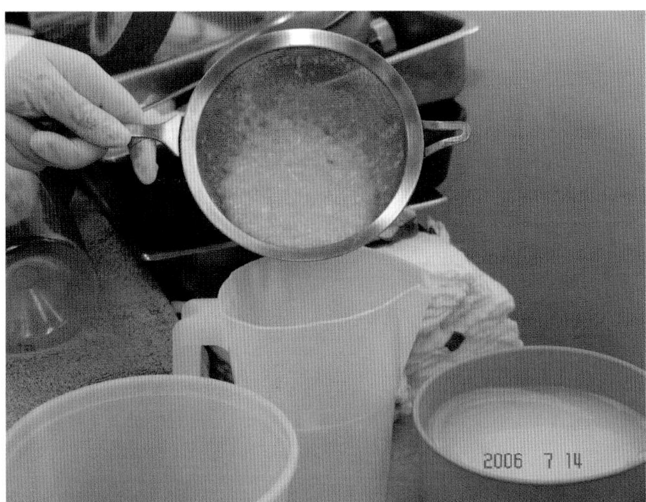

Fig. 13.171 Buttocks Fat Grafting Images This final appearance of the fat is relatively solid.

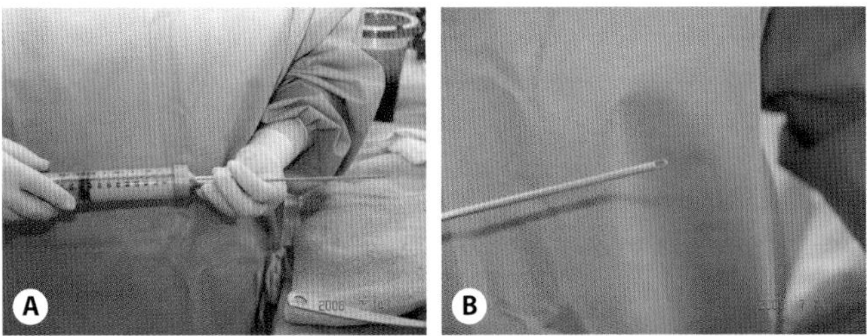

Fig. 13.173 Buttocks Fat Grafting Images A, B A Coleman injecting cannula is connected to the syringe for fat grafting.

The fat is then transferred into 60 mL Toomey syringes (**Fig. 13.172 A–D**), which we connect to a fat grafting cannula designed by Coleman (**Fig. 13.173 A, B**). Fat is injected into the gluteus muscle, the deep fat layer, the superficial fat layer, and several millimeters beneath the skin (**Fig. 13.174 A–G**), but only during cannula withdrawal. This 'all-layer' grafting is essential so that the individual tunnels of grafted fat are maximally surrounded by vascularized tissue, which is important to the overall take of the harvested fat. The entry sites are closed and a light compressive garment is applied.

Postoperative Care

Patients are given prescriptions for pain medication and oral antibiotics for 1 week. No drains are used. Careful

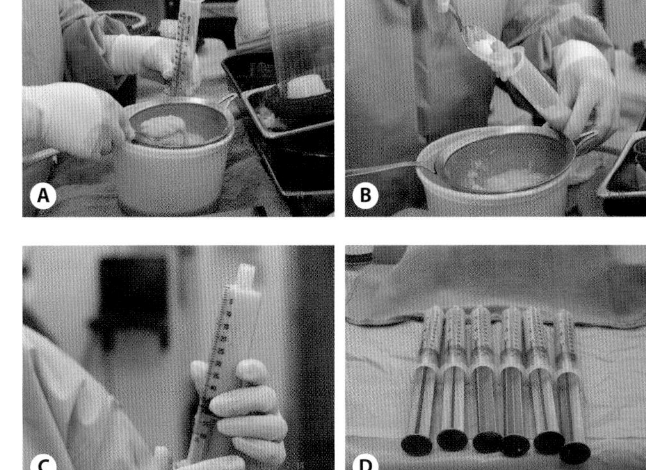

Fig. 13.172 Buttocks Fat Grafting Images A–D The strained fat is placed into 60 mL Toomey syringes.

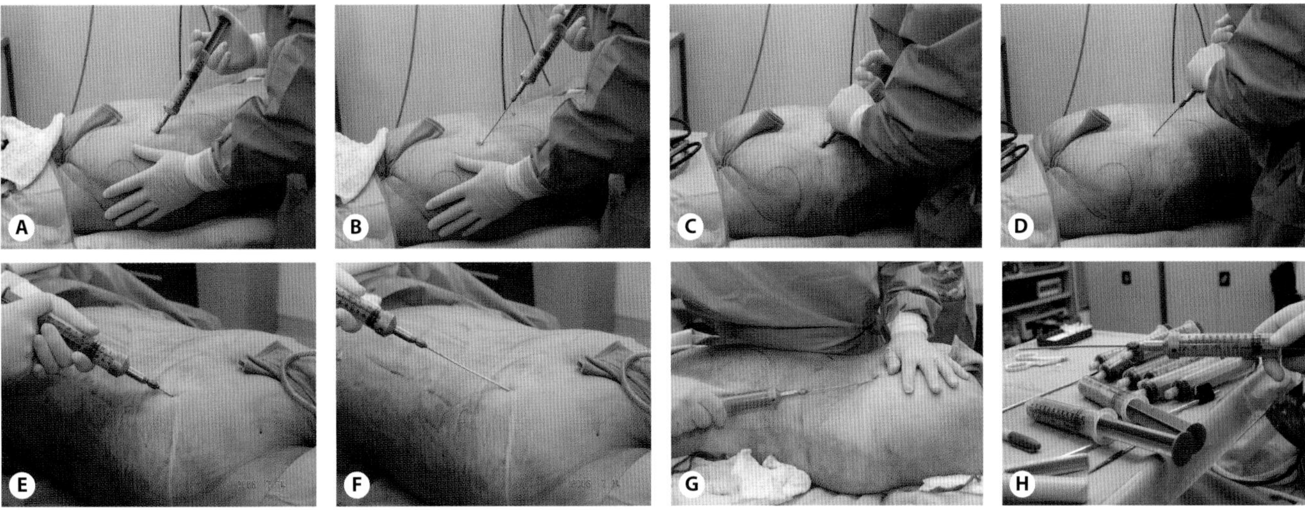

Fig. 13.174 Buttocks Fat Grafting Images A–H Fat grafting is performed in a retrograde filling fashion. The cannula is fully advanced into the tissue to be grafted, and then only on withdrawal is a small amount of fat injected. The concept is to inject small strands of fat that can be surrounded by vascularized tissue, which will promote survival. The fat is injected into the gluteus muscle, the deep fat, the superficial fat, and the subdermal layer. A very even, smooth contour is achieved by placing many strands of fat in all tissue planes.

inspection is performed within a few days to be sure there are no signs of infection. We ask patients to be very gentle when sitting, and to use plenty of padding so as not to displace any of the injected fat.

Before and After Figures for Buttock Fat Grafting (Figs 13.175–13.204)

Mons Remodeling (Box 13.4)

Mons remodeling is a useful technique, particularly in patients who experience mons hypertrophy due to weight gain or significant mons redundancy following weight loss. Liposuction alone for the hypertrophic mons is not always satisfactory,

Box 13.4 Mons correction

- The mons areas is exposed to and affected by the same factors that contribute to abdominal adiposity and soft-tissue laxity
- Excess adiposity should be corrected through liposuction
- Mons laxity is often noted in both the horizontal as well as the vertical dimensions
- Correction of mons laxity should be through resection of skin and underlying soft tissue. The goal is to lift and tighten. The lifting component is usually accomplished through the transverse component of the abdominoplasty. Tightening can be accomplished by resecting a vertical wedge from the midline. A layered closure should be performed

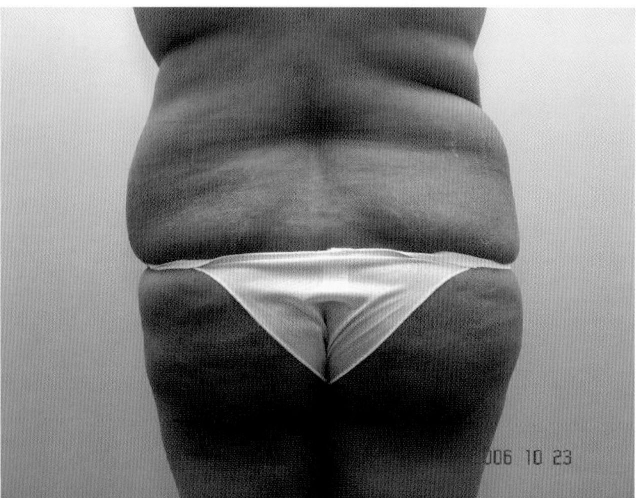

Fig. 13.175

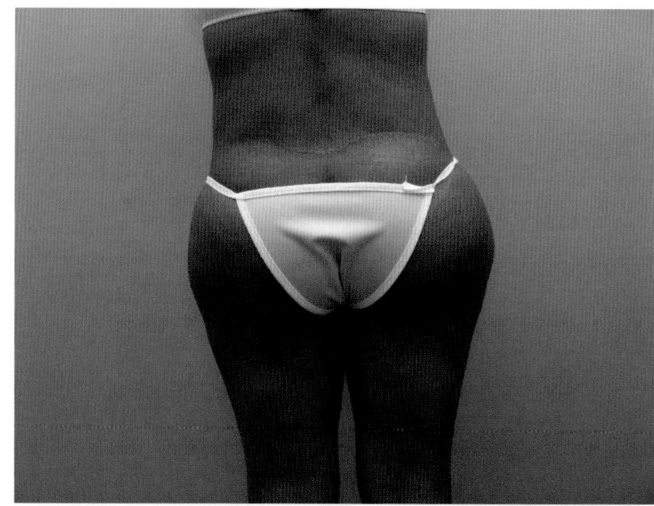

Fig. 13.176

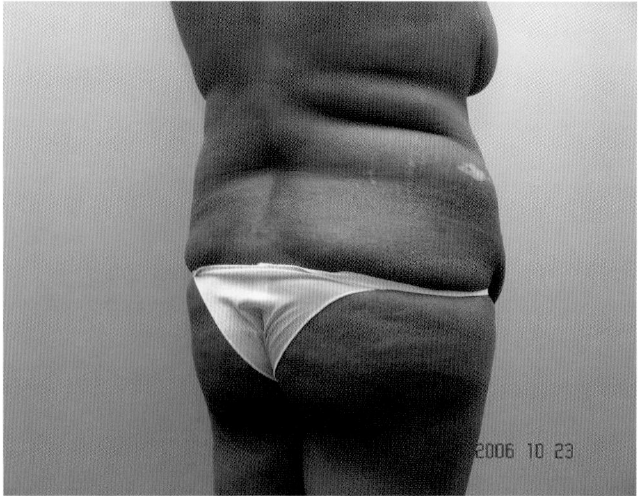

Fig. 13.177

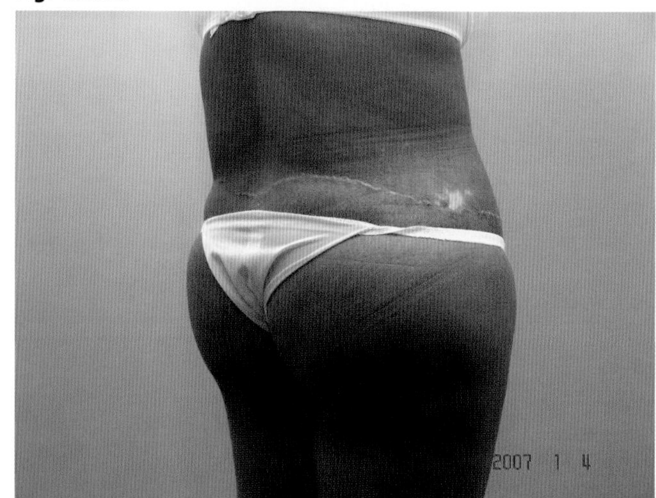

Fig. 13.178

Figs 13.175–13.184 Buttocks Fat Grafting Pre- and Postoperative Images Pre- and postoperative images of a 43-year-old woman who underwent a circumferential abdominoplasty with autologous buttocks fat grafting. The circumferential abdominoplasty and thorough concurrent liposuction of the back greatly improved her overall contour. The augmentation of the buttocks with autologous fat created a smooth, round, enhanced appearance. The combination of tissue resection and liposuction with fat grafting achieved a very balanced, attractive physique.

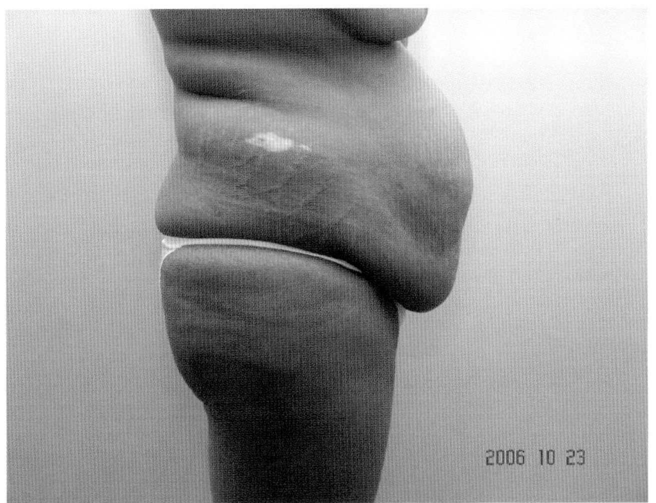

Fig. 13.179

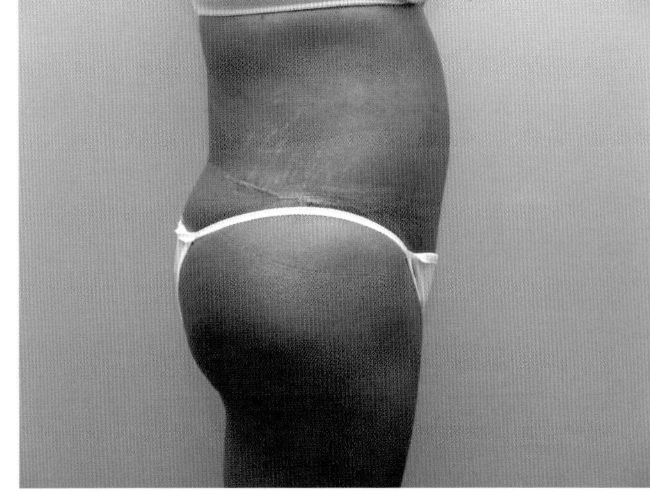

Fig. 13.180

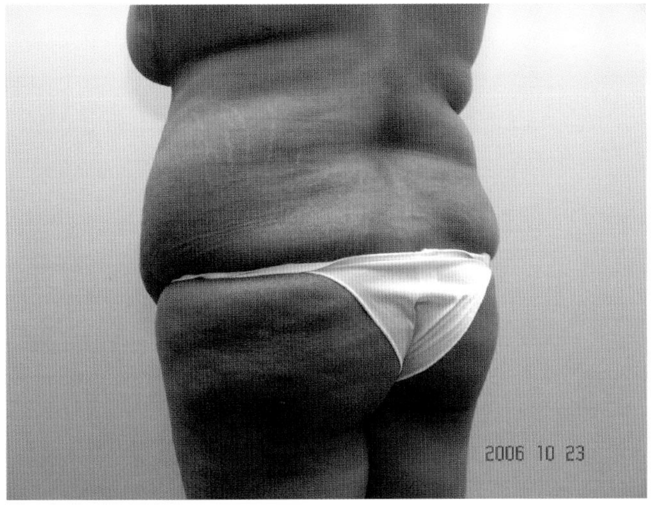

Fig. 13.181

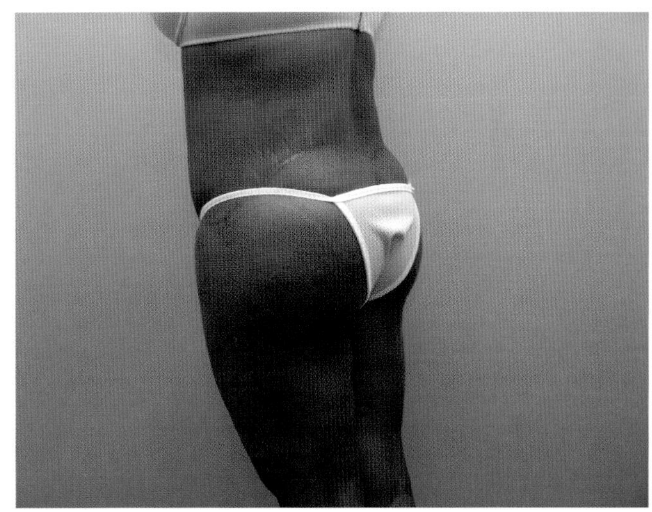

Fig. 13.182

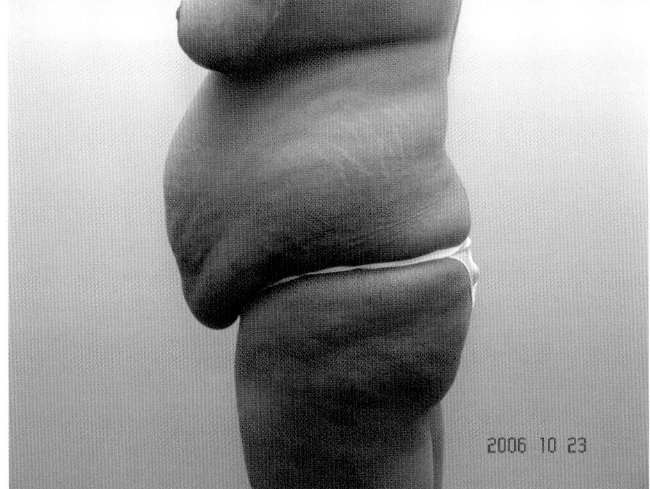

Fig. 13.183

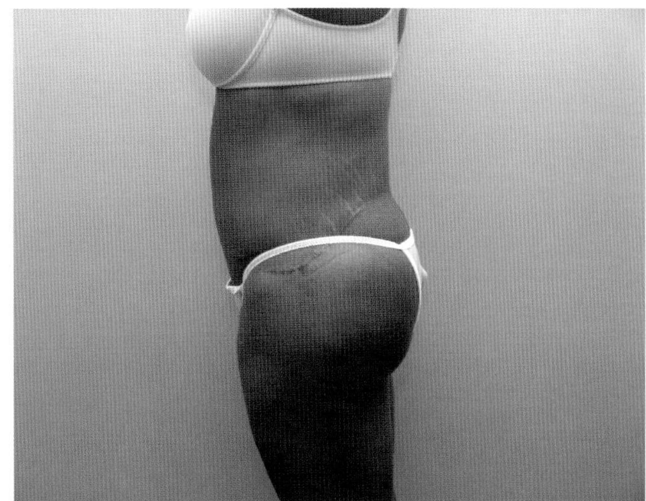

Fig. 13.184

Figs 13.185–13.190

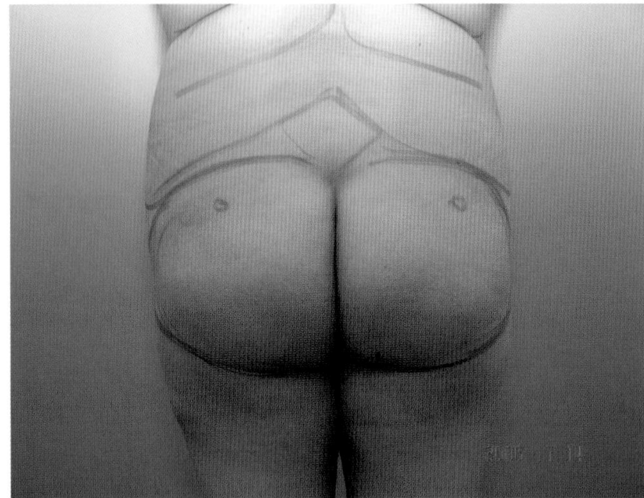

Fig. 13.185

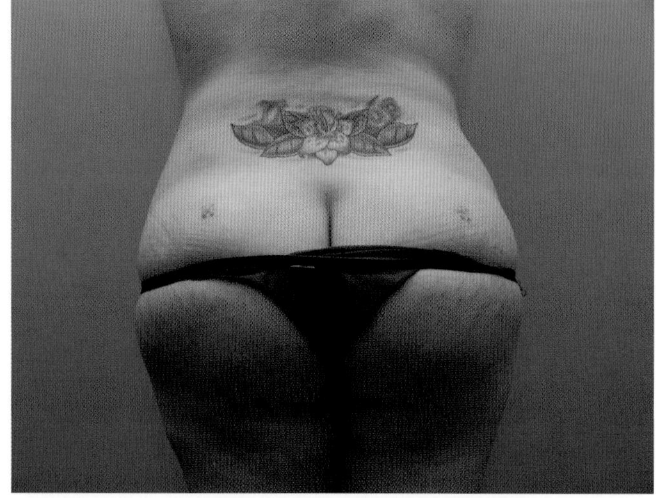

Fig. 13.186

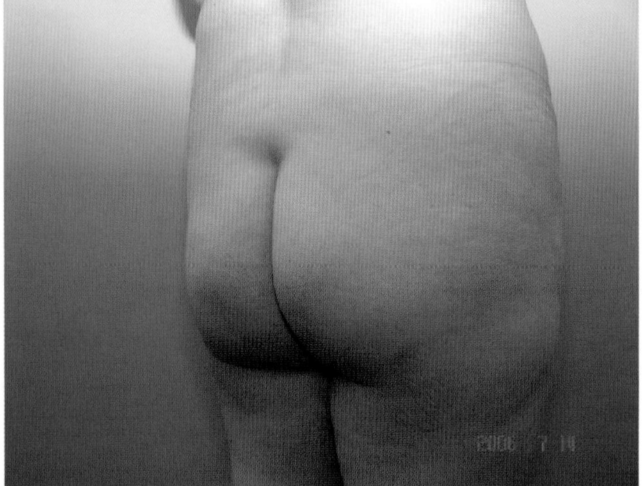

Fig. 13.187

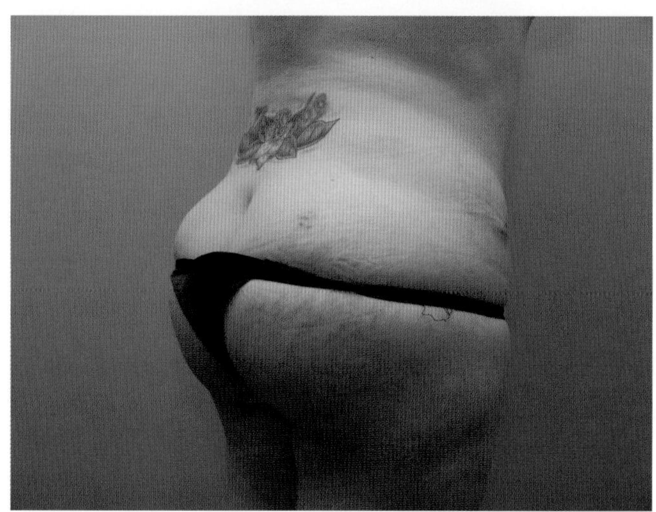

Fig. 13.188

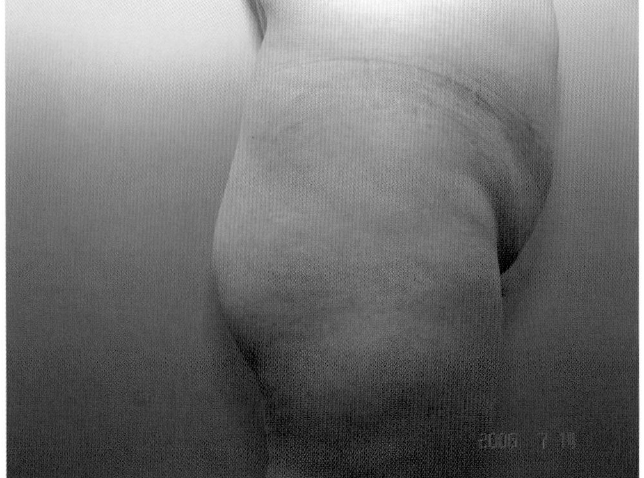

Fig. 13.189

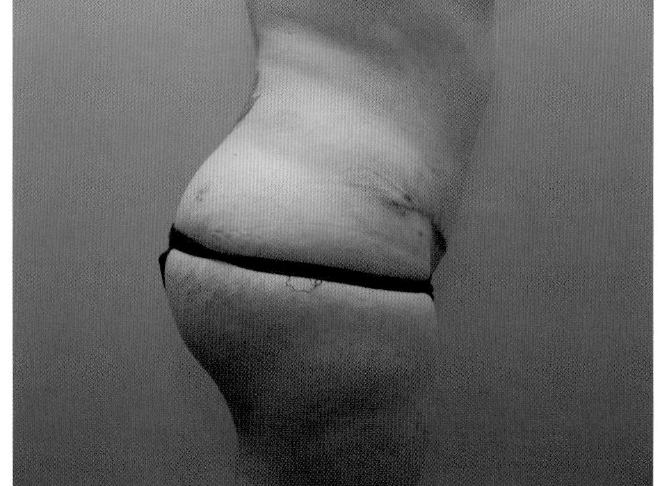

Fig. 13.190

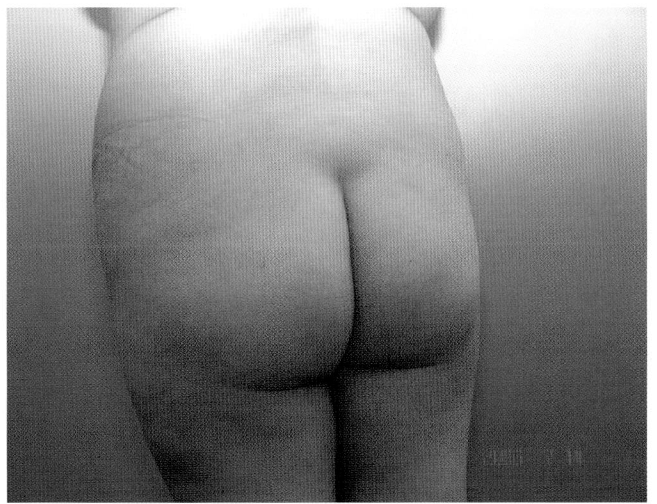

Fig. 13.191

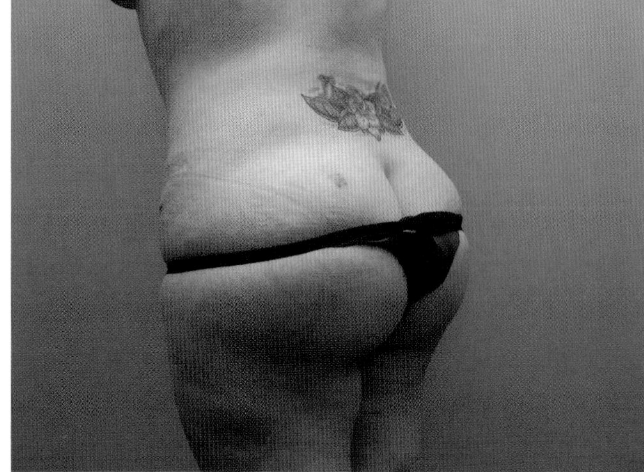

Fig. 13.192

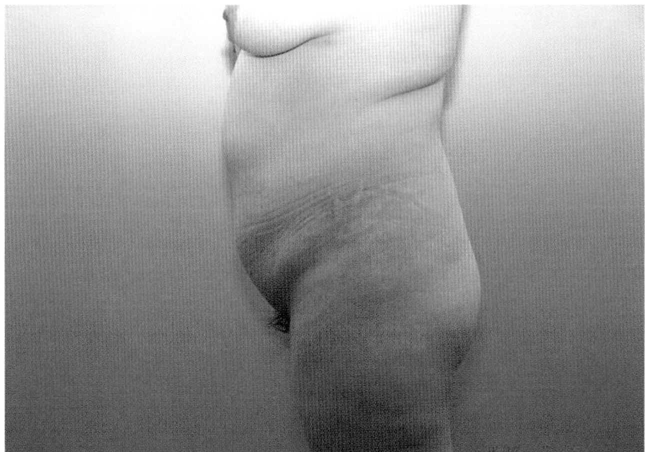

Fig. 13.193

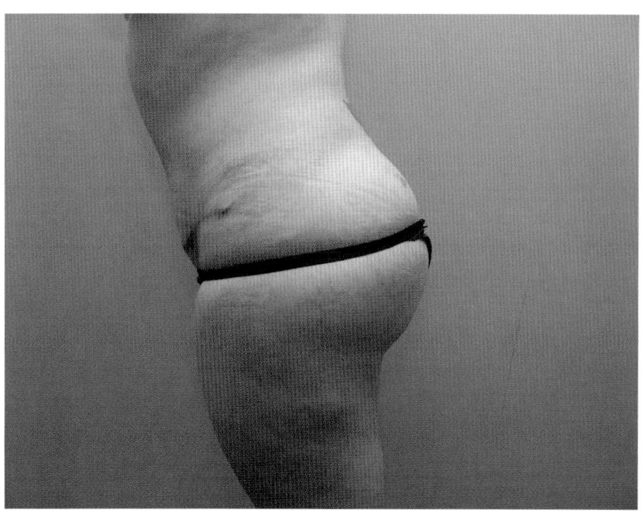

Fig. 13.194

Figs 13.185–13.194 Buttocks Fat Grafting Pre- and Postoperative Images This 41-year-old woman was concerned with her truncal obesity and lack of buttock volume. A full abdominoplasty with concurrent liposuction and liposuction of the hip rolls and back, plus buttocks fat grafting, created a dramatic transformation. The patient was delighted with the resulting thin, tight and flat abdomen, smooth curving waistline, and full round projecting buttocks. She was so pleased that she had a flower tattoo placed on her lower back.

Figs 13.195–13.196

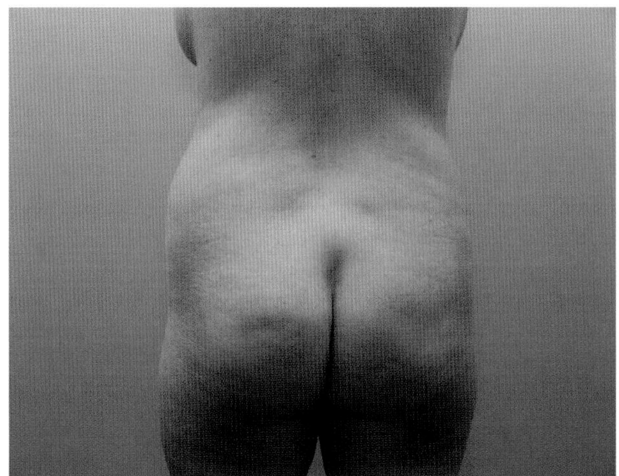

Fig. 13.195

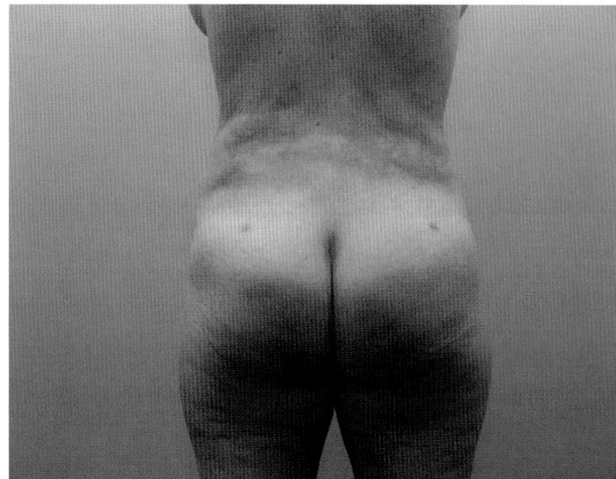

Fig. 13.196

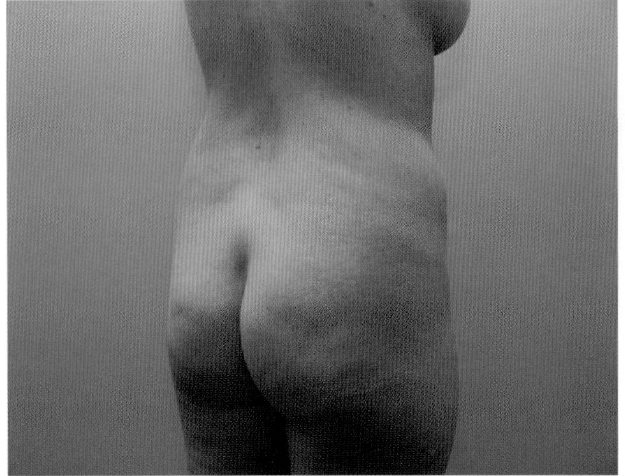

Fig. 13.197

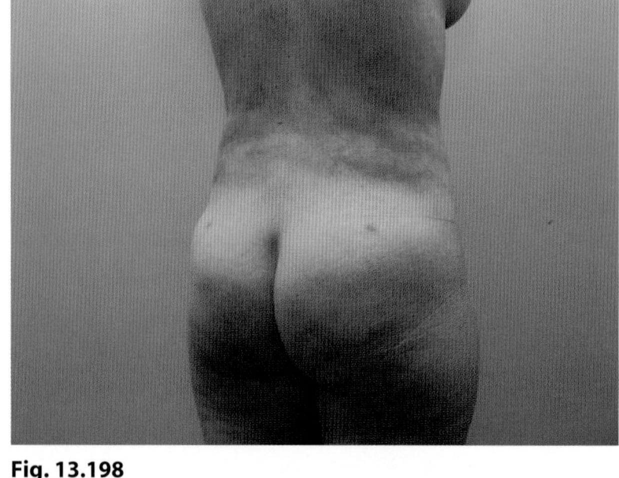

Fig. 13.198

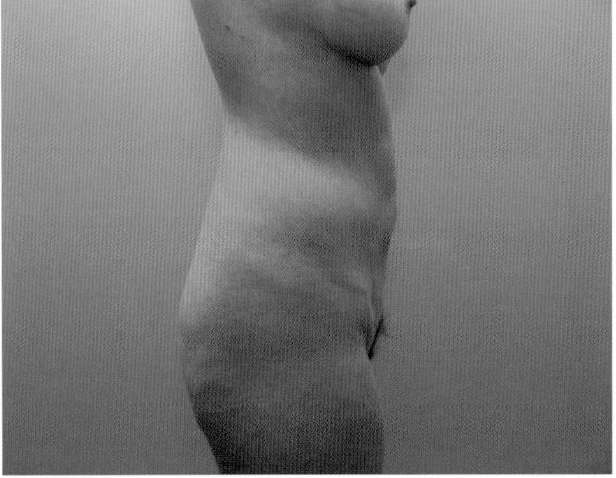

Fig. 13.199

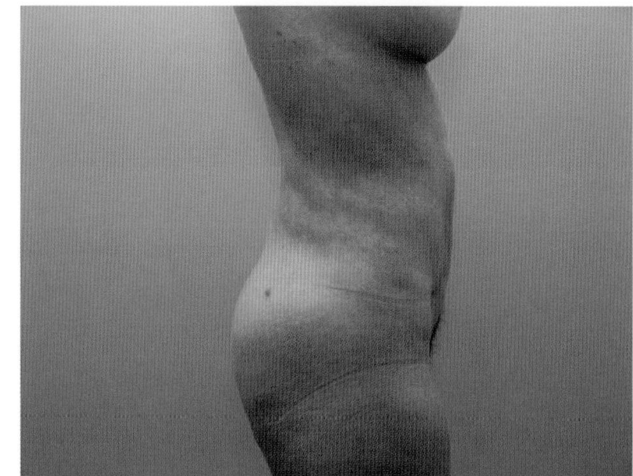

Fig. 13.200

Figs 13.195–13.200 Buttocks Fat Grafting Pre- and Postoperative Images This patient presented with fullness of the hip area and a modest fullness of the abdomen. A full liposuction of the hip rolls, back and abdomen was performed and the suctioned fat was used for autologous fat grafting of the buttocks. A significant enhancement in the waistline and contour is attributable to the liposuction. The buttocks; projection, roundness, and enhanced shape are entirely attributable to the autologous fat grafting.

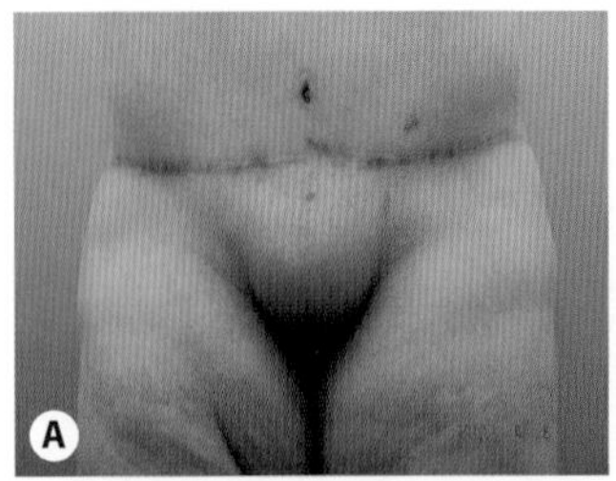

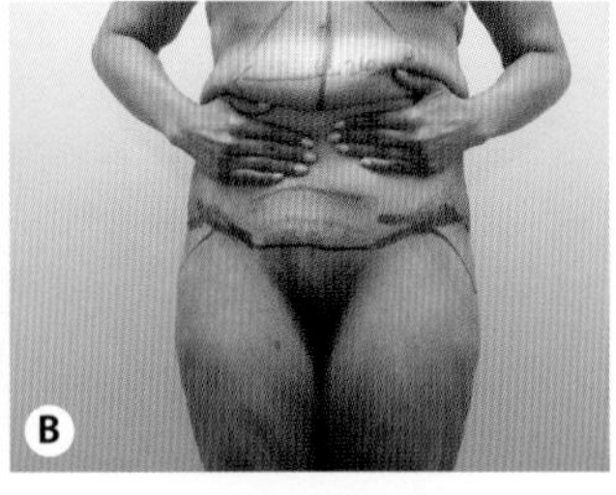

Fig. 13.205 Mons Remodeling Images A Following a circumferential abdominoplasty with mons liposuction mons fullness remains. **B** Following massive weight loss the redundancy of the mons was of great concern to the patient, who felt it made her look aged.

and for these patients mons remodeling via skin and soft-tissue resection can be very helpful (**Fig. 13.205 A, B**).

Mons hypertrophy or redundancy, when present, occurs in both transverse and vertical planes (**Fig. 13.206 A–C**). This should be taken into account during the mons remodeling procedure, and both transverse and vertical resection should be performed if needed. This procedure can be performed in conjunction with an abdominoplasty or as an isolated procedure.

Operative Approach

Patients are marked preoperatively in the standing position. The midline of the mons is marked first, and the amount of redundancy is assessed both transversely and vertically (**Fig. 13.207 A–D**). Once in the operating room and after general anesthesia has been initiated, the incisions are infiltrated with lidocaine containing epinephrine. If the mons area contains a significant amount of subcutaneous tissue liposuction is planned, and therefore tumescent infiltration is performed. When liposuction is planned it is performed first, before the resection component of the procedure. Excess tissue is

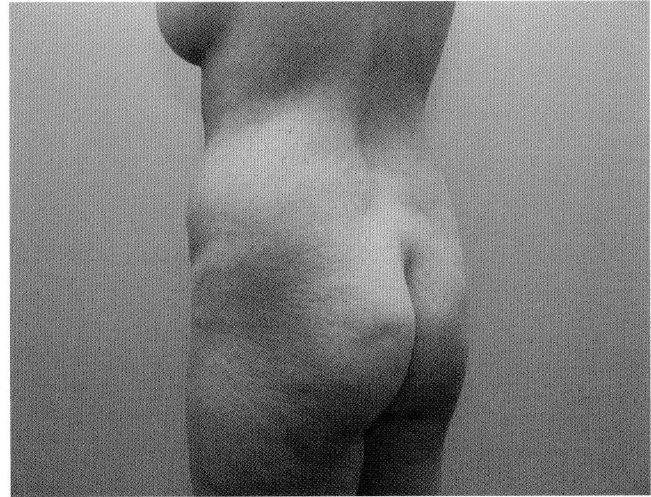

Fig. 13.201

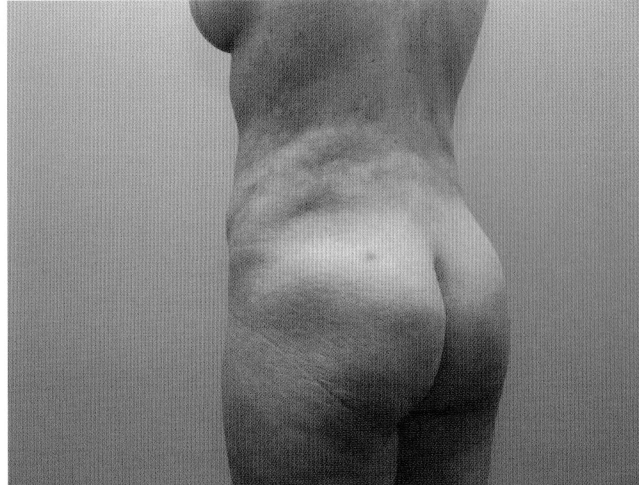

Fig. 13.202

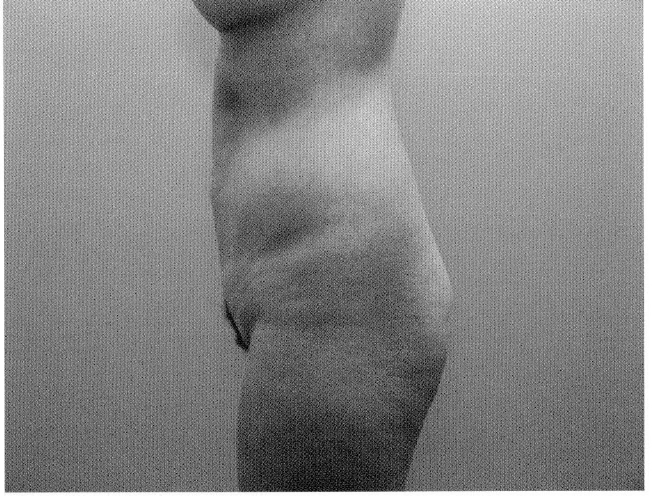

Fig. 13.203

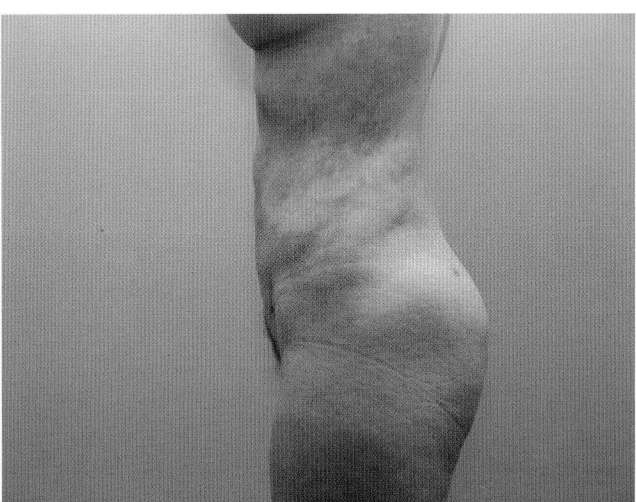

Fig. 13.204

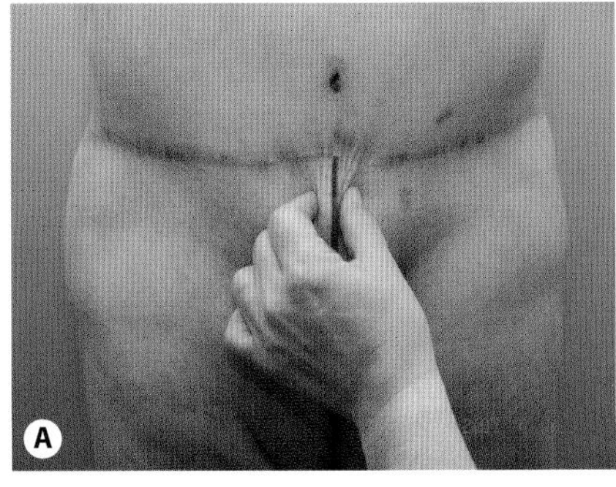

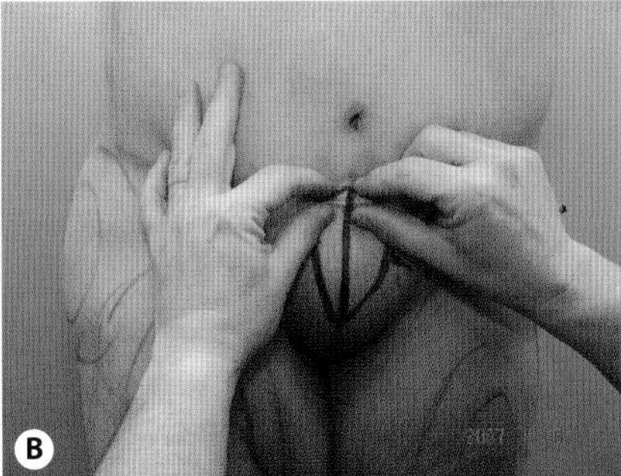

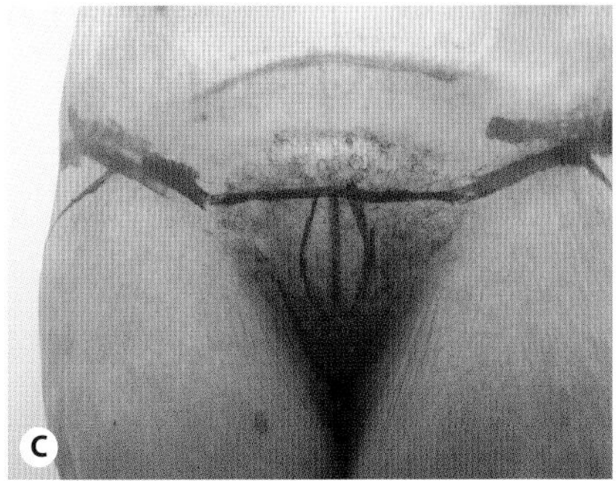

Fig. 13.206 Mons Remodeling Images A–C The mons redundancy is both vertical and transverse. Treatment of the vertical redundancy returns the mons to a more youthful, narrow shape. Treatment of the horizontal by superior excision re-elevates the mons laxity.

resected, including a wedge of subcutaneous tissue, in combination with the abdominoplasty or as a standalone procedure (**Fig. 13.208 A–H**). After achieving hemostasis, closure is performed with interrupted 0 Vicryl sutures placed in the superficial fascia. 2/0 Vicryl sutures are placed in the deep dermis, and a final 4/0 Monocryl intradermal suture is used to achieve formal closure (**Fig. 13.209 A–D**). The incision can be glued, taped, or a simple dressing applied.

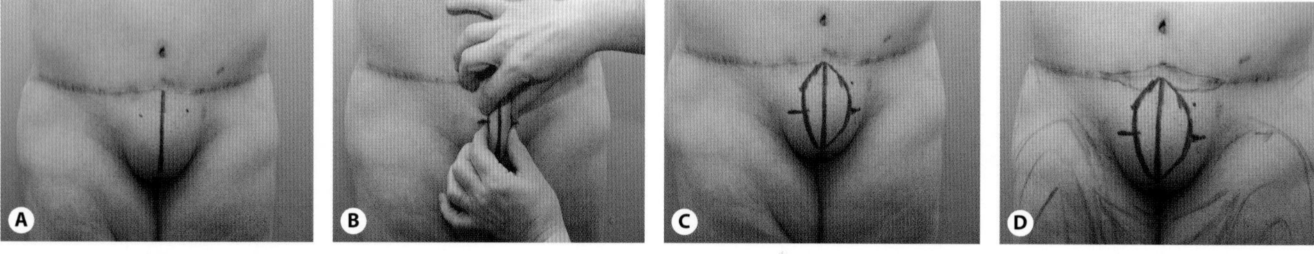

Fig. 13.207 Mons Remodeling Images A–D Preoperative markings are made using bimanual palpation after the midline is marked. Realignment marks are utilized. The horizontal resection is also marked.

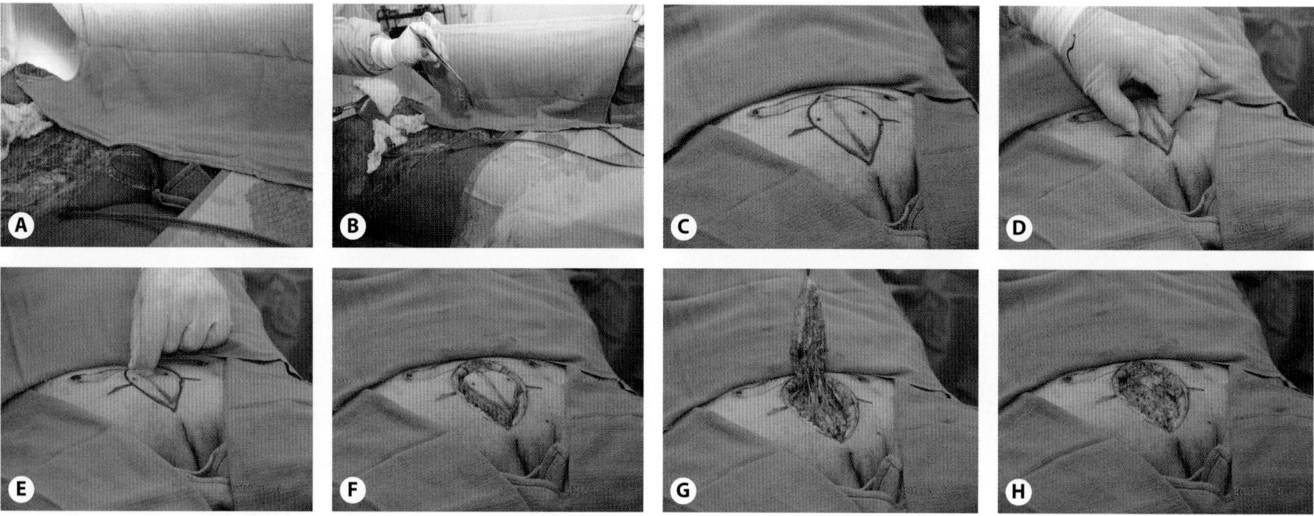

Fig. 13.208 Mons Remodeling Images A, B The vertical resection is performed in a beveling fashion so that closure can be performed without leaving dead space. **C–H** When the mons has residual excess adiposity, vigorous liposuction is performed first to provide maximum thinning of the tissues. The vertical resection is completed at the level of thorough liposuction undermining, leaving the deeper neurovascular and lymphatics structures intact.

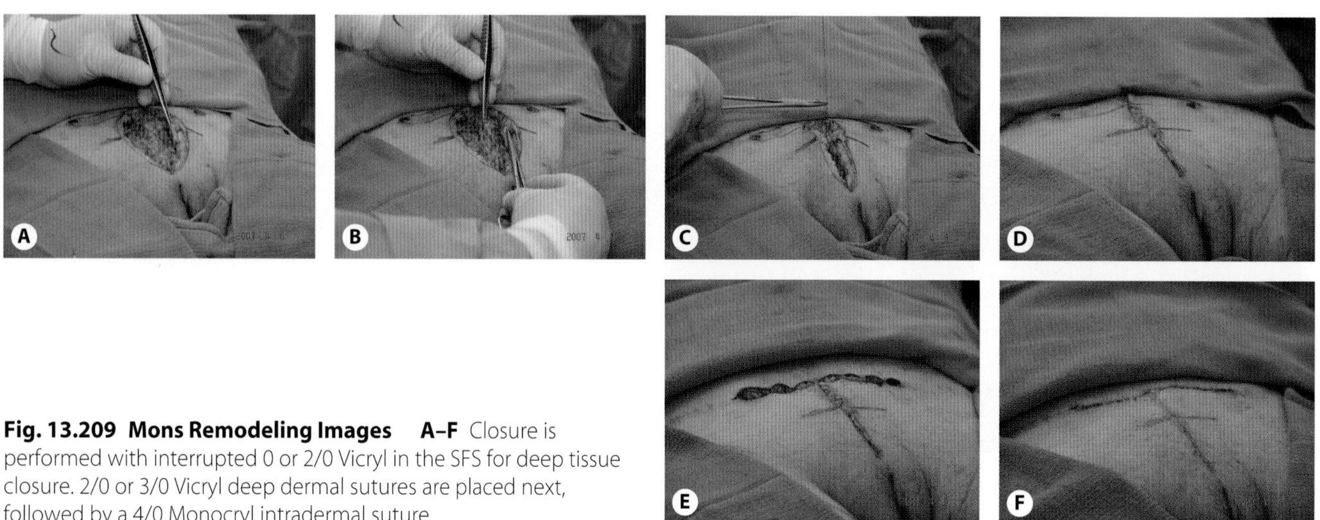

Fig. 13.209 Mons Remodeling Images A–F Closure is performed with interrupted 0 or 2/0 Vicryl in the SFS for deep tissue closure. 2/0 or 3/0 Vicryl deep dermal sutures are placed next, followed by a 4/0 Monocryl intradermal suture.

Postoperative Care

Routine postoperative care instructions are provided. The patient may shower starting on the second postoperative day.

Before and After Figures for Mons Remodelling (Figs 13.210–13.214)

Thigh Lift

Inner Thigh Lift (Box 13.5)

The inner thigh lift is useful for patients with mild to moderate laxity of the inner thighs[8] (**Fig. 13.215**). It can, however, be one of the more problematic procedures in body contouring surgery, because the scar tends to descend caudally from the pubic thigh crease despite firm anchoring to Colles' fascia.[9] It can be performed as an isolated procedure or in combination with abdominal contouring. The key to the procedure is excision of a reasonable amount of inner thigh skin – usually no more than 4 or 5 cm in vertical width. Much more than this can create excessive tension, which adds to the descent and widening of the scar. The superficial fascia of the inferior cut edge of the skin resection is anchored to immobile structures, including the pubic tubercle, the ischiopubic rami, Colles' fascia, and Cooper's

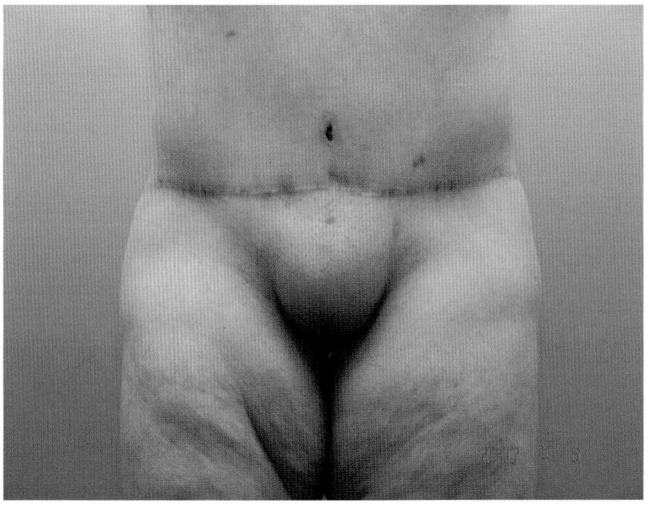

Fig. 13.210 Mons Remodeling Pre- and Postoperative Images Even after a body lift with thorough liposuction residual mons fullness can still be present and of great concern to the patient.

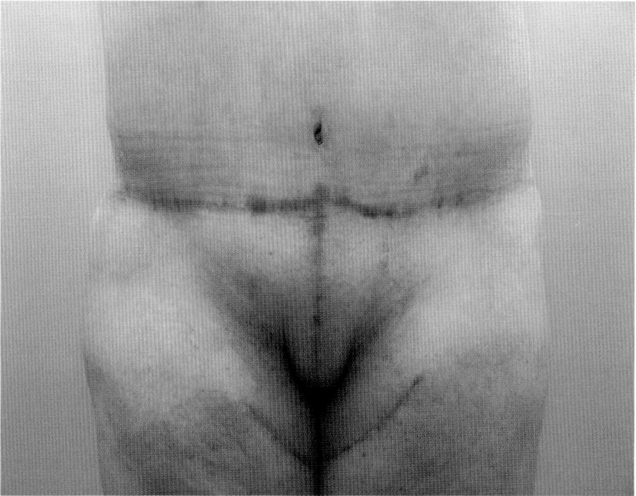

Fig. 13.212 Mons Remodeling Pre- and Postoperative Images Postoperative appearance demonstrates a more youthful, elevated and thinned mons.

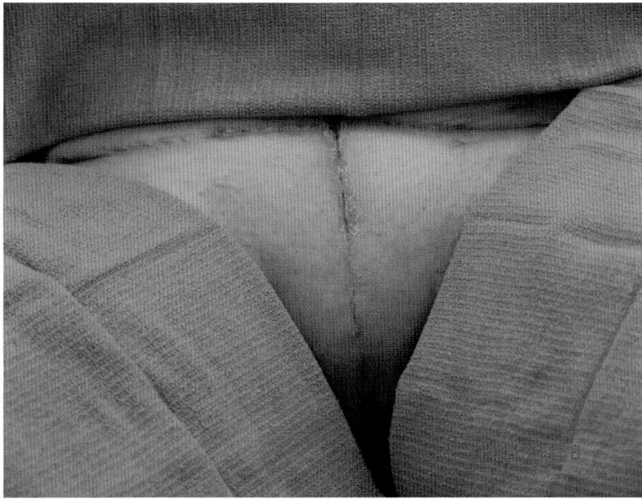

Fig. 13.211 Mons Remodeling Pre- and Postoperative Images Following thorough liposuction and mons remodeling the early postoperative appearance is seen.

Box 13.5 Vertical thigh lift

- The vertical thigh lift is ideal for patients with moderate to significant soft-tissue laxity
- The patient must be willing to accept a long scar in exchange for significantly improved contour of the thigh
- Pre-tunneling using a liposuction cannula will release some of the soft-tissue attachments and help preserve the small veins and lymphatics underneath during removal of the overlying skin
- After dissection down through the superficial fascia circumferentially around the soft-tissue ellipse, the skin can be avulsed off in a *caudal* direction. Countertraction on the soft tissue is helpful during this process
- Reapproximating the wound edges temporarily with staples during the resection process makes closure easier when soft-tissue swelling begins
- Periodic and alternating ambulation and elevation are important postoperatively to reduce the chance of DVT, and also to minimize the effects of soft-tissue swelling

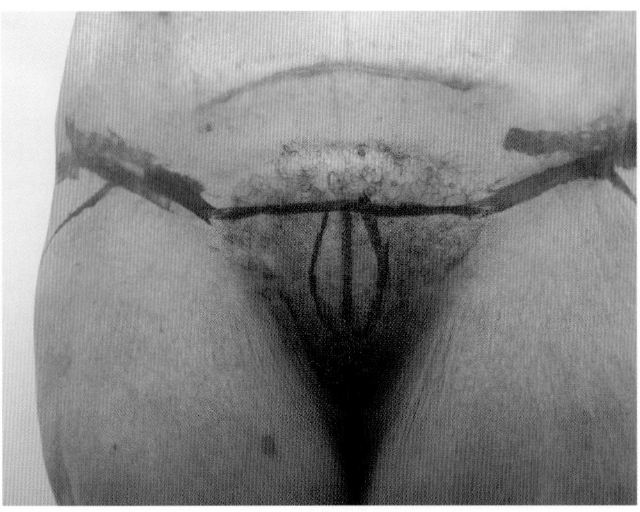

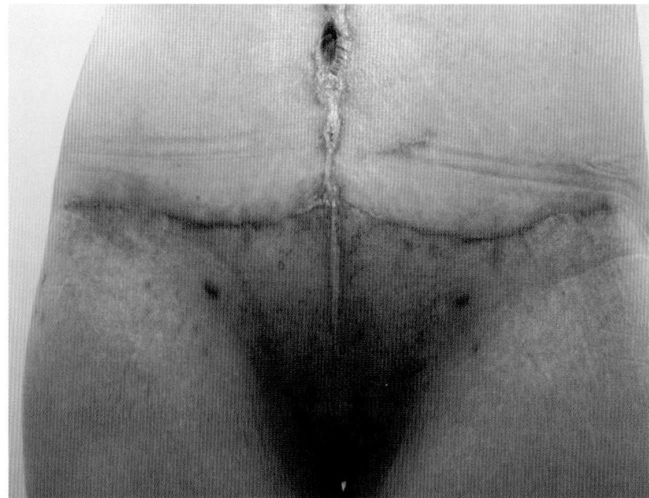

Figs 13.213–13.214 Mons Remodeling Pre- and Postoperative Images Mons reduction in a patient following massive weight loss. The scar associated with wedge resection is usually very well tolerated.

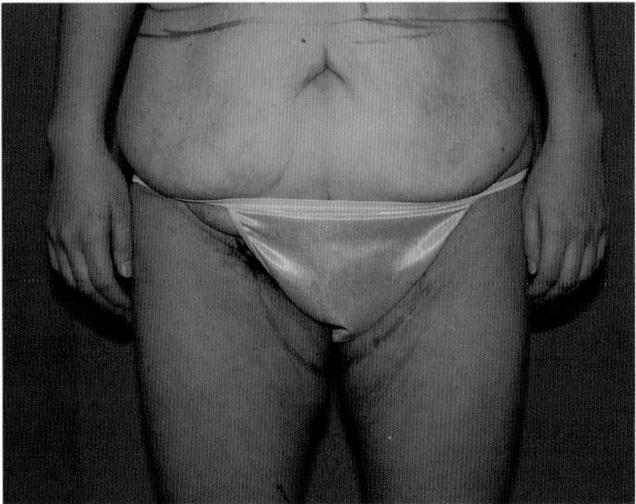

Fig. 13.215 Inner Thigh Lift Preoperative Image This patient experienced a significant weight loss and was very concerned about the laxity of the upper inner thighs. There is also significant laxity of the abdomen and trunk.

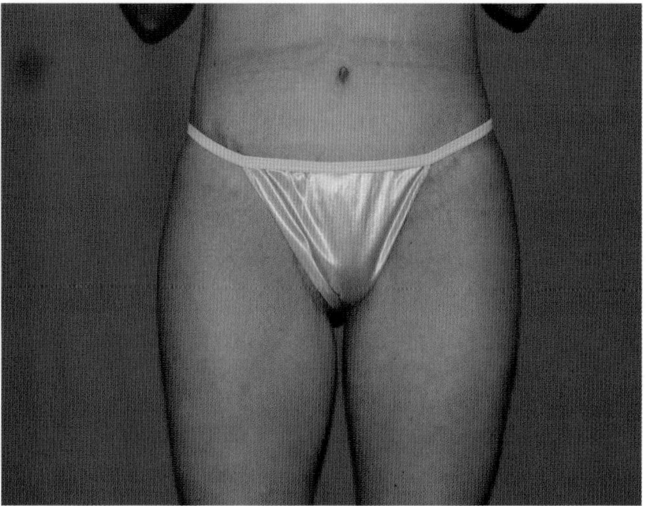

Fig. 13.216 Inner Thigh Lift Postoperative Image The patient underwent circumferential abdominoplasty as well as inner thigh lift. Following the inner thigh lift, a significant improvement in the quality and shape of the thighs is readily apparent.

ligament, using permanent sutures. The skin and soft tissue are then closed in layers with interrupted deep dermal and running intradermal absorbable suture. Care must be taken to strongly advance the inferior cut margin of the skin resection anteriorly to avoid a posterior dog-ear.

Postoperative Care

Leg elevation and gentle ambulation are recommended following this procedure. The patient is instructed to avoid heavy lifting, and vigorous or strenuous activity. Careful inspection of the wound is performed within a few days.

Before and After Figures for Inner Thigh Lift (Figs 13.216–13.218)

Vertical Thigh Lift

The vertical thigh lift has become a very useful method of correcting significant soft-tissue laxity of the thigh, particularly in patients who have experienced massive weight loss,[10] as it can correct the excess laxity all the way down to and including the knees. If necessary, the procedure can be extended to correct soft-tissue laxity in the calves as well, but this is not often required. The

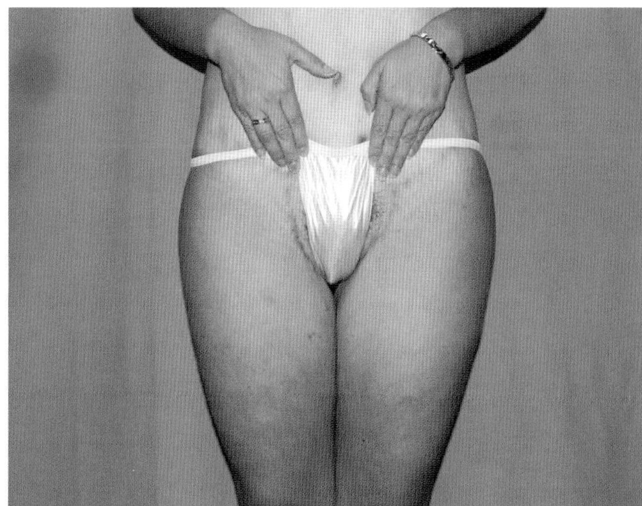

Fig. 13.217 Inner Thigh Lift Postoperative Image The scars have remained concealed within the pubic thigh crease and are easily covered.

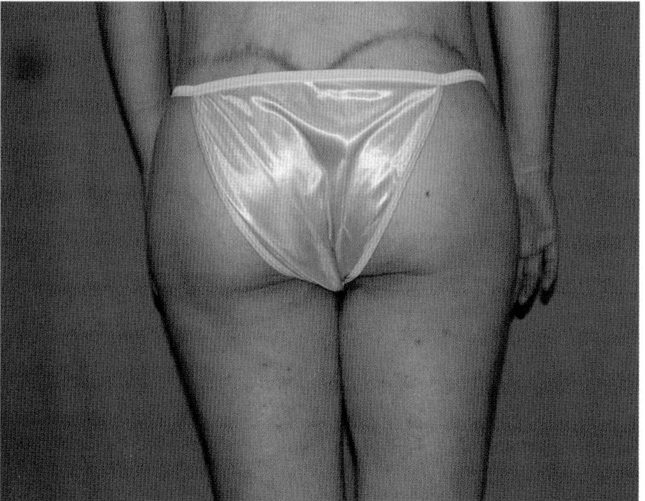

Fig. 13.218 Inner Thigh Lift Pre- and Postoperative Images The inner thigh lift scars are not visible from behind. Preoperative markings should be designed to avoid the scars from being visible or being too posteriorly placed.

scar, although long, usually heals well, and patients gladly exchange this for the dramatic improvement in contour the procedure delivers. Normally we recommend that if there is excess adiposity, a staged procedure should be performed, with thorough liposuction followed in 3–6 months by the vertical thigh lift.

Operative Approach

This procedure begins with preoperative marking performed with the patient standing. Patients will often demonstrate the tissue that they wish to have removed by literally grabbing the redundancy of the inner thigh (**Fig. 13.219 A, B**). The final incision is marked beginning near the origin of the gracilis muscle and terminating at a point that is agreeable to the patient. It is usually preferred to place the final scar slightly more posteriorly than anteriorly (**Fig. 13.220 A–C**). Bimanual palpation determines the amount of tissue to be resected. Realignment marks are placed to facilitate precise closure. The patient should be shown the position and length of the final scar, which can prevent any postoperative concerns. The final incision line should not be visible from the posterior view (**Fig. 13.221**). The incision line can end in the upper thigh or even extend below the knee, as long as the linear scar is broken up with a notch at the knee level (**Fig. 13.222 A–C**).

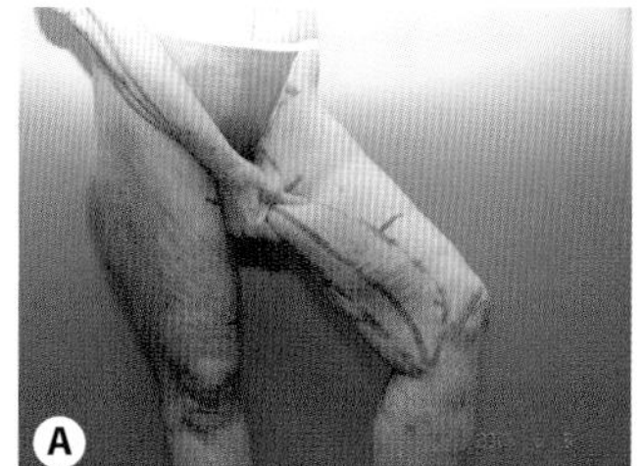

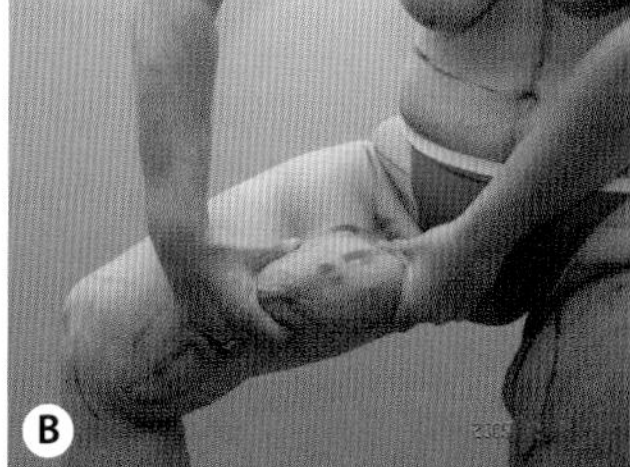

Fig. 13.219 Vertical Thigh Lift Images A-B Patients will often grasp the inner thigh tissue when they discuss what they would like to see corrected. This gives the surgeon a clear idea of what needs to be done, and the vertical thigh lift is the appropriate procedure in this case.

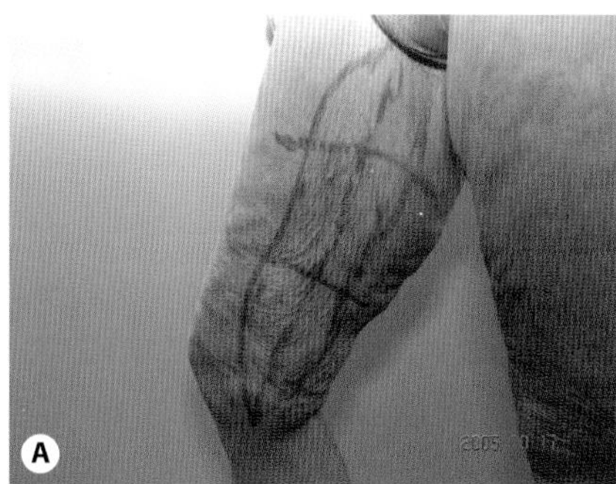

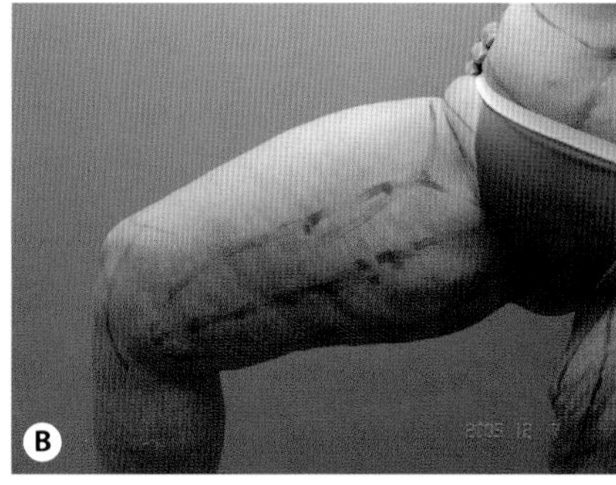

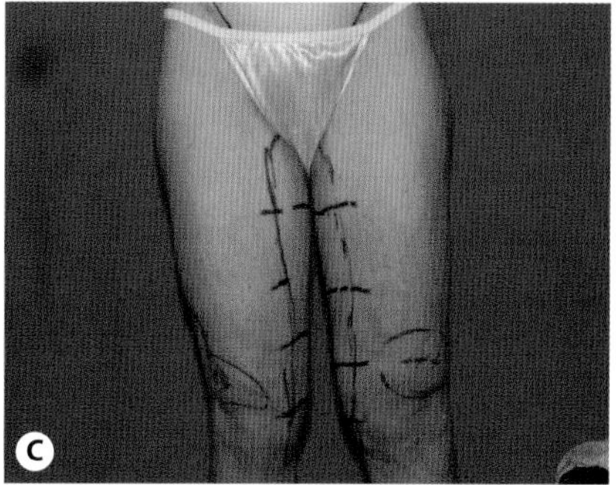

Fig. 13.220 Vertical Thigh Lift Images A–C The markings of the vertical thigh lift are made with the final incision beginning at the insertion of the gracilis and extending distally at a level agreeable to the patient. The width of the resection is determined by bimanual palpation. Realignment marks facilitate closure.

The patient is placed in the supine position with the thighs gently abducted and carefully padded (**Fig. 13.223**). Methylene blue tattoos are placed on the realignment marks for identification following the tissue resection (**Fig. 13.224 A, B**). Penetrating towel clamps are used to ensure there is no excess tension on final closure. If there is any indication that the resection amount is excessive, the markings should be moved inwards for a more conservative resection (**Fig. 13.225 A–D**). Thorough infiltration of the area to be resected is then performed. This is analogous to the tunneling often performed prior to liposuction. The fluid infiltrated is a standard tumescent fluid solution, which helps to minimize bleeding and provides local anesthesia. The infiltration cannula is used vigorously to thoroughly tunnel in the superficial fat several millimetres below the skin. This helps establish the plane of dissection that will be used later (**Fig. 13.226 A, B**) A liposuction cannula can also be used for concurrent liposuction or for additional tunneling (**Fig. 13.226 C**). A number 10 scalpel is used to make the incision partway through the dermis, and the electrocautery device is used to complete the incision and continue the dissection into the superficial fat of the thigh (**Fig. 13.227 A, B**). As the electrocautery dissection deepens, the skin edges

Fig. 13.221 Vertical Thigh Lift Images The posterior aspect of the vertical thigh markings should demonstrate that the final scar is not visible from behind.

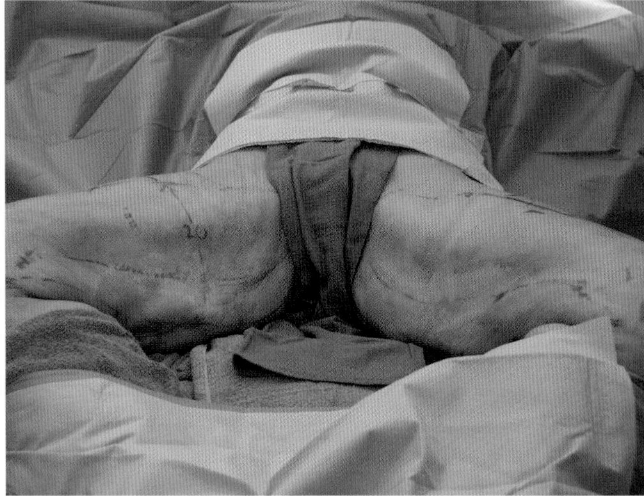

Fig. 13.223 Vertical Thigh Lift Image The patient has been prepped and draped and is placed in the frog-leg position.

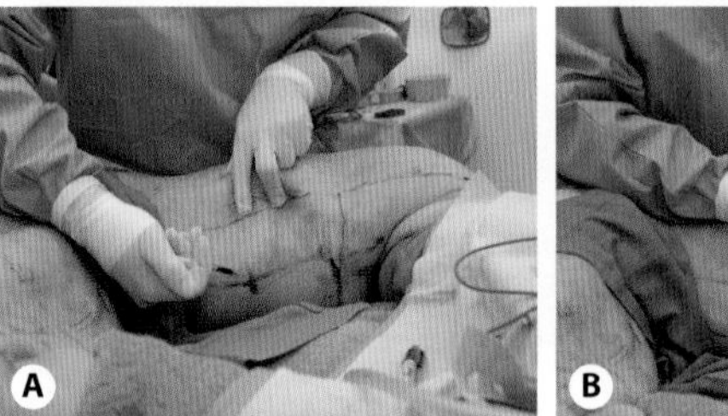

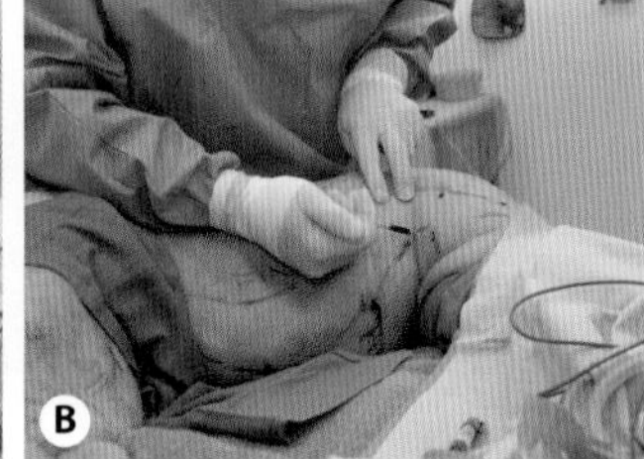

Fig. 13.224 Vertical Thigh Lift Images A, B Methylene blue tattoos are placed on the realignment marks to facilitate subsequent wound closure.

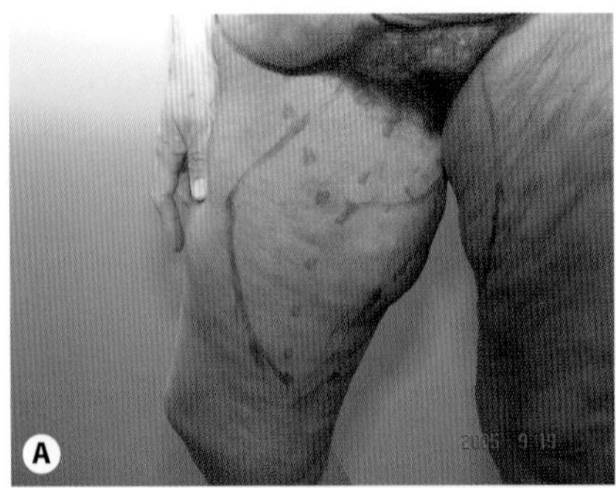

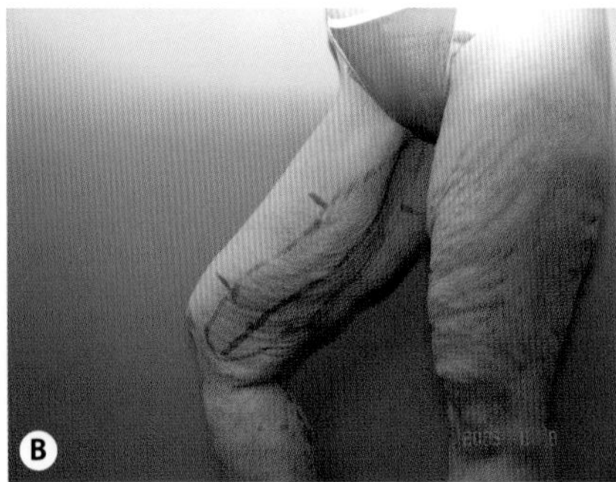

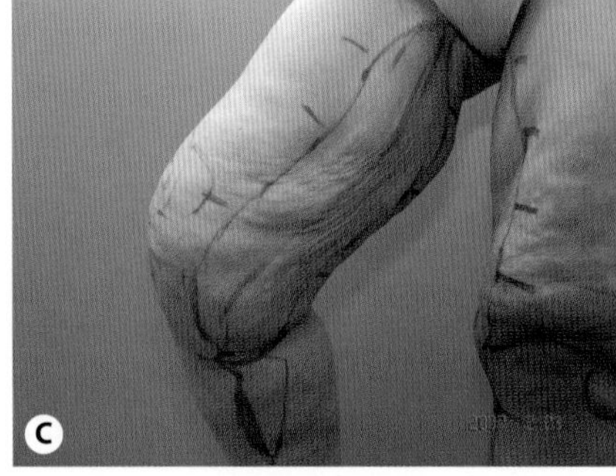

Fig. 13.222 Vertical Thigh Lift Images A–C The extent of the vertical thigh lift is dependent on the patient's deformity and wishes. **A** In this case the inner thigh lift is marked as well as a more limited vertical thigh lift, which was determined by patient preference. **B** The more usual scenario for vertical thigh lift is one that extends down to the level of the knee. This allows tightening and improvement all the way down to and including the knee. **C** In this situation, the extended vertical thigh lift goes beyond the knee to the mid-calf. This patient experienced dramatic weight loss and had significant laxity distal to the knee that she wanted corrected. Note the notch at the level of the knee flexion crease, avoiding a scar band deformity.

suddenly separate, indicating that the superficial fascia has been released and the extent of the sharp dissection reached (**Fig. 13.228**).

At this point, a penetrating towel clamp is placed at the most proximal end of the ellipse of skin to be removed. The assistant supports the surrounding tissue and the entire skin island is slowly and gently avulsed distally (caudally) (**Fig. 13.229 A–F**). This tissue should be removed from proximal to distal to prevent avulsion or undermining of the superficial veins in the area. ***Do not avulse tissue from distal to proximal!***

A drain is frequently used and brought out through the upper thigh or mons area. Final closure is performed with interrupted deep dermal 2/0 PDS (or equivalent) and continuous intradermal 4/0 Monocryl (or equivalent) (**Fig. 13.230 A–D**). It may be wise to staple the wound closed temporarily as the resection proceeds, as soft-tissue swelling may make reapproximation of the skin edges more difficult. The incision line is usually treated with skin adhesive. We routinely use compressive wraps or garments that extend below the knee postoperatively to help reduce the extent of lower extremity edema.

Postoperative Care

Leg elevation and brief but regular ambulation are recommended following this procedure. Prolonged sitting with the legs dependent or standing should be minimized. The wound is inspected after a few days. Scar Guard is useful on the incisions during the healing and maturation process.

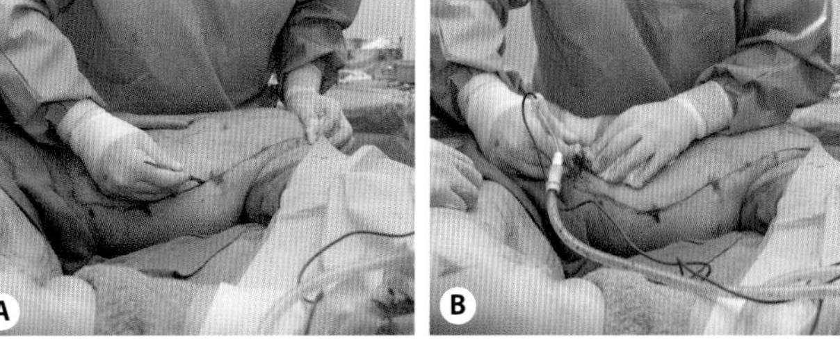

Fig. 13.227 Vertical Thigh Lift Images A, B The incision is made with a number 10 blade into the dermis and then electrocautery deepens the dissection into the subcutaneous tissue.

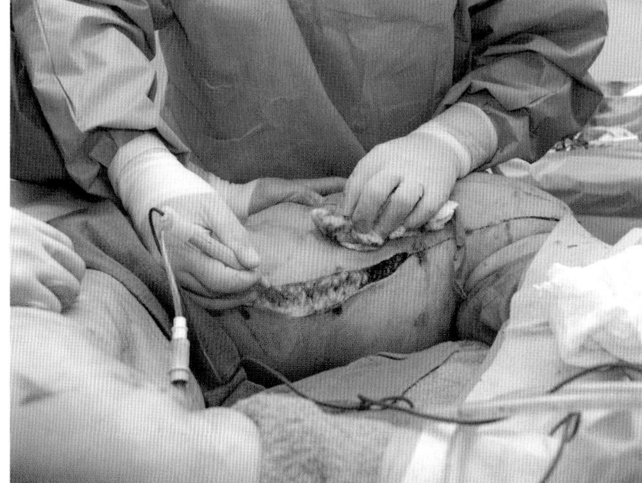

Fig. 13.228 Vertical Thigh Lift Images When the correct plane of tissue dissection is encountered with electrocautery, the wound margins separates indicating release of the superficial foseia.

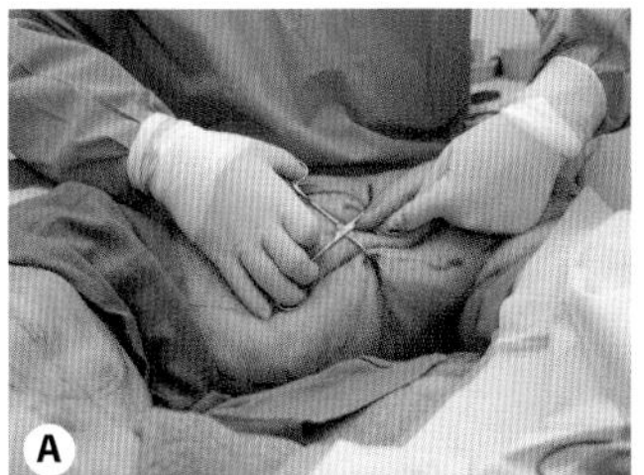
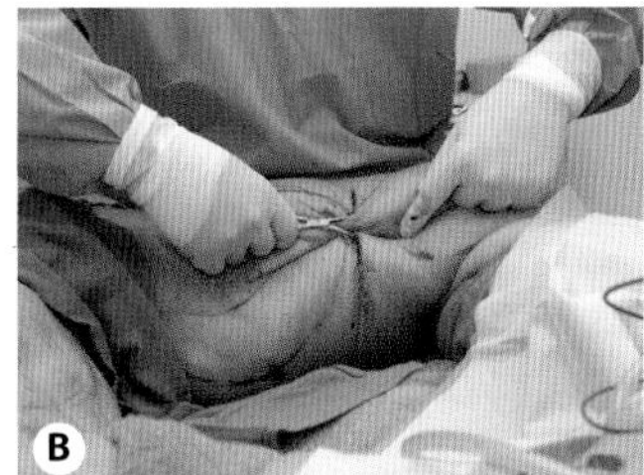
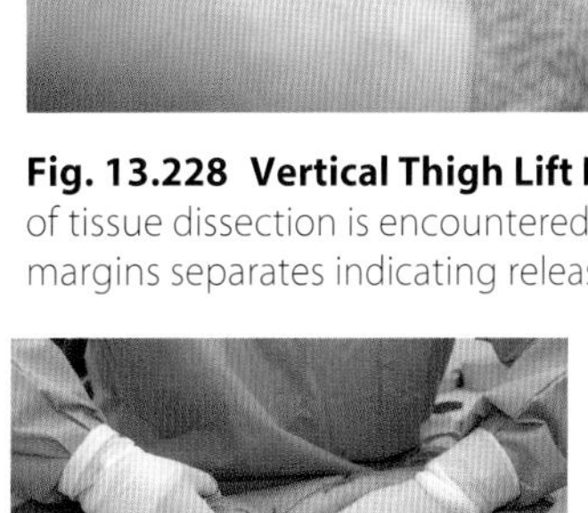
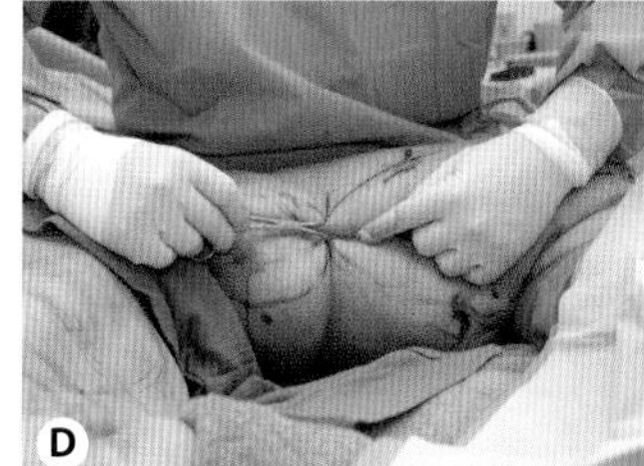

Fig. 13.225 Vertical Thigh Lift Images A–D Penetrating towel clips are used at various levels along the thigh lift to ensure that there is not too much tension on closure. If the tension is excessive the markings are redrawn, reducing the amount of tissue to be excised. This should be done before the infiltration of epinephrine-containing solution because this will increase the thickness of the tissues and make this determination more difficult.

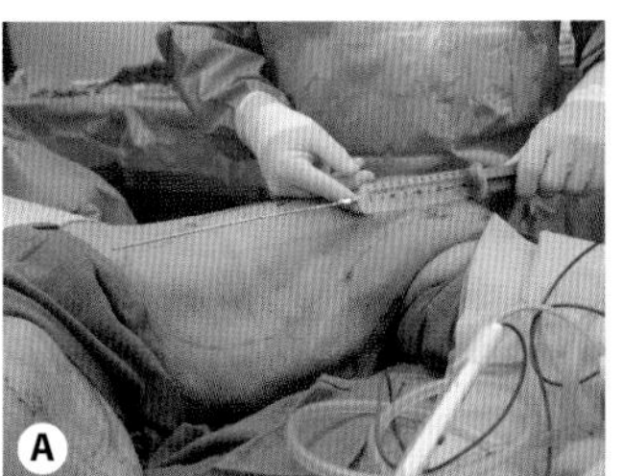
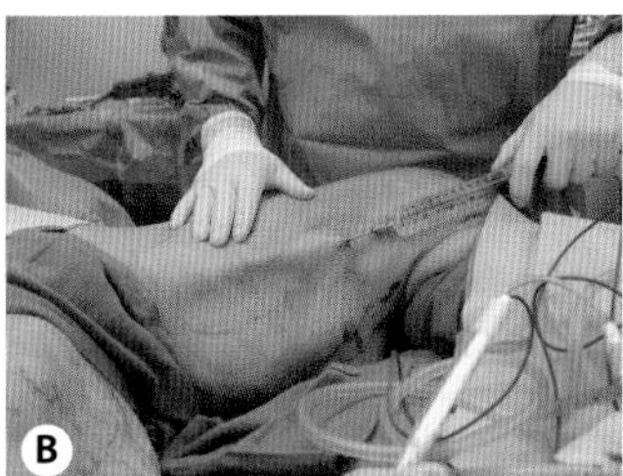
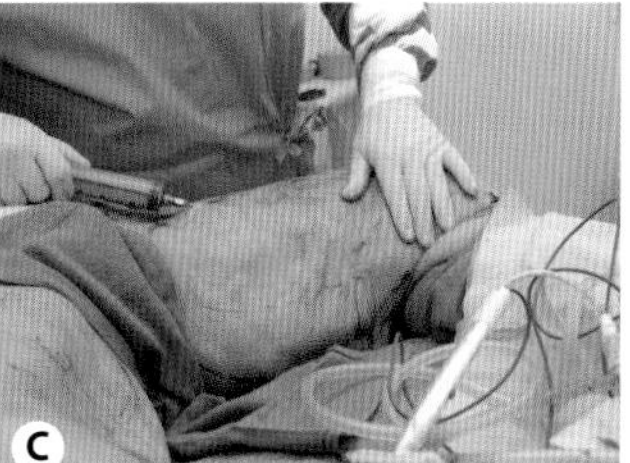
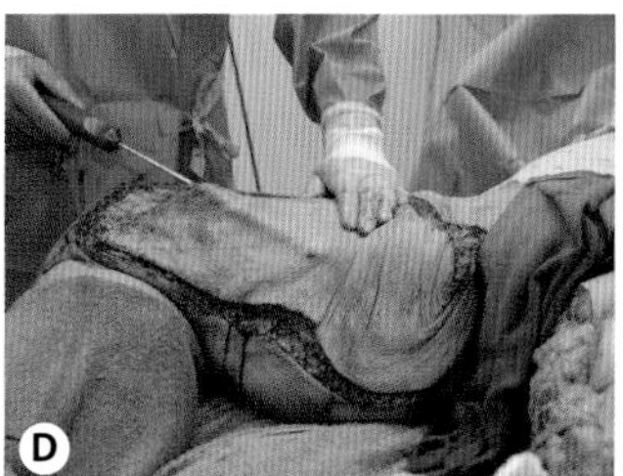

Fig. 13.226 Vertical Thigh Lift Images A–C The dilute lidocaine and epinephrine containing solution is infiltrated to minimize bleeding. The process of infiltration involves tissue tunneling or undermining, defining the plane in which the tissue will be resected. Where there is excess adiposity, thorough liposuction of the subcutaneous fat is performed within the pattern of excision, as well as lateral to the border of resection, which also helps define the plane of resection.

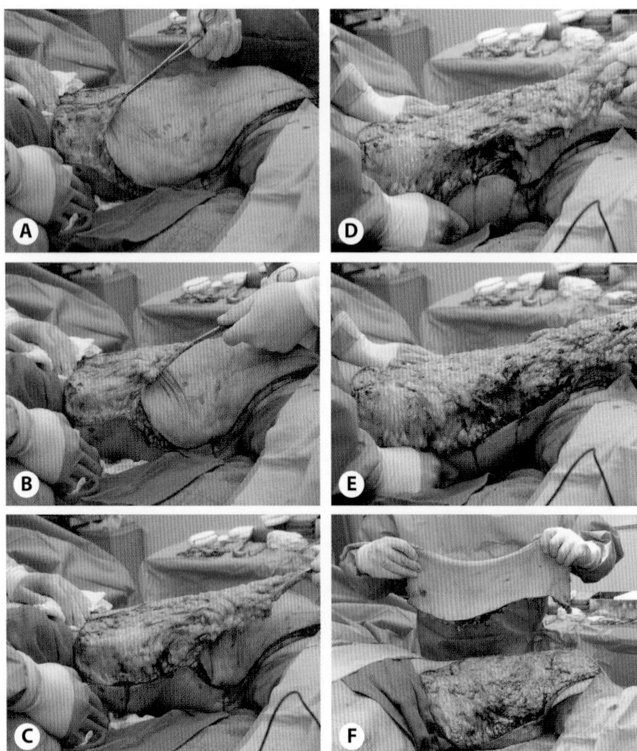

Figs 13.229 Vertical Thigh Lift Images A–F After the subcutaneous tissue has been released circumferentially around the island of skin to be removed by electrocautery, a penetrating towel clamp is placed at the most proximal end of this skin pattern. The assistant supports the surrounding tissues and the surgeon pulls the skin island distally, avulsing the tissue from the underlying subcutaneous fat and vascular structures. The tissue separates smoothly and evenly, leaving behind the latticework of intact veins, nerves, and lymphatics. This technique minimizes the formation of lymphocele, which is not infrequently seen after electrocautery dissection of the vertical inner thigh tissue.

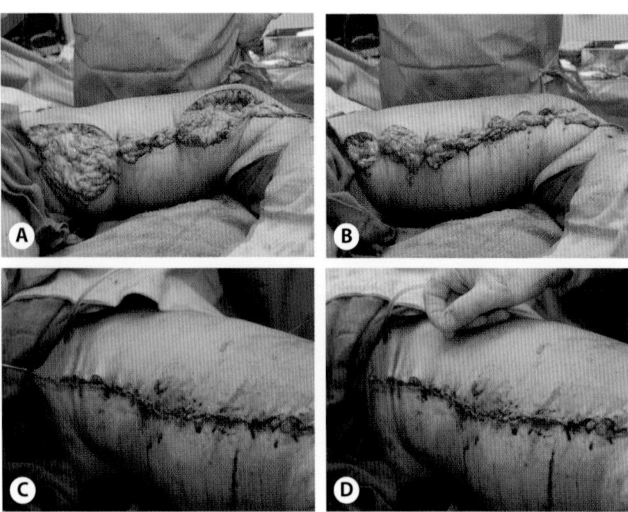

Fig. 13.230 Vertical Thigh Lift Images A, B The wound is closed with interrupted 2/0 or 3/0 PDS or equivalent at the level of the deep dermis. The sutures are placed approximately every centimeter along the course of the incision. A 4/0 Monocryl or equivalent suture is used for final intracuticular closure. **C, D** By placing small bites in the pubic area, the suture can be pulled distally, shortening the final incision.

Before and After Figures (Figs 13.231–13.264)

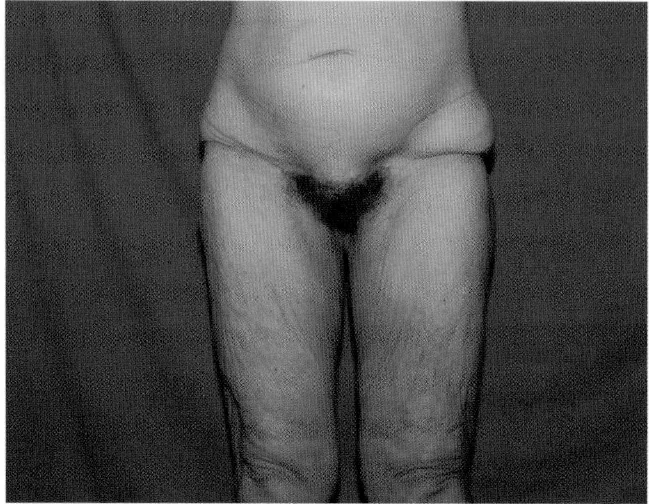

Fig. 13.231

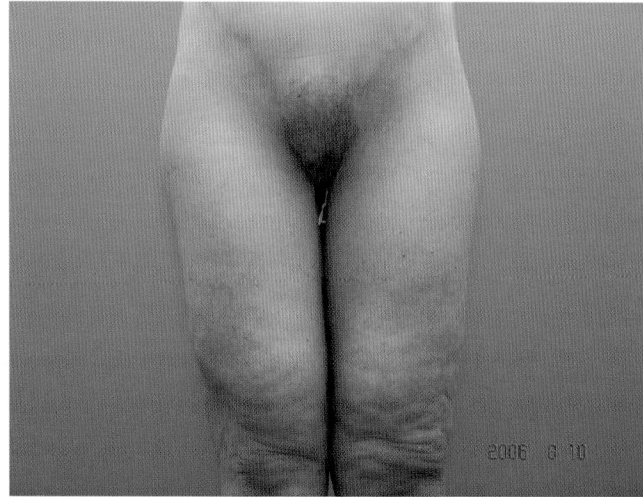

Fig. 13.232

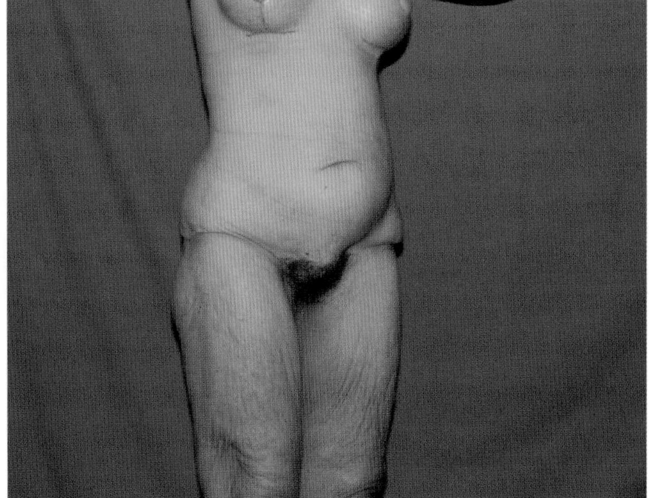

Fig. 13.233

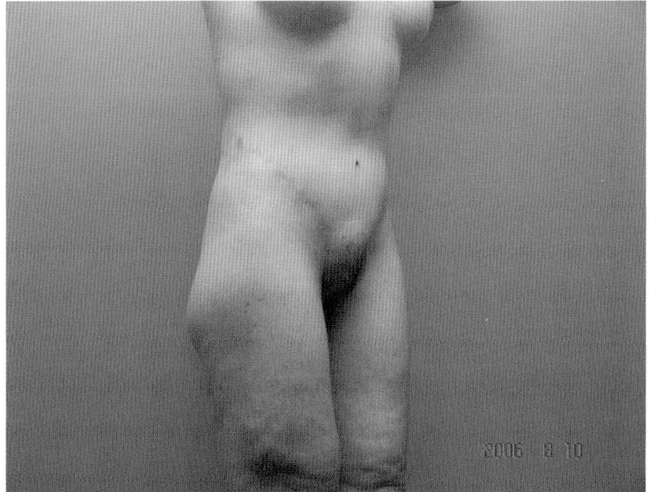

Fig. 13.234

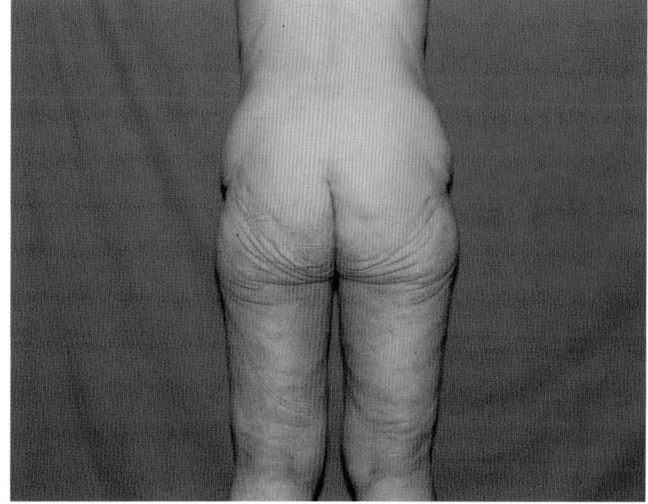

Fig. 13.235

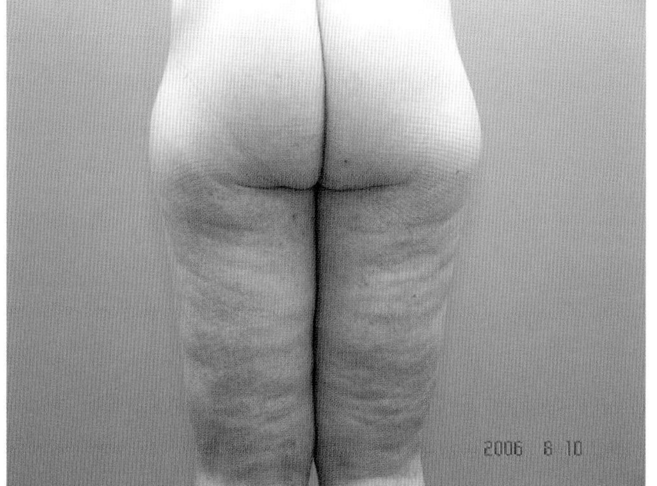

Fig. 13.236

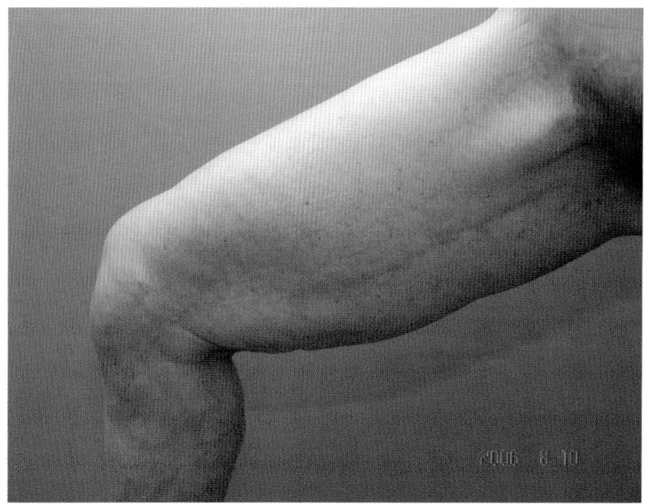

Fig. 13.237

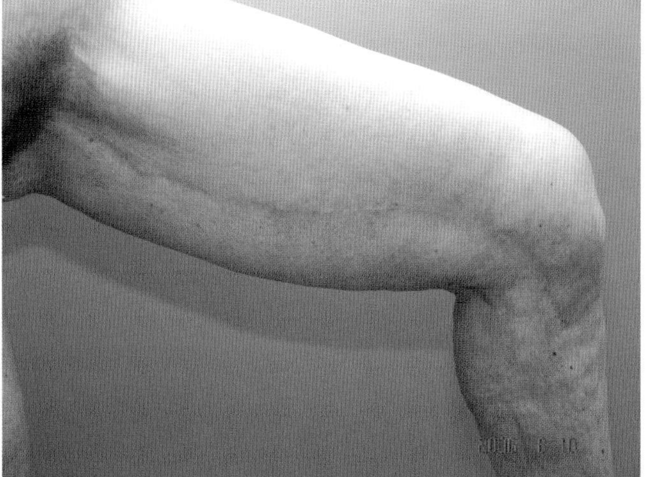

Fig. 13.238

Figs 13.231–13.238 Vertical Thigh Lift Pre- and Postoperative Images The patient has successfully undergone massive weight loss. A vertical thigh lift was an integral component of her post-bariatric rehabilitation. The improvement in the overall laxity of the thighs is dramatic, partly because of the body lift but also due to the vertical thigh lift. Contouring of the leg is evident all the way to the knee. The incisions are not visible anteriorly or posteriorly. The final scar located on the inner side has healed well.

Figs 13.239–13.250

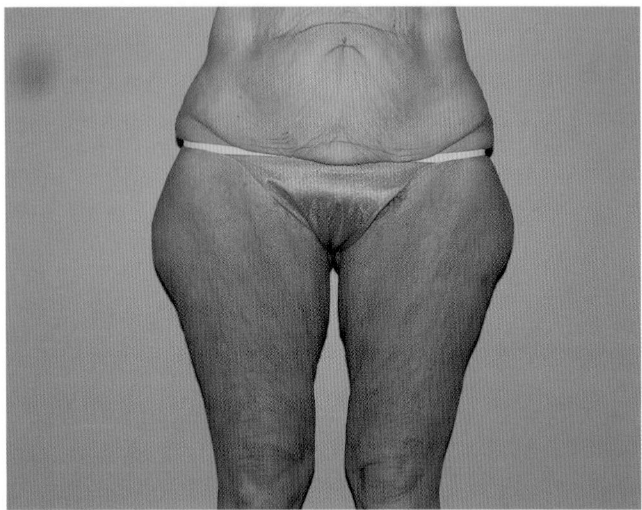

Fig. 13.239

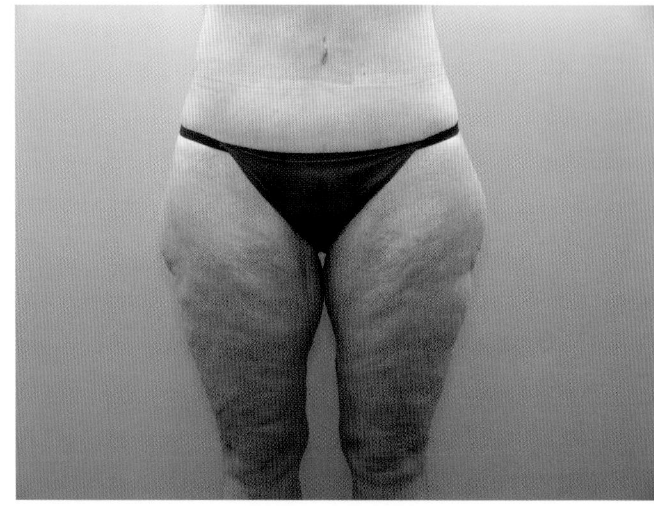

Fig. 13.240

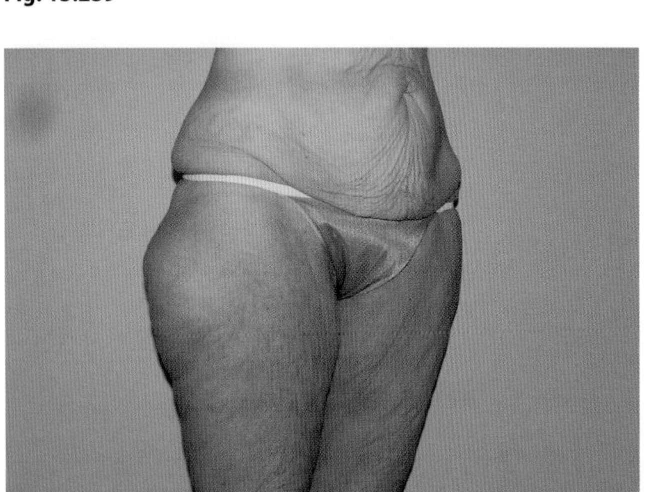

Fig. 13.241

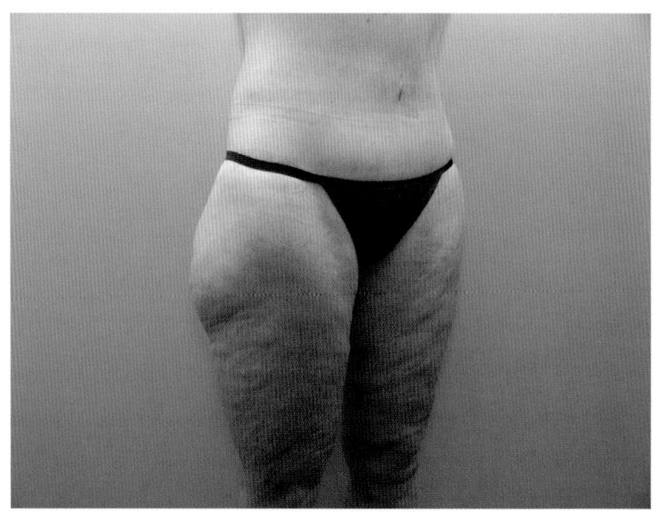

Fig. 13.242

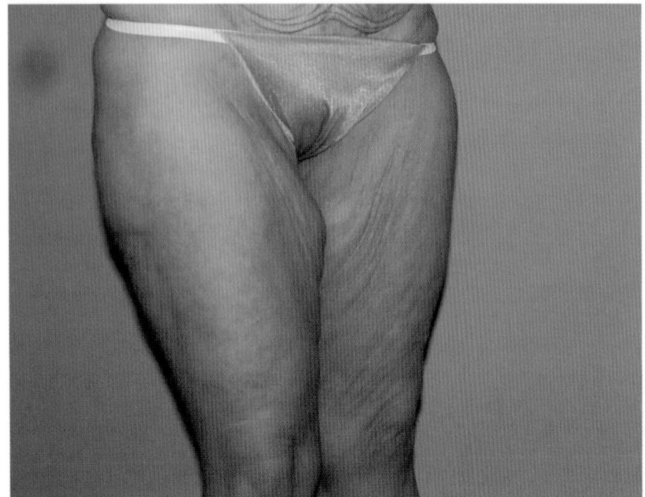

Fig. 13.243

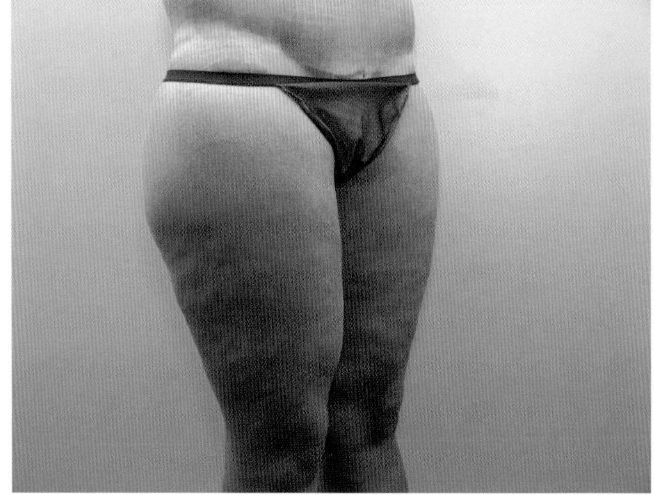

Fig. 13.244

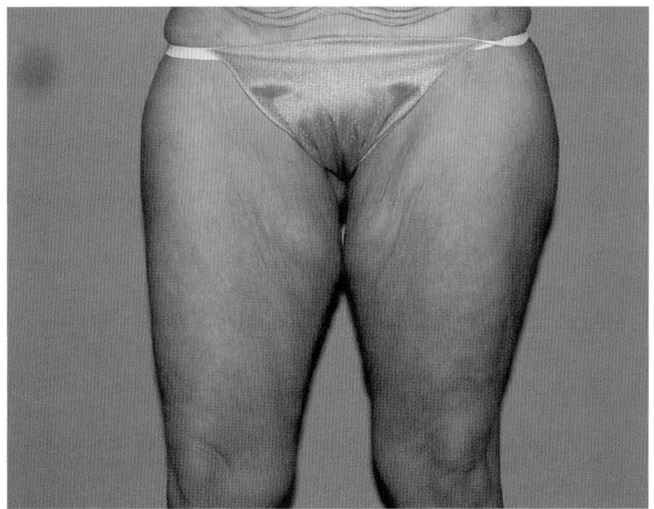

Fig. 13.245

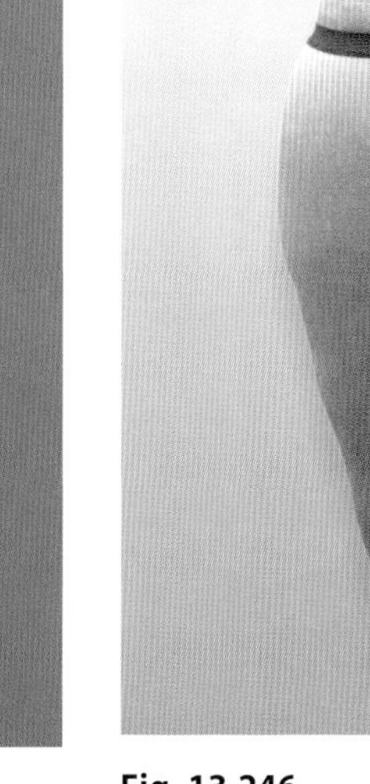

Fig. 13.246

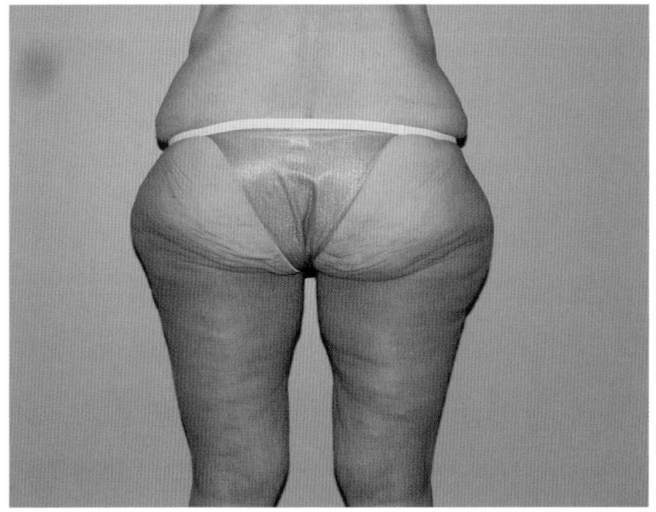

Fig. 13.247

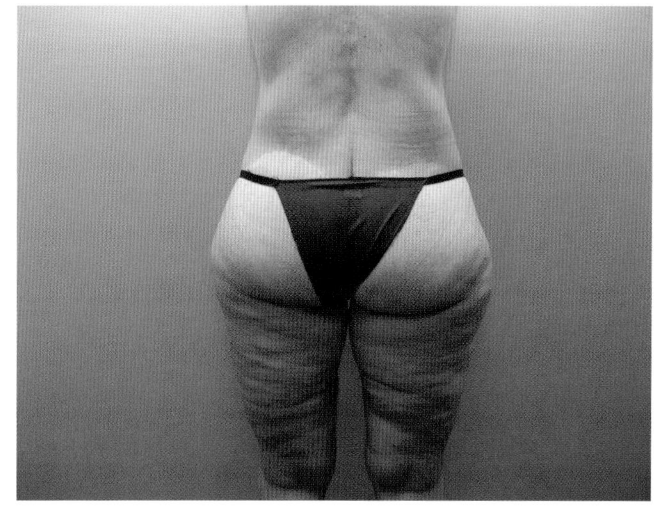

Fig. 13.248

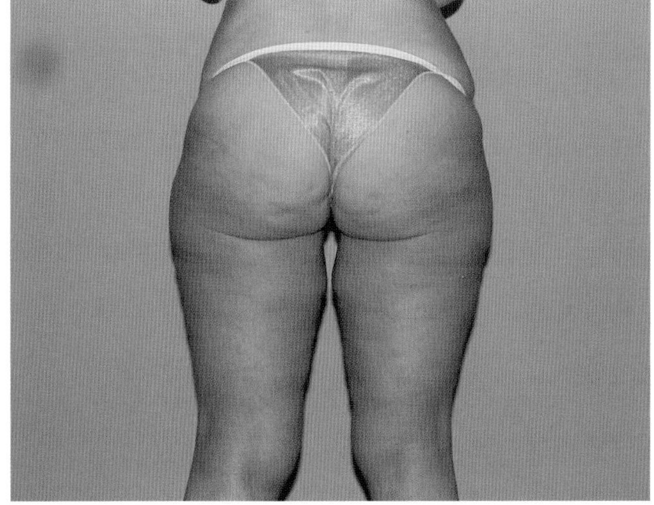

Fig. 13.249

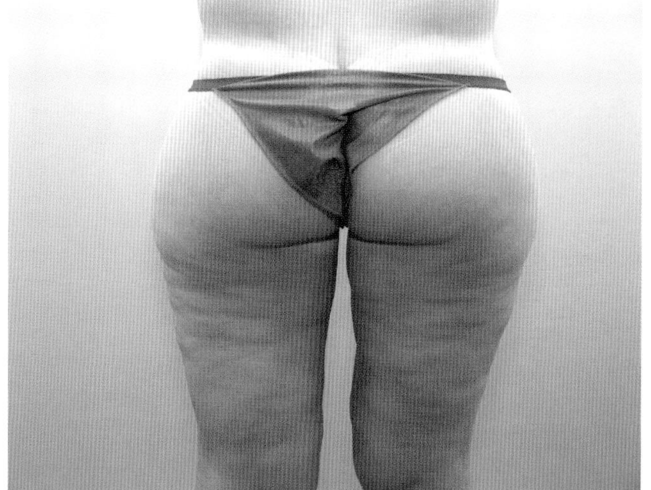

Fig. 13.250

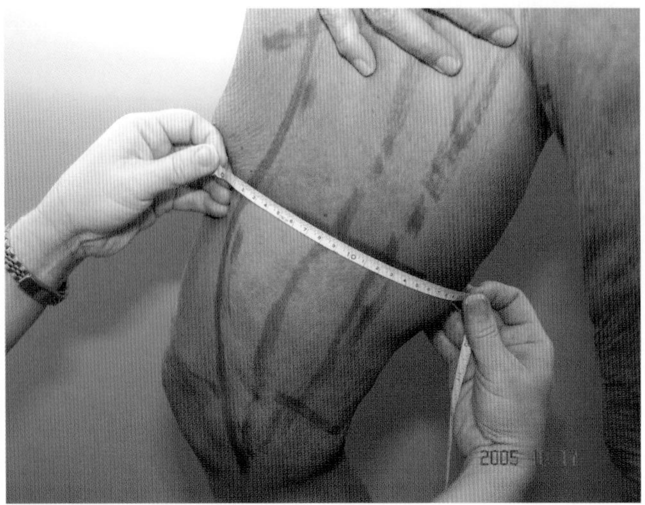

Fig. 13.251

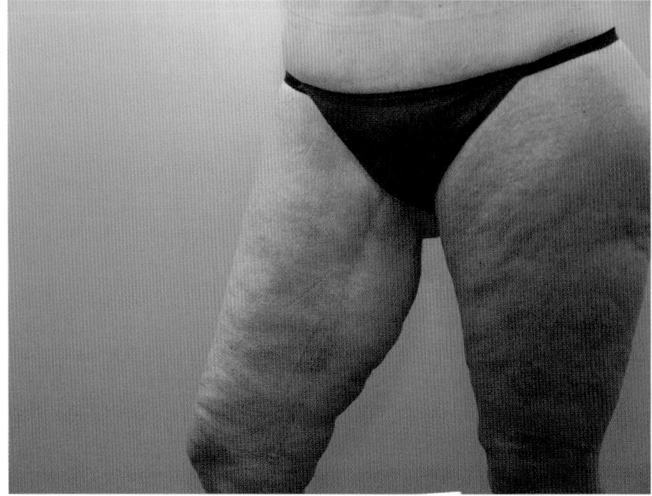

Fig. 13.252

Figs 13.239–13.252 Vertical Thigh Lift Pre- and Postoperative Images This massive weight loss patient has undergone a circumferential abdominoplasty and vertical thigh lift. She developed a lymphocele in the distal thigh but was treated successfully with wound exploration and daily dressings. The wound closed secondarily and the scar was subsequently was revised. She has experienced a significant improvement in overall shape and contour, and has a fine-quality final scar along the posterior aspect of the inner thigh.

Figs 13.253–13.256

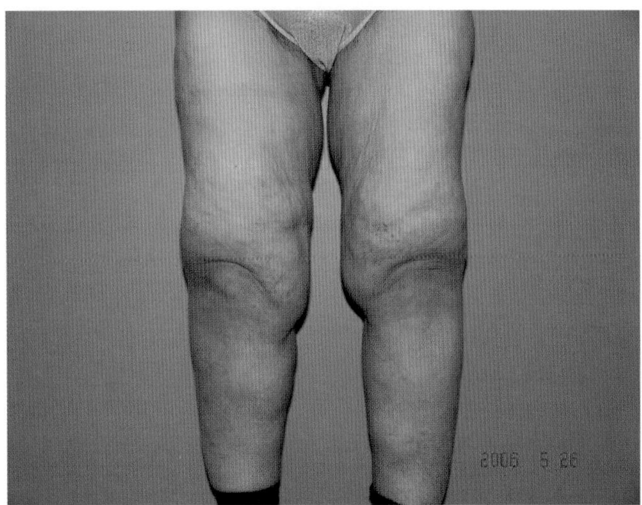

Fig. 13.253

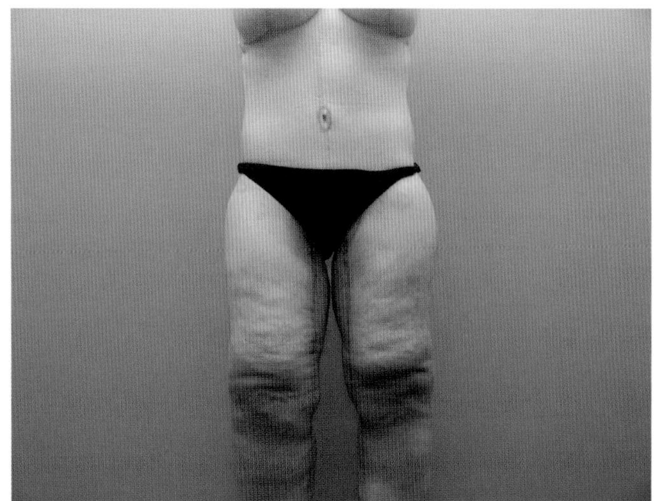

Fig. 13.254

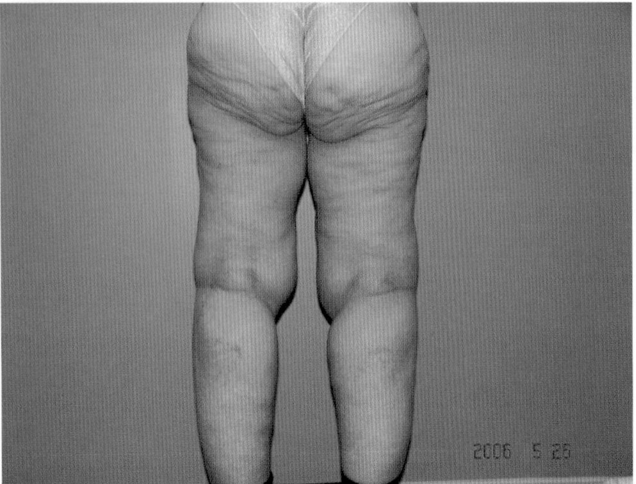

Fig. 13.255

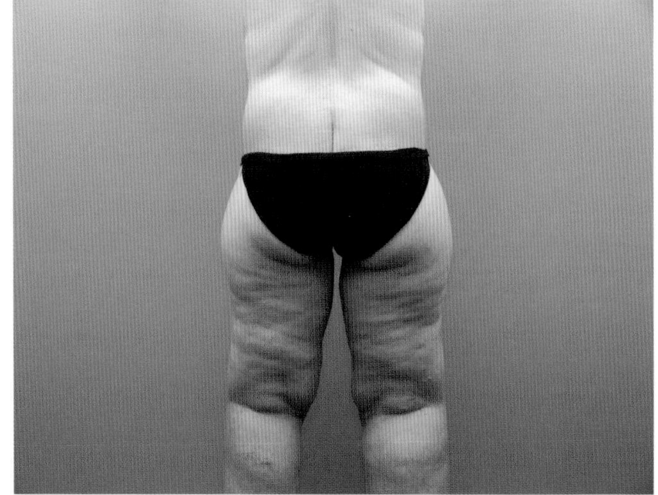

Fig. 13.256

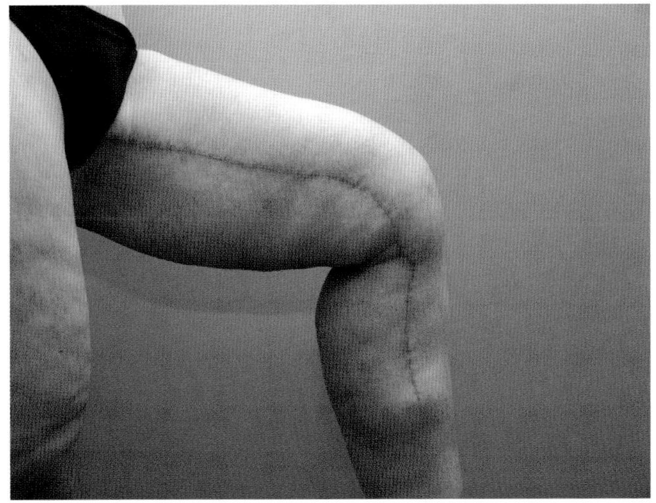

Fig. 13.257

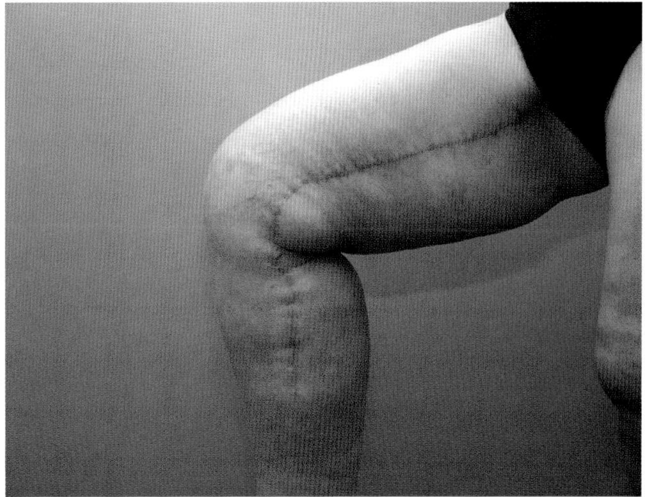

Fig. 13.258

Figs 13.253–13.256 Vertical Thigh Lift Pre-and Postoperative Images This massive weight loss patient underwent an extended vertical thigh lift to the level of the mid-calf, which removed the laxity that was present to this level. The incision healed well without a scar band contracture because of the notching intentionally placed at the level of the knee.

Figs 13.259–13.262

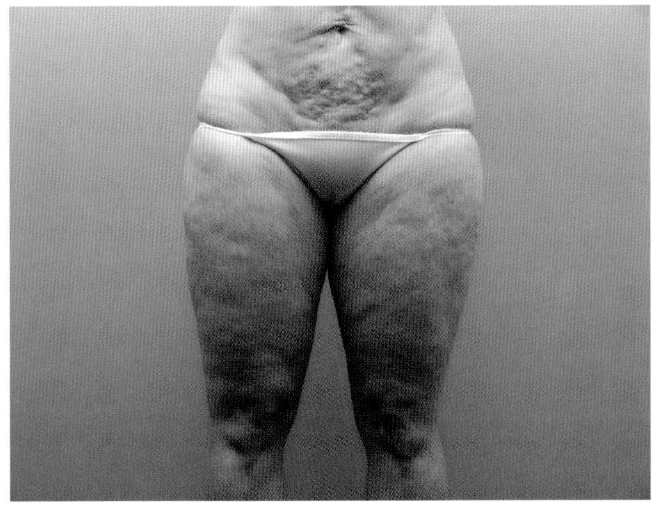

Fig. 13.259

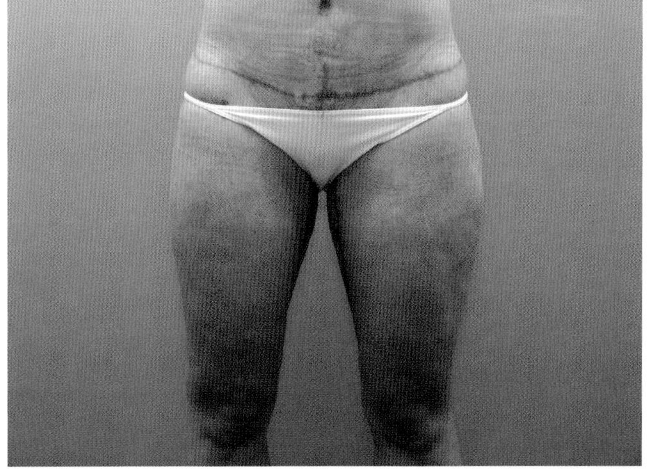

Fig. 13.260

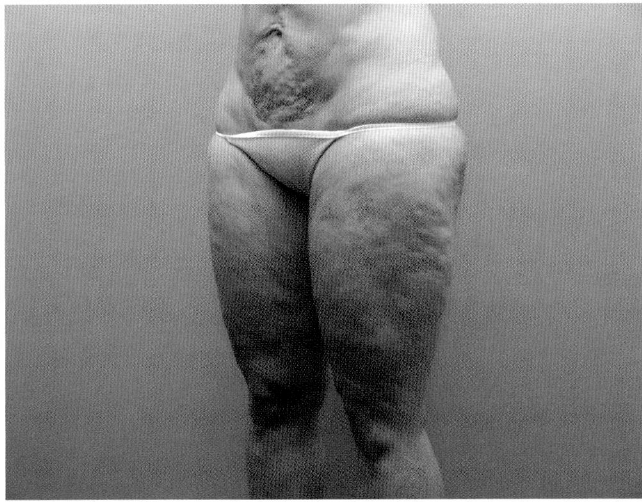

Fig. 13.261

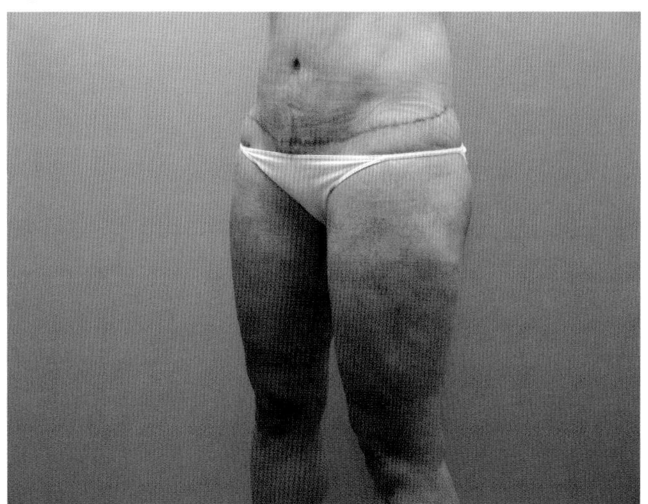

Fig. 13.262

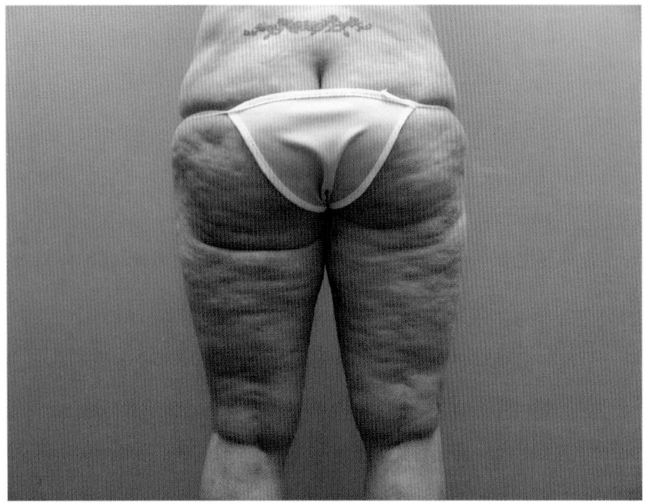

Fig. 13.263

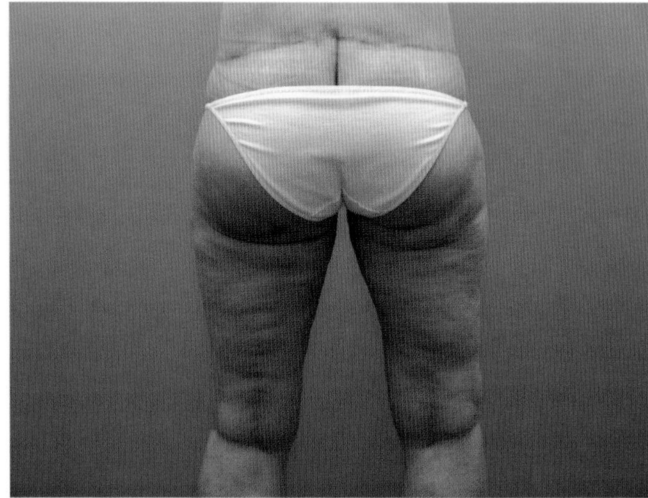

Fig. 13.264

Fig. 13.259–13.264 Vertical Thigh Lift Pre- and Postoperative Images This patient presented following previous abdominal liposuction elsewhere and was treated with a circumferential abdominoplasty, and a vertical thigh lift with concurrent circumferential thigh liposuction. This combination represents a challenge, but when the liposuction is performed thoroughly, and the tissue to be resected is marked again intraoperatively, this can be performed successfully. This patient experienced a dramatic improvement in overall body contour.

Summary

Ancillary procedures are an important and integral part of the body contouring process. They can be performed in conjunction with or following the abdominal contouring procedure. A careful balance should be maintained between allowing the patient to volunteer the desire for correction of certain regions of the body and the surgeon's ability to provide the patient with information and guidance regarding ancillary procedures. When careful discussion and proper evaluation take place, the overall aesthetic result, as well as the level of patient satisfaction, is increased by the addition of these ancillary procedures.

References

1. Trussler AP, Rohrich RJ. Limited incision medial brachioplasty: technical refinements in upper arm contouring. Plast Reconstruct Surg 2008; 121: 305.
2. Regnault P. Brachioplasty, axilloplasty, and pre-axilloplasty. Aesthet Plast Surg 1983; 7: 31.
3. Aly A, Soliman S, Cram A. Brachioplasty in the massive weight loss patient. Clin Plast Surg 2008; 35: 141–147.
4. Hunstad JP, Repta R. Bra-line back lift. Plast Reconstruct Surg 2008; (in press).
5. Hunstad JP, Repta R. Purse-string gluteoplasty. Plast Reconstruct Surg 2008; (in press).
6. Roberts TL III, Weinfeld AB, Bruner TW, Nguyen K. 'Universal' and ethnic ideals of beautiful buttocks are best obtained by autologous micro fat grafting and liposuction. Clin Plast Surg 2006; 33: 371.
7. Cárdenas-Camarena L, Lacouture AM, Tobar-Losada A. Combined gluteoplasty: liposuction and lipoinjection. Plast Reconstruct Surg 1999; 104: 1524.
8. Mathes DW, Kenkel JM. Current concepts in medial thighplasty. Clin Plast Surg 2008; 35: 151.
9. Hodgkinson DJ. Medial thighplasty, prevention of scar migration, and labial flattening. Aesthet Plast Surg 1989; 13: 111.
10. Cram A, Aly A. Thigh reduction in the massive weight loss patient. Clin Plast Surg 2008; 35: 165.

Suggested Reading

Abramson DL. Minibrachioplasty: minimizing scars while maximizing results. Plast Reconstruct Surg 2004; 114: 1631–1634; discussion 1635–1637.

Aly A, Soliman S, Cram A. Brachioplasty in the massive weight loss patient. Augmentation gluteoplasty. Plast Reconstruct Surg 2006; 117: 1781–1788.

Cannistra C, Valero R, Benelli C, Marmuse JP. Brachioplasty after massive weight loss: a simple algorithm for surgical plan. Aesthet Plast Surg 2007; 31: 6–9; discussion 10–11.

Cannistra C, Valero R, Benelli C, Marmuse JP. Thigh and buttock lift after massive weight loss. Aesthet Plast Surg 2007; 31: 233–237.

Cárdenas-Camarena L, Paillet JC. Combined gluteoplasty: liposuction and gluteal implants. Plast Reconstruct Surg 2007; 119: 1067–1074.

Coleman S. Structural fat grafting. St Louis: Quality Medical Publishing, 2004.

Dini GM, Ferreria LM. Augmentation brachioplasty. Plast Reconstruct Surg 2006; 117: 2109–2111.

Ellabban MG, Hart NB. Body contouring by combined abdominoplasty and medial vertical thigh reduction: experience of 14 cases. Br J Plast Surg 2004; 57: 222–227.

Gmür RU, Banic A, Erni D. Is it safe to combine abdominoplasty with other dermolipectomy procedures to correct skin excess after weight loss? Ann Plast Surg 2003; 51: 353–357.

Gonzalez R. Augmentation gluteoplasty: the XYZ method. Aesthet Plast Surg 2004; 28: 417–425.

Gonzalez R. Etiology, definition, and classification of gluteal ptosis. Aesthet Plast Surg 2006; 30: 320–326.

González-Ulloa M. Gluteoplasty: a ten-year report. Aesthet Plast Surg 1991; 15: 85–91.

Hurwitz DJ. Single-staged total body lift after massive weight loss. Ann Plast Surg 2004; 52: 435.

Hunstad JP. Body contouring in the obese patient. Clin Plast Surg 1996; 23: 647–670; PMID: 8906395.

Hurwitz DJ, Holland SW. The L brachioplasty: an innovative approach to correct excess tissue of the upper arm, axilla, and lateral chest. Plast Reconstruct Surg 2006; 117: 403–411; discussion 412–413.

Hurwitz DJ, Neavin T. L brachioplasty correction of excess tissue of the upper arm, axilla, and lateral chest. Clin Plast Surg 2008; 35: 131–140; discussion 149.

Knoetgen J 3rd, Moran SL. Long-term outcomes and complications associated with brachioplasty: a retrospective review and cadaveric study. Plast Reconstruct Surg 2006; 117: 2219–2223.

Lack EB. Contouring the female buttocks. Liposculpting the buttocks. Dermatol Clin 1999; 17: 815–822; vi.

Leitner DW, Sherwood RC. Inguinal lymphocele as a complication of thighplasty. Plast Reconstruct Surg 1983; 72: 878–881.

Lockwood T. Brachioplasty with superficial fascial system suspension. Plast Reconstruct Surg 1995; 96: 912–920.

McGohan LD. Body contouring following major weight loss. J Contin Educ Nurs 2007; 38: 103–104 [Review].

Pascal JF, Le Louarn C. Brachioplasty. Aesthet Plast Surg 2005; 29: 423–429; discussion 430.

Raposo-Amaral CE, Cetrulo CL Jr., Guidi Mde C, et al. Impact of significant weight loss on outcome of body-contouring surgery. Ann Plast Surg 2006; 56: 9–13; discussion 13.

Sozer SO, Agullo FJ, Palladino H. Bilateral lumbar hip dermal fat rotation flaps: a novel technique for autologous augmentation gluteoplasty. Plast Reconstruct Surg 2007; 119: 1126–1127.

Strauch B, Greenspun D, Levine J, Baum T. A technique of brachioplasty. Plast Reconstruct Surg 2004; 113: 1044–1048; discussion 1049.

Strauch B, Herman C, Rohde C, Baum T. Mid-body contouring in the post-bariatric surgery patient. Plast Reconstruct Surg 2006; 117: 2200–2211.

Teimourian B, Malekzadeh S. Rejuvenation of the upper arm. Plast Reconstruct Surg 1998; 102: 545–551; discussion 552–553.

Vergara R, Marcos M. Intramuscular gluteal implants. Aesthet Plast Surg 1996; 20: 259–262.

CHAPTER **14**

Management of Existing Abdominal Scars

Joseph P. Hunstad and Remus Repta

IN THIS CHAPTER

KEY POINTS

Pre-existing abdominal scars can have a significant impact on the safety and final result of abdominoplasty and abdominal contouring procedures. These scars should be judiciously taken into account during the evaluation and planning process. Although safety is the primary focus, pre-existing abdominal scars are not an absolute contraindication to abdominoplasty when the procedure is properly planned and designed. With proper design modification, good aesthetic results can be safely achieved in patients with pre-existing abdominal scars.

Introduction

Abdominal incisions are commonly used for the majority of general, gynecologic, oncologic, urologic, and other surgical operations. Because of this, abdominal scars are frequently encountered in patients presenting for abdominoplasty and abdominal body contouring. Although laparoscopic surgery has reduced the length of the scars associated with many of these common procedures, large surgical scars across important soft-tissue vascular territories are often still encountered. Fortunately, many of these pre-existing scars fall within the area of resection for standard abdominoplasty procedures.

Large scars that do not fall within the abdominoplasty resection segment require careful evaluation and modification of the standard abdominoplasty design. The presence of such scars should not serve as an absolute contraindication to abdominoplasty and abdominal contouring procedures: instead, thoughtful planning should allow a modified design to be tailored to each individual patient so as to reduce the incidence of complications, particularly ischemia and necrosis, and safely achieve the best possible aesthetic result.[1,2]

Patient Selection

Patients seeking abdominal contouring procedures can present with a variety of existing abdominal scars. The significance of these is based on many factors, including size and location of the scar, the amount of abdominal soft-tissue laxity, and the desired aesthetic goal. To simplify the evaluation process as well as selection of the appropriate abdominoplasty procedure, we have categorized those patients whose scars require little modification of the abdominoplasty

Table 14.1 Classification of pre-existing abdominal scars

Category	Scar location/Impact on the abdominoplasty design
I	The scar generally falls within the soft-tissue segment that is resected during a standard abdominoplasty (midline, Pfannensteil, or right/left lower quadrants). Little or no modification of the standard technique is needed
IIA	The subcostal scar (unilateral or bilateral) is near the costal margin. Traditional full abdominoplasty techniques will risk ischemia of the tissue immediately caudal to the scar(s). A reverse abdominoplasty or a lower abdominoplasty (or a staged procedure with both a reverse abdominoplasty and a lower abdominoplasty) can safely be used to resect excess soft-tissue laxity
IIB	The subcostal scar is some distance below the costal margin, either by original design or secondary to soft-tissue descent. Neither a reverse abdominoplasty nor a traditional abdominoplasty can incorporate this scar. A full or circumferential abdominoplasty with a vertical or oblique segment can be used to remove the tissue medial and caudal to the scar that is at highest risk for ischemia. This procedure design is not a safe option for patients in this category who have bilateral subcostal (chevron) scars. A reverse abdominoplasty, either alone or staged with a lower abdominoplasty, is recommended, accepting the fact that the final scar will near the mid-abdomen at the level of the previous scar.

design as category I, and those that require fundamental design alteration as category II (**Table 14.1**). As with most categorizations, some patients fall somewhere in between the groups. Nevertheless, this is an initial step in the evaluation and management of these patients and aids efficient communication among surgeons.

The most common abdominal scars seen are those following laparoscopic surgery. These are usually between three and five in number, between 2 and 4 cm in length, and do not significantly affect the vascular perfusion of the abdominal skin. The traditional 'open' surgical approaches to the abdomen have a greater potential to negatively affect the safety and/or final result of an abdominoplasty procedure. Fortunately, the more common 'open' procedures usually result in a scar in the lower abdomen. These include the traditional right lower quadrant appendectomy approach, infraumbilical midline laparotomy, and the suprapubic Pfannensteil incision (**Fig. 14.1**). Although some caution is warranted in these cases owing to the potential presence of excess scar tissue and abdominal wall incisional hernia, little modification of the standard abdominoplasty technique is usually needed, as these scars usually fall within the soft-tissue segment that is resected. A similar group of patients are those with pre-existing supraumbilical midline scars (**Fig. 14.2**). Because these scars are in the watershed area of the left and right intercostal and subcostal perforators, they are often easily incorporated into standard abdominoplasty techniques. A simple scar revision may be necessary if there is a scar band contracture, or a more sizeable vertical resection can be added if deemed beneficial to the final aesthetic result (**Fig. 14.3**). Patients presenting with these types of scars are classified as category I, as little modification of the standard abdominoplasty procedure is needed.

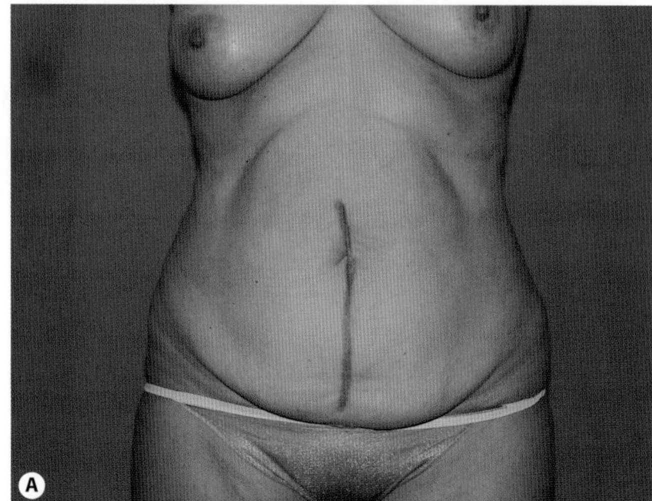

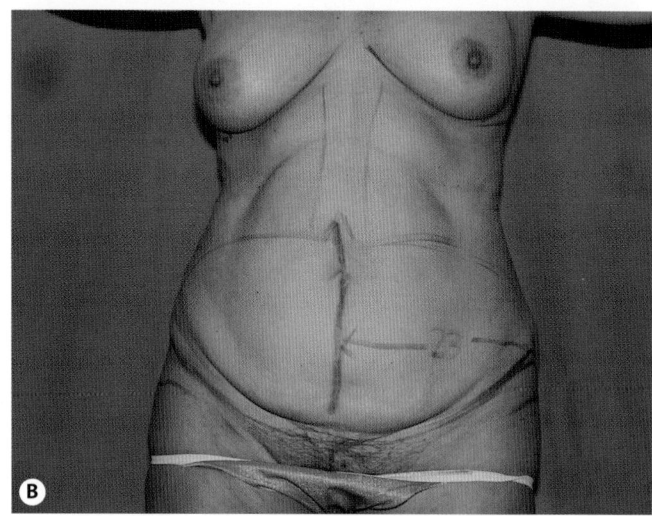

Fig. 14.1 Patients with pre-existing abdominal scars in the lower abdomen (appendectomy, infraumbilical laparotomy, and Pfannensteil incisions) require little modification of the standard full abdominoplasty procedure design because the scar falls within the soft-tissue resection segment.

Abdominal scars that cross important vascular territories and that cannot be incorporated into the resected soft-tissue segment are of greater concern. These include unilateral subcostal incisions (Kocher) or bilateral subcostal incisions connected in the midline (chevron). Patients with these types of scar are classified as category II, as they require significant alteration of the standard abdominoplasty design in order to prevent ischemic complications. These patients can be further subclassified according to the position of the scar relative to the costal margin, because this will in part

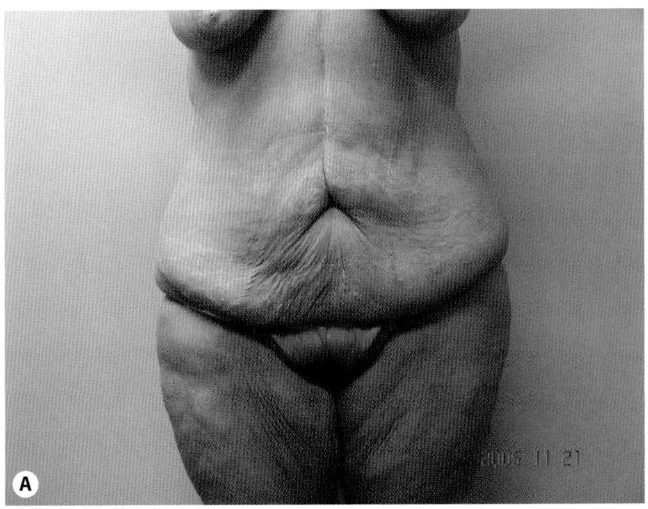

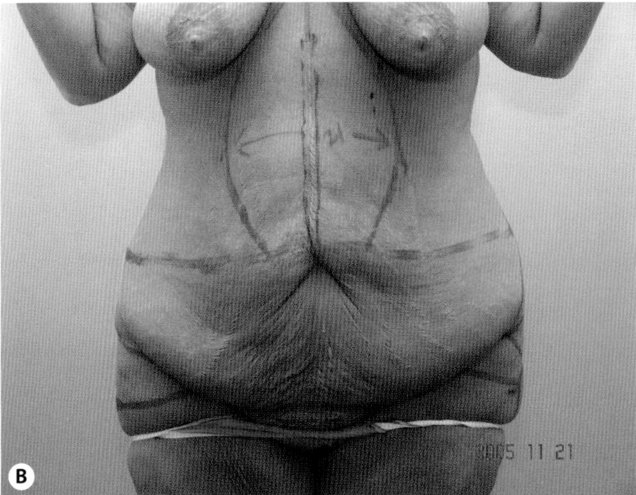

Fig. 14.2 Patients with supraumbilical midline abdominal scars also require little modification of the standard abdominoplasty design, as the pre-existing scars are at the watershed area of the left and right intercostal and subcostal perforators and do not significantly affect the perfusion of the soft-tissue apron.

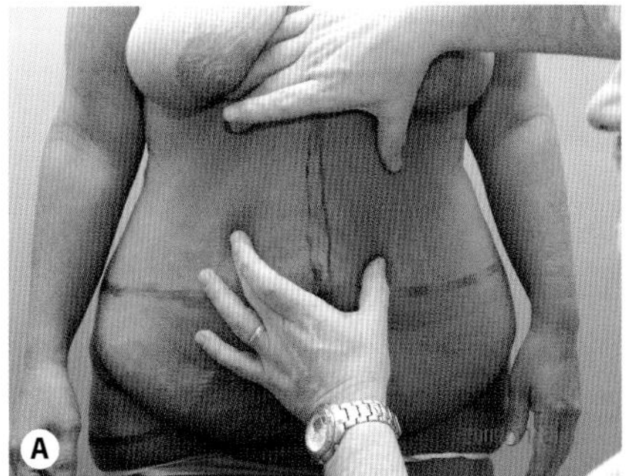

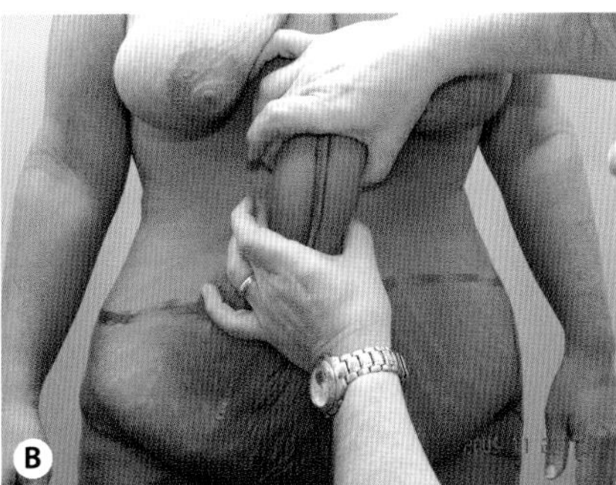

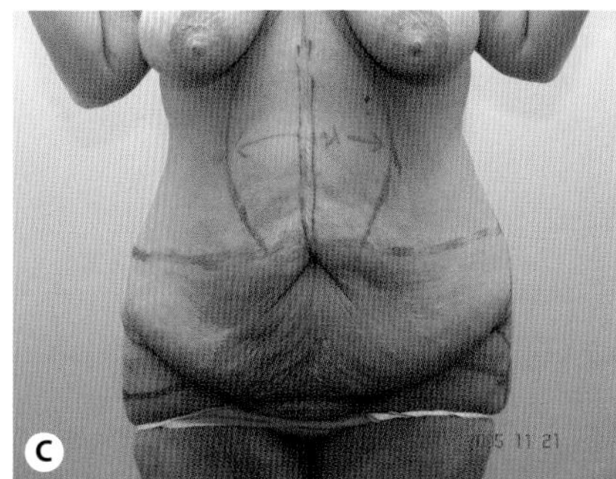

Fig. 14.3 The supraumbilical midline scar in patients undergoing abdominoplasty can be treated with either simple revision, a wider vertical wedge resection, or nothing at all if the scar is of good quality and does not restrict the soft-tissue apron from advancing caudally.

determine the type of abdominoplasty modification needed. Category IIA patients have subcostal scars that are very close to the costal margins, whereas category IIB patients have subcostal scars some distance below the costal margin, either by design or as a result of caudal migration secondary to increasing soft-tissue laxity. This distinction is important, because the abdominoplasty procedures best suited for each of these subgroups are fundamentally different (**Table 14.1**).

Category IIA patients (subcostal scar(s) at or near the costal margin) are at significant risk for ischemia of the abdominal soft tissue immediately distal to the scar (**Fig. 14.4**). The two general options to remove excess soft-tissue laxity in these patients are either a lower abdominoplasty with limited undermining or a reverse abdominoplasty. A lower abdominoplasty is ideally suited for patients with isolated lower abdominal soft-tissue excess. An example of this is the mini abdominoplasty patient (see Chapter 5, Mini Abdominoplasty). The superficial circumflex vessels and the perforators from the deep epigastric arcade above

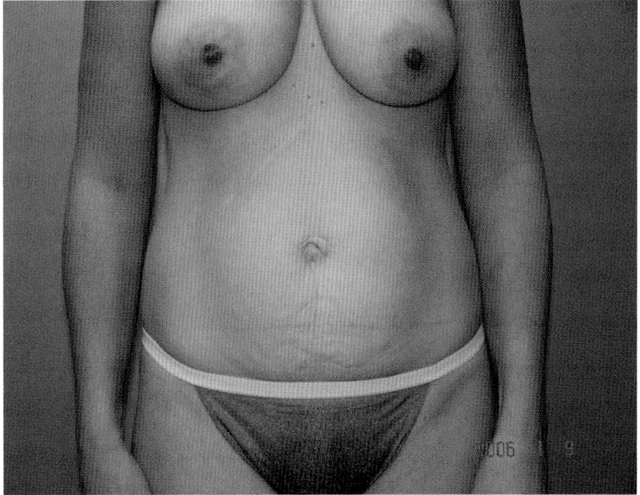

Fig. 14.4 Category IIA patients have a pre-existing subcostal scar at or very near the costal margin. Soft-tissue elevation up to the costal margins as performed in standard abdominoplasty will put the tissue immediately caudal to the pre-existing scar at risk for ischemia.

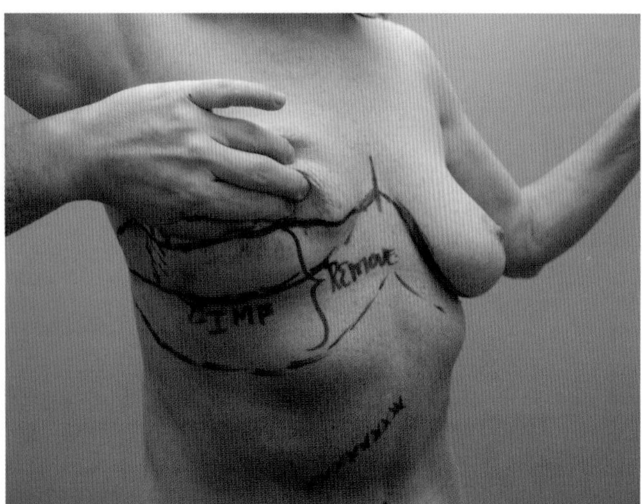

Fig. 14.5 A reverse abdominoplasty corrects some of the abdominal soft-tissue laxity through resection of upper abdominal soft tissue. The subcostal scar can be included within the resection segment or may be left behind, depending on the amount of soft-tissue laxity present.

the umbilicus can be preserved to provide perfusion to the soft-tissue segment immediately caudal to the subcostal scar (see Chapter 2, Anatomic Considerations in Abdominal Contouring). Limited undermining to preserve perforators medial to the existing scar is also recommended to maintain the viability of the abdominal flap.[2] Similarly, a reverse abdominoplasty can be performed for category IIA patients to remove some of the upper abdominal soft-tissue laxity (**Fig. 14.5**). Depending on the amount of laxity and the distance of the scar from the inframammary fold, the resection segment of a reverse abdominoplasty may incorporate the subcostal scar.

It is important to note that with a standard reverse abdominoplasty procedure the final scar should ideally be at the inframammary fold (**Fig. 14.6**).[3] Although this is also the goal of reverse abdominoplasty in category IIA patients, it may be harder to accomplish because the final location of the scar is in part determined by the location of the existing scar. If there is insufficient soft-tissue laxity to enable the skin between the subcostal scar and the inframammary fold to be removed, the final abdominoplasty scar will be placed below the inframammary fold, and this must be pointed out to the patient. Thorough discussion with the patient about these issues will permit them to make an informed decision about the type of abdominal contouring procedure and the type of scar they would prefer to have.

Both the lower and the reverse abdominoplasty procedures individually will help to correct a moderate amount of soft-tissue laxity. For category IIA patients who have more significant soft-tissue laxity, a lower abdominoplasty

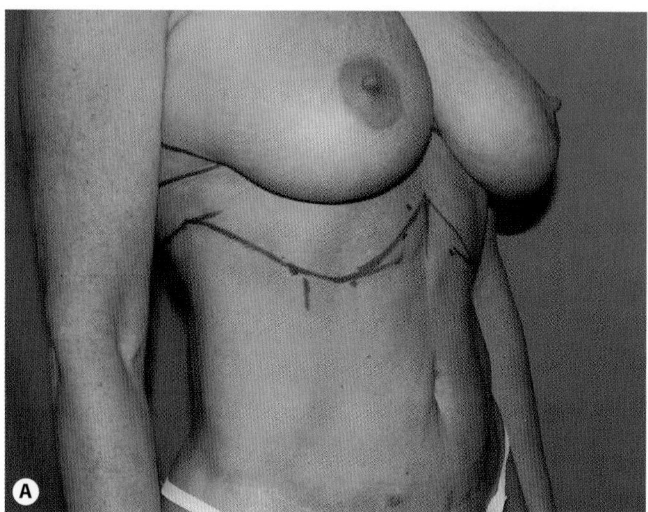

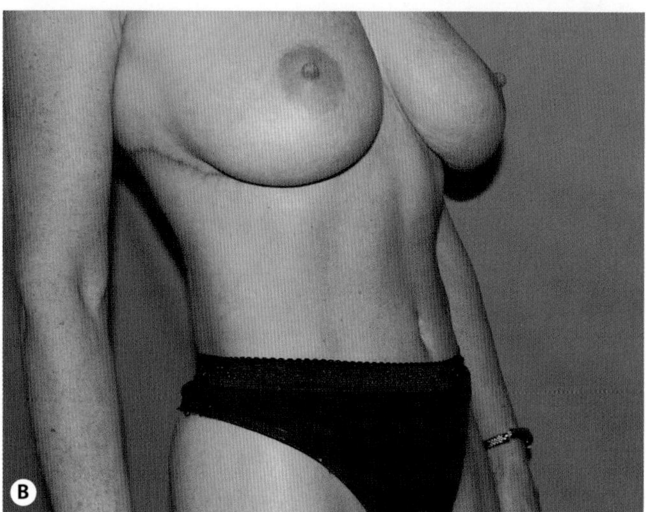

Fig. 14.6 The ideal placement of the final scar for a reverse abdominoplasty should be at the level of the inframammary fold. As the location of the existing scar may influence the level of the final scar, it is important to note and communicate to the patient that this may not be possible.

and a reverse abdominoplasty may be performed in staged fashion to accomplish the desired aesthetic goal safely. The decision to stage these patients is determined largely by the amount of soft-tissue laxity and the amount of correction desired.[4,5]

Category IIB patients (subcostal scar(s) an appreciable distance caudal to the costal margin) may not be good candidates for either lower or reverse abdominoplasty (**Fig. 14.7**). Both of these options often affect only a small portion of the abdominal soft-tissue excess and leave a very poorly positioned scar (positioned too high with lower abdominoplasty, and too low with reverse abdominoplasty). The scars, however, are highly amenable to a formal abdominoplasty with the vertical resection encompassing the scar and

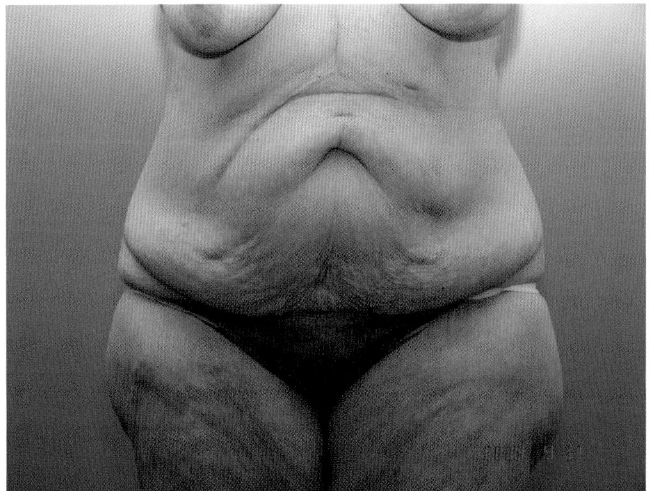

Fig. 14.7 Category IIB patients have a pre-existing subcostal scar some distance caudal to the costal margin. There is often significantly more soft-tissue laxity than in category IIA patients. This is usually the source of the caudal migration of the scar and the reason why a reverse or lower abdominoplasty procedure is less effective in correcting the soft-tissue laxity appropriately.

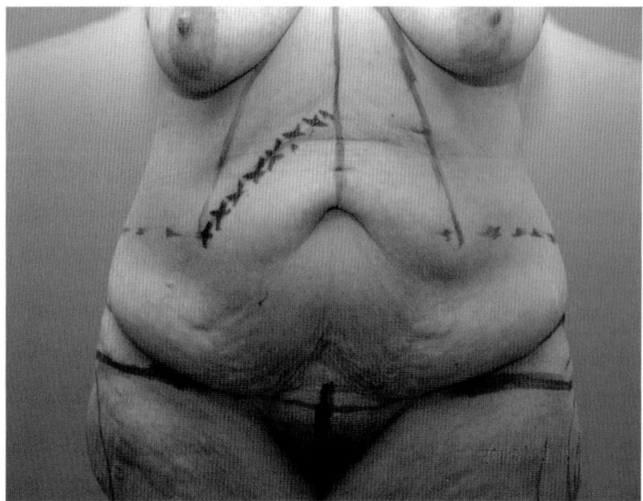

Fig. 14.8 When there is significant soft-tissue laxity, as is the case with most category IIB patients, the scar and the tissue immediately caudal to it at risk for ischemia can be resected through the addition of an anterior vertical segment.

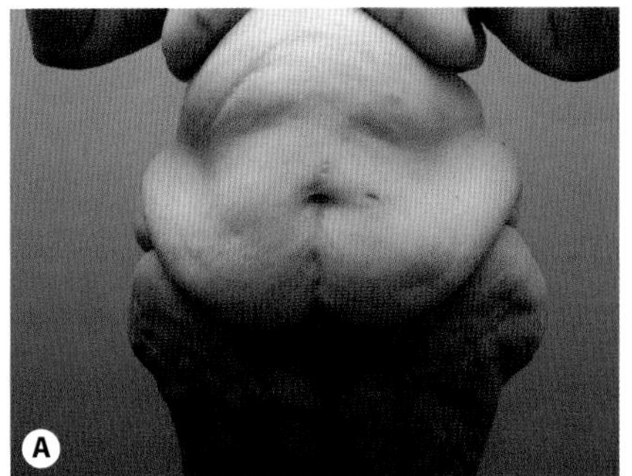

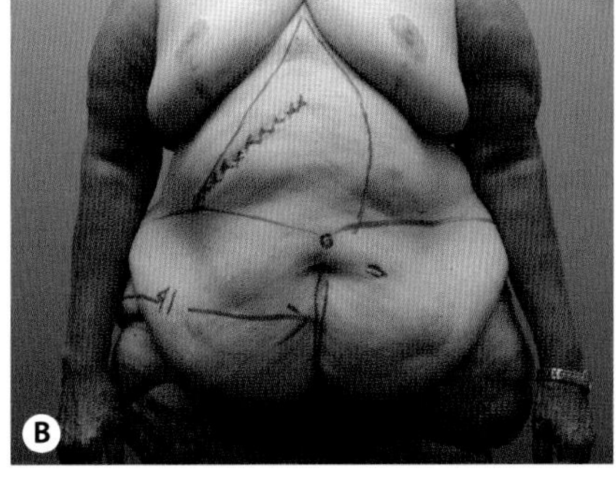

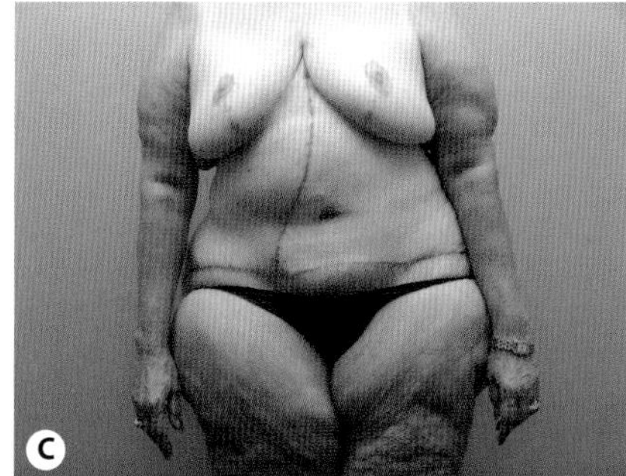

Fig. 14.9 Some category IIB patients have pre-existing scars and soft-tissue laxity that will not allow safe removal with a completely vertical midline closure. For these patients, an anterior 'oblique' resection may be necessary. This allows the preservation of more perforators on the side opposite the pre-existing scar and results in an oblique scar closure.

tissue medial to it, with minimal risk of ischemia and/or necrosis.

Most category IIB patients have caudally located subcostal scars because of gravitational migration secondary to significant soft-tissue laxity. When significant soft-tissue laxity is present in category IIB patients, the addition of a vertical or oblique elliptical resection to a standard abdominoplasty should be strongly considered, as this will allow the scar and the tissue medial to the scar, at risk for ischemia, to be incorporated within the vertical resection. The goal is to remove all of the excess soft-tissue laxity medial to the subcostal scar. If there is significant laxity the subcostal scar can be incorporated in the resection segment and the vertical final scar can still be placed at or near the midline (**Fig. 14.8**). In some patients, however, the size and location of the scar as well as the amount of soft-tissue laxity makes this difficult to accomplish safely. Instead, the dissection and resection are performed asymmetrically to preserve more perforators on the side of the existing scar. This results in a final 'vertical' scar that is oblique, with a position inferior to and sometimes paralleling the path of the previous subcostal scar (**Fig. 14.9**).[6]

This procedure modification is not a safe option for category IIB patients with bilateral subcostal (chevron) scars unless both scars can be incorporated into the vertical resection (**Fig. 14.10**). In return for an improved abdominal contour this select group of patients will have to accept a final scar near or at their existing scar, which may not be

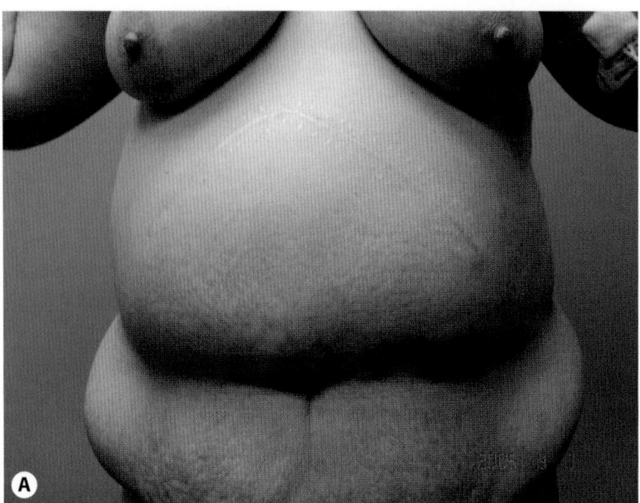

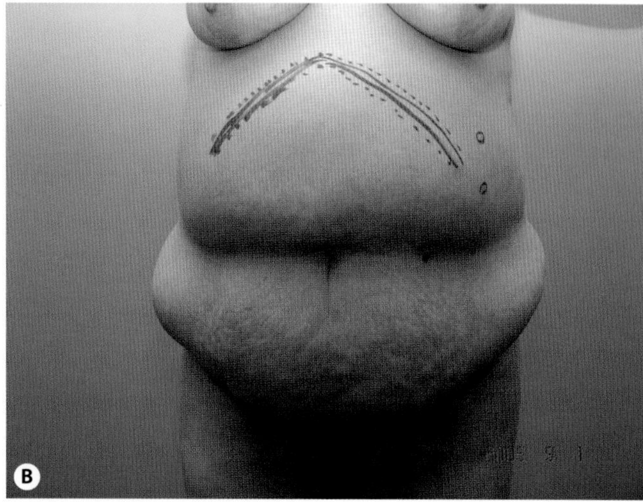

Fig. 14.10 There are some patients in whom a vertical or oblique anterior resection cannot be safely performed. In particular, category IIB patients with long bilateral subcostal (chevron) scars are unlikely to have enough transverse soft-tissue laxity to allow complete resection of tissue immediately caudal to the existing scar.

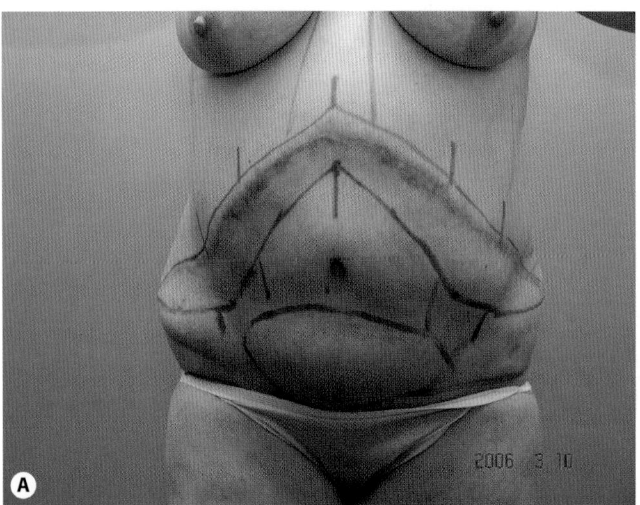

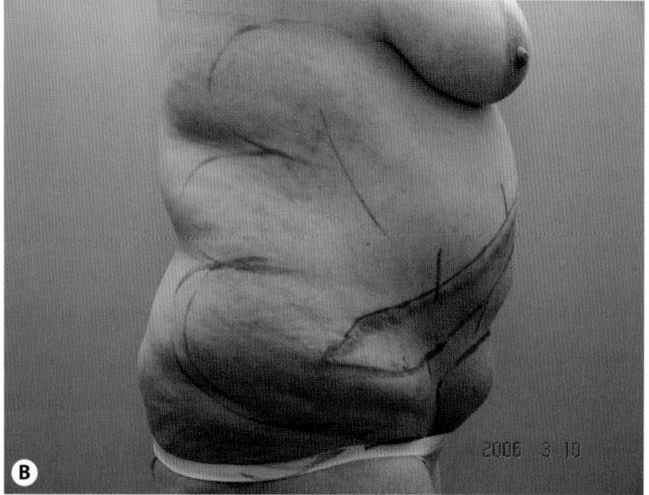

Fig. 14.11 It is often difficult to design an abdominoplasty procedure that places the final scar in a well-concealed location (inframammary fold or bikini line) for patients with pre-existing subcostal scars that are low and bilateral. In these situations the patient may have to accept the location of the final scar in return for improved abdominal contour. This often requires a variation of the reverse abdominoplasty technique whereby the final scar is placed at the location of the previous subcostal scar.

ideal. A reverse abdominoplasty with a final scar well below the inframammary fold can be performed (**Fig. 14.11**). This can be staged with a lower abdominoplasty and/or thorough abdominal liposuction several months later.

Preoperative History and Considerations (Box 14.1)

A focused history and physical examination is particularly important for abdominal contouring patients presenting with abdominal scars. In addition to the potential vascular implications for the soft tissue, the nature of the original abdominal surgery can be associated with various comorbidities that can negatively affect the intra- and postoperative course. These patients may be on medications that can affect blood coagulation, wound healing, pulmonary, gastrointestinal, and cardiac function. Because of this, a thorough understanding of the patient's overall health status, both past and present, is very important.

Smoking is of even greater concern for this patient population because of ischemic issues. We recommend that they stop smoking completely and refrain from exposure to

Box 14.1 Preoperative requirements

- Smoking cessation/avoidance of nicotine exposure for 4–6 weeks prior to surgery
- Multivitamin daily
- Stop aspirin/other blood-thinning products with primary care doctor's permission
- Abstain from all dietary/herbal supplements not approved by the surgeon
- Basic laboratory work should be tailored to each patient. It may include CBC, Chem 7 Factor V Liden, and PT/PTT/INR
- Medical clearance if needed
- Wearing abdominal binder for 2 weeks before surgery
- Shower with a gentle antimicrobial soap the night before and day of surgery

Box 14.2 Category-specific operative approach for abdominoplasty patients with pre-existing scars

- Category I: Little or no modification of the abdominoplasty design is needed. An anterior vertical resection can be added when there is a pre-existing supraumbilical midline scar if deemed beneficial to the final result. However, this is not required to safely complete the abdominoplasty procedure
- Category IIA: A reverse or lower abdominoplasty (or both as a staged procedure) can be performed to help correct a moderate amount of soft-tissue laxity. Patients with more significant laxity may be amenable to an anterior vertical resection if the scar length and orientation are favorable
- Category IIB: These patients often have considerable soft-tissue laxity, which is frequently the source of the caudal migration of the subcostal scar. Because of the amount of laxity, these patients are best served by the addition of an anterior vertical or oblique soft-tissue resection. Patients in this category with bilateral subcostal (chevron) scars, however, may need a two-stage approach involving a modified reverse abdominoplasty followed by a lower abdominal resection. The reverse abdominoplasty in these patients will leave the final scar close to the location of the previous scar.

secondary smoke for a minimum of 6 weeks preoperatively. Even when this is accomplished, it is well known that some long-term negative effects of smoking remain. This issue should be thoroughly discussed with the patient and they should be informed that they remain at an above-normal risk of soft-tissue ischemia and related complications. Appropriate laboratory tests and preoperative health clearances are recommended, as stated in earlier chapters, and should be modified for each patient as needed.

Operative Approach (Box 14.2)

The operative approach for patients with pre-existing abdominal scars varies based partly on the length and location of the scar as well as the amount of soft-tissue laxity. Standard nine-view preoperative photographs with the patient standing are suggested. The surgical marks are made according to the abdominoplasty design modifications selected, and the existing scar(s) is identified and marked. Additional photographs of the markings, the scar area, and other areas of focus are recommended for future reference.

The patient is positioned supine, with padding assured at all pressure points. Preoperative antibiotics, sequential compression devices, a Foley catheter, and a warming blanket are routinely used. Infiltration using the tumescent technique is performed if liposuction is planned. If there is a posterior component of the case, the patient is positioned prone first and then repositioned supine for the anterior component.

The operative sequence for patients with pre-existing abdominal scars vary according to the category of the patient and the abdominoplasty technique selected, and can be found in the operative approach section of the previous chapters. Category I patients do not need significant modification of the standard abdominoplasty design, and the operative approach section of any of the abdominoplasty chapters can be used; the full abdominoplasty chapter (Chapter 7) and the circumferential abdominoplasty chapter (Chapter 9) being most useful. Because category IIA patients are best served by either a reverse abdominoplasty or a lower abdominoplasty or both in a staged fashion, the operative approach sections of the mini abdominoplasty chapter (Chapter 5) and the reverse abdominoplasty chapter (Chapter 10) would be pertinent. Category IIB patients often require the addition of a vertical or oblique anterior elliptical resection to obtain the best results and minimize the risk of ischemia. Chapter 9 (Circumferential Abdominoplasty) contains the operative sequence for an anterior vertical resection.

Preoperative markings are performed by estimating the amount of soft-tissue resection necessary transversely as well as vertically. The vertical or oblique wedge resection is estimated by grasping the excess soft-tissue laxity incorporating the subcostal scar with both hands. The amount of proposed resection should be reassessed intraoperatively, and usually the amount determined to be safely resected is somewhat less than that predicted preoperatively.

Soft-tissue dissection is performed in standard fashion up to the level of the costal margins. The lower abdominal transverse resection is performed as described in the

Chapters 7, 8, and 9 utilizing the Pitanguy demarcator. The vertical or oblique soft-tissue resection is performed last. The soft-tissue laxity is estimated again intraoperatively prior to resection. The goal is to remove all of the excess laxity medial to the subcostal scar. If there is significant laxity, a symmetric resection can be performed which includes the subcostal scar, resulting in a perfectly midline vertical final scar. When the transverse soft-tissue laxity is not sufficient to include the unilateral subcostal scar, an asymmetric resection should be performed which will result in an obliquely oriented final 'vertical' scar. This usually results in the umbilicus being placed outside this oblique scar. If the patient has bilateral subcostal incisions the operative approach of the reverse abdominoplasty will also be useful.

When there is abdominal wall laxity, myofascial plication is performed from xiphoid to pubic symphysis using size 1 or 0 looped nylon in a continuous running fashion, as discussed in the previous chapters. Management of the umbilicus is also performed as previously described (Chapters 9 and 13) by insetting it into the soft tissue directly overlying it, taking care to make sure that it is centered in the midline and at the appropriate vertical height, regardless of the position of the vertical/oblique scar (**Fig. 14.12**). As the perfusion of the abdominal soft-tissue apron can be more tenuous in patients with pre-existing scars, it is recommended that any planned concurrent liposuction should be performed judiciously, and closure accomplished with reduced tension. Pre- and postoperative photographs are shown in **Figs 14.13–14.18**.

Fig. 14.12 Management of the umbilicus is performed in the same fashion as described in the preceding chapters. The umbilicus is brought out and inset into the overlying soft tissue regardless of where the anterior vertical/oblique closure is placed. Care should be taken to ensure that the neoumbilicus is placed in the midline.

Postoperative Care (Box 14.3)

Postoperative instructions for patients with pre-existing abdominal scars who have undergone abdominoplasty are similar to those for the standard abdominoplasty patient. The patient is encouraged to maintain a partially flexed waist position, to drink plenty of fluids and stay appropriately hydrated, to continue appropriate use of the abdominal binder, to manage their drain care, and to take part in regular activity to minimize the incidence of DVT/PE. Because abdominoplasty patients with pre-existing scars may have a more complicated medical history as well as more tenuous perfusion of the soft-tissue apron, extra care, instructions, and more frequent follow-up may be advisable.

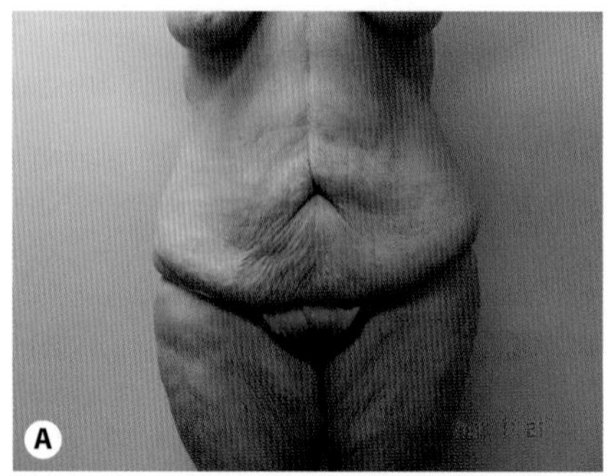

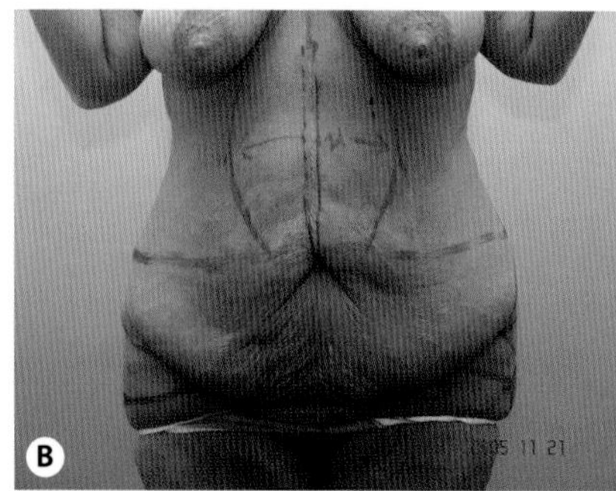

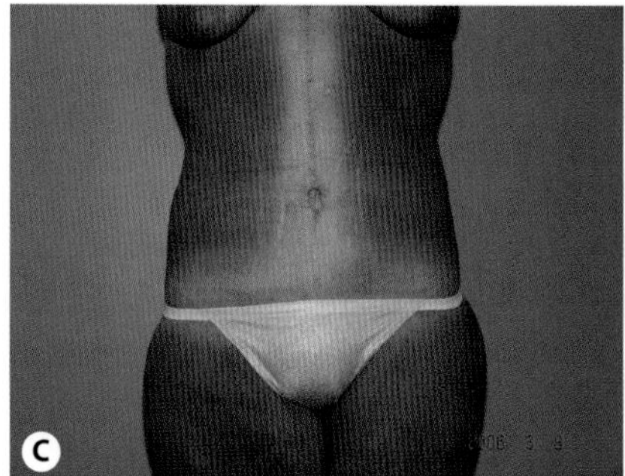

Fig. 14.13 This category I patient had a supraumbilical abdominal scar from a laparotomy. She wanted improved abdominal contour with correction of the abdominal soft-tissue excess. Because she already had a midline incision, a vertical resection component was added to the standard full abdominoplasty. Postoperative results show improved abdominal appearance with reduction in the vertical as well as the transverse amount of soft-tissue laxity.

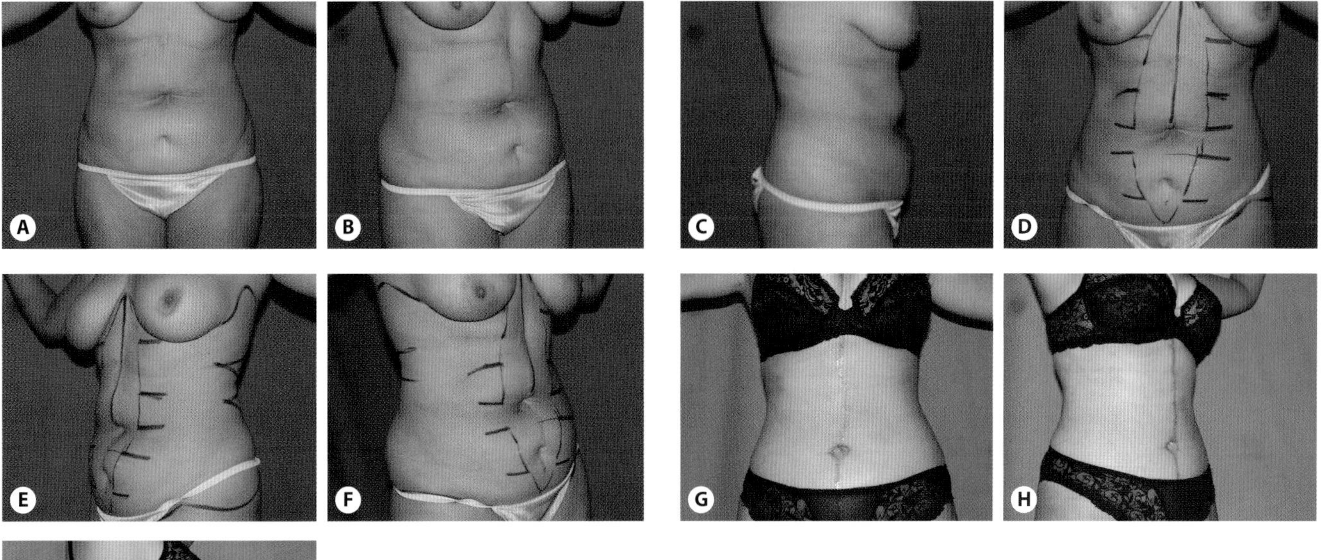

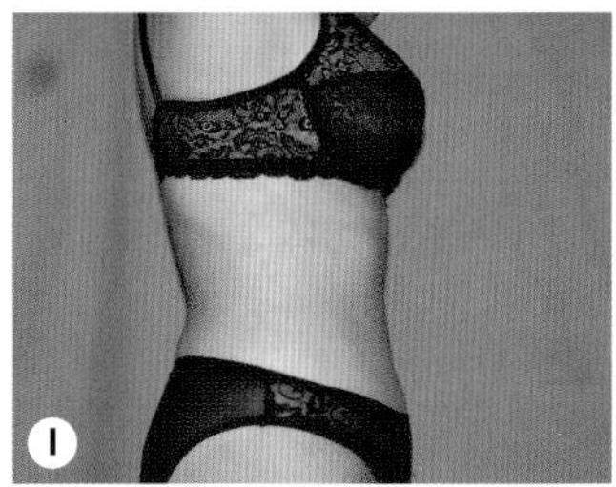

Fig. 14.14 This category I patient underwent an emergency laparotomy secondary to trauma, which left her with a vertical midline abdominal scar from xiphoid to the infraumbilical area. She desired an improved appearance of her abdominal contour and scar. As she had only moderate infraumbilical soft-tissue laxity a vertical wedge resection only was performed as well as through full abdominal liposuction. This provided access to the abdominal wall for plication as well as allowing tightening of the abdominal soft tissue through vertical resection. Significant contour approvement was achieved.

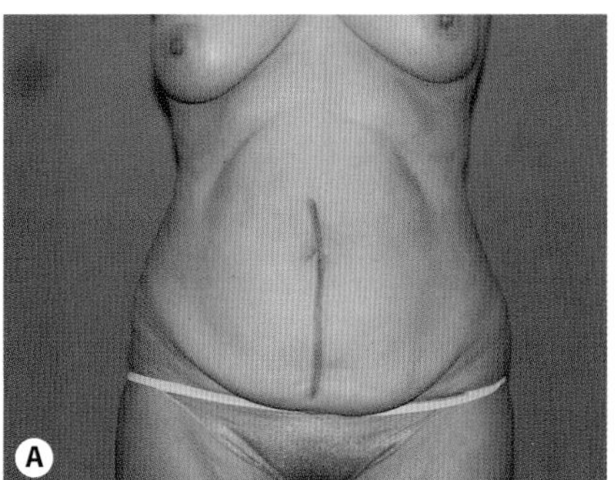

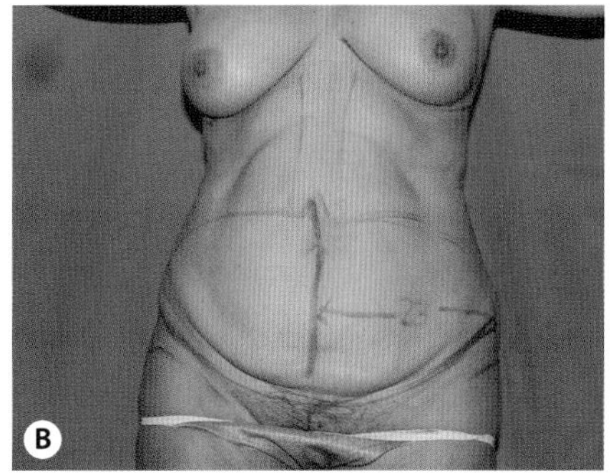

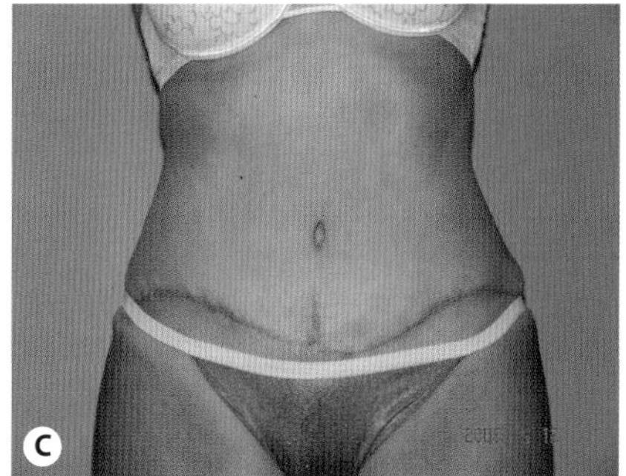

Fig. 14.15 This category I patient had a pre-existing infraumbilical scar. There was also a significant component of this scar above the umbilicus. A full abdominoplasty was performed. Most of the pre-existing scar was removed; however, as only a moderate amount of soft-tissue laxity existed preoperatively, a small inverted 'T' scar was left near the transverse closure. Postoperatively, the patient demonstrates improved abdominal contour secondary to myofascial plication and a significant amount of soft-tissue resection.

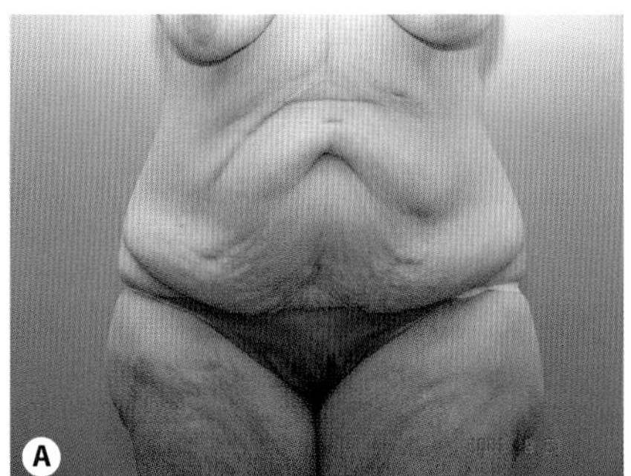

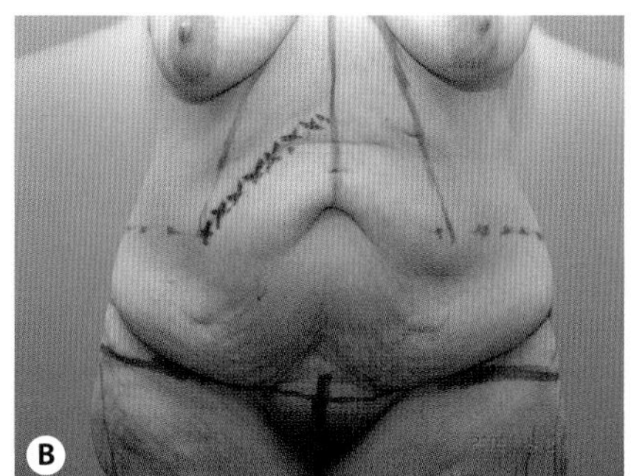

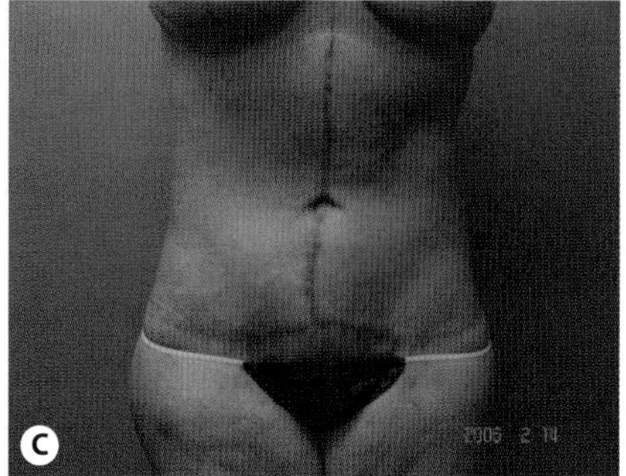

Fig. 14.16 This category IIB patient had a subcostal scar midway between the umbilicus and the costal margin. Through bimanual estimation the amount of transverse soft-tissue laxity at the level of the umbilicus was deemed sufficient to allow complete excision of her subcostal scar and all of the soft tissue caudal to the scar, which is at the greatest risk for ischemia. Postoperatively she demonstrates a significantly improved abdominal appearance. The difference between this patient and the patient in **Fig. 14.13** is that little or no modification of the standard full abdominoplasty design was necessary for the patient in **Fig. 14.13**. For this patient Fig. 14.16 a vertical component was added because it was necessary for the safety of the abdominoplasty procedure and resulting in an enhanced final result. The patient in this figure required modification of the abdominoplasty design by the addition of a vertical component in order to remove the tissue inferior to the subcostal scar. If this had not been done, there would have been an appreciable chance of significant ischemia of that tissue.

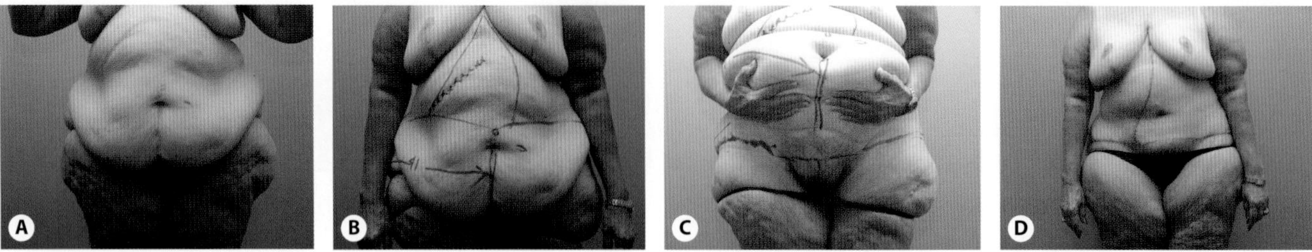

Fig. 14.17 The location and orientation of this patient's subcostal scar made simple vertical wedge excision with a standard abdominoplasty difficult. She had a significant amount of soft-tissue laxity, but most of this was below the subcostal scar. To properly treat this patient it was decided to perform an asymmetric dissection and resection which would spare additional perforators on the left side and result in an oblique 'vertical' scar. The postoperative photographs show a significantly improved abdominal contour with well-perfused tissue and an absence of ischemia-related issues.

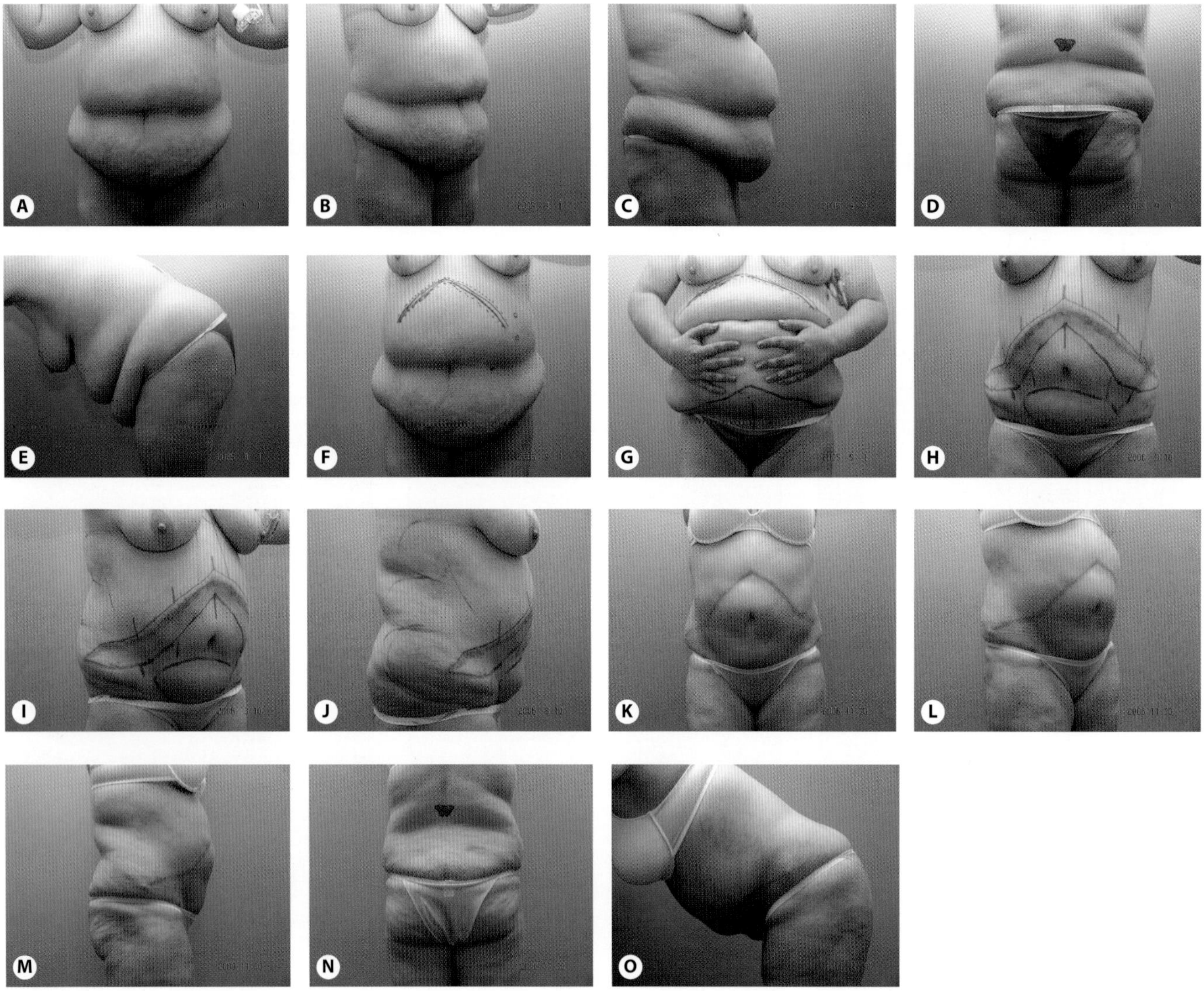

Fig. 14.18 This patient is a unique example of a category IIB. The presence of caudally located bilateral subcostal scars limits which abdominoplasty designs can be used safely. Patients with these types of scar may have to accept a final scar that is not well placed either in the bikini line or at the level of the inframammary fold, in exchange for improved abdominal contour. A modified reverse abdominoplasty was performed for this patient. A significant amount of excess abdominal soft tissue was removed. In addition, myofascial plication was performed and the previous scar was revised. (A–G) A secondary skin excision and additional liposuction was performed to achieve the final result (H–O).

Box 14.3 Postoperative instructions

The postoperative care of abdominoplasty patients with pre-existing abdominal scars is comparable to that of the full abdominoplasty patient.

- Maintain a partially flexed position at the waist for the first 1–2 weeks
- Wear the abdominal binder at all times except for showering
- Make sure the abdominal binder is maintained low enough on the abdomen
- Verify that there are no significant creases, folds, or drain tubes underneath the binder
- Avoid smoking or exposure to nicotine-containing products
- Breathe deeply and use the incentive spirometer frequently
- Drink plenty of fluids: 8 oz/h is the goal
- Move legs frequently while resting, and walk regularly
- Drain care as instructed
- Continue to take multivitamin daily. Resume medications as instructed
- No vigorous activity or heavy lifting for 4–6 weeks

Conclusion

Abdominoplasty and abdominal contouring procedures can be safely performed in patients with pre-existing abdominal scars after proper evaluation, careful planning, and modification of standard abdominoplasty techniques. An understanding of the vascular supply to the abdominal soft tissue and a clear discussion with the patient about risks and expectations are important to achieve the optimal aesthetic result and high patient satisfaction. Category I patients who have scars that will be incorporated into the soft-tissue resection segment require little modification of the standard technique. Category IIA and IIB patients require individualized plans. Category IIA patients are often best served by a reverse abdominoplasty alone or staged with a lower abdominoplasty, whereas category IIB patients usually require the addition of a vertical/oblique anterior resection.

Clinical Caveats: Management of pre-existing abdominal scars

- Pre-existing abdominal scars are not an absolute contraindication to abdominoplasty and abdominal contouring procedures
- Careful evaluation and appropriate selection of the abdominoplasty design is important to safely achieve optimal aesthetic results
- Classification of abdominoplasty patients with pre-existing scars can help simplify the evaluation and decision-making process
- Category I: Little or no modification of the abdominoplasty design is needed
- Category IIA: A reverse abdominoplasty, a lower abdominoplasty or as a staged procedure using both techniques can be useful for this group of patients
- Category IIB: These patients are often best served by the addition of an anterior vertical/oblique soft-tissue resection. Patients in this category with bilateral subcostal scars (chevron design) may need a two-stage approach involving a reverse abdominoplasty and a lower abdominal resection. The reverse abdominoplasty technique in these patients usually leaves the final scar near the location of the previous abdominal scar
- Cessation of smoking is an important component to all abdominoplasty procedures. The patient should understand that they may well remain at an elevated risk of complications even if smoking is stopped several weeks before surgery
- Postoperative care is comparable to that for standard abdominoplasty procedures. The patient's specific medical and surgical history should guide additional postoperative instructions and follow-up intervals

References

1. Sozer SO, Agullo FJ, Santillan AA, Wolf C. Decision making in abdominoplasty. Aesthet Plast Surg 2007; 31: 117.
2. El-Khatib HA, Bener A. Abdominal dermolipectomy in an abdomen with pre-existing scars: a different concept. Plast Reconstruct Surg 2004; 114: 992.
3. Baroudi R, Keppke EM, Carvalho CG. Mammary reduction combined with reverse abdominoplasty. Ann Plast Surg 1979; 2: 368.
4. Rieger UM, Aschwanden M, Schmid D, et al. Perforator-sparing abdominoplasty technique in the presence of bilateral subcostal scars after gastric bypass. Obes Surg 2007; 17: 63.
5. Akbas H, Guneren E, Eroglu L, et al. The combined use of classic and reverse abdominoplasty on the same patient. Plast Reconstruct Surg 2002; 109: 2595.
6. Borud LJ, Warren AG. Modified vertical abdominoplasty in the massive weight loss patient. Plast Reconstruct Surg 2007; 119: 1911.

Suggested Reading

Boyd BJ, Taylor GI. The vascular territories of the superior epigastric and deep inferior epigastric systems. Plast Reconstruct Surg 1984; 73: 1.

Duff CG, Aslam S, Griffiths RW. Fleur-de-lys abdominoplasty – a consecutive case series. Br J Plast Surg 2003; 56: 557–566.

Hamdy EH, Milner RH. The vascular anatomy of the lower anterior abdominal wall: A microdissection study on the deep inferior epigastric vessels and the perforator branches. Plast Reconstruct Surg 2000; 109: 539.

Hunstad JP. Body contouring in the obese patient. Clin Plast Surg 1996; 23: 647.

Lockwood TE. Superficial facial system (SFS) of the trunk and lower extremities: A new concept. Plast Reconstruct Surg 1991; 87: 1009.

Markman B, Barton FE Jr. Anatomy of the subcutaneous tissue of the trunk and lower extremity. Plast Reconstruct Surg 1987; 80: 248.

Matarasso A, Wallach SG, Rankin M, Galiano RD. Secondary abdominal contour surgery: a review of early and late reoperative surgery. Plast Reconstruct Surg 2005; 115: 627–632.

Pitanguy I. Evaluation of body contouring surgery today: a 30-year perspective. Plast Reconstruct Surg 2000; 105: 1499.

CHAPTER 15

Complications

Joseph P. Hunstad and Remus Repta

IN THIS CHAPTER

KEY POINTS

Complications of abdominoplasty are usually minor and may include poor scars, lateral dog-ears, or suture extrusions. More significant complications may include persistent seroma, pseudo-bursae, and small areas of ischemia and wound healing problems. The most worrisome complications are those that are life-threatening or that severely affect the final aesthetic result. These may include large hematomas, significant infection, necrosis, and DVT/PE. The primary goal with all potential complications is to take the proper steps to prevent them. When complications do occur, however, it is important for the surgeon to diagnose the problem accurately and institute the necessary measures to minimize the deleterious effect of the complication and allow the patient to return to the path of healing.

Introduction

Reducing the incidence of complications is an important focus for all surgical procedures. This is especially the case with cosmetic procedures, where relatively healthy and functionally normal patients undergo elective surgery to improve their appearance. Patient selection, preoperative screening, selection of the appropriate surgical procedure, and good surgical technique are all important in avoiding or reducing the incidence of complications. Equally important for overall patient satisfaction, safety, and the final aesthetic result is the proper diagnosis and management of complications when they do occur. As with all problem-solving situations, identifying the existence of the problem, correct diagnosis, and appropriate treatment are all necessary to accomplish this.

For both the surgeon and the patient, the magnitude of complications can range from simple nuisance to potentially lethal. This chapter will address the more common as well as the more significant complications that can occur with abdominoplasty and abdominal contouring procedures. The intention is to provide information that will be useful for the surgeon performing the procedures discussed in this book.

Seroma (Box 15.1)

Technically speaking, 'seroma' formation is an inherent part of the healing process following abdominoplasty procedures. Seroma as a complication is more accurately defined as any collection of fluid that requires repeated percutaneous drainage,

Box 15.1 Seroma

- The formation of seroma fluid is an inherent part of the healing process following an abdominoplasty
- Seroma as a complication is better defined as any clinically detectable fluid that requires repeated or continuous drainage
- The most common site for seroma fluid accumulation is in the midline below the umbilicus, and there may be fullness or a noticeable fluid wave on examination
- Percutaneous aspiration under sterile conditions should be performed at least twice weekly until fluid accumulation ceases. The abdominal binder should be worn continuously (day and night) during this time
- The aspirate should be sent for culture if there is any suspicion of infection

is clinically detectable, and/or affects the final aesthetic result. Many factors have been theoretically attributed to an increased incidence of seroma. In essence, any factor that increases or prolongs the postoperative inflammatory process theoretically increases the chance of seroma.[1] Examples include intraoperative bleeding, excess use of electrocautery, and additional soft-tissue trauma due to concurrent liposuction. Many factors play a role in seroma formation of which we are unaware or cannot confidently identify. Some of these may be patient specific and related to anatomy, physiology, or the presence of certain comorbid conditions.

Minimizing soft-tissue trauma is an important component of seroma prevention. Meticulous surgical technique and proper dissection using an electrocautery setting that is low yet efficient will help minimize the extent of soft-tissue damage. The additional thermal damage to the surrounding soft tissue that occurs with high electrocautery settings is unnecessary and one potential source of increased seroma formation.

Concurrent use of liposuction during abdominoplasty to thin the abdominal soft-tissue apron is common (see Chapter 3, Liposuction in Abdominal Contouring). Although this is a highly useful adjunct in patients with excess adiposity, it does result in a larger surgical surface area.[2] The additional soft-tissue trauma created by the liposuction cannula, as well as the residual tumescent fluid that remains at the end of the procedure, may explain the increased incidence of seroma formation in abdominoplasty procedures when concurrent liposuction is used. The use of smaller-diameter cannulas and proper tumescent infiltration can help minimize the additional trauma.

Proper removal of residual tumescent fluid in the immediate postoperative period is helpful in allowing the process of soft-tissue adherence to begin. Connecting the drains to high-vacuum suction during the early postoperative period evacuates any fluid present and promotes soft-tissue adherence to the underlying abdominal wall (**Fig. 15.1**). The drainage is expected to be significant initially and then to taper off within the first few hours. The drains can be connected to regular drainage bulbs at this time.

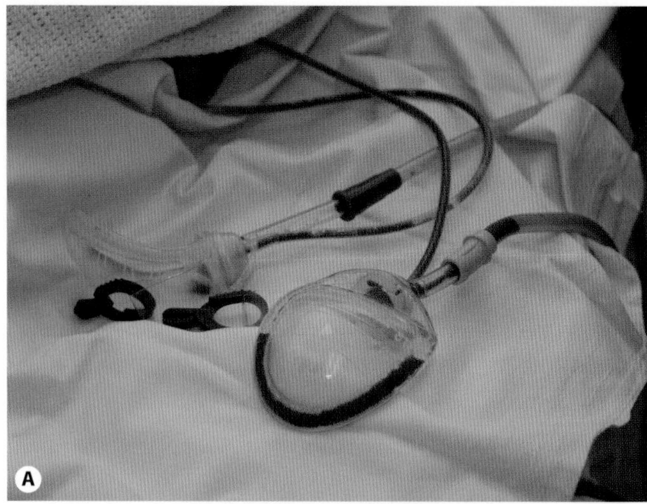

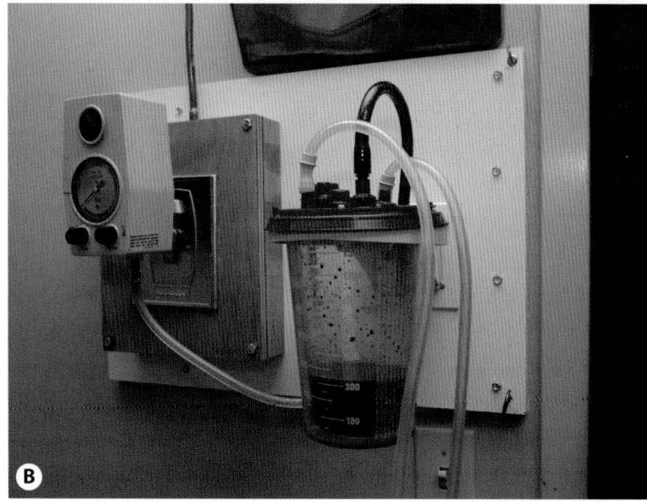

Fig. 15.1 Connecting the abdominoplasty drains to continuous suction (wall suction) during the immediate perioperative period will help remove most of the residual tumescent fluid. It is common for the drain output to be fairly high during the first few hours. After the output decreases and before the patient is sent home, the drains are connected to regular bulb suction. The concurrent use of an abdominal binder will help improve the efficiency of the drains by keeping the soft tissue opposed to the abdominal wall.

An abdominal binder placed at the completion of the procedure also facilitates fluid removal through the drains and promotes the compression of the fluid-filled soft tissue. The binder is an essential part of postoperative seroma management, as it maximizes the efficacy of the drain(s) and promotes adherence of the soft-tissue flap to the underlying abdominal wall fascia.

Re-evaluation of the position and tightness of the abdominal binder during the immediate perioperative period is very important. A binder that is too high or too loose will not compress the soft-tissue apron properly. On the other hand, a binder that is too tight or which applies uneven pressure endangers the blood supply and perfusion to the underlying flap. Careful inspection and discussion with caregivers regarding folds or creases in the binder, as well as the inadvertent presence of a drain tube between the binder and the abdomen, is very important.

Evaluating the capillary refill of the lower portion of the abdominal flap near the midline is a good way to assure that there is adequate soft-tissue perfusion and that the binder is not too tight (**Fig. 15.2**). The binder should be maintained snug but not overly tight until the first postoperative visit, at which time soft-tissue perfusion and drainage are reassessed. The garment can then be worn more tightly during the subsequent days to further promote flap adherence. The drain(s) are removed when the drainage amount is less than 30–50 mL over a 24-hour period.

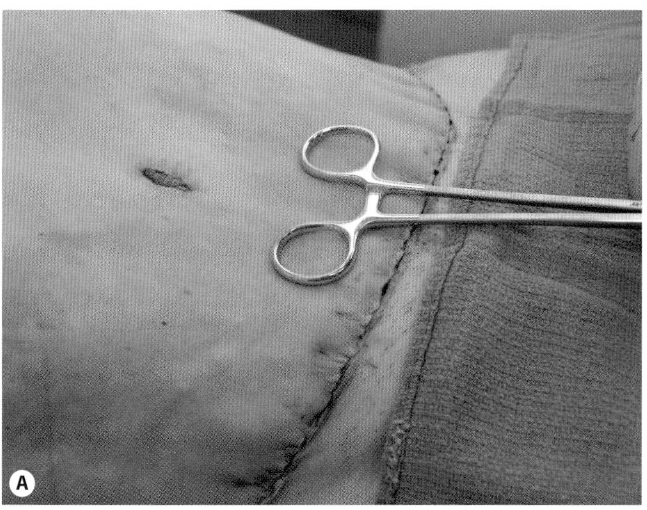

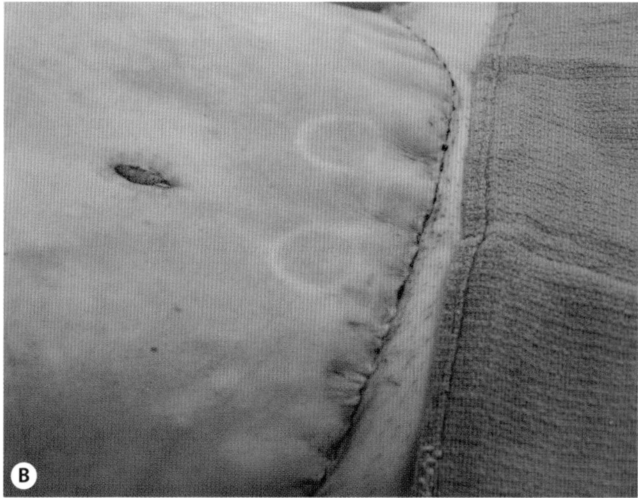

Fig. 15.2 The perfusion of the abdominal flap should be assessed during the perioperative period to ensure that the abdominal binder is not too tight and that there is no accumulation of fluid or other factors that may negatively affect blood flow. The easiest way to do so is to check capillary refill in the midline just above the transverse incision. This area is the furthest away from the blood supply and the most likely area to accumulate fluid.

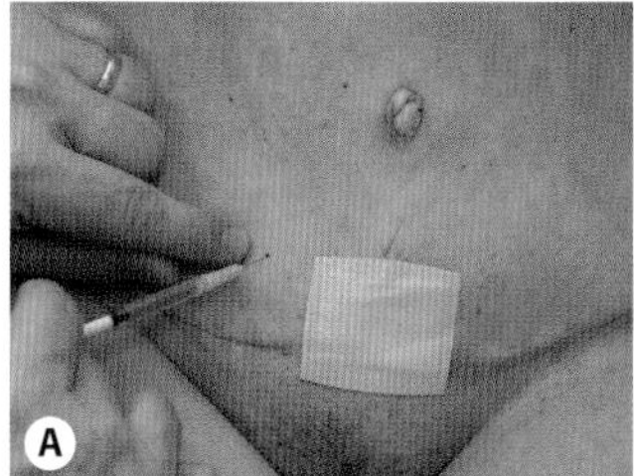

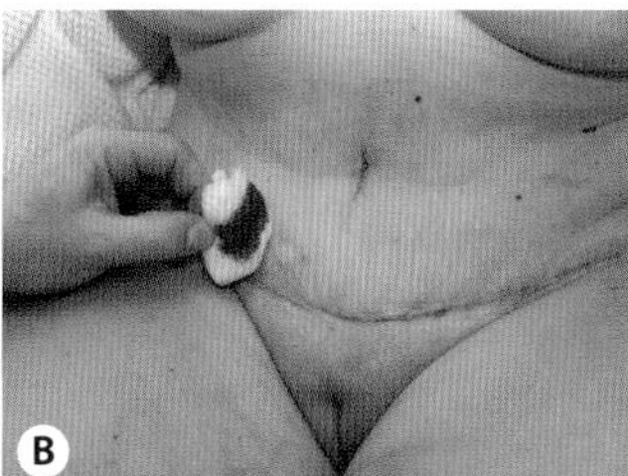

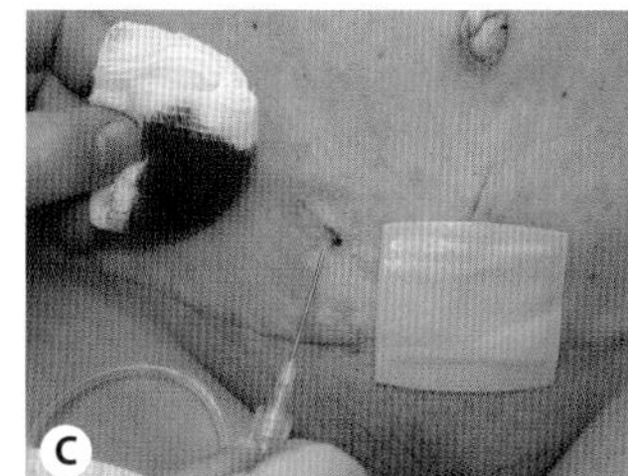

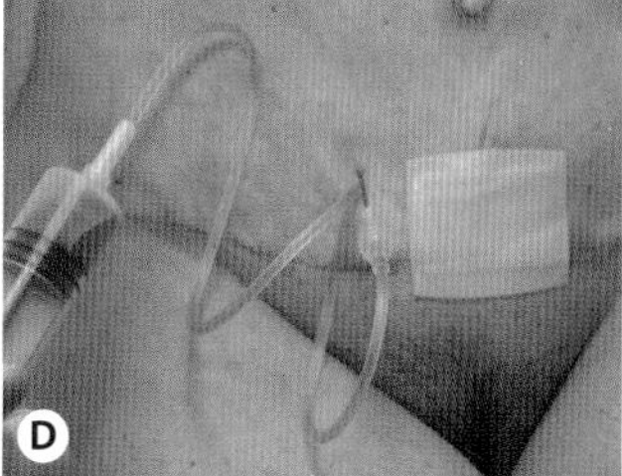

Fig. 15.3 A clinically detectable seroma is often noted after the drain(s) is removed. Frequently, the seroma accumulates at the most dependent portion of the surgical site, which is in the midline below the umbilicus. The presence of a fluid wave is diagnostic. A large amount of fluid may cease to have a fluid wave and may simply present with palpable and visual fullness. The seroma should be aspirated percutaneously twice weekly at first. Lidocaine is frequently used to ensure numbness of the skin entry site. Betadine is used to clean the skin entry site and a sterile 18 gauge needle with a 60 mL syringe is used to aspirate the seroma fluid.

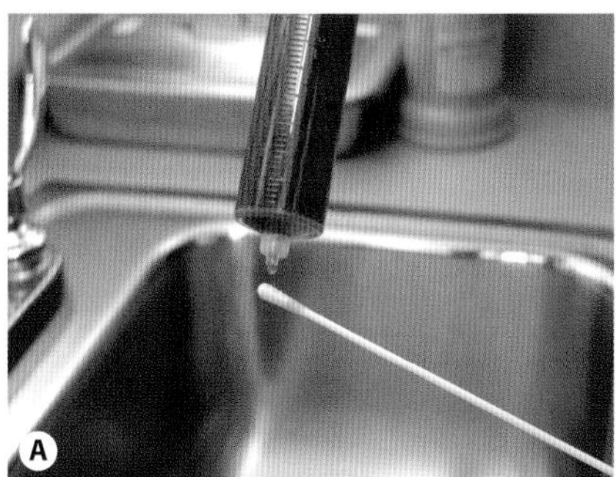

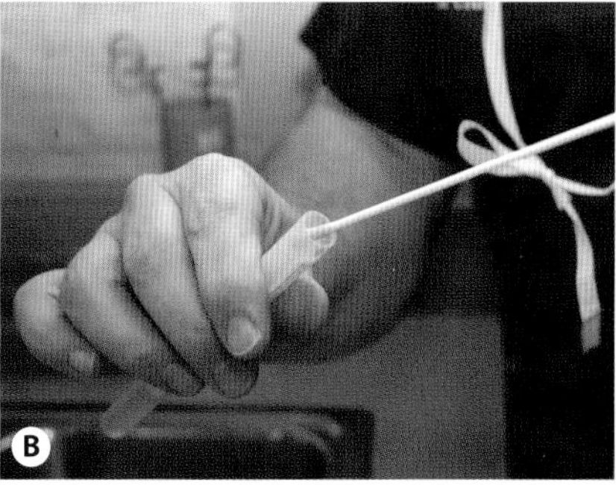

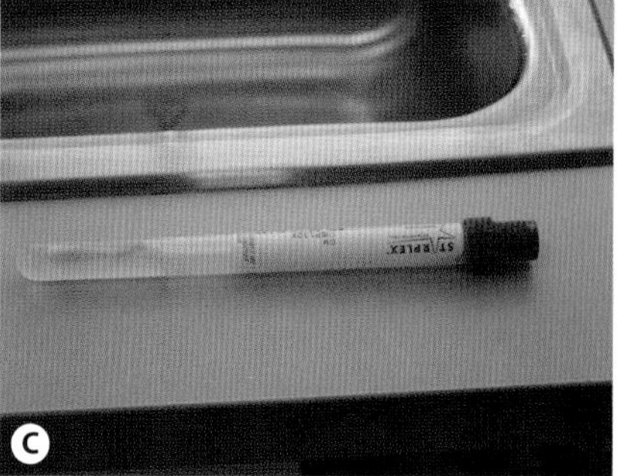

Fig. 15.4 The seroma fluid can be sent for culture if there is suspicion of infection. A cloudy aspirate, fever, or erythema are indications for seroma fluid cultures and restarting oral antibiotics.

Should a seroma be detected following drain removal, percutaneous aspiration should be performed at least twice weekly until the accumulation ceases. During this time we recommend that the abdominal binder be worn continuously day and night. The lower central abdomen superior to the incision is usually a good place to aspirate a seroma because this area is frequently insensate and the fluid is most likely to pool here (**Fig. 15.3**). A Betadine preparation will reduce the risk of introducing bacteria and producing a seroma infection. If the seroma fluid becomes turbid at any point, or there are any signs of infection, culture of the fluid should be considered (**Fig. 15.4**).

Box 15.2 Hematoma

- Despite the large surgical surface area and the release of many perforators, the incidence of hematoma following abdominoplasty is fairly low
- Patients with hematoma will often present within the first or second postoperative day
- Rapid swelling, discomfort, and ecchymosis are indicators of a hematoma
- The quality and quantity of the drain output may also support the diagnosis. The output can also be unremarkable, as the drains easily clog with clot
- Formal operative exploration and evacuation of the hematoma is the safest course of action. This will also expedite the healing process and offer the best aesthetic result
- Although any of the perforators can be a source of postoperative bleeding, we have found that the superficial inferior epigastric and the superficial circumflex vessels are the most frequent culprits

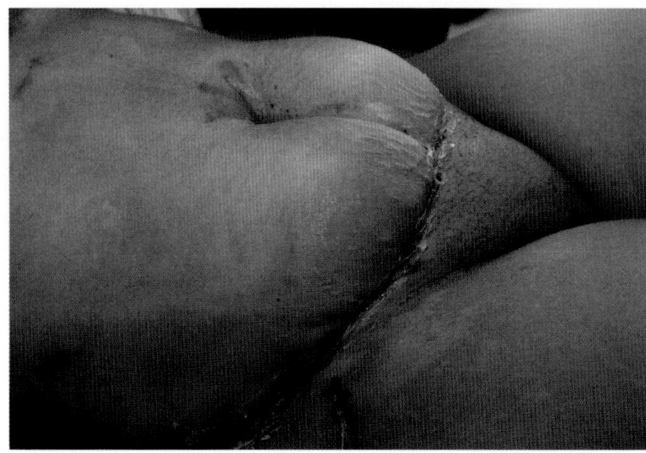

Fig. 15.5 Although relatively rare, hematoma does occur following abdominoplasty. These patients usually present on the first or second postoperative day. Fullness, discomfort, and ecchymosis in the lower abdomen below the umbilicus are usually evident. The drains may show increased bloody output, but frequently clog up with clot and the output may be unimpressive.

Continuous drainage may be indicated for an unusually large or persistent seroma. A percutaneous catheter is placed using sterile technique in the office. It is secured to the skin via suture or tape and connected to an aspiration bulb. A Seromacath or a Jackson Pratt or comparable drain can be used. For seromas that remain recalcitrant despite drain replacement, the incision can be opened and a wick drain, such as a Penrose, can be placed to permit continuous drainage. This will allow the seroma pocket to close from the inside out and reduce the incidence of pseudo-bursa formation.

Hematoma (Box 15.2)

The large undermined area associated with abdominoplasty procedures, as well as the division of multiple perforators, is a good recipe for the creation of a hematoma. It is fortunate – and impressive – that the actual incidence of hematoma in abdominoplasty is quite low.[3] It is a credit to the skill of plastic surgeons, the use of meticulous surgical technique, knowledge of the vascular anatomy of the abdominal soft tissue, and appropriate control of the transected perforators that an inherently 'hematoma-prone' procedure can be performed with little blood loss and with a very low incidence of hematoma.

Most abdominoplasty patients presenting with hematoma do so within the first postoperative day (**Fig. 15.5**). Any of the transected perforators can be the source of the hematoma, but most often the bleeding is from the superficial inferior epigastric or the superficial circumflex vessels. This is why we recommend ligutron or precise electrocautery of these vessels. The reason for this is twofold: first, the midline abdomen where the deep epigastric perforators are found is involved in myofascial plication. The process of myofascial plication invaginates this midline tissue and compresses the cauterized ends of the perforators from the deep epigastric arcade. Nearby perforators from the deep epigastric arcade that are not included in the plicated tissue are likely to be stretched by the plication process, potentially occluding them as well. Second, the source of the superficial inferior epigastric and superficial circumflex perforators maybe outside the boundary of the abdominal binder. The absence of the abdominal binder pressure makes these perforators more prone to postoperative bleeding if not properly controlled.

When hematomas do occur they are often clinically large enough to result in discomfort and contour irregularity. The course of action can be individualized, but it is best to return the patient to the operating room and evacuate the hematoma. Thorough removal of the hematoma fluid and irrigation of the abdominoplasty site should be performed (**Fig. 15.6**). Occasionally the hematoma has solidified to the extent that a sizeable component of the incision needs to be opened in order to physically remove the clot.

Cellulitis (Box 15.3)

Cellulitis must be differentiated from skin hyperemia. Hyperemia is usually seen early during the first few postoperative days and is a normal physiologic reaction to the abdominoplasty procedure. Cellulitis, on the other hand, is unusual in the first few days after surgery: it is more commonly seen in the later part of the first or in the early part of the second postoperative week, usually after the drain(s) has been removed and the prophylactic antibiotics stopped.

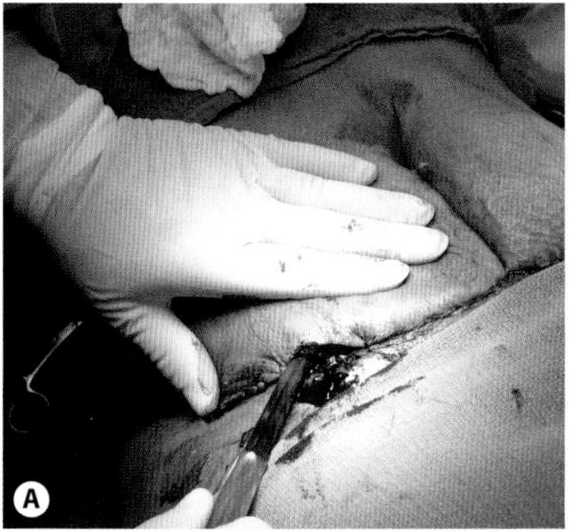

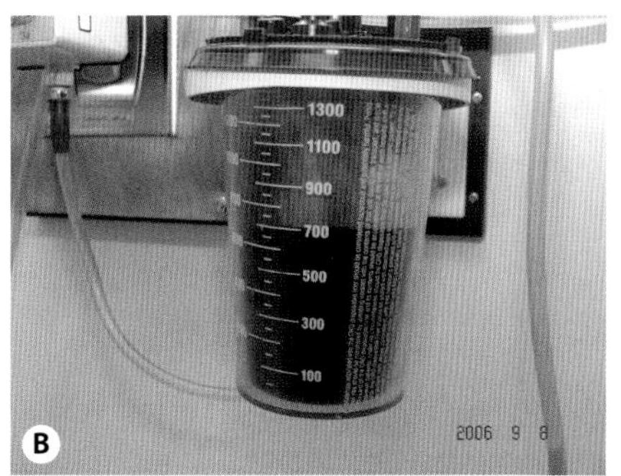

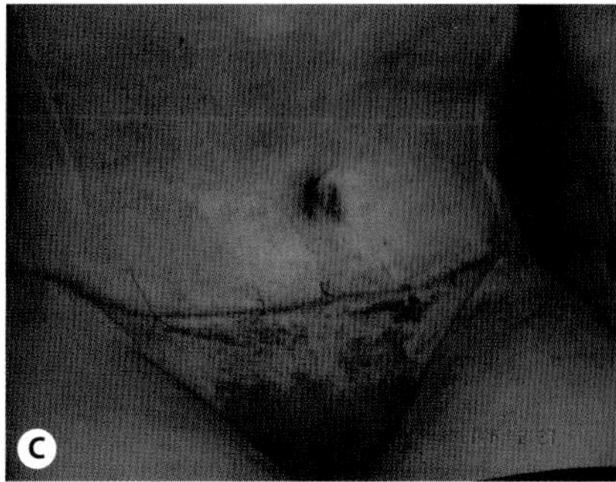

Fig. 15.6 Patients presenting with hematoma should be taken back to the operating room for formal evacuation and attempts to identify the source. If the hematoma has solidified, the incision must be opened generously to remove the clot. This process allows the patient to recover more quickly and with less impact on the final aesthetic result compared to conservative management.

Box 15.3 Cellulitis

- Cellulitis following abdominoplasty is most commonly seen by the end of the first postoperative week. Often, the drain(s) has been removed and the oral antibiotics have been stopped by this time
- Cellulitis is most frequently seen in the midline, just above the transverse incision
- This area is more likely to accumulate seroma fluid and is furthest from the vascular supply
- Initial management of simple cellulitis includes resumption of oral antibiotics, frequent follow-up evaluations, and attempts to aspirate any potential seroma fluid

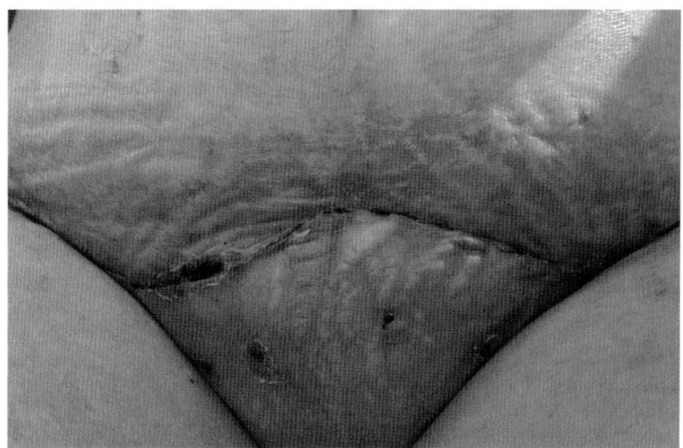

Fig. 15.7 Cellulitis often presents in the midline just above the transverse incision. This area is also the site most likely to accumulate seroma fluid and is the furthest away from the vascular source of the abdominal flap. As this area is numb in the immediate postoperative period, patients may not complain of increased tenderness. Often, erythema and an increase in the soft-tissue edema in the area of the cellulitis may be the only presenting symptoms. It is most common to see cellulitis at the end of the first or the beginning of the second postoperative week following drain removal and cessation of antibodies.

Early cellulitis is often associated with increased skin temperature, erythema, localized discomfort, and increased edema of the skin and underlying soft tissue. The most common location for cellulitis is in the midline just above the transverse incision (**Fig. 15.7**), which is the most prone to fluid accumulation and by design is the furthest away from the vascular supply of the abdominal soft-tissue apron. There may be no pain associated with the cellulitic area, as it is usually insensate. The initial management of early cellulitis is conservative and includes outlining the extent of the erythema, more frequent follow-up evaluations, and restarting or continuing standard oral antibiotics.

Later signs of cellulitis may also include clear drainage from the incision line. This is frequently also associated with an underlying seroma. In these cases, the incision line should be opened at the bedside where drainage is occurring. The fluid can be sent for cultures and the site can be kept open by using wet-to-dry dressings with normal saline. This will assist the body in expelling the underlying infected seroma. Oral antibiotics can be initiated and should be modified according to the results of the culture.

More extensive cellulitis, especially when the patient has developed constitutional symptoms of fever and malaise, may be a sign of underlying fat necrosis with more extensive infection. These patients also usually present in the first or second week. The severity of the symptoms may not be fully appreciated until the drain is removed and the prophylactic oral antibiotics are discontinued. For these patients, formal wound exploration is often the safest and most appropriate action, as it will allow proper diagnosis and treatment with debridement of non-viable fat (**Fig. 15.8**).

Pseudo-Bursa

A pseudo-bursa usually presents as a firm mass, usually in the lower central or upper central abdomen (**Fig. 15.9**).

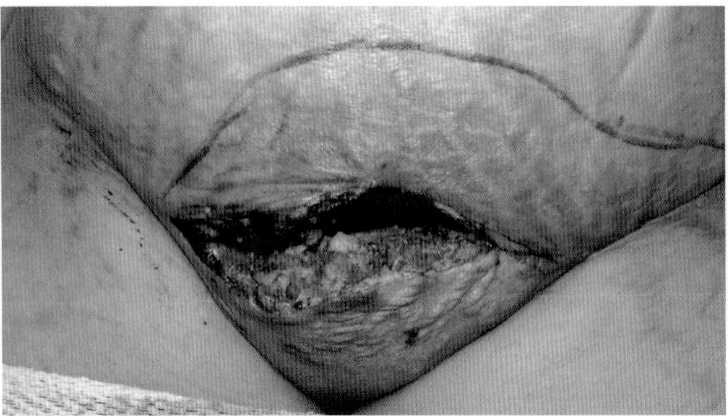

Fig. 15.8 Cellulitis that does not respond to oral antibiotics, is associated with soft-tissue firmness, or presents with constitutional symptoms, including fever and malaise, should be given extra attention. These patients are likely to have ischemic or necrotic fat that functions as a continued nidus for infection. Formal exploration with debridement of the necrotic fat will expedite the healing process and eliminate the source of the infection.

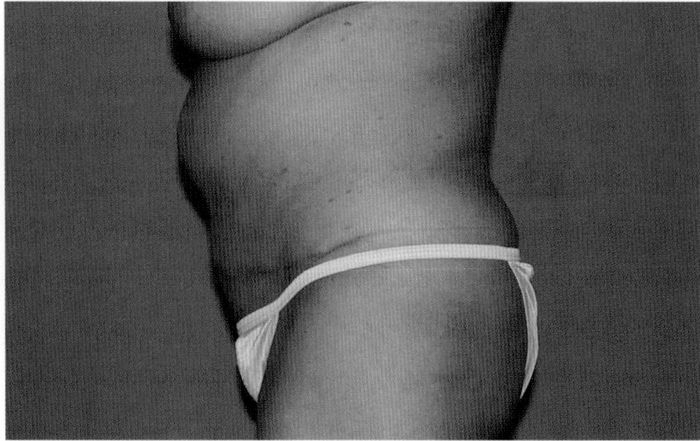

Fig. 15.9 Localized fullness that develops weeks after an abdominoplasty is likely to be a pseudo-bursa. This is especially true if the patient has had a postoperative history of recurrent or persistent seroma.

Often the patient has a postoperative history of a persistent seroma. With time, the body has created a fibrous capsule surrounding the seroma site. This pseudo-bursa may be clinically detectable as a palpable firmness, or it can be noted visually as fullness if the capsule is relatively thick compared to the abdominal soft tissue, or if the pseudo-bursa accumulates fluid. Percutaneous aspiration of clear fluid from this area is diagnostic.

Unfortunately, simple aspiration is not an effective option for these patients as reaccumulation of the fluid is almost guaranteed, and the capsule walls are often thick enough to be a source of contour irregularity as well. Injection of triamcinolone acetate or tetracycline into the bursa to scarify and obliterate the space can be attempted but is usually unsuccessful. Direct surgical removal of the pseudo-bursa is usually the best method to correct the contour irregularity.[4] This often requires re-elevating the abdominal soft tissue to allow access. It may be necessary to use the full extent of the abdominoplasty scar and recreate the soft-tissue dissection to access the pseudo-bursa. This is particularly the case when the pseudo-bursa is located above the umbilicus (**Fig. 15.10**). Partial (anterior wall only) or complete removal of the pseudo-bursa is usually necessary (**Fig. 15.11**).

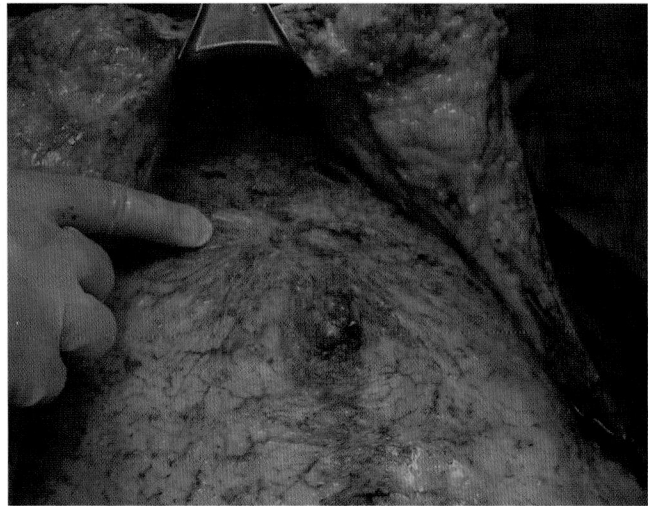

Fig. 15.10 Removal of the pseudo-bursa usually requires the use of most or all of the transverse length of the abdominoplasty incision for proper access. This is especially the case when the pseudo-bursa is located above the umbilicus. In these cases, the entire abdominal soft-tissue apron must be re-elevated to allow sufficient access to the supraumbilical pseudo-bursa.

If there was an appreciable amount of fluid in the pseudo-bursa, there may be some atrophy of the overlying fat. Complete removal of the pseudo-bursa (anterior and posterior wall) may result in a contour depression. This is usually temporary, but may take some time to correct fully. Thorough preoperative discussion with the patient is critical to avoid misunderstanding and dissatisfaction. Partial capsulectomy with removal of the anterior wall only and scarification of the remaining posterior wall is another option. Placement of space-obliterating sutures is a reasonable consideration to help promote adherence of the abdominal soft tissue to the posterior wall of the pseudo-bursa.[5–7] The use of a drain, abdominal binder, and perioperative antibiotics is important to prevent secondary seroma-related complications.

Dog-Ears (Box 15.4)

Lateral dog-ears are often a preventable complication. The source of the dog-ear may be secondary to the design of the soft-tissue resection, the presence of excess adiposity at the lateral corners, or lack of medial advancement of the upper tissue during closure. Often, prominent lateral dog-ears result from the design of the soft-tissue resection. However, even with the appropriate design small lateral

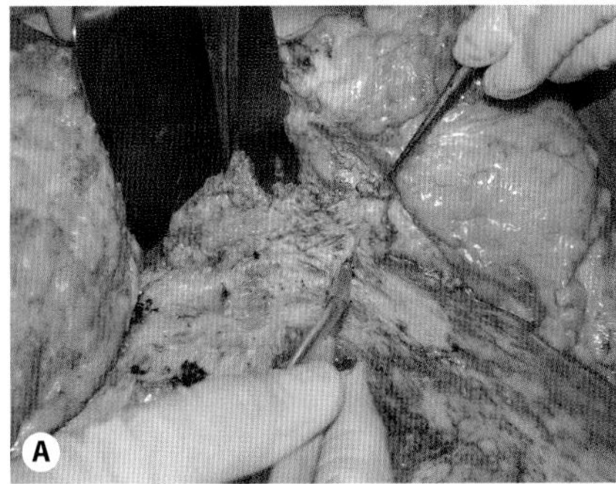
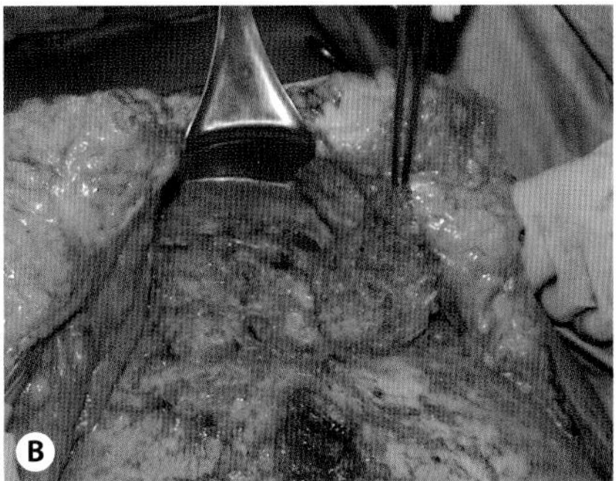
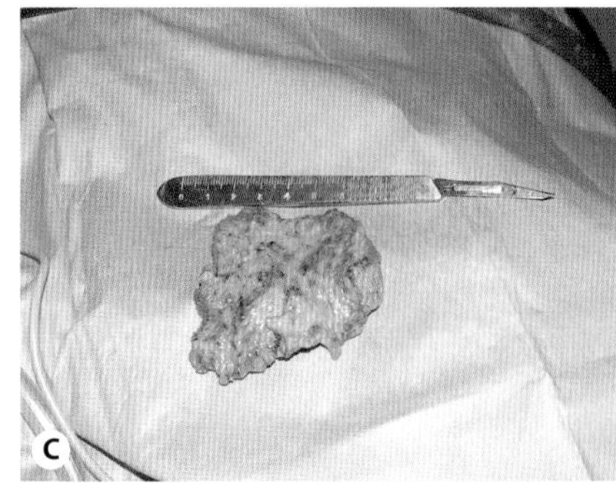

Fig. 15.11 A pseudo-bursa is removed with sharp dissection using electrocautery. Often, both the anterior and posterior walls of the pseudo-bursa are removed. This will allow the normal abdominal soft tissue and the abdominal wall to come into contact to facilitate healing. Occasionally, the pseudo-bursa compresses the overlying adipose tissue, and its removal may result in a slight contour depression in this area. The patient should be told this beforehand. Alternately, only the anterior portion of the pseudo-bursa can be removed.

Box 15.4 Lateral dog-ears

- The presence of lateral dog-ears is usually avoidable complication
- Often it is a result of the procedure design
- Even with a well-designed procedure, small lateral dog-ears may still exist if the upper tissue is not sufficiently advanced towards the midline during closure of each layer
- Lateral-dog ears present at the completion of the case will remain, especially if adipose tissue is present
- Midline pleats or folds of tissue at the completion of the case invariably smooth out with time

dog-ears may exist if the upper tissue is not strongly advanced medially. The incision should be closed from lateral to medial, taking care to advance each layer strongly towards the midline, which will help reduce the incidence of dog-ear formation (**Fig. 15.12**). If the lateral dog-ear is secondary to residual fullness or excess adiposity, thorough superficial liposuction at the end of the procedure will help correct this.

Postoperative correction of lateral dog-ears depends on the amount of tissue present and whether concurrent liposuction of the dog-ear and/or surrounding area is needed. The presence of a small amount of residual skin laterally can be easily corrected by simple excision under local anesthesia. More prominent dog-ears and excess adiposity may be treated with the addition of IV sedation or general anesthesia. In these cases, the patient should be warned that lengthening of the scar will probably be necessary.

Excess soft-tissue laxity in the midline as a result of the medial advancement of the upper tissue during closure may also be seen at the completion of the case. Often this scenario exists when the patient is relatively thin and a maximum amount of tissue is removed to eliminate striae while keeping the incision relatively short. An important caveat to consider regarding central soft-tissue laxity or pleating is that it usually smoothes out with time. Whereas lateral dog-ears at the

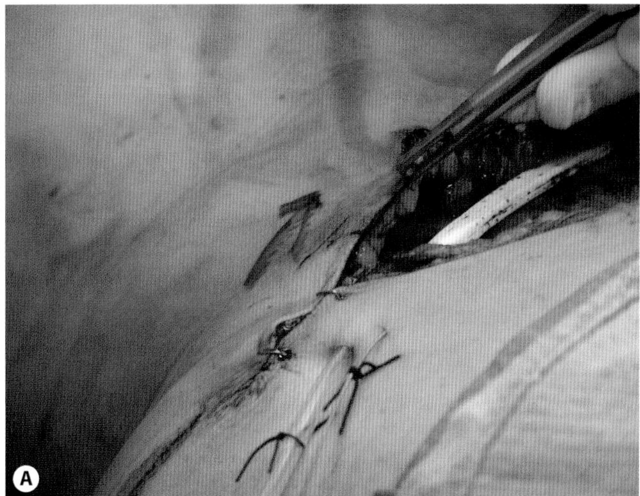
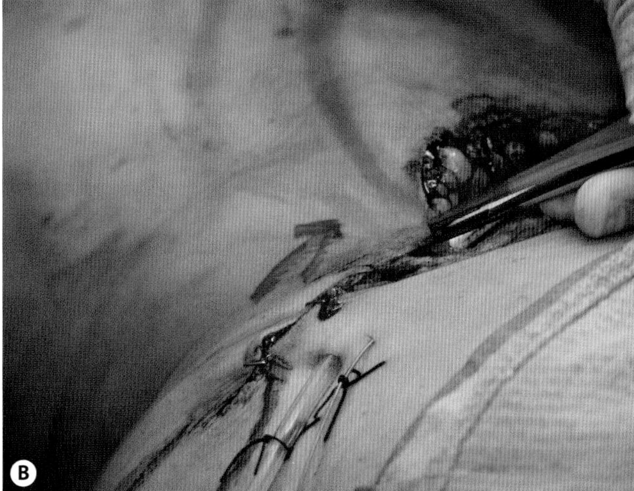

Fig. 15.12 The possibility of small lateral-dog ears forming can be seen even with a properly designed abdominoplasty resection. During closure of the transverse incision of an abdominoplasty, advancement of the upper tissue towards the midline with each of the layers will significantly help reduce the incidence of dog-ears.

completion of the case will persist, central pleating will eventually smooth out and disappear. This is also commonly seen in breast surgery, where moderate pleating around the areola resolves with time, whereas dog-ears at the ends of the transverse incision tend to persist.

Scar Placement

The location of the final transverse scar is partly determined by the characteristics of the patient's body and the desired aesthetic result. The ideal location of the final scar is at or near the upper border of the pubic symphysis. The goal of abdominoplasty is to improve the shape and contour of the abdomen with surgical scars that can be easily hidden, allowing the patient to look good in clothes as well as swimwear and revealing undergarments. To achieve this, the transverse scar should be kept low enough to be hidden within the border of these garments.

The location of the final scar can be determined during the preoperative markings by having the patient lift their lower abdominal skin upwards. Marking the upper border of the pubic symphysis with the patient pulling upwards will result in placement of the transverse incision within the hair-bearing mons (**Fig. 15.13**). At the completion of the abdominoplasty and in the days that follow, the tension generated during closure will pull the incision slightly cephalad, resulting in a final transverse scar that is near the top of the pubic symphysis. In essence, having the patient pull superiorly on the lower abdominal soft tissue replicates the pull that the abdominoplasty closure will generate. Another method for determining the ideal location of the abdominoplasty incision is to have the patient wear their most revealing swimwear or lingerie. The patient then lifts their redundant abdominal tissues upward and the garment outline is marked. Placing the lower incision line within these borders will help keep the final scar low and easily hidden (**Fig. 15.14**).

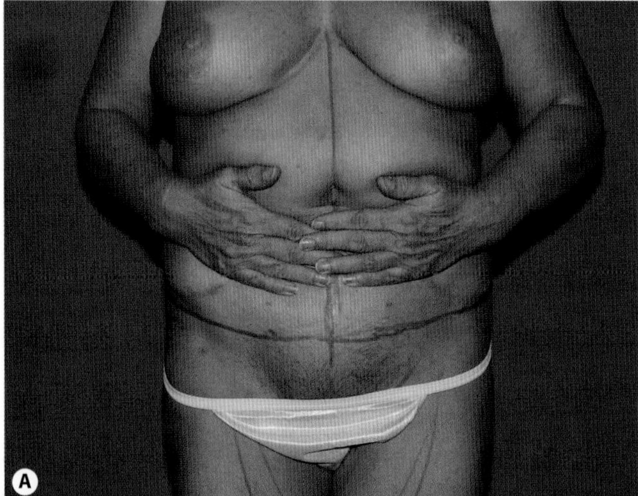

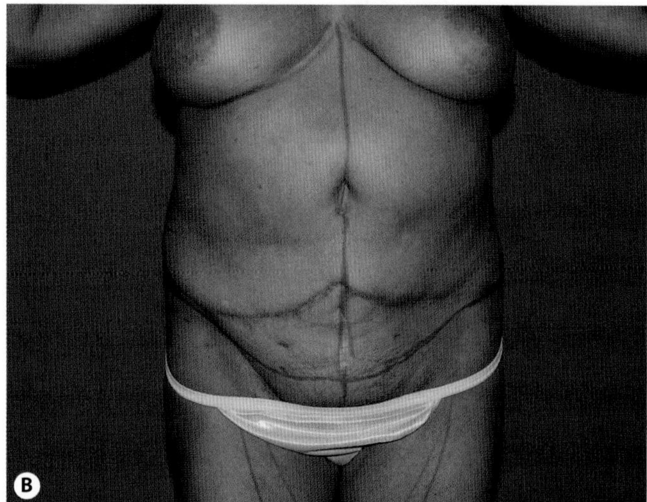

Fig. 15.13 The ideal location of the final transverse scar is at the upper border of the pubic symphysis. The upward force generated during closure will result in the final transverse scar migrating superiorly. This should be taken into account when marking the ideal placement of the initial transverse incision. The patient is asked to pull up (cephalad) on their abdominal soft tissue to replicate the force generated during closure of the transverse incision. With the patient pulling up, the superior border of the pubic symphysis is marked. This will be the center of the lower transverse incision and the expected location of the final scar.

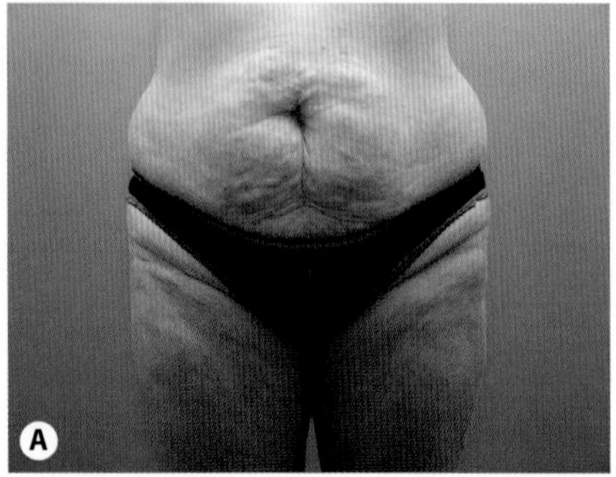

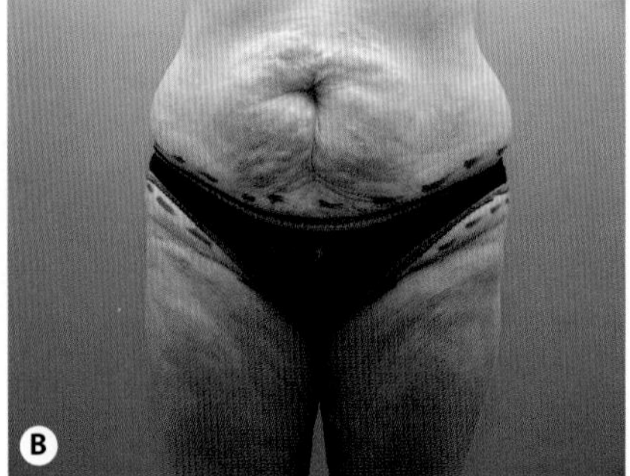

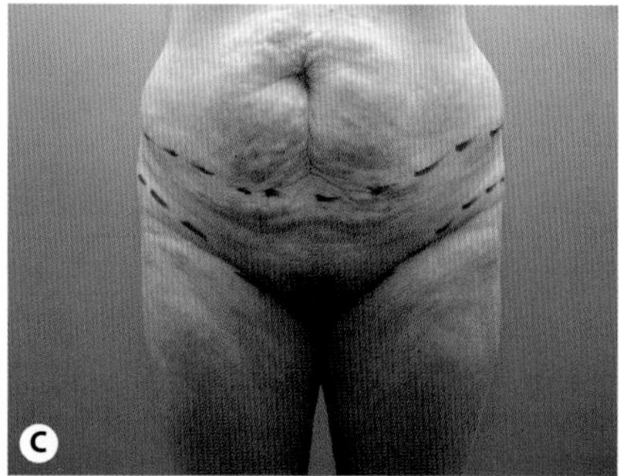

Fig. 15.14 An alternate method to assure that the final transverse scar will be low enough is to ask the patient to bring in revealing swimwear or underwear. The patient is asked to pull up on their abdominal soft tissue and the outline of their underwear is drawn. Placing the transverse incision within the outline of the underwear will ensure the final scar will be easily concealed by even the most revealing garments.

Great care should be taken to evaluate the incision laterally for both length and position. Length can be measured from the midline to each end of the proposed incision to ensure symmetry. Careful examination of the final preoperative markings will also help ensure symmetry of the height of the incision laterally as well.

A final scar that is too high may be lowered with additional soft-tissue resection if there is sufficient residual laxity. However, for a high scar to be lowered appropriately, the abdominal soft tissue may need to be fully re-elevated (see Chapter 11, Complete Revision Abdominoplasty). Abdominoplasty scars that are wide or aesthetically poor are often a result of poor healing secondary to ischemia, infection, or dehiscence. These scars, as well as those that are irregular or asymmetric, can be revised by simple excision and multilayer closure using delicate tissue handling techniques.

Umbilical Complications

The umbilicus is the focal point of the central abdomen. Malposition, stenosis, or ischemia and necrosis with umbilical loss can be very disturbing for both the patient and the surgeon. Careful planning and delicate surgical technique will prevent or reduce the incidence of many of these problems. Avoiding and managing complications related to the umbilicus is discussed in Chapter 13, The Umbilicus in Body Contouring.

Ischemia

The blood supply to the abdominal soft tissue is extensive (see Chapter 2, Anatomical Considerations in Abdominal Contouring). During a full, extended, or circumferential abdominoplasty the perforators from the deep epigastric arcade as well as the superficial inferior perforators (superficial inferior epigastric and superficial circumflex vessels) are divided.[8] As a result, the abdominal soft-tissue apron remains supplied primarily by the intercostal and subcostal perforators bilaterally. A thorough understanding of anatomy and proper intraoperative technique are most important in avoiding ischemic complications.

Additional factors also play a part in soft-tissue perfusion following abdominoplasty. Significant tension during closure, especially on the skin, smoking, dehydration, incorrect use of the abdominal binder, and a number of pre-existing comorbidities can further stress the balance between perfusion and the metabolic demand of the abdominal soft-tissue flap. The tissue in the midline just above the transverse incision is the watershed area and is the furthest away from the intercostals and subcostal vascular source. Therefore, careful and frequent evaluation of tension and perfusion in this area both intraoperatively and in the immediate postoperative period is very important (**Fig. 15.15**).

Venous congestion of this area may be evidence of impending ischemia. The tissue will appear dusky or cyanotic, and

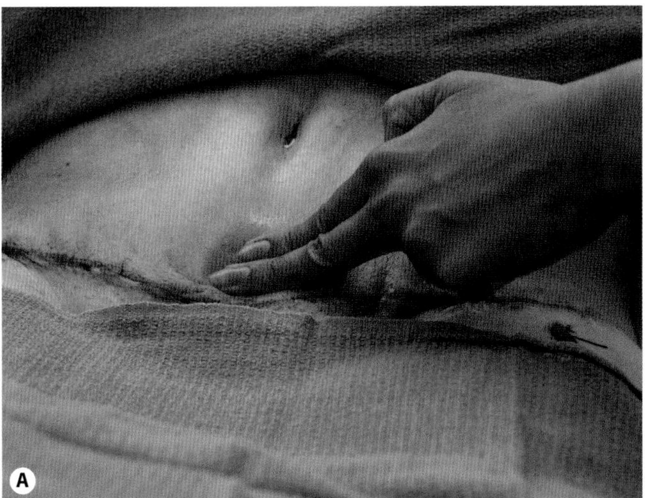

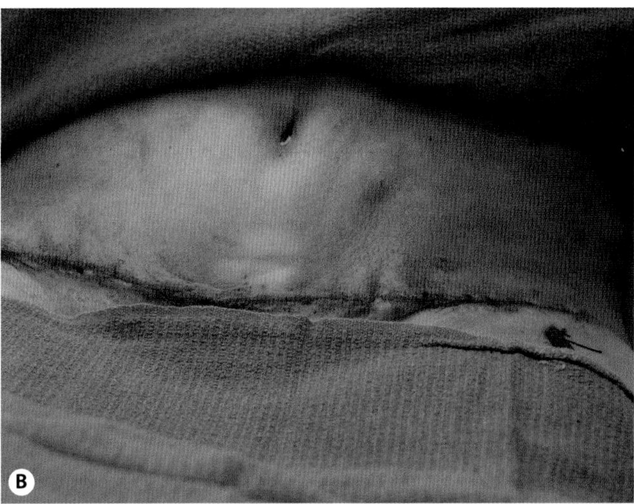

Fig. 15.15 The perfusion of the abdominal flap should be checked at the time of closure and in the immediate perioperative period. This is best done in the midline above the transverse incision. Any number of factors, some that can be controlled or reversed and others that cannot, can result in vascular embarrassment of the abdominal soft tissue. Excessive tension during closure, an overly tight abdominal binder, and fluid accumulation may all negatively affect perfusion. Venous congestion as indicated by cyanotic or dusky skin is most worrisome for perioperative ischemia. Skin that is uniformly blanched is often secondary to the continued effect of epinephrine. As time passes, the effect of the epinephrine wears off and capillary dilation occurs, a slight hint of hyperemia can often be detected.

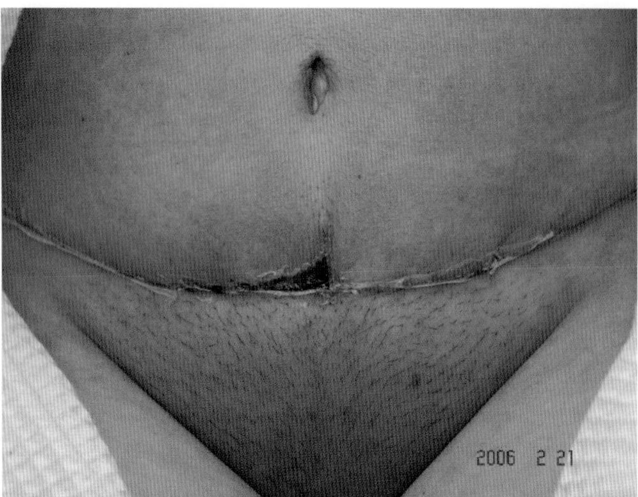

Fig. 15.16 Small areas of dry eschar can be managed conservatively. The body will release the eschar as secondary healing occurs from the periphery.

Box 15.5 Fat necrosis

- The dissection process of standard abdominoplasty techniques leaves the abdominal soft-tissue apron vascularized by the intercostal and subcostal perforators
- The center of the abdominoplasty flap just above the final transverse scar is the furthest away from the vascular supply and therefore most susceptible to ischemia or necrosis
- Ischemic or necrotic fat may present in various ways but is often not noticed in the first few postoperative days. When it does present, there is frequently firm fullness of the lower midline area of the abdominal flap
- Observation and frequent follow-up may be attempted if the area is small. Oral antibiotics should be maintained or restarted to prevent reduce the chance of infection
- More commonly, the area in question is clinically significant in size and formal debridement of the non-viable fat is the safest course of action
- Sharp debridement, copious irrigation, oral antibiotics, and closure with external sutures over a drain are recommended

can be associated with sluggish capillary refill. Impending ischemia is much more common with these findings than with skin pallor. Skin pallor is often an indication of a persistent epinephrine effect secondary to tumescent infiltration. With postoperative patient warming and proper positioning relieving abdominal soft-tissue tension, the skin pallor usually resolves and the skin becomes pink, with rapid capillary refill.

Evaluation for evidence of excessive tension or underlying fluid accumulation should be sought if the lower abdominal skin appears ischemic or congested in the perioperative period. Constricting garments or binders should be immediately removed and the patient should be placed in a maximally flexed position to minimize tension on the abdominal flap. If there is not a correctable source of tissue ischemia, the application of topical nitroglycerin ointment to the affected area can be attempted. To minimize tissue trauma, the ointment should be applied to a non-adherent dressing that is then applied to the skin. This should be reapplied two or three times a day, and the patient should be warned about the possibility of a headache as a side-effect. The affected area should be carefully inspected frequently following the recognition of ischemia. The effectiveness of nitroglycerin should be reviewed and, if not effective, it should discontinued.

If epidermolysis occurs, the area should be kept clean and protected from desiccation and infection, which may lead to further tissue injury. The formation of eschar is often a sign that deeper tissue injury has occurred. The extent of the injury may still not be fully appreciated at this time, and sharp surgical resection should be avoided until the non-viable tissue is clearly demarcated. Relatively small areas of dry eschar can be managed conservatively (**Fig. 15.16**). The body will release portions of the eschar from the periphery as healing progresses. Wet eschar can be surgically or mechanically debrided, depending on the size of the affected area, tissue characteristics, and patient compliance. In the interim, the wet eschar should be treated with betadine or Silvadene cream to keep the bacterial count low until it is ready for removal.

Necrosis (Box 15.5)

As opposed to ischemia, where the extent of tissue injury is still unknown, soft-tissue necrosis is a clear indication that surgical intervention is needed. Necrosis can present in various ways, depending on the tissue involved. The skin is usually metabolically more resistant to vascular embarrassment than the underlying fat. Because of this, necrosis can present as full-thickness tissue death involving skin and soft tissue, or it can present with fat necrosis only. Full-thickness soft-tissue necrosis is easy to diagnose once the tissue has fully demarcated. The very early stages of this process, however, may be a little harder to predict (**Fig. 15.17**). Once full demarcation of the necrotic tissue has occurred, surgical resection should be performed. These wounds are usually treated with daily dressing changes and allowed to heal, at least temporarily, by secondary intention. Larger areas can be treated with negative pressure therapy following debridement. This will help expedite the healing process as well as making wound management simpler for the patient.

Some patients may present with viable skin but underlying fat necrosis. The signs and symptoms will vary and will depend on the amount of fat necrosis present and whether

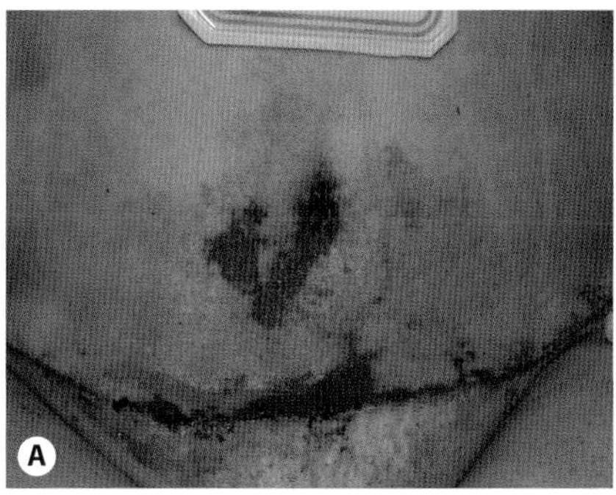

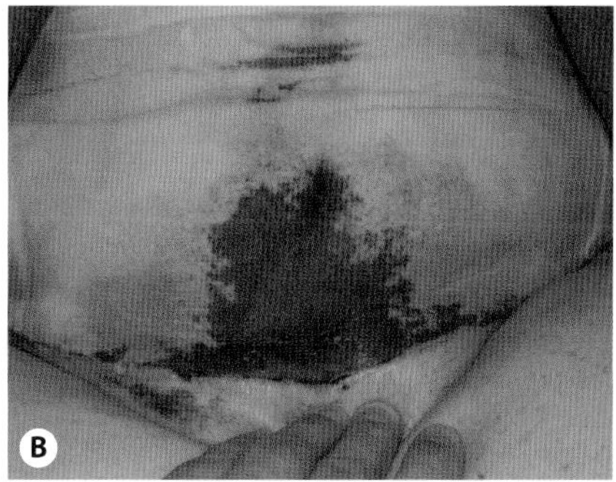

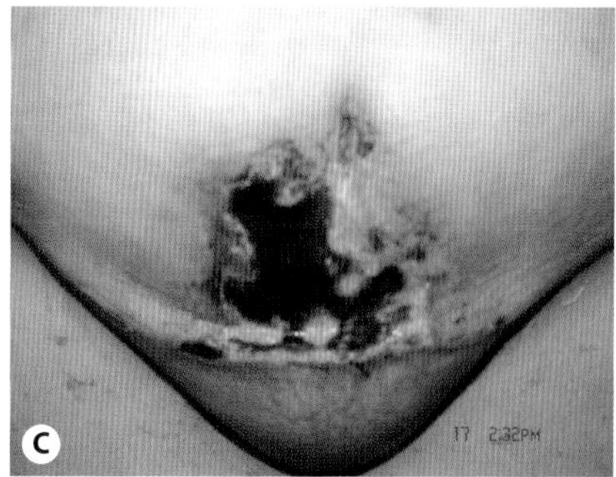

Fig. 15.17 Full-thickness soft-tissue necrosis is easy to diagnose once demarcation is complete. The early stages of this process are often a large area of dusky or cyanotic skin. Similar to a second degree burn, the tissue at the periphery of the dusky skin will probably survive if no further metabolic or vascular insults occur. The amount of the actual tissue in the center that will be full-thickness necrosis cannot be reliably predicted through clinical examination and must be allowed to demarcate fully prior to debridement.

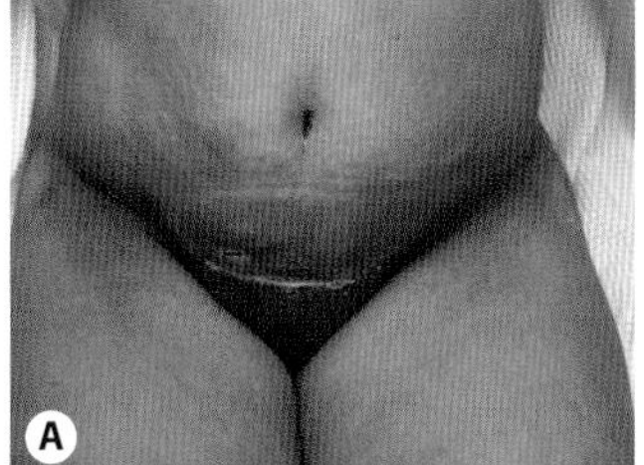

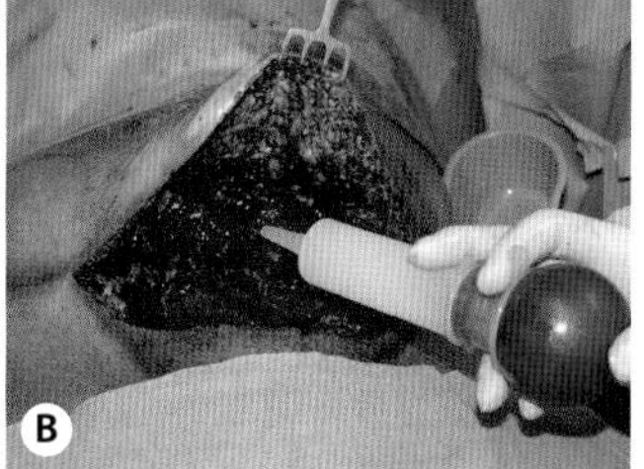

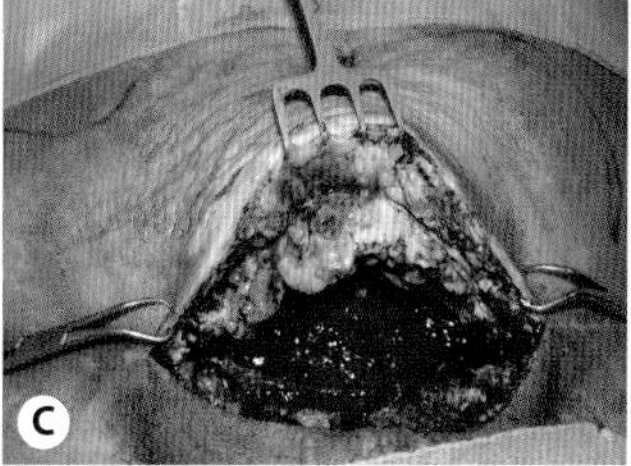

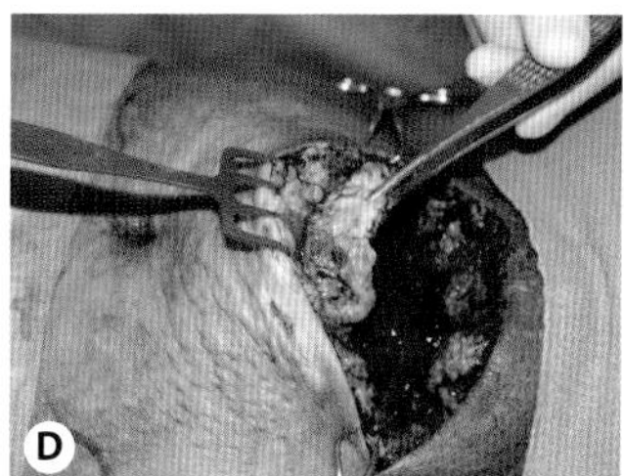

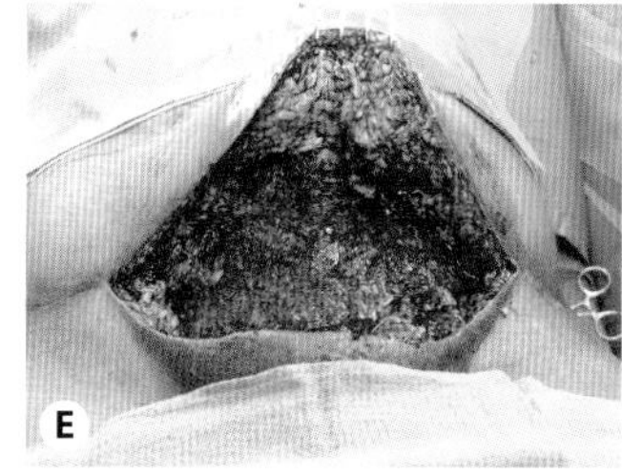

Fig. 15.18 Extensive fat necrosis will usually present with firmness and swelling. The most likely site of fat necrosis is in the midline just above the transverse incision, as this is the area furthest away from the vascular supply. Because the non-viable fat is a potential nidus of infection, patients may also present with erythema and developing cellulitis. Patients with extensive fat necrosis should be formally explored and debrided. Doing so eliminates the nidus of infection and allows the patient to heal more rapidly. Sharp debridement, copious irrigation, closure of the wound with external sutures over a drain, and resumption of oral antibiotics until final tissue cultures are available is recommended.

there is concurrent infection. These patients may present with skin hyperemia, incision site drainage, cellulitis, and/or wound dehiscence. The extent of surgical intervention required depends on the amount of fat necrosis present as well as the magnitude of the symptoms. Often, the best course is to formally explore these patients. Removal of the necrotic fat will expedite the healing process and prevent further sequelae, such as infection (**Fig. 15.18**).

Surgical exploration can be performed under IV sedation or general anesthesia. The wound is opened generously and the necrotic fat debrided until bright red bleeding is noted or the color of the fat signifies viability. Although the skin is still viable, the wound edges may benefit from being trimmed. Copious irrigation with antibiotic solution is performed, and hemostasis is achieved prior to completion of the case. In the past, surgical doctrine taught that wound necrosis and infection must be debrided and left open to heal secondarily. For small areas, particularly along the skin edge, this is still a reasonable option. For larger areas, however, an open wound significantly prolongs the healing phase and can be painful, inconvenient, and psychologically disturbing. Our philosophy regarding these wounds is that once the necrotic tissue is removed the nidus of infection is also removed. We commonly treat these wounds after debridement by placing drains, closing the surgical site with external sutures only, and starting the patient on standard oral antibiotics until cultures have returned. To date we have had very positive results with this technique.

Patients with open wounds that have been treated with dressing changes can be treated with delayed primary closure after sufficient healing and granulation has occurred. The tissue at this point has effectively undergone the process of vascular delay and usually has sufficient vascularity to permit delayed primary closure. Patient response to this process is understandably positive, as it eliminates the unpleasantness and inconvenience of an open wound (**Fig. 15.19**).

Infection

Infection is fairly rare with abdominoplasty or other abdominal contouring procedures.[9,10] The combination of

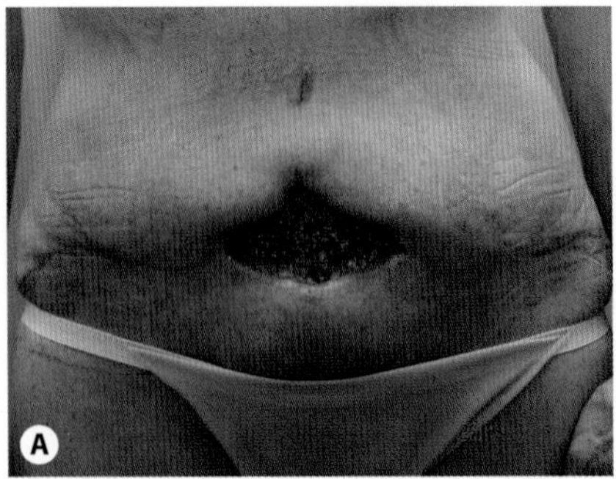
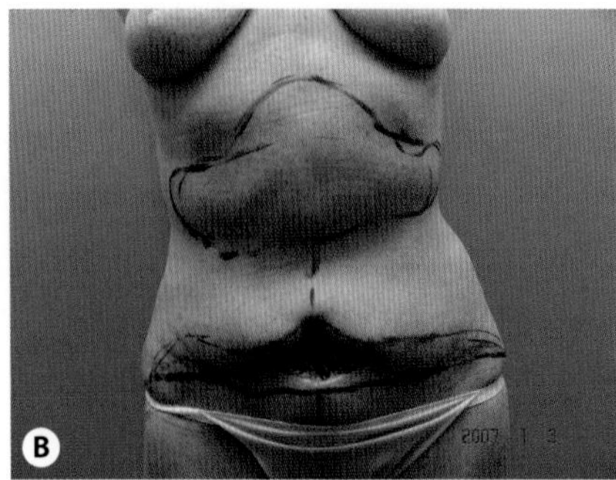
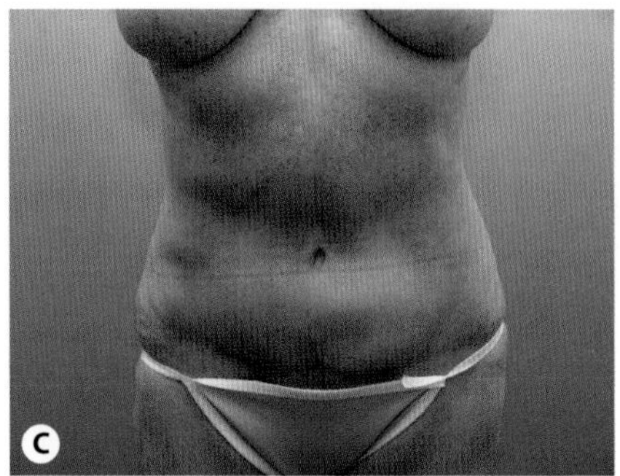

Fig. 15.19 Patients who have experienced full-thickness soft-tissue necrosis and have required debridement have also experienced the discomfort and psychological stress of an open wound. Delayed primary closure can be a tremendous service to these patients, and can be performed once the wound has formed sufficient granulation tissue and has reduced in size to the point where it can be closed with moderate undermining. The time elapsed during this process has also served as a vascular delay which facilitates undermining and closure of the wound.

prophylactic perioperative antibiotics, gentle tissue handling, obliteration of dead space, and postoperative drainage in an otherwise clean procedure results in a very low incidence of infection. When infection does occur it is often associated with the presence of a seroma or nonviable tissue. Mild signs of infection, including a small area of cellulitis, can be treated with oral antibiotics. If there is a seroma this should be drained percutaneously and the aspirate sent for culture. If this does not resolve the problem, a small area of the transverse incision nearest the area of erythema or fullness can be opened, and cultures should be taken. The wound is usually packed open with daily dressing changes and expected to heal secondarily.

Recurrent or persistent infection, especially with clinical signs of fullness that cannot be aspirated, should be surgically explored. In such cases a focus of infection is usually present, such as a seroma, pseudo-bursa, hematoma, fat necrosis, or a significant amount of retained suture. Appropriate formal treatment in these more recalcitrant or persistent cases will return the patient to the path of healing sooner, with a better final aesthetic result compared to repeated small incision and drainage procedures and long-term oral antibiotics.

Suture Extrusion (Box 15.6)

When a large number of sutures are used, as is the case with abdominoplasty procedures, it is not unexpected that some of them, especially those in the deep dermal layer, may extrude or 'spit.' The likelihood of suture extrusion depends on several factors, including the material used, surgical technique, and the individual's skin quality and healing ability. Suture extrusions often present as small localized incision line abscesses. These can be managed expectantly at first, until the overlying skin show signs that it will open. At this point the suture should be removed, and the site can be treated with a simple dressing, such as antibiotic ointment, to keep it protected and free from desiccation or excessive bacterial contamination. If running intradermal sutures, such as barbed sutures, are used, there is an increased chance that the entire suture may need to be removed once one part of it is exposed. Frequent follow-up in these cases is beneficial, as spreading erythema along the incision line can occur following partial wound dehiscence or extrusion of one segment of the suture.

Box 15.6 **Suture extrusion**

- Suture extrusion is a nuisance to both the patient and the surgeon
- It is an inevitable part of any surgical procedure that involves the placement of hundreds of sutures
- The individual buried deep dermal sutures are the main source of extrusion
- The potential for suture extrusion is increased by the type and caliber of the suture, the thickness of the dermis, surgical technique, tension on the closure, and healing characteristics of the tissue
- Most cases can be treated with removal of the suture if detectable, conservative care, and patient education and reassurance
- Certain types of suture, including barbed suture, may be more problematic. Exposure of one part of the suture may necessitate removal of the entire suture strand. Frequent follow-up and removal of the suture is recommended if the incision line shows evidence of spreading infection

DVT/PE

The most dreaded complication in abdominal contouring procedures is DVT/PE. The above-mentioned complications are unwanted and care must be taken to prevent them, but they are not life-threatening and all can be corrected. Deep venous thrombosis and pulmonary embolism are potentially life threatening complications that require hospitalization and treatment by physicians other than the plastic surgeon.

Table 15.1 Perioperative measures that aid in decreasing the incidence of DVT/PE

Intraoperative positioning	The knees are kept flexed using a pillow
Sequential compression device	The device is placed and activated prior to general anesthesia
Hydration	Intravenous fluids are administered and hydration is maintained by monitoring urine output
Perioperative medication	Lovenox is used
Postoperative activity	Ambulation several hours after the procedure and routinely thereafter is encouraged

Patient and family/caregiver education regarding the signs and symptoms of DVT/PE is essential for prompt evaluation and treatment. We instruct all patients and their carers that shortness of breath, dizziness, elevated heart rate, and lower extremity swelling/pain must be evaluated immediately. When there is concern of DVT/PE the patient is sent to the emergency room immediately.

Treatment of DVT/PE will necessitate anticoagulation. Anticoagulation can result in a hematoma or prolonged seroma, but these can be addressed by the surgeon during hospitalization. It is imperative that surgeons do everything possible to prevent DVT/PE. Such measures include proper patient positioning, sequential compression devices, perioperative anticoagulation, adequate hydration, efficient use of intraoperative time, and early postoperative ambulation (**Table 15.1**).

Conclusion

Complications can occur with any surgical procedure. Fortunately, with good patient and procedure selection, careful planning, and proper surgical technique, many potential complications of abdominal contouring can be avoided. When they do occur, however, it is important for the surgeon to intervene, either surgically or through medical treatment, to prevent further injury and to return the patient back to the normal healing process. Extra care and attention is advised for patients who have experienced a complication, as they will undoubtedly have fear and uncertainty about their health and their decision to undergo cosmetic surgery, as well as the final aesthetic appearance.

Clinical Caveats: Complications

- The first goal is to avoid complications. The second is to reduce the incidence of complications. The third goal is proper identification and treatment of complications when they do occur
- Most abdominoplasty complications are not life-threatening and can be treated by the surgeon. Carefully addressing both the psychological and surgical components of the complication will help the patient through this sometimes difficult process
- The most dreaded complication is death secondary to DVT/PE or other cardiopulmonary events
- Careful patient selection may be the most important component in avoiding DVT/PE or other significant complications
- Appropriate pre-, intra-, and postoperative precautions will help reduce the incidence of DVT/PE
- Patient education regarding the signs and symptoms will help expedite medical evaluation and treatment if DVT/PE does occur

References

1. Andrades P, Prado A, Danilla S, et al. Progressive tension sutures in the prevention of postabdominoplasty seroma: a prospective, randomized, double-blind clinical trial. Plast Reconstruct Surg 2007; 120: 935.
2. Pascal JF. Risk of seroma with simultaneous liposuction and abdominoplasty and the role of progressive tension sutures. Aesthet Plast Surg 2008; 32: 100.
3. Spiegelman JI, Levine RH. Abdominoplasty: a comparison of outpatient and inpatient procedures shows that it is a safe and effective procedure for outpatients in an office-based surgery clinic. Plast Reconstruct Surg 2006; 118: 517.
4. Roje Z, Roje Z, Karanovic N, Utrobicic I. Abdominoplasty complications: a comprehensive approach for the treatment of chronic seroma with pseudobursa. Aesthet Plast Surg 2006; 30: 611.
5. Nahas FX, Ferreira LM, Ghelfond C. Does quilting suture prevent seroma in abdominoplasty? Plast Reconstruct Surg 2007; 119: 1060.
6. Andrades P, Prado A. Composition of postabdominoplasty seroma. Aesthet Plast Surg 2007; 31: 514.
7. Khan S, Teotia SS, Mullis WF, et al. Do progressive tension sutures really decrease complications in abdominoplasty? Ann Plast Surg 2006; 56: 14.

8. Mayr M, Holm C, Höfter E, et al. Effects of aesthetic abdominoplasty on abdominal wall perfusion: a quantitative evaluation. Plast Reconstruct Surg 2004; 114: 1586.
9. Stewart KJ, Stewart DA, Coghlan B, et al. Complications of 278 consecutive abdominoplasties. J Plast Reconstruct Aesthet Surg 2006; 59: 1152.
10. Hansen JE, Neaman KC. Analysis of complications from abdominoplasty: a review of 206 cases at a university hospital. Ann Plast Surg 2007; 58: 292.

Suggested Reading

Broughton G 2nd, Rios JL, Rohrich RJ, Brown SA. Deep venous thrombosis prophylaxis practice and treatment strategies among plastic surgeons: survey results. Plast Reconstruct Surg 2007; 119: 157–174.

Matarasso A, Swift RW, Rankin M. Abdominoplasty and abdominal contour surgery: a national plastic surgery survey. Plast Reconstruct Surg 2006; 117: 1797–1808.

Matarasso A, Wallach SG, Rankin M, Galiano RD. Secondary abdominal contour surgery: a review of early and late reoperative surgery. Plast Reconstruct Surg 2005; 115: 627–632.

Hunstad J. Revision abdominoplasty: complications and their management operative techniques in plastic and reconstructive surgery, Vol 3, No. 1, February 1996.

Ozgenel Ege GY, Ozcan M. Heating-pad burn as a complication of abdominoplasty. Br J Plast Surg 2003; 56: 52–53.

Index

Note: Page numbers in **bold** refer to figures and tables.

ELSEVIER DVD-ROM LICENCE AGREEMENT

PLEASE READ THE FOLLOWING AGREEMENT CAREFULLY BEFORE USING THIS DVD-ROM PRODUCT. THIS DVD-ROM PRODUCT IS LICENSED UNDER THE TERMS CONTAINED IN THIS DVD-ROM LICENSE AGREEMENT ("Agreement"). BY USING THIS DVD-ROM PRODUCT, YOU, AN INDIVIDUAL OR ENTITY INCLUDING EMPLOYEES, AGENTS AND REPRESENTATIVES ("You" or "Your"), ACKNOWLEDGE THAT YOU HAVE READ THIS AGREEMENT, THAT YOU UNDERSTAND IT, AND THAT YOU AGREE TO BE BOUND BY THE TERMS AND CONDITIONS OF THIS AGREEMENT. ELSEVIER INC. ("Elsevier") EXPRESSLY DOES NOT AGREE TO LICENSE THIS DVD-ROM PRODUCT TO YOU UNLESS YOU ASSENT TO THIS AGREEMENT. IF YOU DO NOT AGREE WITH ANY OF THE FOLLOWING TERMS, YOU MAY, WITHIN THIRTY (30) DAYS AFTER YOUR RECEIPT OF THIS DVD-ROM PRODUCT RETURN THE UNUSED, PIN NUMBER PROTECTED, DVD-ROM PRODUCT, ALL ACCOMPANYING DOCUMENTATION TO ELSEVIER FOR A FULL REFUND.

DEFINITIONS As used in this Agreement, these terms shall have the following meanings:

"Proprietary Material" means the valuable and proprietary information content of this DVD-ROM Product including all indexes and graphic materials and software used to access, index, search and retrieve the information content from this DVD-ROM Product developed or licensed by Elsevier and/or its affiliates, suppliers and licensors.

"DVD-ROM Product" means the copy of the Proprietary Material and any other material delivered on DVD-ROM and any other human-readable or machine-readable materials enclosed with this Agreement, including without limitation documentation relating to the same.

OWNERSHIP This DVD-ROM Product has been supplied by and is proprietary to Elsevier and/or its affiliates, suppliers and licensors. The copyright in the DVD-ROM Product belongs to Elsevier and/or its affiliates, suppliers and licensors and is protected by the national and state copyright, trademark, trade secret and other intellectual property laws of the United States and international treaty provisions, including without limitation the Universal Copyright Convention and the Berne Copyright Convention. You have no ownership rights in this DVD-ROM Product. Except as expressly set forth herein, no part of this DVD-ROM Product, including without limitation the Proprietary Material, may be modified, copied or distributed in hardcopy or machine-readable form without prior written consent from Elsevier. All rights not expressly granted to You herein are expressly reserved. Any other use of this DVD-ROM Product by any person or entity is strictly prohibited and a violation of this Agreement.

SCOPE OF RIGHTS LICENSED (PERMITTED USES) Elsevier is granting to You a limited, non-exclusive, non-transferable license to use this DVD-ROM Product in accordance with the terms of this Agreement. You may use or provide access to this DVD-ROM Product on a single computer or terminal physically located at Your premises and in a secure network or move this DVD-ROM Product to and use it on another single computer or terminal at the same location for personal use only, but under no circumstances may You use or provide access to any part or parts of this DVD-ROM Product on more than one computer or terminal simultaneously.

You shall not (a) copy, download, or otherwise reproduce the DVD-ROM Product in any medium, including, without limitation, online transmissions, local area networks, wide area networks, intranets, extranets and the Internet, or in any way, in whole or in part, except for printing out or downloading nonsubstantial portions of the text and images in the DVD-ROM Product for Your own personal use; (b) alter, modify, or adapt the DVD-ROM Product, including but not limited to decompiling, disassembling, reverse engineering, or creating derivative works, without the prior written approval of Elsevier; (c) sell, license or otherwise distribute to third parties the DVD-ROM Product or any part or parts thereof; or (d) alter, remove, obscure or obstruct the display of any copyright, trademark or other proprietary notice on or in the DVD-ROM Product or on any printout or download of portions of the Proprietary Materials.

RESTRICTIONS ON TRANSFER This License is personal to You, and neither Your rights hereunder nor the tangible embodiments of this DVD-ROM Product, including without limitation the Proprietary Material, may be sold, assigned, transferred or sublicensed to any other person, including without limitation by operation of law, without the prior written consent of Elsevier. Any purported sale, assignment, transfer or sublicense without the prior written consent of Elsevier will be void and will automatically terminate the License granted hereunder.

TERM This Agreement will remain in effect until terminated pursuant to the terms of this Agreement. You may terminate this Agreement at any time by removing from Your system and destroying the DVD-ROM Product. Unauthorized copying of the DVD-ROM Product, including without limitation, the Proprietary Material and documentation, or otherwise failing to comply with the terms and conditions of this Agreement shall result in automatic termination of this license and will make available to Elsevier legal remedies. Upon termination of this Agreement, the license granted herein will terminate and You must immediately destroy the DVD-ROM Product and accompanying documentation. All provisions relating to proprietary rights shall survive termination of this Agreement.

LIMITED WARRANTY AND LIMITATION OF LIABILITY NEITHER ELSEVIER NOR ITS LICENSORS REPRESENT OR WARRANT THAT THE DVD-ROM PRODUCT WILL MEET YOUR REQUIREMENTS OR THAT ITS OPERATION WILL BE UNINTERRUPTED OR ERROR-FREE. WE EXCLUDE AND EXPRESSLY DISCLAIM ALL EXPRESS AND IMPLIED WARRANTIES NOT STATED HEREIN, INCLUDING THE IMPLIED WARRANTIES OF MERCHANTABILITY AND FITNESS FOR A PARTICULAR PURPOSE. IN ADDITION, NEITHER ELSEVIER NOR ITS LICENSORS MAKE ANY REPRESENTATIONS OR WARRANTIES, EITHER EXPRESS OR IMPLIED, REGARDING THE PERFORMANCE OF YOUR NETWORK OR COMPUTER SYSTEM WHEN USED IN CONJUNCTION WITH THE DVD-ROM PRODUCT. WE SHALL NOT BE LIABLE FOR ANY DAMAGE OR LOSS OF ANY KIND ARISING OUT OF OR RESULTING FROM YOUR POSSESSION OR USE OF THE SOFTWARE PRODUCT CAUSED BY ERRORS

OR OMISSIONS, DATA LOSS OR CORRUPTION, ERRORS OR OMISSIONS IN THE PROPRIETARY MATERIAL, REGARDLESS OF WHETHER SUCH LIABILITY IS BASED IN TORT, CONTRACT OR OTHERWISE AND INCLUDING, BUT NOT LIMITED TO, ACTUAL, SPECIAL, INDIRECT, INCIDENTAL OR CONSEQUENTIAL DAMAGES. IF THE FOREGOING LIMITATION IS HELD TO BE UNENFORCEABLE, OUR MAXIMUM LIABILITY TO YOU SHALL NOT EXCEED THE AMOUNT OF THE LICENSE FEE PAID BY YOU FOR THE SOFTWARE PRODUCT. THE REMEDIES AVAILABLE TO YOU AGAINST US AND THE LICENSORS OF MATERIALS INCLUDED IN THE SOFTWARE PRODUCT ARE EXCLUSIVE.

If this DVD-ROM Product is defective, Elsevier will replace it at no charge if the defective DVD-ROM Product is returned to Elsevier within sixty (60) days (or the greatest period allowable by applicable law) from the date of shipment.

Elsevier warrants that the software embodied in this DVD-ROM Product will perform in substantial compliance with the documentation supplied in this DVD-ROM Product. If You report a significant defect in performance in writing to Elsevier, and Elsevier is not able to correct same within sixty (60) days after its receipt of Your notification, You may return this DVD-ROM Product, including all copies and documentation, to Elsevier and Elsevier will refund Your money.

YOU UNDERSTAND THAT, EXCEPT FOR THE 60-DAY LIMITED WARRANTY RECITED ABOVE, ELSEVIER, ITS AFFILIATES, LICENSORS, SUPPLIERS AND AGENTS, MAKE NO WARRANTIES, EXPRESSED OR IMPLIED, WITH RESPECT TO THE DVD-ROM PRODUCT, INCLUDING, WITHOUT LIMITATION THE PROPRIETARY MATERIAL, AND SPECIFICALLY DISCLAIM ANY WARRANTY OF MERCHANTABILITY OR FITNESS FOR A PARTICULAR PURPOSE.

If the information provided on this DVD-ROM Product contains medical or health sciences information, it is intended for professional use within the medical field. Information about medical treatment or drug dosages is intended strictly for professional use, and because of rapid advances in the medical sciences, independent verification of diagnosis and drug dosages should be made.

IN NO EVENT WILL ELSEVIER, ITS AFFILIATES, LICENSORS, SUPPLIERS OR AGENTS, BE LIABLE TO YOU FOR ANY DAMAGES, INCLUDING, WITHOUT LIMITATION, ANY LOST PROFITS, LOST SAVINGS OR OTHER INCIDENTAL OR CONSEQUENTIAL DAMAGES, ARISING OUT OF YOUR USE OR INABILITY TO USE THE DVD-ROM PRODUCT REGARDLESS OF WHETHER SUCH DAMAGES ARE FORESEEABLE OR WHETHER SUCH DAMAGES ARE DEEMED TO RESULT FROM THE FAILURE OR INADEQUACY OF ANY EXCLUSIVE OR OTHER REMEDY.

U.S. GOVERNMENT RESTRICTED RIGHTS The DVD-ROM Product and documentation are provided with restricted rights. Use, duplication or disclosure by the U.S. Government is subject to restrictions as set forth in subparagraphs (a) through (d) of the Commercial Computer Restricted Rights clause at FAR 52.22719 or in subparagraph (c)(1)(ii) of the Rights in Technical Data and Computer Software clause at DFARS 252.2277013, or at 252.2117015, as applicable. Contractor/Manufacturer is Elsevier Inc., 360 Park Avenue South, New York, NY 10010 USA.

GOVERNING LAW This Agreement shall be governed by the laws of the State of New York, USA. In any dispute arising out of this Agreement, You and Elsevier each consent to the exclusive personal jurisdiction and venue in the state and federal courts within New York County, New York, USA.